D1082749

VASCULAR DISEASE

DIAGNOSTIC AND THERAPEUTIC APPROACHES

VASCULAR DISEASE

DIAGNOSTIC AND THERAPEUTIC APPROACHES

EDITED BY

Michael R. Jaff DO, FACP, FACC, FAHA
Associate Professor of Medicine, Harvard Medical School; Medical Director,
Vascular Center, Massachusetts General Hospital, Boston, Massachusetts

AND

Christopher J. White MD, FSCAI, FACC, FAHA, FESC
Professor of Medicine, System Chairman for Cardiovascular Diseases,
The John Ochsner Heart and Vascular Institute, Ochsner Medical Institutions,
New Orleans, Louisiana

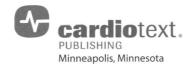

cardiotext.
PUBLISHING
Minneapolis, Minnesota

Cardiotext Publishing, LLC
3405 W. 44th Street
Minneapolis, MN 55410
USA

www.cardiotextpublishing.com

Any updates to this book may be found at: www.cardiotextpublishing.com/titles/detail/9781935395164

Cover image courtesy of NASA/JPL/UCSD/JSC (Ganges River Delta photo details taken by the space shuttle *Atlantis* on January 13, 1997).

Comments, inquiries, and requests for bulk sales can be directed to the publisher at: info@cardiotextpublishing.com.

♾ Printed on acid-free paper.

This book's text pages are printed on 100% FSC-certified paper from well-managed forests, where people, wildlife, and the environment benefit from the forestry practices. Forest Stewardship Council certification is globally recognized for ensuring well-managed forests.

Cover and book design by Zan Ceeley, Trio Bookworks

Library of Congress Control Number: 2011920097

ISBN-13: 978-1-935395-16-4

Printed in the United States of America

16   15   14   13   12   11   1   2   3   4   5   6   7   8   9   10

Contents

About the Contributors

About the Editors

Michael R. Jaff DO, FACP, FACC, FAHA
Associate Professor of Medicine, Harvard Medical School; Medical Director, Vascular Center, Massachusetts General Hospital, Boston, Massachusetts

Christopher J. White MD, FSCAI, FACC, FAHA, FESC
Professor of Medicine, System Chairman for Cardiovascular Diseases, The John Ochsner Heart and Vascular Institute, Ochsner Medical Institutions, New Orleans, Louisiana

About the Contributors

Julia A. M. Anderson MD, BSc(Hons), MBChB, FRCPEdin, FRCPath
Consultant Hematologist and Honorary Senior Lecturer, College of Medicine and Veterinary Medicine, University of Edinburgh; Department of Clinical and Laboratory Hematology, Royal Infirmary of Edinburgh, Scotland, United Kingdom; Associate Professor (P/T), Department of Medicine, McMaster University, Hamilton, Ontario, Canada

Gary M. Ansel MD, FACC
Director, Critical Limb Care Center, Riverside Methodist Hospital; Associate Director, MidWest Cardiology Research Foundation, Division of the Ohio Health Research Institute, Columbus, Ohio; Assistant Clinical Professor of Medicine, Medical University of Ohio, Toledo, Ohio

John R. Bartholomew MD, FACC

Section Head, Vascular Medicine, Department of Cardiovascular Medicine, Professor of Medicine, Cleveland Clinic Lerner College of Medicine, Cleveland, Ohio

Joshua A. Beckman MD, MS, FACC, FAHA, FSVM

Assistant Professor of Medicine, Cardiovascular Division, Brigham and Women's Hospital, Harvard Medical School, Boston, Massachusetts

John A. Bittl MD

Interventional Cardiologist, Ocala Heart Institute, Munroe Regional Medical Center, Ocala, Florida

Richard P. Cambria MD

Chief, Division of Vascular and Endovascular Surgery, Massachusetts General Hospital; Professor of Surgery, Harvard Medical School, Boston, Massachusetts

Tyrone J. Collins MD, FACC, FSCAI

Section Head, Interventional Cardiology, The John Ochsner Heart and Vascular Institute, New Orleans, Louisiana

Mark F. Conrad MD, MMSc

Assistant Professor in Surgery, Division of Vascular and Endovascular Surgery, Massachusetts General Hospital, Harvard Medical School, Boston, Massachusetts

Steven M. Dean DO, FACP, RPVI

Associate Professor of Clinical Internal Medicine, Program Director-Vascular Medicine, Division of Cardiovascular Medicine, The Ohio State University College of Medicine, Columbus, Ohio

Andrew C. Eisenhauer MD

Director, Interventional Cardiovascular Medicine Service; Associate Director, Cardiac Catheterization Laboratory, Brigham and Women's Hospital; Assistant Professor of Medicine, Harvard Medical School, Boston, Massachusetts

Jeffrey A. Goldstein MD

Prairie Cardiovascular Consultants, Assistant Professor of Medicine, Southern Illinois School of Medicine, Springfield, Illinois

Bruce H. Gray DO

Professor of Surgery, University of South Carolina School of Medicine, Greenville; Director of Endovascular Services, Greenville Memorial Hospital, Greenville, South Carolina

Ashequl M. Islam MD, MPH, FACC, FSCAI

Division of Cardiology, Baystate Medical Center, Springfield, Massachusetts; Assistant Professor of Medicine, Tufts University School of Medicine, Boston, Massachusetts

Tikva S. Jacobs MD

Assistant Clinical Professor of Surgery, Division of Vascular Surgery, Department of Surgery, Mount Sinai School of Medicine, New York, New York

J. Stephen Jenkins MD, FACC, FSCAI
Associate Section Head Interventional Cardiology, Director Interventional Cardiology Research, The John Ochsner Heart and Vascular Institute, New Orleans, Louisiana

Vikram S. Kashyap MD, FACS
Staff, Departments of Vascular Surgery and Cell Biology, Associate Professor of Surgery, Cleveland Clinic Lerner College of Medicine, Cleveland, Ohio

Thomas J. Kiernan MD, FESC
Consultant Cardiologist, Senior Clinical Lecturer in Medicine, Department of Cardiology, Cork University Hospital, University College Cork Medical School, Cork, Ireland

Raghu Kolluri MD, RVT, FACC, FACP
Director, Vascular Medicine and Non-Invasive Vascular Laboratory; Clinical Assistant Professor, Southern Illinois School of Medicine, Springfield, Illinois

Juzar Lokhandwala MD, RVT, RPVI
Interventional Cardiologist, First Coast Cardiovascular Institute, Jacksonville, Florida

Michael L. Marin MD, FACS
The Julius H. Jacobson II MD Professor of Surgery, Chairman, Department of Surgery, Mount Sinai School of Medicine, New York, New York

Jessica Nevins Morse MD
Academic Department of Internal Medicine, Greenville Hospital System, University Medical Center, Greenville, South Carolina

Stephen O'Connor MD
Department of Cardiology, Cork University Hospital, Cork, Ireland

John A. O'Dea MD
Centre for Research in Vascular Biology, University College Cork, Cork, Ireland

Jeffrey W. Olin DO
Professor of Medicine, Director Vascular Medicine, Zena and Michael A. Wiener Cardiovascular Institute and Marie-Josee and Henry R. Kravis Center of Cardiovascular Health, Mount Sinai School of Medicine, New York, New York

Kenneth Ouriel MD
Vascular Surgery, Columbia University Medical Center, New York, New York

Reena L. Pande MD
Associate Physician, Cardiovascular Division, Brigham and Women's Hospital; Instructor, Harvard Medical School, Boston, Massachusetts

Stephen R. Ramee MD, FACC
Medical Director, Structural and Valvular Heart Center, Interventional Cardiology, Ochsner Medical Center, New Orleans, Louisiana.

John P. Reilly MD
Associate Director, Cardiac Catheterization Laboratory, Interventional Cardiology, The John Ochsner Heart and Vascular Institute, Ochsner Medical Center, New Orleans, Louisiana

Joseph J. Ricotta II MD, FACS
Assistant Professor of Surgery, Division of Vascular Surgery and Endovascular Therapy, Emory University School of Medicine, Atlanta, Georgia

Krishna Rocha-Singh MD
Medical Director, Prairie Vascular Institute and Prairie Education and Research Cooperative, Prairie Cardiovascular Consultants, Springfield, Illinois

Kenneth Rosenfield MD, FACC
Associate Physician in Medicine, Section Head, Vascular Medicine and Intervention, Cardiology Division, Massachusetts General Hospital; Lecturer on Medicine, Harvard Medical School, Boston, Massachusetts

Jose A. Silva MD, FACC
Tchefuncte Cardiovascular Associates and TCA Research, Covington, Louisiana

Mitchell J. Silver DO, FACC, FABVM
Director, Vascular Imaging, McConnell Heart Hospital, Riverside Methodist, Columbus, Ohio

John A. Spittell Jr. MD, MACP, FACC
Emeritus Consultant in Internal Medicine, Mayo Clinic; Emeritus Professor of Medicine, Mayo Medical School, Rochester, Minnesota

Peter C. Spittell MD, FACC
Division of Cardiovascular Diseases, Mayo Clinic, Rochester, Minnesota

Saundra S. Spruiell DO, FACPh, RPVI
Medical Director, Oklahoma Vein Specialists, Oklahoma City, Oklahoma

Timothy M. Sullivan MD, FACS, FSVM, FACC
Chairman, Vascular/Endovascular Surgery, Minneapolis Heart Institute at Abbott Northwestern Hospital; Clinical Professor of Surgery, University of Minnesota, Minneapolis, Minnesota

Jeffrey I. Weitz MD
Professor of Medicine & Biochemistry, McMaster University, HSFO/J.F. Mustard Chair in Cardiovascular Research, Canada Research Chair (Tier 1) in Thrombosis; Executive Director, Thrombosis and Atherosclerosis Research Institute, Hamilton General Hospital Campus, Hamilton, Ontario

Foreword

Jess R. Young MD

Emeritus Chairman of the Vascular Medicine Department, Cleveland Clinic, Cleveland, Ohio

It was with some reluctance that I agreed to write this foreword. Since I retired as Chairman of the Vascular Medicine Department at the Cleveland Clinic twelve years ago, I have been busy enjoying my leisure time and working on my golf game. However, I could not refuse Michael Jaff. He is an outstanding graduate of our program, and I knew that any project involving him would be both worthwhile and significant. I was not mistaken. Michael has teamed with Christopher White and many distinguished contributors to bring us a splendid new text on vascular diseases.

A new publication in this field is most welcome. Vascular diseases are common and have a major impact on health. Their incidence is rapidly increasing in our aging population. Unfortunately, training in the diagnosis and treatment of these conditions has not been emphasized or even included in most medical schools or postgraduate training programs. *Vascular Disease: Diagnostic and Therapeutic Approaches* helps keep us current in this dynamic and growing field. The reader is offered the latest options for dealing with commonly and uncommonly encountered vascular problems. The book has a clinically oriented approach and is written mainly by practicing physicians. The entire spectrum of arterial, venous, and lymphatic diseases is addressed in a practical and topical manner. Percutaneous therapy for many vascular problems has been of increasing interest, and this approach is discussed thoroughly when appropriate. I would like to thank Dr. Jaff and Dr. White for interrupting my leisure time and giving me the opportunity to read this major contribution to the diagnosis and treatment of vascular diseases.

Preface

As the US population grows older in the midst of unprecedented epidemics of obesity and diabetes, we must prepare for the epidemic of vascular disorders that will likely overwhelm the relatively few specialist physicians trained to diagnose and treat them. We believe there is a need for a comprehensive approach to vascular diseases—not limited to atherosclerotic artery disease—that bridges vascular and endovascular medicine. *Vascular Disease: Diagnostic and Therapeutic Approaches,* written by recognized experts in the diagnosis and treatment of a broad array of vascular diseases, successfully spans both disciplines.

We have integrated vascular medicine—the diagnosis and medical management of vascular diseases—where appropriate, with endovascular medicine—the percutaneous therapy of vascular diseases. With the rapid advances in noninvasive imaging technology and the emergence of novel revascularization strategies, the practicing clinician is faced with the daunting task of remaining current on all aspects of care.

The book begins with the practice of office-based vascular medicine in Part 1, followed by an overview of the assessment of peripheral artery disease in Part 2. Next, in Parts 3, 4, and 5, the critical aspects of diagnosis and management of aortic arch and supraclavicular artery disease; aortic, visceral, and renal artery disease; and lower-extremity artery disease are explored. The book concludes with careful attention to nonatherosclerotic artery disease (Part 6), venous disease (Part 7), and hypercoagulability and uncommon vascular diseases (Part 8).

We are confident that this approach to vascular and endovascular medicine addresses an educational need for students, physicians-in-training, and practicing clinicians. It is our hope that the knowledge derived from this book will benefit a population of patients who need effective, compassionate, and collaborative vascular care.

—Michael R. Jaff and
Christopher J. White

Part 1

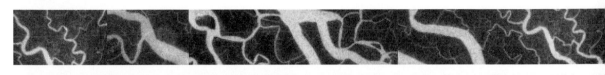

Evaluation of the Patient with Peripheral Vascular Disorders

Taking a Vascular History and Physical Examination

Peter C. Spittell and John A. Spittell Jr.

Introduction

Since peripheral vascular disorders can be due to either local or systemic disease, and significantly affected by comorbid conditions (eg, diabetes mellitus and cardiopulmonary disease), it is essential that a complete medical history be reviewed in addition to the specific details of the vascular complaint. Attention to demographic data—family history, occupation, current or previous illness, surgery, and/or medication—can facilitate prompt and accurate diagnosis, even of complaints or clinical findings that are unusual or perplexing. Questionnaires are useful in providing the patient time to think and record such demographic information and can facilitate this part of the medical history.

The growing availability and reliance on "high-tech" medicine in place of "high-touch" medicine[1] should not limit attention paid to inquiring about specific historical points when evaluating any symptom or symptom complex. Time relationships of the complaint (onset, progression) should be established as accurately as possible. Exact location and severity of the symptom(s) and any modifying factors, as well as the degree of disability imposed by the symptom(s), are essential details. Results of pre-

vious investigations of the complaint(s)—noninvasive laboratory studies, imaging procedures, and biopsies of various types—and of treatment are basic to a complete vascular history.

Evaluating Pain

Painful extremities are not necessarily the result of a peripheral vascular disorder. Pain due to circulatory problems can be persistent or intermittent.

Persistent severe pain in any extremity is the hallmark of severe ischemia of that extremity—sudden arterial occlusion, ischemic ulceration, and severe chronic limb ischemia, all conditions readily confirmed and distinguished from neurologic and orthopedic disorders by the vascular examination. The pain of sudden arterial occlusion may be associated with, or even replaced by, other symptoms of acute ischemia—numbness, tingling, coldness, and/or paresis. Pain due to severe chronic ischemia is constant, worse at night, and difficult to control with medication; at times dependency on the extremity will give partial relief of the pain due to severe ischemia, and if prolonged

Vascular Disease: Diagnostic and Therapeutic Approaches. © 2011 Michael R. Jaff and Christopher J. White, editors. Cardiotext Publishing, ISBN: 978-1-935395-16-4.

in an attempt to get some relief, may result in an edematous, ruborous cold foot (Figure 1.1). Ulceration due to ischemia is characteristically severely painful, distinguishing it readily from the other common types of ulceration of the extremity (Table 1.1). The pain due to acute venous thrombosis is generally mild and relieved by local heat and analgesics. Lymphedema is painless unless complicated by acute lymphangitis/cellulitis, with the pain being proportionate to the extent of the inflammation and relieved by local heat and control of the infection.

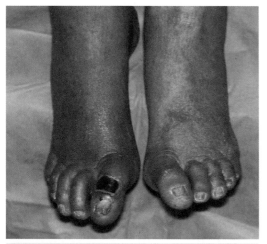

Figure 1.1 Dependent edema and an ischemic ulcer of the toe in a patient with critical limb ischemia and ischemic rest pain. (Reproduced from Spittell A Jr., *Peripheral Vascular Disease for Cardiologists. A Clinical Approach.* Elmsford, NY, and Oxford, UK: Blackwell Publishing/Futura Division; 2004. By permission of Blackwell Publishing.)

The principal intermittent pain in peripheral vascular disorders is *intermittent claudication*, which always indicates an inadequate arterial blood supply (usually evident on physical examination) to contracting muscles. While patients use various terms to describe their intermittent claudication—eg, "aching," "cramping," "tightness"—it is brought on only by exercise and is relieved promptly by rest; in the case of occlusive arterial disease of a lower extremity, whatever its cause, intermittent claudication occurs with walking and is relieved promptly by standing still. A significant number of patients will be asymptomatic or have atypical leg symptoms, therefore a typical history of intermittent claudication has a high specificity but a low sensitivity.[2] Determining the amount of walking that causes the person's intermittent claudication provides an estimate of the severity of the occlusive arterial disease, although the degree of functional limitation can vary depending on the collateral circulation, exercise capacity, and comorbid conditions. Furthermore, the location of the distress of intermittent claudication is a rough indication of the level of the occlusive arterial disease in the affected part. Thus, intermittent claudication in the arch of the foot as may be seen in Buerger's disease suggests occlusive arterial disease at or above the ankle, while intermittent claudication located in the thigh or buttock indicates occlusive arterial disease of the iliac artery or aorta. Unusual locations of intermittent claudication,

	Ischemic (major arterial)	Ischemic (arteriolar)	Venous	Neurotrophic
Onset	Trauma	Spontaneous	Trauma	Trauma
Location	Foot, toes, heel	Posterolateral Lower leg	Medial leg	Plantar
Pain Level	Severe	Severe	None, unless infected	None
Skin	Atrophic	Normal	Stasis change	Callous
Ulcer Edges	Discrete	Serpiginous	Shaggy	Discrete
Ulcer Base	Pale; eschar	Eschar; ischemic	Healthy	Normal or pale

Table 1.1 Common Leg and Foot Ulceration

Intermittent Claudication	Neurogenic Etiologies	Musculoskeletal Etiologies
Atherosclerosis	Lumbosacral spine/disc disease	Arthritis
Popliteal artery entrapment syndrome	Peripheral neuropathy	Bursitis
Cystic adventitial disease of the popliteal artery	Venous claudication	Tendonitis
Fibromuscular dysplasia	Extensive iliofemoral occlusive deep venous thrombosis	Hamstring/quadriceps tightness
Giant cell arteritis		Plantar fasciitis
Endofibrosis of the iliac artery		

Table 1.2 Differential Diagnosis of Limb Pain

such as *jaw claudication*, which may occur in giant cell arteritis, or *arm claudication*, which can occur with occlusion of the subclavian artery, are useful indicators of the location of the occlusive arterial disease.

An intermittent type of pain that mimics true intermittent claudication is *pseudoclaudication* due to lumbar spinal stenosis. When symptomatic lumbar spinal stenosis exists in the absence of symptomatic occlusive arterial disease, clinical differentiation of true intermittent claudication from pseudoclaudication is not difficult (Table 1.2); but, when both occlusive arterial disease of the lower extremities and lumbar spinal stenosis coexist and are symptomatic, historical differentiation may not be possible so that evaluation with exercise tests in the vascular laboratory,[3] imaging of the lumbar spine by computed tomography angiography (CTA) or magnetic resonance angiography (MRA) may be necessary to determine which is the more serious and symptomatic of the 2 conditions.

The occurrence of muscle cramps during rest, often during sleep ("nocturnal leg cramps"), does not indicate occlusive arterial disease in the extremity though patients may consider them such and seek evaluation because of them.

Color change of the extremity(s) or digit(s), both permanent and intermittent, are usually easy to diagnose clinically if sufficient details are elicited historically. For example, some questions useful clinically in the differential diagnosis of primary Raynaud's phenomenon

(Raynaud's disease) from secondary Raynaud's phenomenon are shown in Table 1.3. Another vasospastic disorder, livedo reticularis, can be primary or secondary to a variety of disorders, but as a rule, the secondary types of livedo reticularis are of recent onset. The constant discoloration of the hands and occasionally the feet that occurs in the benign vasospastic acrocyanosis, seen in some young women, distinguishes it from Raynaud's phenomenon.

Primary Raynaud's Disease	Secondary Raynaud's Phenomenon
Painless	Painful
No skin changes	Sclerodactyly, digital ulcers
No associated medical issues	GERD, + pulmonary hypertension
Antinuclear antibody negative	Antinuclear antibody positive

Table 1.3 Differential Diagnosis of Primary Raynaud's Disease from Secondary Raynaud's Phenomenon

Since leg edema has many different causes, both systemic and regional, it is useful to have an organized historical approach to categorize its type; the answers to the following 8 questions usually differentiate regional from systemic types of edema[4]:

1. When did the edema begin?
2. Is the swollen extremity painful?
3. Does the edema recede overnight?
4. Are there associated cardiac symptoms?
5. Is there any evidence of renal disease?

6. Is there evidence of chronic hepatic disease?

7. Are there any bowel or significant weight changes?

8. What medications, if any, is the person taking?

Important to keep in mind are the frequent causes of drug-induced edema, such as dihydropyridine calcium channel blockers. The regional types of edema of vascular origin—venous and lymphatic—are usually easy to differentiate from lipedema (Figure 1.2), a leg enlargement that is lipodystrophic in origin (Table 1.4).

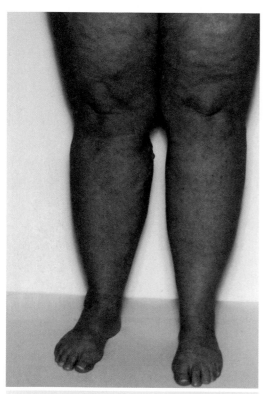

Figure 1.2 Lipedema

The Vascular Examination

The vascular examination should include examination of the ocular fundus and the skin as well as the arterial, venous, and lymphatic systems. These will be covered in order.

The *ocular fundus* provides a unique opportunity to view and assess arteries and veins. Findings that are relevant to vascular disorders include the cholesterol plaque (Figure 1.3), which indicates atherosclerosis of the ascending, or arch, portion of the thoracic aorta or the ipsilateral carotid artery; there is an increased frequency of stroke in persons with asymptomatic retinal cholesterol emboli.[5] Noting engorged retinal veins (Figure 1.4), seen in polycythemia vera, may explain the occurrence of a patient's arterial or venous thrombosis. A rare heritable disorder of elastic tissue frequently associated with occlusive peripheral, coronary, and cerebral arterial disease, pseudoxanthoma elasticum, has a classic ocular fundus finding of angioid streaks (Figure 1.5). The important secondary and correctible cause of hypertension, coarctation of the aorta, may be "tipped off" by very tortuous retinal arterioles (Figure 1.6), though this is not an absolute association.

Like the ocular fundus, the skin can be a valuable source of clinical diagnostic findings. After noting the color, temperature, and hair growth of the skin, attention to some other specific "vascular" points is useful. Venous stars (Figure 1.7) in the skin of the upper arm or anterior chest indicate occlusion or obstruction of a major mediastinal vein[6] (which may also present with nonpulsatile distention of a jugular vein). A useful maneuver in the evaluation

Characteristics			
	Venous	Lymph	Lipedema
Bilateral	Occasionally	±	Always
Stasis change	+	0	0
Thickened skin	0	+	0
Foot involved	+	+	0
Toes involved	0	+	0

Table 1.4 Edema, regional types

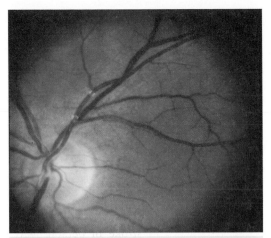

Figure 1.3 Cholesterol emboli in a retinal arteriole.

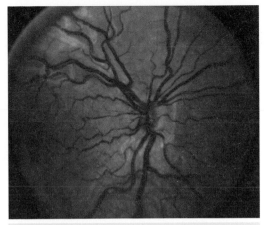

Figure 1.4 Engorged retinal veins in a patient with polycythemia vera. (Reproduced from Spittell A Jr. *Peripheral Vascular Disease for Cardiologists. A Clinical Approach.* Elmsford, NY, and Oxford, UK: Blackwell Publishing/Futura Division; 2004. By permission of Blackwell Publishing.)

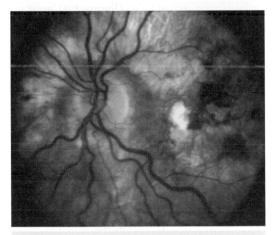

Figure 1.5 Pseudoxanthoma elasticum. Angioid streaks in the retina. (Reproduced from Spittell A Jr. *Peripheral Vascular Disease for Cardiologists. A Clinical Approach.* Elmsford, NY, and Oxford, UK: Blackwell Publishing/Futura Division; 2004. By permission of Blackwell Publishing.)

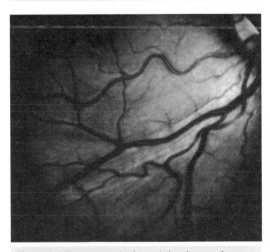

Figure 1.6 Tortuous retinal arterioles that can be seen in some patients with coarctation of the aorta. (Reproduced from Spittell A Jr. *Peripheral Vascular Disease for Cardiologists. A Clinical Approach.* Elmsford, NY, and Oxford, UK: Blackwell Publishing/Futura Division; 2004. By permission of Blackwell Publishing.)

of a swollen limb is comparing the texture of the skin of the back of one's hand (Figure 1.8) to the texture of the skin of the swollen limb; the skin in lymphedema is palpably thickened. Other diagnostically valuable skin lesions are the xanthomata in lipid disorders, telangiectasia in scleroderma (Figure 1.9), and the "plucked chicken" skin in the face, neck, and axilla in pseudoxanthoma elasticum (Figure 1.10). Four common types of ulceration of the skin of the extremity are seen in persons with vascular disease, and each has enough characteristic features to readily allow identification on examination (see Table 1.1).

Evaluation of the peripheral arterial system should include palpation of the carotid arteries and of the subclavian, brachial, radial, and ulnar arteries in the upper extremity, and the abdominal aorta and femoral, popliteal, posterior tibial, and dorsal pedis arteries in the lower extremity. Having a system of grading of each artery's pulsation is useful—eg, 0 indicates absence of pulsation, 4 indicates normal pulsation, and 1, 2, and 3 indicate degrees of impairment of

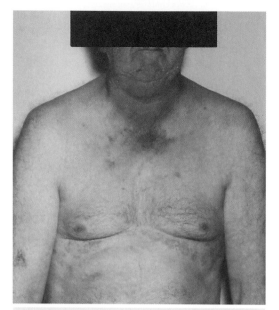

Figure 1.7 Venous "stars" on anterior chest and right arm in a patient with chronic superior vena cava obstruction. (Reproduced from Spittell A Jr. *Peripheral Vascular Disease for Cardiologists. A Clinical Approach.* Elmsford, NY, and Oxford, UK: Blackwell Publishing/Futura Division; 2004. By permission of Blackwell Publishing.)

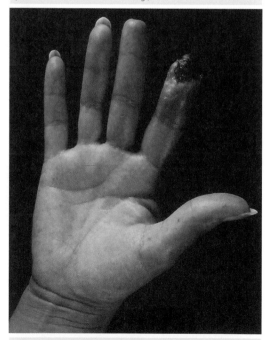

Figure 1.9 Gangrene on tip of index finger due to digital artery thrombosis in a patient with scleroderma. Note typical telangiectatic spot on third finger. (Reproduced from Spittell A Jr. *Peripheral Vascular Disease for Cardiologists. A Clinical Approach.* Elmsford, NY, and Oxford, UK: Blackwell Publishing/Futura Division; 2004. By permission of Blackwell Publishing.)

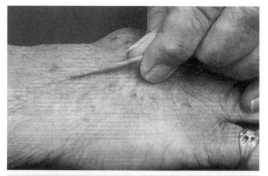

Figure 1.8 Normal skin texture demonstrated on dorsum of examiner's hand. (Reproduced from Spittell A Jr. *Peripheral Vascular Disease for Cardiologists. A Clinical Approach.* Elmsford, NY, and Oxford, UK: Blackwell Publishing/Futura Division; 2004. By permission of Blackwell Publishing.)

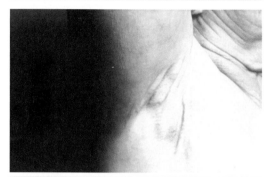

Figure 1.10 Pseudoxanthoma elasticum. "Plucked chicken" appearance of the skin in the axilla. (Reproduced from Spittell A Jr. *Peripheral Vascular Disease for Cardiologists. A Clinical Approach.* Elmsford, NY, and Oxford, UK: Blackwell Publishing/Futura Division; 2004. By permission of Blackwell Publishing.)

pulsation. There are many other grading scales, with some advocating 0 being absent, 1 being palpable but diminished, and 2 being normal. A widened or aneurysmal pulse should be described as such, and not be given a number. The abdominal aorta should be examined and if a palpable pulsatile mass is evident, further screening tests for abdominal aortic aneurysm are warranted. Routinely palpating and comparing the timing of the pulsation of the radial arteries simultaneously will prevent missing the "delayed pulsation" of the radial artery ipsilateral to an occluded subclavian artery, so-called *subclavian steal* (Figure 1.11); identifying the subclavian steal can be quite important in the potential coronary bypass patient since the ipsilateral internal mammary artery would not

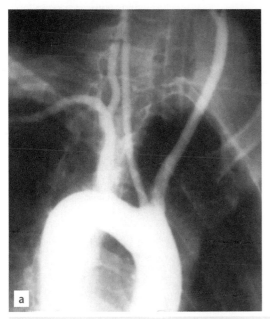
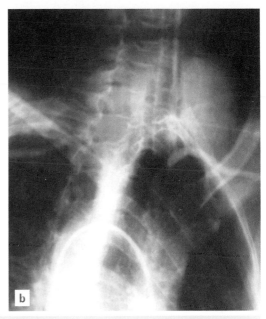

Figure 1.11 Subclavian "steal." (a) Arch aortogram in a 65-year-old woman, a veteran smoker, demonstrating stenosis of the proximal left subclavian artery (a "smoker's lesion"). (b) Latter phase of arch aortogram showing opacification of left vertebral artery—the subclavian "steal." (Modified from Spittell JA Jr. Peripheral arterial disease. *Disease-A-Month*. 1994;40(12):641-704. With permission from Elsevier.)

be a good choice for revascularizing a coronary artery unless the subclavian artery lesion is corrected prior to coronary artery surgery. A similar and important "delay" of a femoral artery pulsation compared to a radial artery pulsation in the person with coarctation of the aorta will be evident if simultaneous palpation of the radial and femoral arteries is always included in the arterial examination.

Following the peripheral arterial examination, a clinically useful maneuver is elevation of the lower extremities to 60° above the level and observing any change in color of the skin of the soles of the feet. If no pallor develops in 60 seconds of elevation the arterial circulation is normal or minimally occluded; however, if definite pallor of the skin of the sole of the foot develops within 60 seconds of elevation (Figure 1.12) of the extremity, there is significant occlusive arterial disease in the extremity. Confirmation can be obtained by having the patient hang the extremities dependent to observe the time for color to return to the skin (normal, 10 seconds; ischemia, 15 or more seconds), and for the superficial veins to fill (normal, 15 seconds; ischemia, 20 or more seconds). When the extremity

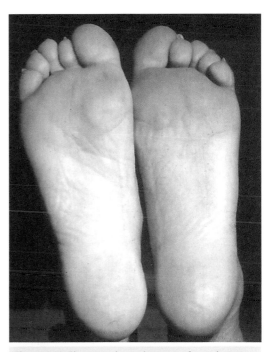

Figure 1.12 Elevation-dependency test for occlusive peripheral arterial disease. Pallor of the right foot on elevation. Patient had an ankle-brachial index (ABI) of 0.32 in the right leg and 0.80 in the left leg. (From Spittell JA Jr. Office and bedside. Diagnosis of occlusive arterial disease. *Curr Prob Cardiol.* 1983;8:3-34. With permission from Elsevier.)

is severely ischemic, with dependency a deep rubrous color—dependent rubor (see Figure 1.1)—will develop. These elevation-dependency tests provide a rapid office or bedside clinical evaluation of the peripheral arterial circulation.

Since the radial artery is at times being considered for access or use as a conduit, for percutaneous coronary angiography or interventional procedures, the adequacy of the collateral circulation in the hand can be reliably evaluated with the Allen test (Figure 1.13).[7] The Allen test has been modified to provide a timed end point to evaluate the adequacy of the collateral circulation in the hand by the ulnar artery; timing of the return of color to the thenar eminence and thumb while the radial artery compression is maintained and the compression of the ulnar artery is released is the end point of this modification.[8] The Allen test is also useful for the diagnosis of thromboangiitis obliterans (Buerger's

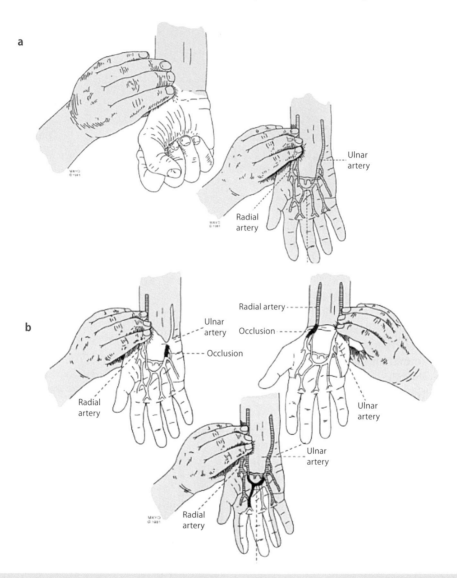

Figure 1.13 The Allen test. (a) Normal (negative) result, indicating patency of ulnar artery and superficial palmar arch. (b) Abnormal (positive) results due to occlusion of ulnar artery (left), radial artery (right), and superficial palmar arch (center). (From Spittell JA Jr. Occlusive peripheral arterial disease: Guidelines for office management. *Postgrad Med.* 1982;71:137-151. *Postgraduate Medicine* is a registered trademark of JTE Multimedia, LLC, 1235 Westlakes Drive Suite 320, Berwyn, PA 19312, 610-889-3730.)

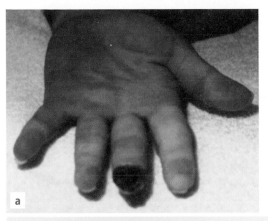
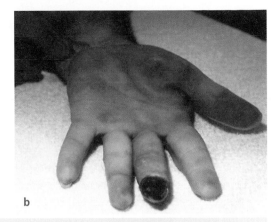

Figure 1.14 Occlusion of palmar arch in a man with thromboangiitis obliterans, demonstrated by persistence of pallor of radial side of hand and second and third fingers whether radial (a) or ulnar (b) arterial inflow is blocked by examiner's finger. (Reproduced from Spittell JA Jr. Introduction to the use of noninvasive techniques in vascular disease. In: Bernstein EF. *Noninvasive Techniques in Vascular Diseases.* St. Louis, MO: C.V. Mosby;1978.)

disease) (Figure 1.14), the purpose for which the test was originally described by Allen.[9]

Auscultation for *bruits* over large arteries (carotid, subclavian, renal and femoral, and the abdominal aorta) is an essential part of a complete arterial examination. Bruits usually indicate turbulence of flow due to stenosis upstream; most bruits are systolic but occasionally the systolic bruit will extend into diastole as a result of an arterial stenosis in the range of 80%—a significant clinical finding (Figure 1.15).

Many physicians have included performance of the *ankle-brachial index (ABI)* in their offices or clinic evaluations since the ABI has become the objective standard for diagnosis; furthermore, the ABI detects clinically occult disease in a significant number of patients. A normal ABI (at rest) is 1.0 to 1.4, an ABI ≤ 0.9 is abnormal and not only confirms the diagnosis of lower-extremity arterial occlusive disease but an abnormal ABI is also associated with a higher risk of mortality (BARI trial), future cardiovascular morbidity and mortality (HOPE trial), and increased risk of stroke.[10]

Determining the ABI before and after standard exercise (eg, active pedal plantar flexion, an office-based exercise study, or treadmill walking[3]) provides an accurate estimate of any arterial insufficiency and the functional impairment it is imposing.

Severe stenosis without collateral circulation

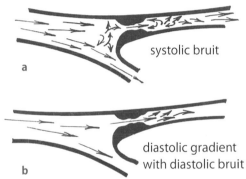

systolic bruit

diastolic gradient with diastolic bruit

Figure 1.15 Arterial bruits in occlusive arterial disease. (a) Systolic bruit with slight to moderate stenosis upstream. (b) Systolic bruit flowing into diastole in severe (≥ 80%) arterial stenosis upstream. (Reproduced from Spittell A Jr. *Peripheral Vascular Disease for Cardiologists. Clinical Approach.* Elmsford, NY, and Oxford, UK: Blackwell Publishing/Futura Division; 2004. By permission of Blackwell Publishing.)

Many examiners have difficulty adequately examining the popliteal artery, so some useful points about this aspect of the vascular examination are warranted. From a clinical point of view, the popliteal artery begins in the lower medial thigh at the point where the superficial femoral artery exits the adductor tendon, and it then extends distally to the level of the knee joint, where it is located at the junction of the lateral and medial vertical thirds of the knee. The "clinical" popliteal artery ends where it trifurcates, about 1 inch below the knee joint in the middle of the upper calf. The reason for emphasizing the "clinical" popliteal artery is that popliteal artery aneurysm can occur at the upper, middle, and/or lower portions of the artery (Figure 1.16) and could be overlooked unless all portions of the artery are examined.

The subclavian vessels can be compressed in the thoracic outlet, most often in the space between the uppermost rib (a cervical rib or the first rib) and the clavicle (Figure 1.17), resulting in variable symptoms and complications. Compression of the subclavian artery can be demonstrated by performance of the thoracic outlet maneuvers (active and passive costoclavicular, hyperabduction, and scalene maneuvers[11]) and noting a change in the amplitude of the radial artery on the side of the maneuver. Ultrasonography of the subclavian artery during thoracic outlet maneuvers can document compression of the subclavian artery and of the subclavian vein.

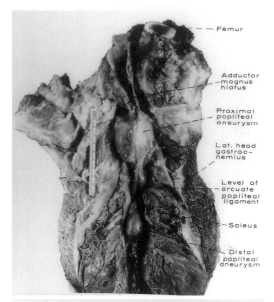

Figure 1.16 Photograph of popliteal fossa in dissected amputated limb of patient having proximal and distal popliteal aneurysms. (From Gedge SW, Spittell JA Jr, Ivins JC, et al. Aneurysm of the distal popliteal artery and its relationship to the arcuate popliteal ligament. *Circulation*. 1961;24:270-273. With permission from Lippincott Williams and Wilkins.)

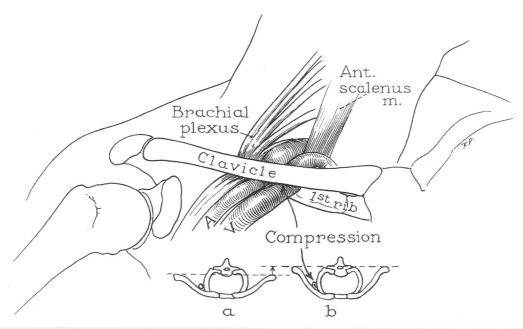

Figure 1.17 Costoclavicular syndrome. Compression of the subclavian vessels very commonly occurs between the clavicle and the uppermost (first and/or cervical) rib. (From Fairbairn JF II, Campbell K, Payne WS. Neurovascular compression syndromes of the thoracic outlet. In: Juergens JF, Spittell JA Jr, Fairbairn JF II. *Peripheral Vascular Diseases*. 5th ed. Philadelphia: WB Saunders; 1980. By permission of Mayo Foundation.)

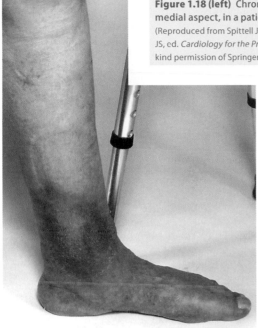

Figure 1.18 (left) Chronic indurated cellulitis (lipodermatosclerosis) of lower leg, medial aspect, in a patient with uncontrolled chronic deep venous insufficiency. (Reproduced from Spittell JA Jr, Spittell PC. Diseases of the peripheral arteries and veins. In: Alpert JS, ed. *Cardiology for the Primary Care Physician*. 3rd ed. Philadelphia: Current Medicine, 2001. With kind permission of Springer Science-Business Media.)

Many venous disorders of the extremities are easy to evaluate and/or diagnose by careful physical examination (eg, varicose veins and chronic deep venous insufficiency) while others, particularly acute deep venous thrombosis, require noninvasive or venographic procedures for accurate diagnosis.

Examination for varicose veins should be done with the patient standing. The competency and course of superficial veins can be determined by compressing the vein at various levels while simultaneously palpating the vein distally for any impulse; transmission of the impulse distally for 20 cm indicates venous valvular incompetence. The presence of deep venous valvular incompetence is suggested by the presence of dependent edema, stasis pigmentation, and chronic indurated cellulitis (Figure 1.18), but in their absence deep venous valvular insufficiency can be detected by noninvasive vascular laboratory studies. Varicose veins and other signs of localized increased venous pressure can be a sign of arteriovenous fistula. In the case of congenital arteriovenous fistula in the extremity, the clinical signs can vary from the presence of a birthmark to increased size of the extremity, varicose veins, and "hot" venous ulceration (Figure 1.19). Acquired arteriovenous fistula in extremity vessels can produce signs of increased venous pressure in the extremity (Figure 1.20) in addition to pulsatile varicose veins and the typical multiple pitched bruit on auscultation near or over the fistula.

Superficial thrombophlebitis is usually quite easily recognized by its reddened linear course, which is palpably hardened and tender, but if it does not present these classic findings, Doppler ultrasonography can readily confirm the diagnosis. Acute lymphangitis is usually easily differentiated by its associated high fever, frequently accompanied by chills, from superficial thrombophlebitis.

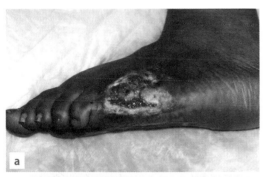

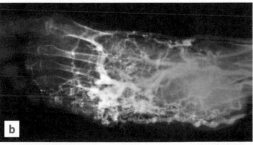

Figure 1.19 (above) (a) "Hot" venous ulceration of the foot. (b) Angiogram demonstrating congenital arteriovenous fistula of patient shown in a. (Reproduced from Spittell A Jr. *Peripheral Vascular Disease for Cardiologists. A Clinical Approach*. Elmsford, NY, and Oxford, UK: Blackwell Publishing/Futura Division; 2004. By permission of Blackwell Publishing.)

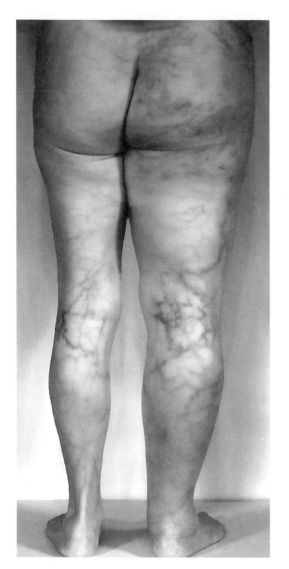

Figure 1.20 (left) Infrared photograph of right lower extremity showing edema and increased venous pattern. Cause is an arteriovenous fistula of iliac vessels created at time of subject's lumbar disc surgery. (Reproduced from Spittell A Jr. *Peripheral Vascular Disease for Cardiologists. A Clinical Approach.* Elmsford, NY, and Oxford, UK: Blackwell Publishing/Futura Division; 2004. By permission of Blackwell Publishing.)

Unlike superficial thrombophlebitis, acute deep venous thrombosis is often not diagnosed with confidence by physical examination alone since the findings are nonspecific and similar to those of musculoskeletal conditions. An exception, however, is the classic but rare phlegmasia cerulea dolens (Figure 1.21). Consequently, in most cases of suspected acute deep venous thrombosis, objective testing is needed to confirm or exclude the diagnosis; duplex ultrasonography is currently the test of choice for the diagnosis of acute deep venous thrombosis, but venography or magnetic resonance direct thrombus imaging has the advantage of diagnosing calf vein as well as proximal deep venous thrombosis.

Lymphedema, which can be primary or secondary, is the type of regional leg edema that is

Figure 1.21 (below) Phlegmasia cerulea dolens in right lower extremity. Note discoloration of right foot. (Reproduced from Spittell JA Jr, Spittell PC. Diseases of the peripheral arteries and veins. In: Alpert JS, ed. *Cardiology for the Primary Care Physician.* 3rd ed. Philadelphia: Current Medicine, 2001. With kind permission of Springer Science-Business Media.)

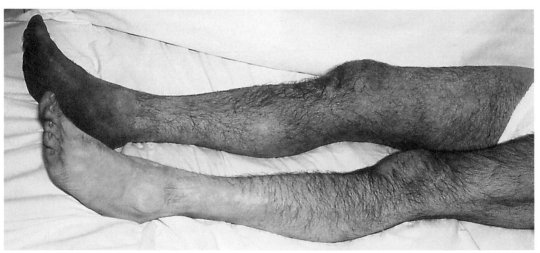

difficult diagnostically for many clinicians. The clinical features of lymphedema include a predominance of location on the dorsum of the foot and toes, with a firm, woody appearance associated with cobblestoning of the skin. One particular feature of lymphedema is involvement of the toes, which differentiates it from venous edema and lipedema. As noted earlier, because lymphedema causes thickening of the skin, using the skin of the back of the hand of the examiner (see Figure 1.8) as normal skin texture in comparison to the skin of the swollen extremity is useful to identify lymphedema. Clinical features that differentiate the common type of primary lymphedema, lymphedema precox, from secondary obstructive lymphedema due to neoplasm is the age of the patient; lymphedema precox virtually always starts before the age of 40 years, while obstructive lymphedema due to neoplasm, usually pelvic in origin, has its onset after the age of 40.

Summary

This chapter addresses the traditional diagnostic approaches that are available to the clinician for patients with peripheral vascular disease. In an age of advanced diagnostic tools and cutting edge technology, there is still also immense value, efficiency, and reliability in the eyes, ears, and hands of the skilled physician.

References

1. Fred HL. Hyposkillia. Deficiency of clinical skills. *Texas Heart Inst J*. 2005;32:255-257.
2. Hirsch AT, Criqui MH, Treat-Jacobson D, et al. Peripheral arterial disease detection, awareness, and treatment in primary care. *JAMA*. 2001;286:1317-1324.
3. McPhail IR, Spittell PC, Weston SA, et al. Intermittent claudication: an office-based assessment. *J Am Coll Cardiol*. 2001;37(5):1381-1385.
4. Spittell JA Jr. Leg edema. In: Spittell JA Jr. *Peripheral Vascular Disease for Cardiologists. A Clinical Approach*. Elmsford, NY, and Oxford, UK: Blackwell Publishing/Futura Division; 2004;92-99.
5. Bruno A, Jones WL, Austin JK, et al. Vascular outcome in men with asymptomatic retinal cholesterol emboli. *Ann Intern Med*. 1995;122:249-253.
6. Fred HL, Castle CH, Cancilla PA, et al. Venous stars in mediastinal disease. *AMA Arch Int Med*. 1962;109:290-296.
7. Greenwood MJ, Della-Siega AJ, Fretz EB, et al. Vascular communication in the hand in patients considered for transradial coronary angiography: is the Allen's test accurate? *J Am Coll Cardiol*. 2005;46:2013-2017.
8. Conklin LD, Fergeson ER, and Reardon MJ. The technical aspects of radial artery harvesting. *Texas Heart Inst J*. 2001;28:129-131.
9. Allen EV. Thromboangiitis obliterans: methods of diagnosis of chronic occlusive arterial lesions distal to the wrist with illustrative cases. *Am J Med Sci*. 1929;78:237-244.
10. Murabito JM, Evans JC, Larson MG, et al. The ankle-brachial index in the elderly and risk of stroke, coronary disease, and death: the Framingham Study. *Arch Intern Med*. 2003;163(16):1939-1942.
11. Spittell JA Jr. Some uncommon peripheral vascular disorders. In: Spittell JA Jr. *Peripheral Vascular Disease for Cardiologists. A Clinical Approach*. Elmsford, NY, and Oxford, UK: Blackwell Publishing/Futura Division; 2004; 117-124.

Part 2

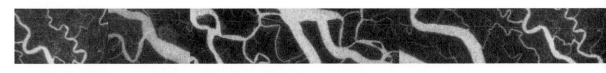

The Assessment of Peripheral Artery Disease

2

The Diagnosis of Peripheral Artery Disease

Stephen O'Connor, Thomas J. Kiernan, and Michael R. Jaff

A number of diagnostic tools are available for the practicing clinician seeing patients with suspected *peripheral artery disease (PAD)*. These tests are commonly performed in the consultant's examination room and the noninvasive vascular laboratory, and a thorough knowledge of the strengths, weaknesses, and clinical applicability of each test is essential to effectively diagnose patients with PAD.

There are 2 components to the diagnosis of PAD: (1) *physiologic testing* to determine the presence, severity, and functional impact of PAD, and (2) *anatomic assessment* to determine optimal medical and revascularization strategies. The initial modality used depends largely on the clinical presentation. For example, patients at risk for PAD, or those who have no known cardiovascular disease and multiple cardiovascular risk factors, may benefit from assessment with the ankle-brachial index. Symptomatic patients with findings suggestive of intermittent claudication may undergo ankle-brachial index assessment, segmental limb pressures, pulse volume recordings, and treadmill exercise testing. Those patients who have already been diagnosed with PAD and who have been treated with revascularization (either surgical or endovascular) commonly are followed with duplex ultrasonography surveillance.

Physiologic Testing

The physiologic tests for PAD include the ankle-brachial index, segmental limb pressures, Doppler waveforms, pulse volume recordings, and exercise treadmill testing.

Ankle-Brachial Index

The *ankle-brachial index (ABI)* serves as the standard for the diagnosis of lower-extremity PAD. In clinical practice, the ABI is the most simple, inexpensive, reliable, and reproducible method of identifying PAD. There are specific patient populations in whom ABI testing should be considered, including those patients who:

- are age 50 to 69 years with a history of smoking or diabetes;
- are > 70 years of age;
- are experiencing limb symptoms with exertion (suggestive of intermittent claudication);

Vascular Disease: Diagnostic and Therapeutic Approaches. © 2011 Michael R. Jaff and Christopher J. White, editors. Cardiotext Publishing, ISBN: 978-1-935395-16-4.

- are suffering ischemic rest pain, non-healing ulcerations, or gangrene;
- have an abnormal lower-extremity pulse examination.

The ABI is performed by determining the ratio of systolic blood pressure of the ankle arteries relative to that of the brachial arteries using a hand-held, continuous-wave Doppler device with a 5- to 10-MHz transducer. This test requires a blood pressure cuff and acoustic gel. Measurements for the ABI should be obtained after the patient has been supine for 5 to 10 minutes. The test requires that the systolic blood pressure be recorded in both brachial arteries and in both the dorsalis pedis and posterior tibial arteries of each limb. The ABI is calculated for each leg by dividing the highest ankle systolic pressure by the highest brachial systolic pressure, recording the value to 2 decimal places. In general, the ankle pressure will exceed the brachial pressure by 10 to 15 mm Hg in healthy individuals as a result of higher peripheral resistance at the ankles. The ABI was initially interpreted according to practice guidelines for PAD management from the American College of Cardiology and the American Heart Association (ACC/AHA).[1] However, a more recent publication of the Ankle Brachial Index Collaboration, analyzing 16 studies, redefined the ABI grading and relation to PAD severity. A normal ABI is 1.0-1.39. Borderline values are between 0.90-1.0, and an abnormal ABI is <0.90.[2] The lower the ABI, the more severe the peripheral artery disease. An ABI < 0.4 suggests critical limb ischemia, and likely represents atherosclerotic disease of multiple arterial segments of the limb. Vascular diagnostic laboratories perform ABIs in similar fashion, however, these laboratories also provide waveform assessments, either with pulse volume recordings or Doppler waveforms (Figure 2.1).

The overall accuracy of the ABI to establish the lower-extremity PAD diagnosis has been well established. An ABI of 0.9 or less has a sensitivity of 95% and a specificity of 100%, relative to the gold standard, contrast angiography, for detecting a stenosis of at least 50%.[3] There is low measurement variance with an overall reproducibility of approximately 0.1.[1]

An abnormal ABI is a potent predictor of cardiovascular events and premature mortality. More recently, deterioration in the ABI over time has been shown to be associated with increased mortality. Criqui et al[4] demonstrated that patients who had > 0.15 deterioration of the ABI over a 1- to 2-year period had an over 2-fold increase in all-cause and cardiovascular mortality.

The ABI has also been used to assess efficacy of antiplatelet therapy in patients with a low as compared to normal ABI and no clinical evidence of cardiovascular disease.[5]

Significant medial artery calcification will prevent arterial compression and can result in elevated ABI values. This finding is most commonly seen in patients with diabetes but may also be present in elderly individuals, patients with chronic kidney disease who require dialysis, and patients receiving chronic corticosteroid therapy. This group of patients also has an increased rate of cardiovascular events.[6]

In addition, a falsely normal ABI can occur. This phenomenon is most often found among patients with aortoiliac atherosclerosis and moderate arterial stenosis, which, at rest, does not result in hemodynamically significant stenosis. However, with exercise, where the musculature is distal to the fixed stenosis, there is an increased requirement for oxygenated blood, and a translesional pressure gradient develops. This results in a reduction in the ankle pressure and the ABI. Therefore, if a patient's clinical picture is very suggestive of peripheral artery disease and they have a normal resting ABI, the clinician should pursue the diagnosis of PAD using other noninvasive testing modalities such as exercise treadmill testing.

One final limitation of the ABI is the inability to identify the specific location of the arterial disease, to define whether or not an arterial stenosis or occlusion is present, and to determine the true length of the atherosclerotic lesion. If this information is desired, anatomic imaging is necessary.

Exercise Treadmill Testing

Exercise treadmill ABI measurements can help diagnose PAD in patients who have nor-

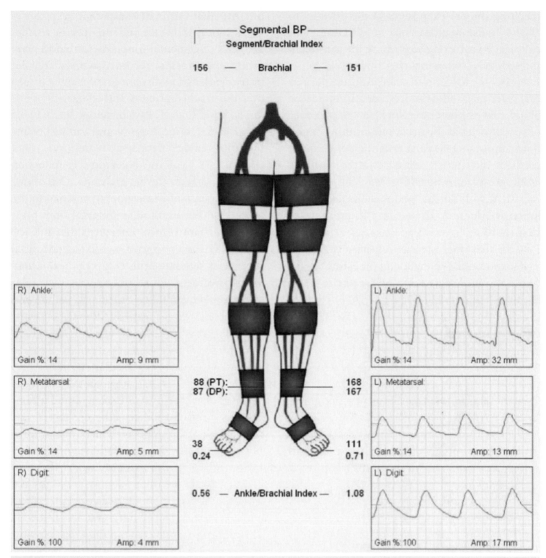

Figure 2.1 Vascular laboratory measurement of ankle-brachial index at rest. Note the normal left leg ABI, 1.08, abnormal right leg ABI, 0.56.

mal measurements at rest. In addition, this is often the most important test to document whether exertional limb discomfort is due to arterial occlusive disease or nonvascular *pseudoclaudication*. Exercise treadmill testing can also serve as a functional assessment for newly diagnosed patients and for monitoring response to medical and revascularization therapies (eg, surveillance following aortoiliac and infrainguinal percutaneous transluminal angioplasty [PTA]).

Once a baseline ABI is obtained, the individual is placed on a treadmill using a preset speed and grade (commonly 2 mph at a 10% or 12% incline). Variable-grade testing can also be used. The patient's limb symptoms, their intensity, and their location should be recorded at symptom-onset, with changes during the examination, and at the time of maximal discomfort when the patient must stop ambulating. When the patient has walked until maximal discomfort or the test has reached a predefined end point (eg, 5 minutes) the ABI is measured immediately following cessation of exercise. Some vascular laboratories continue measuring ankle pressures at 1-minute intervals until reaching the pre-exercise baseline, referred to as the "pulse reappearance time." Other labs perform a post-exercise pressure measurement immediately following cessation of exercise. Exercise normally produces significant peripheral arterial vasodilation resulting in increased blood flow to the extremities. In the presence of fixed arterial obstruction, arterial blood flow cannot increase and a significant pressure gradient develops, resulting in a reduction in ankle pressure compared to brachial pressure. A patient with normal peripheral artery circulation will have no change or a slight increase in the ABI.

An abnormal exercise response is defined as a post-exercise reduction in the ABI of > 0.2 *or* an absolute decrease in post-exercise ankle pressure > 20 mm Hg (Figure 2.2).

Segmental Limb Pressures

The location and extent of PAD can be further defined by segmental limb systolic blood pressure measurements, recorded with a Doppler instrument, and plethysmographic cuffs placed over the brachial arteries and at various points on the lower limb. These commonly include the upper thigh, lower thigh, upper calf just below the knee, ankle, metatarsal region, and digit (Figure 2.3). Typically, a 20-mm Hg reduction between adjacent levels indicates underlying arterial disease of the segment proximal to the lower cuff. For example, segmental limb pressures of 120 mm Hg at the lower thigh and 100 mm Hg at the upper calf would suggest distal superficial femoral artery or popliteal artery disease. Segmental limb pressure measurements have the same limitation as the ABI with regard

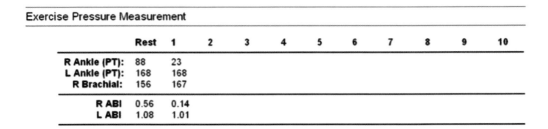

Exercise Pressure Measurement											
	Rest	1	2	3	4	5	6	7	8	9	10
R Ankle (PT):	88	23									
L Ankle (PT):	168	168									
R Brachial:	156	167									
R ABI	0.56	0.14									
L ABI	1.08	1.01									

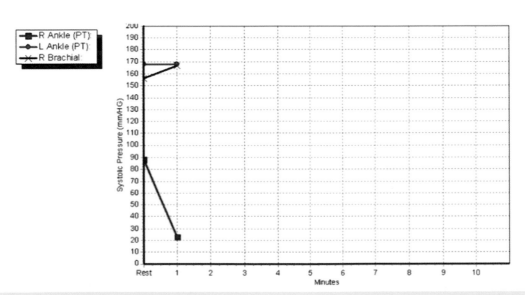

Figure 2.2 Post-exercise pressure results in the same patient as Figure 2.1. Note that the left leg pressure remains unchanged following exercise, but the right ankle pressure drops significantly.

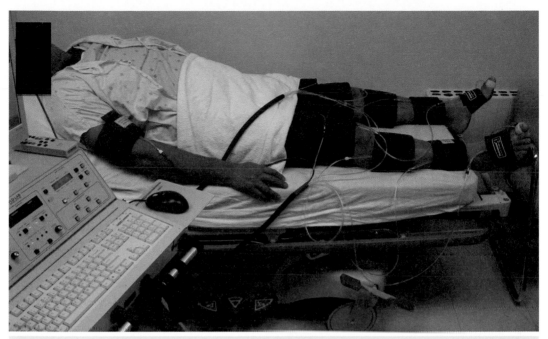

Figure 2.3 Vascular laboratory setup for segmental limb pressures and pulse volume recordings at rest.

to noncompressible vessels. Although segmental limb pressures can be measured alone, they are more commonly obtained with pulse volume recordings.

Pulse Volume Recording

A *pulse volume recording (PVR)* is obtained with a cuff system that incorporates pneumoplethysmography to detect volume changes in the limb throughout the cardiac cycle. Changes in pulse contour and amplitude can be analyzed, providing additional information on the status of the limb arteries. Cuffs are inflated to ~65 mm Hg, and with each pulse of arterial blood passing beneath the cuff, the volume of the cuff surrounding the limb at this point will increase; this change is detected and recorded as a waveform, or PVR. A normal waveform mirrors that of an intra-arterial pressure waveform, with a steep upstroke, a sharp systolic peak, a narrow pulse width, a dicrotic notch, and a downslope bowing to the baseline[7] (Figure 2.4). In the presence of PAD, the slope of the upstroke flattens, the peak becomes more rounded and has a wider pulse width, the dicrotic notch disappears, and

the downslope bows away from the baseline. PVR is effective at evaluating small-vessel disease when applied to the feet.

The combination of PVR and segmental pressures has a reported diagnostic accuracy of 97%.[8] The PVR-segmental pressure technique accurately predicts the severity of iliac and superficial femoral artery disease. It is less accurate in the assessment of more distal disease, particularly in the face of upstream "inflow" PAD.[9] PVRs are also useful to assess limb perfusion after revascularization procedures, and can predict risk of critical limb ischemia and limb prognosis.[10]

Noninvasive Anatomical Assessment

Duplex Ultrasonography

Arterial *duplex ultrasonography* of the lower extremities is commonly used to diagnose PAD. It is reproducible, accurate, and relatively

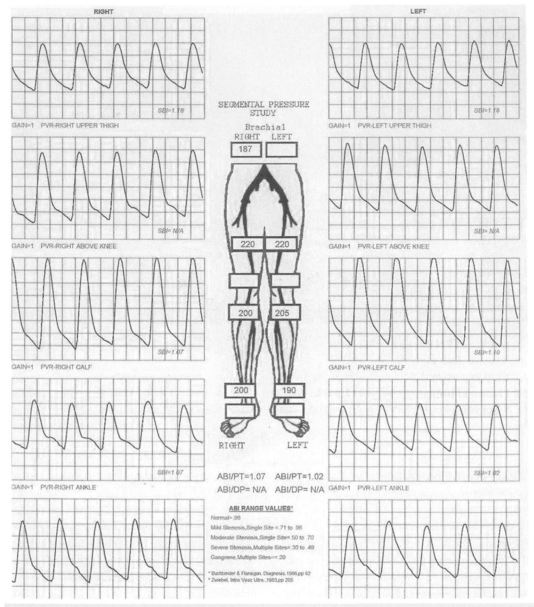

Figure 2.4 Normal pulse volume recordings at rest.

inexpensive. It allows for direct visualization of the vessel and is thus useful in determining the location of disease and in delineating between stenotic and occlusive lesions. Duplex ultrasonography combines color imaging, Doppler spectral waveform analysis, and Doppler-derived systolic and diastolic velocities. A normal peripheral arterial Doppler waveform is triphasic. Cardiac systole results in initial forward flow of blood, followed by a brief period of flow reversal in early diastole and subsequent forward flow in late diastole. The flow-reversal component, a result of high peripheral vascular resistance, is absent in the presence of hemodynamically significant stenosis due to dampening of pulse wave reflection. Stenoses are also identified quantitatively based on peak systolic velocity ratios within the lesion and in the normal artery segment proximal to the stenosis. A ratio of greater than 2.0 is generally accepted to diagnose a stenosis greater than 50% in severity.[9,11] Doppler waveform analysis can be used to identify other indicators of disease, including the presence of turbulence.

In one meta-analysis, the sensitivity and specificity of duplex ultrasonography was 86% and 97%, respectively, for the aortoiliac arteries; 80% and 96% for the femoropopliteal arteries; and 83% and 84% for the infrageniculate arteries.[12] Duplex ultrasonography is widely accepted and recommended for surveillance of surgical vein grafts despite mixed results in published studies of its clinical utility.[1] Although surveillance duplex ultrasonography of synthetic grafts or arteries after angioplasty are often performed, their value remains unproven. Despite accuracy, some limitations exist (Figure 2.5).

Duplex ultrasonography is an accurate noninvasive test for PAD, though it requires technical expertise that may be lacking in some centers. Other limitations include assessment of the aortoiliac vessels due to body habitus and overlying bowel gas, signal "dropout" in heavily calcified vessels, and reduced sensitivity for significant stenosis in the presence of multiple lesions within close proximity (tandem lesions). In addition, multiple stenoses may be difficult to assess with duplex ultrasonography.

Magnetic Resonance Angiography

Magnetic resonance angiography (MRA) is a rapidly evolving technique that facilitates noninvasive assessment of the peripheral arteries without sedation, catheterization, ionizing radiation, or potentially nephrotoxic iodinated contrast agents. Rapid advances in MRA technology in the past several years have led to improvements in resolution, anatomic coverage, and speed of image acquisition.[13]

MRA is based on the combination of rapid 3D imaging and the T1-shortening effect of intravenously infused paramagnetic contrast. These agents greatly shorten the T1 of blood resulting in very bright signal intensity in T1-

weighted images. Data acquisition needs to be precisely timed to the arterial phase of the contrast when the intraluminal signal is maximal, and be fast enough to minimize motion artifacts and to avoid venous contamination that may hamper image interpretation. To facilitate this, there have been continuing advancements including continuous table motion, whole-body

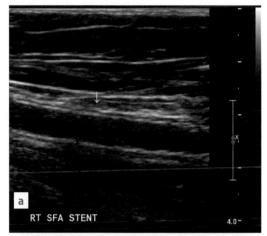

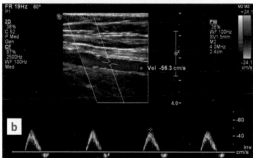

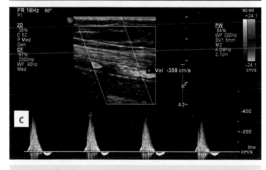

Figure 2.5 (a) Gray scale ultrasonography image of stent within the superficial femoral artery. (b) Color Doppler image of a normal right superficial femoral artery stent. (c) Color Duplex image demonstrating significant increase in peak systolic velocity within stent, suggestive of > 50% stenosis.

MRA techniques, high performance gradients, and new MRA-compatible contrast agents.[14] Multiple acquisition techniques successfully cover long fields of view, such as the suprarenal aorta to the toes. The large field of view required to image the lower extremities requires 3 to 4 overlapping stations with separate contrast boluses. Alternatively, use of "bolus chase" techniques with floating tables is possible. The addition of parallel imaging technologies has made peripheral runoff MRA significantly more robust, with fewer failed studies and with vastly improved image quality.[15]

Contrast-enhanced MRA has replaced conventional catheter-based contrast angiography for diagnosis and procedural planning at many institutions (Figure 2.6). Early experience comparing contrast-enhanced MRA with duplex ultrasonography suggested MRA to be accurate in planning peripheral arterial revascularization. A retrospective series of 100 patients who underwent both imaging methods found that MRA was more effective than duplex ultrasonography in planning revascularization.[16] The ACC/AHA guidelines on PAD sug-

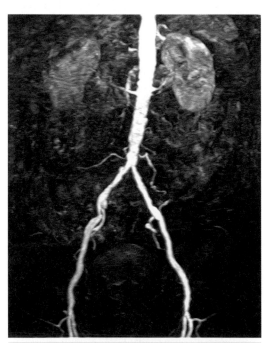

Figure 2.6 Contrast-enhanced MRA of the aortoiliac segments.

gest that MRA may be useful in determining the location and severity of stenosis and may aid in decisions between endovascular and surgical revascularization.[1]

In a meta-analysis of 34 studies (1090 patients) between January 1985 and May 2000, researchers reported high accuracy for the assessment of the lower-extremity arteries using MRA.[17] Furthermore, 3D gadolinium-enhanced MRA improved diagnostic performance compared with 2D MRA; the estimated points of equal sensitivity and specificity were 94% and 90% for 3D gadolinium-enhanced MRA and 2D MRA, respectively.

The predominant criticism of MRA is centered on the misclassification of moderate stenoses as severe, and severe stenoses as occlusions. This tendency to overestimate the extent of stenosis may be avoided by meticulous postprocessing of images and by improved timing of contrast agent administration. When areas of stenosis are seen on 3-dimensionally reconstructed images, cross-sectional source images should be examined recognizing that the Fourier transformations required to generate 3D images degrade spatial resolution. In addition, MRA cannot reliably detect arterial calcification, which is a potential limitation when revascularization options are being considered. Finally, the metal alloys used in current endovascular stents result in signal dropout, which precludes imaging of the arterial segments within stents. MRA can reliably determine the presence of flow proximal and distal to a stent. With newer alloys, imaging within stents using MRA may become a reality in the future.

Other limitations of MRA center on patient factors and technology issues. Patients with implantable defibrillators and permanent pacemakers may not undergo MRA studies, for fear of causing these devices to malfunction.[18,19] Patients with intracranial aneurysm clips also are at high risk if exposed to the magnetic environment. Claustrophobia also is a major issue, precluding approximately 10% of patients from completing MRA studies. Finally, the US Food and Drug Administration (FDA) has issued a warning on the use of gadolinium in patients with advanced chronic kidney disease because it has been linked to the development of nephrogenic systemic fibrosis, also known as nephrogenic fibrosing dermopathy,[11] a rare but devastating, debilitating, and deadly complication of gadolinium exposure in these patients.

Computed Tomography Angiography

Computed tomography angiography (CTA) is increasingly attractive due to rapid technological developments. Shorter acquisition times, thinner slices, higher spatial resolution, and improvement of multidetector row computed tomography (MDCT) scanners enable scanning of the entire vascular tree in a limited period with a decreasing (but still substantial) required amount of contrast medium (Figure 2.7). Recent studies[19,20] evaluating CTA for the diagnosis of PAD report sensitivity and specificity rates of 98%. Advantages of CTA over MRA include better patient acceptance, speed of examination, better spatial resolution, identification of arterial calcification, and the ability to

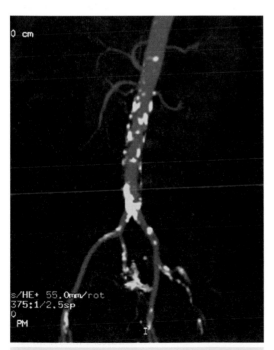

0 cm

s/HE+ 55.0mm/rot
375:1/2.5sp
0
 PM   I

Figure 2.7 CTA of the aortoiliac segment, demonstrating diffuse arterial calcification.

evaluate arteries with indwelling endoluminal stents. The diagnostic accuracy of CTA seems to compare well with MRA,[21,22] although studies directly comparing these imaging modalities are limited. The added advantage of CTA is the ability to image patients with pacemakers and defibrillators.

A recent meta-analysis by Met et al[23] analyzed 957 patients with symptoms of peripheral arterial disease. Overall, the sensitivity of CTA for detecting more than 50% stenosis or occlusion was 95% (95% confidence interval [CI], 92%–97%) and specificity was 96% (95% CI, 93%–97%) when compared with digital subtraction angiography. Computed tomography angiography correctly identified occlusions in 94% of segments, the presence of more than 50% stenosis in 87% of segments, and absence of significant stenosis in 96% of segments. Overstaging occurred in 8% of segments and understaging in 15%.

Venous opacification and asymmetric filling of the arteries in the legs may degrade arterial detail. Evaluation of peripheral arterial stents can be performed with CTA, as there is no signal dropout during CTA scanning. However, the true degree of in-stent stenosis has not been adequately quantified with current technology and scanning algorithms.

Because of the need for large volumes of iodinated contrast media administered via a peripheral intravenous cannula, CTA cannot be performed in patients with azotemia or in individuals at increased risk of contrast-induced acute tubular necrosis. In addition, repetitive CTA studies are not recommended, as they result in patients receiving considerable doses of ionizing radiation.

Contrast Angiography

Contrast angiography, the gold standard for the diagnosis of PAD, is now used less as a diagnostic tool. It is currently reserved for patients in whom revascularization is planned or for those situations in which the results from noninvasive imaging are ambiguous or contradictory. Multiple studies suggest that contrast-enhanced

MRA obviates the need for contrast angiography in most cases. Similar data are emerging with CTA.[24] In many centers, however, it remains the standard that a diagnostic angiogram is obtained with digital subtraction techniques before an intervention is planned. A detailed review of contrast arteriography appears in Chapter 3 of this textbook.

Summary

Currently, a number of noninvasive and invasive imaging tools and techniques can be offered to the patient with suspected PAD. These methods of evaluation are vital in diagnosing and planning future management of patients. Strategies begin with the confirmation of the presence of PAD with the ABI, followed by an assessment of the physiologic significance of the disease by using treadmill exercise testing, segmental limb pressures, and pulse volume recordings. For anatomic assessments of PAD, MRA and CTA are commonly used, with catheter-based contrast arteriography reserved for those patients who are considered candidates for endovascular intervention. Surveillance of revascularization, either surgical or endovascular, is achieved with duplex ultrasonography at specific time intervals.

References

1. Hirsch AT, Haskal ZJ, Hertzer NR, et al. ACC/AHA 2005 Practice Guidelines for the management of patients with peripheral arterial disease (lower extremity, renal, mesenteric, and abdominal aortic): a collaborative report from the American Association for Vascular Surgery/Society for Vascular Surgery, Society for Cardiovascular Angiography and Interventions, Society for Vascular Medicine and Biology, Society of Interventional Radiology, and the ACC/AHA Task Force on Practice Guidelines (Writing Committee to Develop Guidelines for the Management of Patients with Peripheral Arterial Disease): endorsed by the American Association of Cardiovascular and Pulmonary Rehabilitation; National Heart, Lung, and Blood Institute; Society for Vascular Nursing; TransAtlantic Inter-Society Consensus; and Vascular Disease Foundation. *Circulation*. 2006;113(11):e463-654.

2. Fowkes FG, Murray GD, Butcher I, et al. Ankle brachial index combined with Framingham risk score to predict cardiovascular events and mortality. *JAMA* 2008;300:197-208.

3. Bernstein EF, Fronek A. Current status of noninvasive tests in the diagnosis of peripheral arterial disease. *Surg Clin North Am*. 1982;62(3):473-487.

4. Criqui MH, Ninomiya JK, Wingard DL, et al. Progression of peripheral arterial disease predicts cardiovascular disease morbidity and mortality. *J Am Coll Cardiol*. 2008;52(21):1736-1742.

5. Fowkes FG, Price JF, Stewart MC, et al. Aspirin for the prevention of cardiovascular events in a general population screened for a low ankle brachial index: a randomized controlled trial. *JAMA*. 2010;303:841-848.

6. Resnick HE, Lindsay RS, McDermott MM, et al. Relationship of high and low ankle brachial index to all-cause and cardiovascular disease mortality: the Strong Heart Study. *Circulation*. 2004;109(6):733-739.

7. Darling RC, Raines JK, Brener BJ, Austen WG. Quantitative segmental pulse volume recorder: a clinical tool. *Surgery*. 1972;72(6):873-877.

8. Rutherford RB, Lowenstein DH, Klein MF. Combining segmental systolic pressures and plethysmography to diagnose arterial occlusive disease of the legs. *Am J Surg*. 1979;138(2):211-218.

9. Symes JF, Graham AM, Mousseau M. Doppler waveform analysis versus segmental pressure and pulse-volume recording: assessment of occlusive disease in the lower extremity. *Can J Surg*. 1984;27(4):345-347.

10. Kaufman JL, Fitzgerald KM, Shah DM, Corson JD, Leather RP. The fate of extremities with flat lower calf pulse volume recordings. *J Cardiovasc Surg*. (Torino). 1989;30(2):216-219.

11. Moneta GL, Yeager RA, Lee RW, Porter JM. Noninvasive localization of arterial occlusive disease: a comparison of segmental Doppler pressures and arterial duplex mapping. *J Vasc Surg.* 1993;17(3):578-582.

12. Koelemay MJ, den Hartog D, Prins MH, Kromhout JG, Legemate DA, Jacobs MJ. Diagnosis of arterial disease of the lower extremities with duplex ultrasonography. *Br J Surg.* 1996;83(3):404-409.

13. Wardlaw JM, Chappell FM, Best JJ, et al. Noninvasive imaging compared with intra-arterial angiography in the diagnosis of symptomatic carotid stenosis: a meta-analysis. *Lancet.* 2006;367(9521):1503-1512.

14. Ersoy H, Rybicki FJ. MR angiography of the lower extremities. *AJR Am J Roentgenol.* 2008;190(6):1675-1684.

15. Bezooijen R, van den Bosch HC, Tielbeek AV, et al. Peripheral arterial disease: sensitivity-encoded multiposition MR angiography compared with intraarterial angiography and conventional multiposition MR angiography. *Radiology.* 2004;231(1):263-271.

16. Leiner T, Tordoir JH, Kessels AG, et al. Comparison of treatment plans for peripheral arterial disease made with multi-station contrast medium-enhanced magnetic resonance angiography and duplex ultrasound scanning. *J Vasc Surg.* 2003;37(6):1255-1262.

17. Koelemay MJ, Lijmer JG, Stoker J, Legemate DA, Bossuyt PM. Magnetic resonance angiography for the evaluation of lower extremity arterial disease: a meta-analysis. *JAMA.* 2001;285(10):1338-1345.

18. Martin ET, Coman JA, Shellock FG, Pulling CC, Fair R, Jenkins K. Magnetic resonance imaging and cardiac pacemaker safety at 1.5-Tesla. *J Am Coll Cardiol.* 2004;43(7):1315-1324.

19. Nazarian S, Roguin A, Zviman MM, et al. Clinical utility and safety of a protocol for noncardiac and cardiac magnetic resonance imaging of patients with permanent pacemakers and implantable-cardioverter defibrillators at 1.5 tesla. *Circulation.* 2006;114(12):1277-1284.

20. Laswed T, Rizzo E, Guntern D, et al. Assessment of occlusive arterial disease of abdominal aorta and lower extremities arteries: value of multidetector CT angiography using an adaptive acquisition method. *Eur Radiol.* 2008;18(2):263-272.

21. Schernthaner R, Stadler A, Lomoschitz F, et al. Multidetector CT angiography in the assessment of peripheral arterial occlusive disease: accuracy in detecting the severity, number, and length of stenoses. *Eur Radiol.* 2008;18(4):665-671.

22. Nelemans PJ, Leiner T, de Vet HC, van Engelshoven JM. Peripheral arterial disease: meta-analysis of the diagnostic performance of MR angiography. *Radiology.* 2000;217(1):105-114.

23. Met R, Bipat S, Legemate DA, Reekers JA, Koelemay MJ. Diagnostic performance of computed tomography angiography in peripheral arterial disease: a systematic review and meta-analysis. *JAMA.* 2009;301(4):415-424.

24. Kock MC, Adriaensen ME, Pattynama PM, et al. DSA versus multi-detector row CT angiography in peripheral arterial disease: randomized controlled trial. *Radiology.* 2005;237(2):727-737.

3

Peripheral Vascular Angiography

Jose A. Silva and Christopher J. White

The age-adjusted prevalence of peripheral artery disease (PAD) is approximately 12%.[1] However, patients with established risk factors for this condition, such as diabetes mellitus, or patients with known coronary artery disease have a much higher prevalence of PAD. In a prospective study, it was found that compared to patients without significant coronary disease, patients with > 50% stenosis in at least one coronary artery have a significantly higher prevalence of atherosclerosis (intimal-medial thickness > 1 mm by ultrasonography) in the descending aorta (91% vs. 32%, $P < 0.00001$), carotid circulation (72% vs. 47%, $P < 0.01$), and femoral arteries (77% vs. 42%, $P < 0.0003$).[2] Despite these facts, PAD remains poorly recognized, as recently demonstrated by the Peripheral Arterial Disease Awareness, Risk, and Treatment: New Resources for Survival (PARTNERS) investigators, who in a US survey of almost 7000 patients seen in 320 primary care clinics showed that only 45% of the patients with PAD had been diagnosed with this condition prior to the PARTNERS Program.[3]

Consequently, patients with known risk factors for PAD or with established coronary artery disease must undergo a detailed history and physical examination as well as noninvasive tests such as the ankle-brachial index and/or arterial duplex ultrasonography to rule out the presence of PAD. In those with significant symptoms, assessment of the peripheral vascular anatomy is necessary if intervention is being considered.[4]

Despite major advances in noninvasive imaging techniques such as duplex ultrasonography, computerized tomography angiography (CTA), and magnetic resonance angiography (MRA) (Figure 3.1), contrast angiography remains the gold standard for diagnosing PAD. It provides the anatomic details necessary to plan percutaneous or surgical revascularization. In this chapter, we will address the basic anatomy and angiographic procedure of the vascular territories, which more commonly undergo percutaneous or surgical intervention.

General Considerations

High-quality angiography of the aorta, its primary branches, and the peripheral vasculature requires that the operator be familiar with a

Vascular Disease: Diagnostic and Therapeutic Approaches. © 2011 Michael R. Jaff and Christopher J. White, editors. Cardiotext Publishing, ISBN: 978-1-935395-16-4.

variety of arterial vascular access sites, eg, common femoral, brachial, and radial (Table 3.1). To obtain high-quality angiographic images, a radiographic gantry with angulation capability in both the axial and sagittal planes as well as a large-field (14- to 16-in, or 36- to 41-cm) image intensifier capable of capturing the larger regions of interest such as the entire aortic arch, entire pelvic vasculature, and both legs is abso-

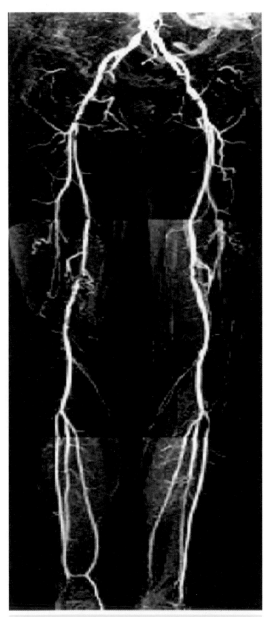

Figure 3.1 MRA of the aortic bifurcation, iliac, femoral, popliteal, and infrapopliteal arteries.

lutely essential.[5] While a coronary-sized image intensifier (9-in) serves to guide interventions, it is not adequate for diagnostic imaging.

Image recording of peripheral studies has conventionally been obtained using film-screen radiographic techniques and mechanical rapid-cut film changers. This has been replaced by digital angiography, which allows immediate monitor display of the acquired image, as well as electronic processing to enhance contrast, reduce noise, and subtract bony and soft-tissue density. Digital subtraction angiography (DSA) significantly enhances the angiographic anatomical detail and allows less contrast to be used, thereby shortening procedure time. A preliminary image (mask) is recorded immediately prior to the contrast injection, so that any background density (bone, calcification, radiopaque objects, soft tissue, and air densities) can be subtracted from subsequent images (Figure 3.2). Quantitative online, angiographic analysis is available and often helpful to provide an objective method of measurement.[5] In Table 3.1 we have summarized some of the most useful angiographic views for the performance of angiography of different vascular territories.

Regarding contrast agents, the use of low/iso-osmolar agents is preferred to high osmolar agents. These more modern and more expensive agents are better tolerated by patients as they cause fewer side effects such as nausea, vomiting, light-headedness, or pain.[6] In addition, low/iso-osmolar agents carry a lower osmotic load and promote less fluid retention, which is desirable in patients with impaired left ventricular and/or renal function.

Alternatives to iodinated contrast, carbon dioxide (CO_2) and gadolinium (gadopentetate dimeglumine), are available to patients with severely impaired renal function and/or a history of life-threatening contrast allergy. Carbon dioxide has been used in many vascular beds, but as a general rule, its use should be avoided for angiograms above the diaphragm, to minimize the risk of distal embolization and stroke.[7-9] Gadolinium use has been significantly constrained in patients with renal insufficiency due to the possibility of nephrogenic systemic

Vascular Territory	Optimal Angiographic View
Aortic arch	30°–60° LAO
Brachiocephalic vessels (origin)	30°–60° LAO
Subclavian	AP, ipsilateral oblique with caudal angulation
Vertebral origin	AP, ipsilateral oblique with cranial angulation
Carotid extracranial	Lateral, AP, ipsilateral oblique
Renal arteries (origin)	5°–10° LAO
Mesenteric arteries (origin)	Lateral, AP
Iliac artery	Contralateral 20° oblique and 20° caudal
CFA, SFA, and PFA arteries	Ipsilateral 20°–40° oblique
Femoro-popliteal	AP
Infrapopliteal trifurcation and runoff	AP

Table 3.1 Most Useful Angiographic Views for Different Vascular Territories. AP: anteroposterior; LAO: left anterior oblique; CFA: common femoral artery, SFA: superficial femoral artery, PFA: profunda femoris artery.

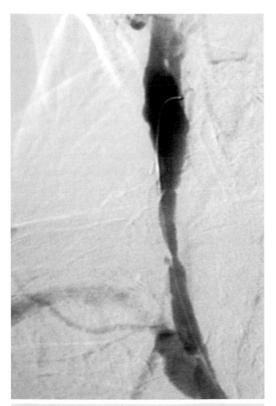

Figure 3.2 DSA of a severely diseased right common carotid artery. The spine and jaw have been subtracted allowing a better visualization of the common carotid artery.

fibrosis, which can affect 2.4% of patients with end stage renal disease (ESRD).[10]

A wide variety of diagnostic catheters and guide wires are available for vascular angiography. Standard guide wires vary in diameter from 0.012 to 0.052 inch, but the most commonly used sizes are 0.035 and 0.038 inch. The length of most standard guide wires is between 100 and 180 cm, and the longer-exchange guide wires measure between 260 and 300 cm. Tip configurations include straight or angled tip and J shape. Varying degrees of shaft stiffness allow advancement of rigid devices through tortuous vessels, and low-friction, hydrophilic-coated wires allow passage in tortuous or difficult-to-cross lesions.

Aortic Arch and Thoracic Aorta

Anatomy

The *aortic arch* and *thoracic aorta* include the ascending, transverse, and descending aorta to the diaphragm. The ascending aorta begins just distal to the sinus of Valsalva and courses from anterior to posterior in the chest. The transverse portion begins as the aorta crosses the main pulmonary artery and the left main stem bronchus and stretches to the ligamentum arteriosum (remnant of the fetal ductus arteriosum). The descending portion begins distal to the ligamentum arteriosum and continues to the diaphragm.[11] The normal aortic diameter ranges from 2.2 to 3.8 cm.[12]

The transverse portion of the thoracic aorta courses posteriorly and gives rise to the brachiocephalic trunk proximally, the left common carotid artery in the midportion, and the left subclavian artery in its distal portion. In 10% to 20% the left common carotid artery may originate from a common ostium with the brachiocephalic trunk or from the brachiocephalic trunk itself, an anatomic variation also known as a *bovine arch* (Figure 3.3).[13] Other less common variations include the left vertebral artery originating directly from the aortic arch, between the left common carotid artery and the left subclavian artery, and the right subclavian artery originating from the aortic arch distal to the origin of the left subclavian artery.[13] The descending aorta courses anterior to the spine and gives origin to 9 pairs of intercostal arteries (T3–T11).

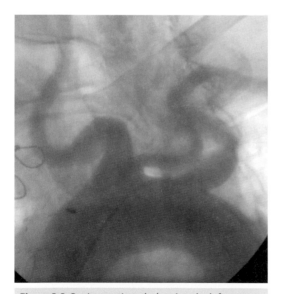

Figure 3.3 Bovine aortic arch showing the left common carotid artery arising from the brachiocephalic trunk.

Thoracic Aortography

Thoracic aortography is performed for the diagnosis of pathologic entities such as aneurysms, aortic dissection, coarctation of the aorta, patent ductus arteriosus, and vascular rings, as well as for the evaluation of vascular injuries such as blunt or penetrating chest trauma and stenoses in the origin of the great vessels. It is also useful prior to planning cerebrovascular intervention, to plan which access site (arm or leg) is most beneficial. However, most of this pathology may also be diagnosed with high accuracy with noninvasive tests such as CTA, MRA, ultrasonography, and transesophageal echocardiography.[14]

Vascular access is usually obtained at the common femoral artery, although the brachial or radial approaches are also useful. A 4- to 6-French (Fr) pigtail catheter is advanced into the ascending aorta and positioned just above the sinus of Valsalva. Using a power injector, a total of 40 to 60 cc of contrast is injected at 20 to 30 cc/sec. For cine imaging 15 to 30 frames/sec is commonly used. For cut films or digital imaging 3 frames/sec or faster should be used, asking the patient to remain still and hold his or her breath to avoid motion artifact. The left anterior oblique (LAO) projection (30°–60°) best separates the ascending from the descending aorta and allows visualization of the origin of the great vessels. The anteroposterior (AP) and right anterior oblique (RAO) views may be helpful to assess the cervical branching vessels (vertebral, subclavian, common carotid).

The aortic arch has recently been classified into 3 types according to the relationship between the origin of the great vessels and a transverse line drawn at the level of the apex of the aortic arch. The type I aortic arch is characterized by origin of all 3 great vessels in the same horizontal plane as the outer curvature of the aortic arch. In the type II aortic arch, the innominate artery originates between the horizontal planes of the outer and inner curvatures of the aortic arch. In the type III aortic arch, the innominate artery originates below the horizontal plane of the inner curvature of the aortic arch (Figure 3.4).[15] This classification has practical clinical applications since the degree of dif-

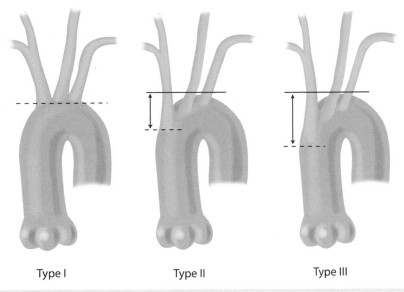

Type I   Type II   Type III

Figure 3.4 Aortic arch types I, II, and III.

ficulty and complication rates for performing selective cervical and cerebrovascular angiography and intervention are related to the aortic arch type (III > II > I).

Cervical Vessels

Anatomy

The *brachiocephalic trunk, left common carotid,* and *subclavian arteries* originate in the transverse portion of the thoracic aorta. The brachiocephalic trunk, or "innominate artery," divides into the right common carotid artery and the right subclavian artery.[11] Although the left common carotid and left subclavian artery most commonly originate separately from the aortic arch, in 10% to 20% of individuals the left common carotid artery arises from a common ostium or from the proximal portion of the innominate artery and is termed a *bovine arch.*[13]

In the AP view, the common carotid arteries run lateral to the cervical vertebral bodies and bifurcate into the external and the internal carotid arteries at the level of the fourth cervi

cal vertebrae.[11] The major distinguishing feature between external and internal carotid arteries is that the internal carotid artery has no branches. The internal carotid artery enters the skull in the petrous portion of the temporal bone, after which it becomes very tortuous in a portion known as the carotid siphon, which courses within the cavernous sinus and the supraclinoid segment. Thereafter, it terminates into the anterior cerebral artery (ACA) and middle cerebral artery (MCA).

The most important branches of the subclavian artery are the internal mammary and the vertebral arteries, which arise at the inferior and the superior aspects of this vessel, respectively, opposite to each other. The vertebral artery is the first and usually the largest branch of the subclavian artery, arising from the upper and posterior surface of the vessel. It angles backward to the transverse process of the sixth cervical vertebra and courses cephalad through the foramina of the transverse processes of the upper 5 cervical vertebrae, where it enters the skull. After penetrating the foramen of the atlas, it turns medially and posteriorly to enter the skull through the foramen magnum. It then gives origin to the posterior inferior cerebellar artery (PICA), and subsequently joins the contralateral vertebral artery to form the basilar artery.

The vertebral artery is divided into 4 segments, V_1 to V_4 (Figure 3.5). This division is of clinical importance because atherosclerotic disease is commonly located in the most proximal 2-cm segment, sometimes called V_0 and within the first 2 segments of the vertebral artery (V_1 and V_2). V_1 begins after the ostial (V_0) portion and continues to the vertebral artery's entrance into the foramen of the sixth transverse process (88% of the cases). V_2 courses cephalad through the foramina of the transverse processes, until it reaches the transverse process of the axis. V_3 continues to its entrance into the spinal canal, and it courses laterally and posteriorly to pass through the transverse foramen of the atlas, approaching the midline and then cephalad to perforate the posterior atlanto-occipital membrane to enter the vertebral canal. V_4 perforates the dura mater and passes thorough the foramen magnum, joining then the contralateral vertebral artery to form the basilar artery.

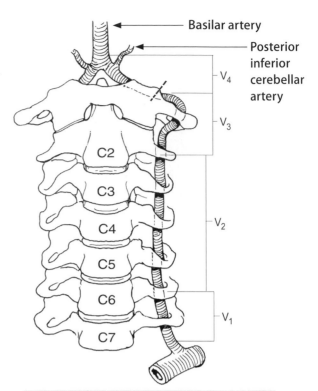

Figure 3.5 Diagrammatic representation of the 4 segments of the vertebral artery. (Reproduced with permission from Elsevier: Silva JA, White CJ. Peripheral vascular intervention. In: Kern MJ. *The Interventional Cardiac Catheterization Handbook.* 2nd ed. Philadelphia: Mosby; 2004:386-440.)

Angiography of the Brachiocephalic and Cervical Arteries

Vascular access may be obtained at the common femoral artery, the brachial artery, or the radial artery. An aortic arch aortogram (30°–60° LAO) is performed prior to selective angiography. This nonselective angiogram allows the operator to identify ostial disease in any of the brachycephalic vessels and significant tortuosity, and to visualize any anatomic variations.

Carotid angiography

Despite major advances in noninvasive diagnostic imaging techniques such as duplex ultrasonography, MRA, and computed tomography angiography (CTA) in recent years,[16-19] *carotid angiography* remains the gold standard for diagnosis and quantitation of stenoses of the carotid arteries.[14] Selective carotid angiography is performed after obtaining an aortic arch aortogram in the LAO (30°–60°) view, which allows the operator to visualize the level at which the

brachiocephalic trunk and left common carotid artery originate from the aortic arch. Using the same LAO angle, the brachiocephalic trunk may be easily engaged from the femoral access with a variety of shaped catheters (4-Fr or 6-Fr angled catheters, eg, right Judkins-4, internal mammary, Berenstein; or shepherd's crook shapes, eg, Vitek, Headhunter, Simmons [I, II, III]). From the arm access, selective angiography may be performed with the shepherd's crook shapes, particularly the Simmons catheters.

For selective angiography, after the ostium of the primary branch vessel has been cannulated, a 0.035-in J-tip or soft-tip guide wire (Wholey wire, Mallinckrodt) is steered into the proximal portion of the common carotid artery and the catheter advanced over the guide wire, positioning it at the origin of the common carotid artery. The catheter is then aspirated and cleared to minimize the risk of embolization.

Hand injections of contrast are preferred to power injections for selective angiography (Figures 3.6 and 3.7). When using small catheters and digital subtraction angiography, iodinated contrast may be diluted with saline 1:1 or 1:2 to enable better filling of the vessels.

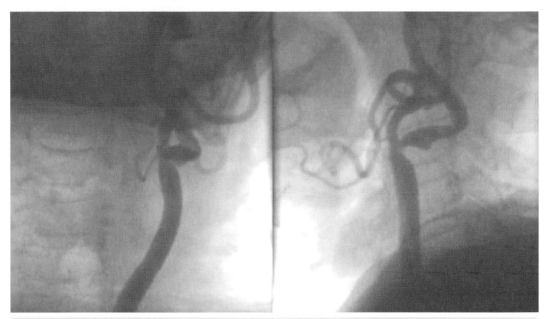

Figure 3.6 Unsubtracted angiography of a carotid stenosis affecting the distal portion of the left common carotid artery and ostium of the internal carotid artery in (left) the AP view and (right) left lateral view.

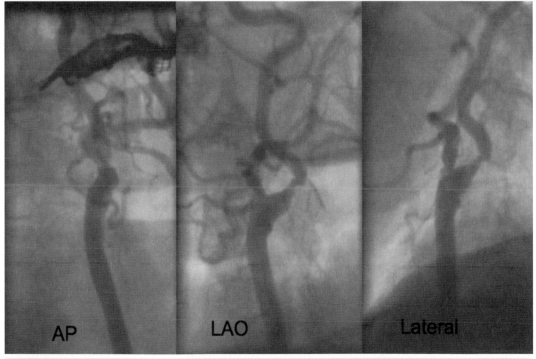

Figure 3.7 Unsubtracted angiography of a carotid stenosis of the proximal portion of the left internal carotid artery better visualized in the LAO and lateral views than in the AP view.

For angiography of the intracranial portion of the internal carotid artery and its branches, orthogonal views should be obtained. This allows visualization of any anomalous vessels or collateral circulation from the ipsilateral external carotid artery and/or the Circle of Willis (Figure 3.8).

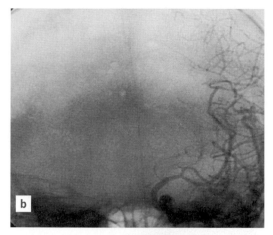

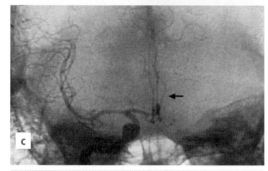

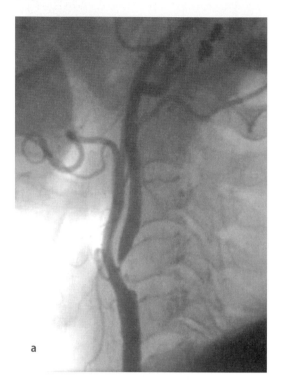

Figure 3.8 (a) Critical stenosis of the ostium of the left internal carotid artery. (b) Baseline intracranial angiography shows that the anterior cerebral artery (ACA) is occluded. (c) Left anterior cerebral artery (ACA, arrow) filling from the contralateral carotid circulation through the anterior communicating artery (ACom).

Subclavian and vertebral angiography

After obtaining an aortic arch arteriogram, the right or left subclavian arteries are selectively engaged using a 4-Fr or 6-Fr catheter with the same guide wires and in a similar fashion as previously described for the carotid arteries. When a subclavian stenosis is suspected based upon the history and physical examination—that is, a significant pressure gradient exists between the arms, claudication, or steal syndrome—selective *subclavian angiography* is performed using hand injections. The AP view with or without shallow oblique views will usually demonstrate the area of stenosis. In those with a tortuous proximal left subclavian artery (the left subclavian artery is affected with athero-occlusive

disease, 3 to 4 times as frequently as the right subclavian artery),[20] a steep caudal or RAO view with steep caudal views is very useful for showing the proximal vessel that may not be obvious in the AP view (Figure 3.9). If the area of interest is the ostium of the right subclavian artery, the AP view may not show the stenosis due to overlapping of the origin of the right common carotid artery. A steep RAO caudal (40°–60° RAO with 10°–20° caudal) or RAO cranial view may be necessary to separate the origin of the right subclavian artery from the right common carotid artery (Figure 3.10).

Vertebral artery angiography is usually performed with a nonselective injection of contrast in the subclavian artery close to the origin

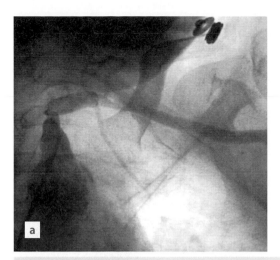
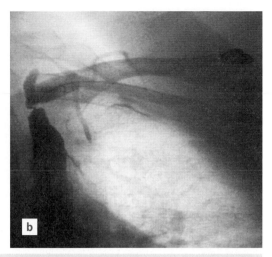

Figure 3.9 (a) AP view may obscure a significant stenosis in the proximal portion of the subclavian artery. (b) Same patient with caudal angulation in the AP projection demonstrates a significant proximal subclavian stenosis.

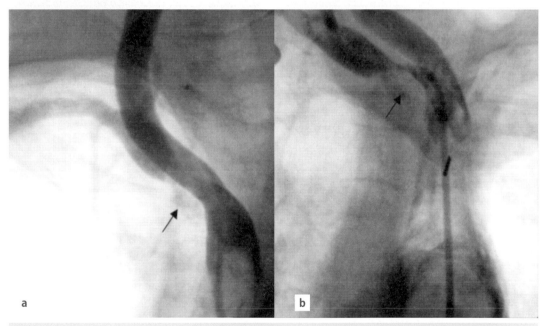

Figure 3.10 (a) AP view overlaps the origin (arrow) of the right subclavian artery and the right common carotid artery. (b) The RAO caudal view separates these 2 vessels and allows visualization of the stenosis (arrow).

of vertebral artery. The vertebral artery arises from the superior aspect of the subclavian artery. Not infrequently, the vertebral artery may arise posteriorly. Since the ostium of this vessel is the most commonly affected area (> 90% of the cases),[21] the AP view may not show the stenosis best. A shallow cranial oblique (RAO or LAO with cranial angulation, 10°–30°) often is needed to demonstrate the stenosis (Figure 3.11).

When necessary, selective engagement of the vertebral artery can be performed with angled tip catheters (4-Fr to 6-Fr internal mammary, Berenstein, or right Judkins-4 diagnostic catheter). The catheter is manipulated in a very similar fashion as when trying to engage the

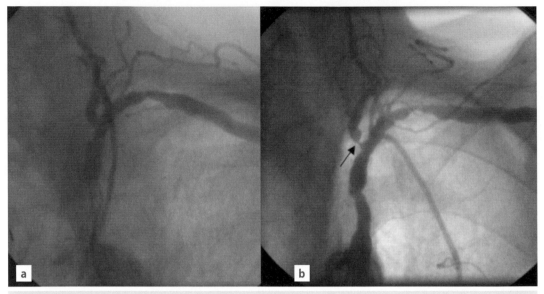

Figure 3.11 Vertebral artery stenosis at the ostium not well seen in (a) the AP view, but becomes very clear in (b) the AP cranial view.

internal mammary artery, however, it is torqued in the opposite direction than that used to engage the mammary artery (ie, clockwise for the left vertebral artery and counterclockwise for the right vertebral artery).

Abdominal Aorta

Anatomy

The *abdominal aorta* begins at the level of the diaphragm at the twelfth thoracic vertebra. At this level the aorta is anterior and leftward of the spine before its bifurcation into the common iliac arteries at the fourth lumbar vertebra.[11] The normal diameter of the abdominal aorta ranges between 1.5 and 2.15 cm.[22] Three main branches originate from the anterior aspect of the abdominal aorta: The first is the celiac trunk or celiac artery, which arises at the level of T12 to L1. Next, the superior mesenteric artery (SMA), which originates above the renal arteries, between L1 and L2. The final branch, the inferior mesenteric artery (IMA), takes off in a left anterolateral direction at the

level of L3 to L4. The renal arteries originate from the lateral aspect of the abdominal aorta at the level of L1 to L2 taking a lateral and posterior direction. Below the main renal arteries, 4 pairs of lumbar arteries arise in a posterolateral direction.[11]

Abdominal Aortogram

Vascular access may be obtained from the arm or leg. A 4-Fr to 6-Fr pigtail catheter is positioned in the abdominal aorta so that the side holes are directly adjacent to the ostia of renal arteries. With a breath hold and subtraction angiogram a power injection of contrast at 15 to 20 cc/sec, for a total of 30 to 40 cc of contrast, is usually adequate for good-quality angiograms. It is important that the upper, lower, and lateral margins of both kidneys are visualized. This usually requires an image intensifier of 12 in or larger. Two views should be obtained: the AP view allows good visualization of the renal arteries, and the lateral view enables assessment of the origin of the celiac and mesenteric arteries (Figures 3.11 and 3.12). It is important obtain images through the venous phase to visualize any late-filling collaterals. Of particular impor-

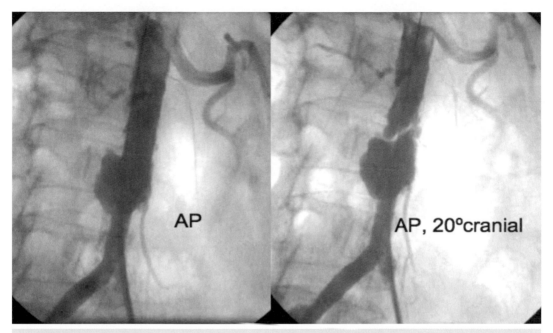

Figure 3.12 Abdominal aortogram showing an abdominal aortic aneurysm in the AP view. With mild cranial angulation it can also be appreciated as a significant stenosis.

tance are pelvic collaterals that may be filling the mesenteric vessels.

Renal Arteries

Anatomy

The *renal arteries* arise from the lateral aspect of the abdominal aorta usually between L1 and L2. They course laterally and posteriorly, and may take a caudal, horizontal, or cranial orientation.[11] In about one-quarter of the normal population an accessory renal artery will be present, which may originate anywhere from the suprarenal aorta down to the iliac arteries.[13] Identifying these accessory branches is a major reason to perform an abdominal aortogram first, rather than proceeding immediately to selective renal angiography.

Renal Angiography

An abdominal aortogram should be obtained prior to selective *renal angiography*. This identifies the origin of the renal arteries, the presence of accessory renal arteries and their location, and the presence of renal artery stenosis. Selective renal angiography is indicated, if the aortogram demonstrates a renal artery stenosis of questionable hemodynamic significance, or detailed images are required or there is a need for pressure gradient measurement. Selective renal angiography is indicated if intrarenal vascular disease is suspected, as in fibromuscular dysplasia (FMD), vasculitis, or aneurysmal disease.

Selective engagement of the renal arteries is done with 4-Fr to 6-Fr angled diagnostic catheters, although shepherd's crook shapes (Sos, or Simmons) may be helpful. Selective renal angiography is performed with hand injection of contrast in a shallow LAO angulation (5°–10°) for both renal arteries (Figure 3.13). The shallow LAO view has been shown to be the best view for the assessment of the ostium and proximal portions of both the right and the left renal arteries.[23] Occasionally some caudal or cranial angulation (15°–20°) may be helpful for tortuous vessels.

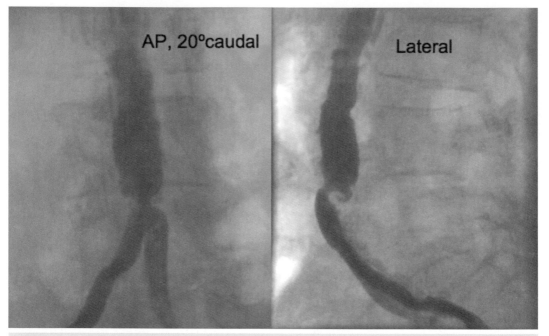

Figure 3.13 Significant stenosis of the terminal aorta immediately below the abdominal aortic aneurysm shown in Figure 3.12, which is evident with mild caudal angulation in the AP caudal view and in the lateral view.

Mesenteric Arteries

Anatomy

The mesenteric circulation includes 3 arteries that originate from the anterior aspect of the abdominal aorta: the *celiac artery, the superior mesenteric artery (SMA),* and the *inferior mesenteric artery (IMA).* The celiac artery arises at the level of T12 to L1 and supplies blood to the stomach and half of the duodenum (foregut); the SMA originates at the level of L1 to L2 and provides blood flow to the lower half of the duodenum, ileum, cecum-appendix, ascending colon, and proximal two-thirds of the transverse colon (midgut); and the IMA takes off in a left anterolateral direction at the level of L3 to L4 and supplies blood to the distal third of the transverse colon, descending colon, sigmoid colon, rectum, and upper part of the anal canal (hindgut).[24]

Angiography

Angiography of the mesenteric arteries is the gold standard to assess the anatomy of this vascular system. As is the case for the renal arteries, before selective angiography is performed, an abdominal aortogram should be obtained in the AP and lateral projections (Figure 3.14). After the origin of the mesenteric vessels has been identified, selective angiography if indicated may be performed in the lateral view using angled diagnostic catheters (Figure 3.15). The IMA often arises in a very acute inferior angle on the anterior portion of the abdominal aorta, for which a Simmons-1 or Sos catheter is very useful for engagement.

Selective engagement of the mesenteric arteries allows measurement of translesional pressure gradients, since, as is the case for the renal arteries, the majority of stenoses in these vessels are located in their ostium or their very proximal portion.[25] Using hand injections, selective angiography is performed in the lateral and oblique views.

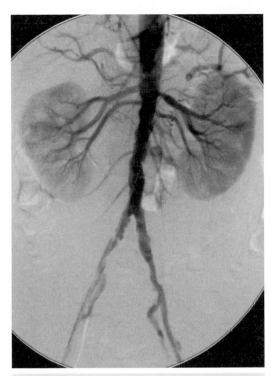

Figure 3.14 Digital subtraction of an abdominal aortogram demonstrating a mild stenosis of the proximal left renal artery, bilateral renal artery accessory branches are visible, and bilateral iliac (R > L) disease is present.

Pelvic and Lower-Extremity Arterial Circulation

Anatomy

The abdominal aorta bifurcates into the *common iliac arteries (CIA)* at the level of L4 to L5.[26] The CIA bifurcates into the *internal iliac artery (IIC;* ie, hypogastric artery) and *external iliac artery (EIA)* at the level of the lumbosacral junction. At the level of the inguinal ligament, 2 small branches originate from the EIA: the *inferior epigastric artery,* which follows a medial and superior direction, and the *deep iliac circumflex artery,* which takes a lateral and superior direction. These vessels are important to visualize as they may be the source of postprocedure access site bleeding.

Once the EIA crosses the inguinal ligament, it becomes the *common femoral artery (CFA),* which courses medially over the femoral head. When it reaches the lower edge of the femoral head, the CFA divides into the *superficial femoral artery (SFA)* and *profunda femoris artery (PFA,* ie, deep femoral artery). The PFA

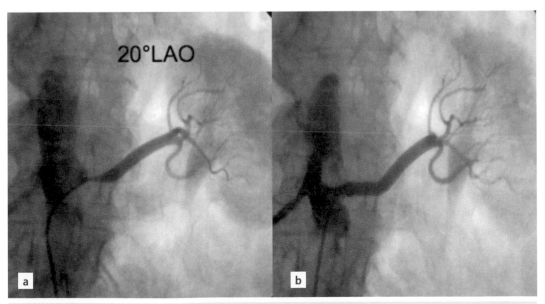

Figure 3.15 (a) Baseline angiogram of a tight stenosis of the ostial left renal artery. (b) Angiogram following stent placement.

runs posterior and lateral along the internal aspect of the femur. A few centimeters after its origin, the PFA gives origin to 2 small branches: the *lateral femoral circumflex,* and the *medial femoral circumflex arteries* and subsequently to several small perforating arteries. The SFA continues down the anteromedial thigh, and in its distal portion runs deeper to cross the adductor (ie, Hunter's) canal where it becomes the *popliteal artery.* The popliteal artery crosses the knee and gives origin to small muscular branches, 2 *sural branches*, and 3 *geniculate arteries* (superior, medial, and inferior).[27]

Below the knee, the popliteal artery gives rise to the *anterior tibial (AT) artery* and continues as the *tibioperoneal trunk (TPT).* The AT artery runs laterally and anterior to the tibia to the foot, and as it passes over the ankle onto the dorsum of the foot, it becomes the *dorsalis pedis (DP) artery.* The TPT bifurcates into the *posterior tibial (PT)* and the *peroneal arteries.* The PT artery courses posteromedially in the calf, while the peroneal artery runs near the fibula between the AT and PT arteries. The peroneal artery then rejoins the PT above the ankle via the posterior division, and the anterior tibial through the anterior division. On the dorsum of the foot, the DP artery has lateral and medial tarsal branches. After the PT artery passes behind the medial malleolus, it divides into medial and lateral plantar arteries. The lateral plantar and distal DP arteries join to form the plantar arch.[27]

Angiography

Vascular access from the arm or femoral arteries is equally effective for diagnostic angiography. If the CFA is chosen, the extremity that is less symptomatic is preferred. A 4-Fr to 6-Fr pigtail catheter is positioned in the terminal aorta, below the IMA and above the aortic bifurcation at L4 or L5. A power injection of 8 to 10 cc/sec for a total 80 to 100 cc is needed to image both legs (from the CIA to the feet) using a stepping table and digital subtraction.

Selective angiograms in different angulations of a particular artery or arterial segment are useful when the nonselective angiogram shows possible stenoses or when further anatomic clarification is needed. If access has been obtained in the CFA and the arterial segment in question is located in the contralateral extremity, a diagnostic internal mammary catheter (or a Simmons-1 or -2 in case of significant acute angulation between the origin of both CIAs) is positioned at the origin of the contralateral CIA. A soft-tip straight steerable 0.035-in guide wire such as a Wholey wire (Mallinckrodt) or an angled Glidewire (Terumo, BSC) is advanced to the CFA. The angiographic catheter is advanced over the guide wire to the area of interest, and angiography is obtained.

Specific angiographic views are important to mention because they help to improve anatomical detail. In the AP view there is significant overlapping of the origin of the EIA and the IIA, and ostial lesions in either vessel may be missed. To "separate" these 2 segments, the contralateral oblique 20° with 20° caudal view is very useful (Figures 3.16 and 3.17). The proximal portions of SFA and the PFA are overlapping in the AP view.[28] They are separated best with a 30° lateral angulation (Figure 3.18).[29] Finally, it is desirable to avoid overlapping of the SFA, popliteal artery, or infrapopliteal artery with the dense cortical

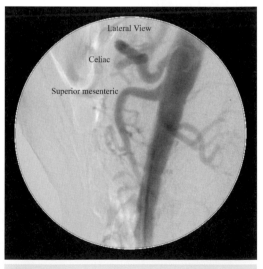

Figure 3.16 Subtracted abdominal aortogram in the lateral view to assess the ostium and proximal portion of the celiac trunk and the superior mesenteric arteries.

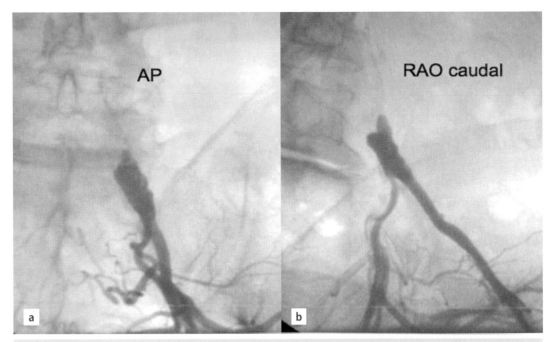

Figure 3.17 (a) AP view and (b) RAO caudal view demonstrating the internal iliac artery with an occlusion of the left common iliac artery.

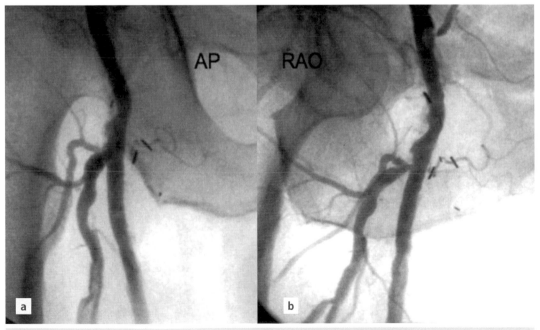

Figure 3.18 (a) Angiography of the right common femoral artery (CFA) bifurcation in the AP view. (b) A stenosis at the ostium of the profunda femoris artery (PFA) is noted in the ipsilateral oblique (20° RAO) view, which was missed in the AP view.

leg bones. Lateral oblique angulation (30°) with digital subtraction images offers an excellent separation of the vessels (Figures 3.19 to 3.21).

Complications of Peripheral Vascular Angiography

With the advent of new technology such smaller catheter profiles and newer contrast agents, peripheral angiography has become safer than in the past. Complications leading to significant morbidity or mortality, although unusual, do occur, and the operator must remain vigilant

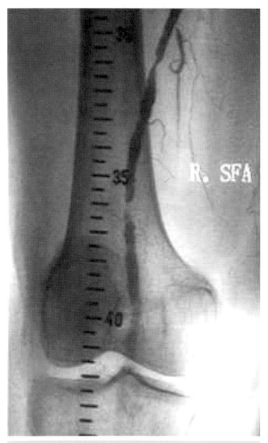

Figure 3.19 AP view of the distal superficial femoral artery (SFA) and popliteal artery with stenoses at the level of the Hunter's canal and in the proximal portion of the popliteal artery.

during and after angiography in order to minimize them.

In the registry of the Society for Cardiovascular Angiography and Interventions (SCAI), the incidence of vascular complications for diagnostic angiography was 0.5% to 0.6%.[30] With CFA access, the most common vascular complication is hematoma, which usually resolves within several weeks after the procedure. If the hematoma remains in continuity with the arterial lumen due to inadequate sealing of the puncture site, a pseudoaneurysm may develop. This is usually manifested as a painful pulsatile mass, with an audible bruit. The diagnosis is easily confirmed with duplex ultrasonography. When the femoral arterial puncture (front or back wall) is above the inguinal ligament, a hematoma may extend into the retroperitoneal space, with bleeding not evident from the surface examination.

The diagnosis of retroperitoneal bleeding must be strongly suspected when a postangiogram patient becomes hypotensive, with or without flank pain. Aggressive volume replacement with normal saline is indicated. If there is recurrent or sustained hemodynamic embarrassment, the patient is taken for angiography of the access, with the idea of stopping the bleeding. Although the majority of retroperitoneal hematomas resolve spontaneously, some require treatment. Percutaneous, catheter-based modalities may be effective for treating retroperitoneal bleeding in selected patients.[31-33] Other less-frequent vascular complications include arterial laceration, which requires a covered stent or surgical repair, and symptomatic arteriovenous fistulas, which usually require surgical treatment.

Stroke is an unusual but potentially devastating complication of catheter placement in the aortic arch. The SCAI registry described an incidence of 0.07% for stroke during cardiac catheterization.[34] The incidence of neurologic events during carotid angiography is substantially higher. In a review of 8 prospective studies, there was a 1% incidence of stroke following angiography,[35] and in the patients who entered the North American Symptomatic Carotid End-

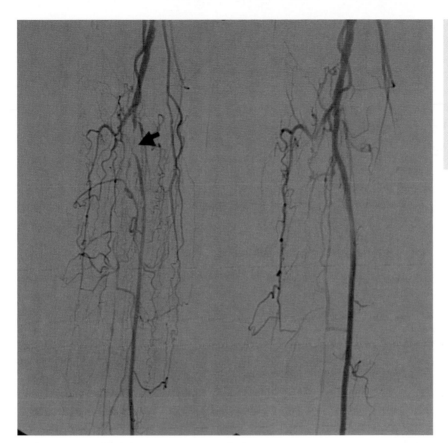

Figure 3.20 Digital subtraction angiography (left) of the right popliteal artery showing occlusion of the anterior tibial (AT) artery and the tibioperoneal trunk (TPT) (arrow). Following stent placement (right).

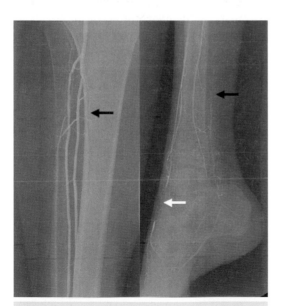

Figure 3.21 Occlusion of the right posterior tibial artery (black arrow) in its proximal portion (left) and distal segment (right) (black arrow). There is also occlusion of the dorsalis pedis artery (white arrow). Notice that cortical bone can obscure the vessel.

arterectomy Trial (NASCET) it was 0.78%.[36] In general, asymptomatic patients have a lower risk, whereas patients who undergo angiography in the setting of transient ischemic events have a slightly higher complication rate.[37-39] The neurologic complication rate for patients with severe bilateral carotid stenoses is 12.5%.[39] In a review of cerebral angiography performed by cardiologists, the risk of angiography was 0.05%.

Allergic and anaphylactoid reactions are related to the use of iodinated contrast agents, which have decreased with the use of low/iso-osmolar contrast agents. The current reported rate of allergic and anaphylactoid reactions with these new agents is less than 1%.[40]

The risk to develop contrast-induced nephropathy (CIN) is highest in those with baseline chronic renal insufficiency (creatinine > 2.1 mL/dL), diabetes mellitus, multiple myeloma, and those who are receiving other nephrotoxic drugs such as aminoglycosides, nonsteroidal anti-inflammatory drugs, and angiotensin-converting enzyme inhibitors.[41,42] Patients at higher risk for CIN must be well hydrated (before and after) the procedure, and the volume of contrast administered must be minimized.[43,44] Data regarding the efficacy of the dopamine-1 receptor antagonist, fenoldopam, in preventing contrast nephropathy is inconsistent and conflicting.[45] There is also inconsistent evidence that the use of N-acetylcysteine (Mucomyst) may be of benefit for preventing CIN.[46,47] In addition, one small, randomized trial showed that the use of hydration with sodium bicarbonate can prevent this complication, however, this needs to be confirmed in larger studies.[48] At present, it is recommended that patients with a glomerular filtration rate of < 50 mL/1.73 m^2 should avoid iodinated contrast agents if possible. If conventional angiography is required, a low/iso-osmolar agent should be used at the minimal dose, nonsteroidal anti-inflammatory drugs and diuretics withheld, and ~ 1 mL/kg of 0.9% saline be started at least 3 hours prior to the procedure and continuing 12 hours after the procedure.[49]

Summary

Invasive contrast angiography is the standard method for diagnosing peripheral arterial disease (PAD) and against which all other methods are compared for accuracy. Angiography provides the "road map" on which therapeutic decisions are based. Knowledge of the vascular anatomy and its normal variations is a core element in the skill set required to safely perform peripheral vascular angiography and intervention.

References

1. Criqui MH, Fronek A, Barrett-Connor E, et al. The prevalence of peripheral arterial disease in a defined population. *Circulation.* 1985;71:510-515.

2. Khoury Z, Schwartz R, Gottlieb S, Chenzbraun A, Shlomo S, Keren A. Relation of coronary artery disease to atherosclerotic disease in the aorta, carotid, and femoral arteries evaluated by ultraswound. *Am J Cardiol.* 1997;80:1429-1433.

3. Hirsh A, Criqui MH, Treat-Jacobson D, et al. The PARTNERS Program: a national survey of peripheral arterial disease prevalence, awareness, and ischemic risk. *JAMA.* 2001;286:1317-1324.

4. Pentecost MJ, Criqui MH, Dorros G, et al. Guidelines for peripheral percutaneous trans-luminal angioplasty of the abdominal aorta and lower extremity vessels. A statement for health professionals from a special writing group of the councils on cardiovascular radiology, arteriosclerosis, cardio-thoracic and vascular surgery, clinical cardiology, and epidemiology and prevention, the American Heart Association. *Circulation.* 1994;89:511-531.

5. Cardella JF, Casarella WJ, DeWeese JA, et al. Optimal resources for the examination and endovascular treatment of the peripheral and visceral vascular systems. AHA Intercouncil Report on Peripheral and Visceral Angiographic and Interventional Laboratories. *Circulation.* 1994;89:1481-1493.

6. Krouwels MM, Overbach EH, Guit GL. Iohexol vs. ioxaglate in lower extremity angiography: a comparative randomized double-blind study in 80 patients. *Eur J Radiol.* 1996;22:133-138.

7. Hawkins IF. Carbon dioxide digital subtraction arteriography. *Am J Roentgenol.* 1982;139:19-27.

8. Kerns SR, Hawkins IF. Carbon dioxide digital subtraction angiography: expanding applications and technical evolution. *Am J Radiol.* 1995;164:735-743.

9. Caridi JG, Hawkins IF. CO_2 digital subtraction angiography: potential complications and their prevention. *J Vasc Interv Radiol.* 1997;8:383-391.

10. Yerram P, Saab G, Karuparthi PR, Hayden MR, Khanna R. Nephrogenic systemic fibrosis: a mysterious disease in patients with renal failure—role of gadolinium-based contrast media in causation and the beneficial effect of intravenous sodium thiosulfate. *Clin J Am Soc Nephrol.* 2007;22:258-263.

11. Gabella G, ed. Cardiovascular system. In: Williams PL, Bannister LH, Berry MM, et al, eds. *Gray's Anatomy*. 38th ed. New York: Churchill Livingstone; 1995:1505.

12. Aronberg DJ, Glazer HS, Madsen K, et al. Normal thoracic aortic diameters by computed tomography. *J Comput Assist Tomogr*.1984:8:247-252.

13. Kadir S. Regional anatomy of the thoracic aorta. In: Kadir S, ed. *Atlas of Normal and Variant Angiographic Anatomy*. Philadelphia: WB Saunders; 1991:19.

14. Schainfield RM, Jaff MR. Angiography of the aorta and peripheral arteries. In: Baim DS, Grossman W, eds. *Grossman's Cardiac Catheterization, Angiography and Intervention*. 6th ed. Philadelphia: Lippincott Williams & Wilkins; 2000:293-322.

15. Myla S. Controversies in carotid stenting: an editorial perspective. *J Interv Cardiol*. 2001;14:459-463.

16. Ratliffe D, Hames T, Humphries K, Birtch S, Chant A. The reliability of Doppler ultrasound techniques in the assessment of carotid disease. *Angiology*. 1985;36:333-340.

17. Heiserman JE, Drayer BP, Fram EK, et al. Carotid artery stenosis: clinical efficacy of two-dimensional time-of-flight MR angiography. *Radiology*. 1992;182:761-768.

18. Huston J, Lewis BD, Wiebers DO, et al. Carotid artery: prospective blinded comparison of two-dimensional time-of-flight angiography with conventional angiography and duplex US. *Radiology*. 1993;186:339-344.

19. Beauchamp NJ. Spiral CT angiography: a new technique for evaluating the neurovasculature. *App Radiol*. 1995;(Suppl 14):15-20.

20. Zelenock GB, Cronenwett JL, Graham LM, et al. Brachiocephalic arterial occlusive and stenosis. Manifestations and management of complex lesions. *Arch Surg*. 1985;120:370-376.

21. Courtheaux P, Tournade A, Theron J, et al. Transcutaneous angioplasty of vertebral artery athromatous ostial stricture. *Neuroradiology*. 1984;27:259-264.

22. Horejs D, Gilbert PM, Burnstein S, et al. Normal aortoiliac diameters by CT. *J Comput Assist Tomogr*. 1988;12:602-606.

23. Bates MC, Crotty B, Kavasmaneck C, et al. Renal artery angiography: "The right ipsilateral oblique" myth. *Cath Cardiovasc Intervent*. 2006;67:283-287.

24. Uflacker R. Abdominal aorta and its branches. In: Uflacker R, ed. *Atlas of Vascular Anatomy. An Angiographic Approach*. Philadelphia: Lippincott Williams & Wilkins; 1997:405-604.

25. Derrick JR, Pollard HS, Moore RM. The pattern of atherosclerotic narrowing of the celiac and superior mesenteric arteries. *Ann Surg*. 1959;149:684-689.

26. Uflacker R. Arteries of the pelvis. In: Uflacker R, ed. *Atlas of Vascular Anatomy. An Angiographic Approach*. Philadelphia: Lippincott Williams & Wilkins; 1997:605-634.

27. Uflacker R. Arteries of the lower extremities. In: Uflacker R, ed. *Atlas of Vascular Anatomy. An Angiographic Approach*. Philadelphia: Lippincott Williams & Wilkins; 1997:743-778.

28. Silva JA, White CJ, Ramee SR, et al. Percutaneous profundoplasty in the treatment of lower extremity ischemia: results of long-term surveillance. *J Endovasc Ther*. 2001;8:75-82.

29. Beales JS, Adcock FA, Frawley JS, et al. The radiological assessment of the disease of the profunda femoris artery. *Br J Radiol*. 1971;44:854-859.

30. Noto TJ, Johnson LW, Krone R, et al. Cardiac catheterization 1990: a report of the registry of the Society for Cardiac Angiography and Interventions. *Cath Cardiovasc Diagn*. 1991;24:75.

31. Mak GYK, Daly B, Chan W, et al. Percutaneous treatment of post catheterization massive retroperitoneal hemorrhage. *Cathet Cardiovasc Diagn*. 1993;29:40.

32. Silva JA, Stant J, Ramee SR. Endovascular treatment of a massive retroperitoneal bleeding: successful balloon-catheter delivery of intra-arterial thrombin. *Catheter Cardiovasc Intervent*. 2005;64:218-222.

33. Silva JA, White CJ. Femoral vascular access and vascular bleeding complications (chapter 4). In: Eeckhout E, Carlier S, Lerman A, Kern M, eds. *Handbook of Complications During Percutaneous Coronary Interventions*. London: Taylor & Francis: Informa Healthcare; 2007.

34. Johnson LW, Lozner EC, Johnson S, et al. Coronary angiography 1984-1987: a report of the registry of the Society for Cardiac Angiography and Interventions. I. Results and complications. *Cath Cardiovasc Diagn.* 1989;17:5.

35. Hankey GJ, Warlow CP, Sellar RJ. Cerebral angiographic risk in mild cerebrovascular disease. *Stroke.* 1990;21:209-222.

36. Moneta GL, Edwards JM, Chitwood RW, et al. Correlation of North American Symptomatic Carotid Endarterectomy Trial (NASCET) angiographic definition of 70% to 99% internal carotid artery stenosis with duplex scanning. *J Vasc Surg.* 1993;17:152-159.

37. Earnest F, Forbes G, Sandok BA, et al. Complications of cerebral angiography: prospective assessment of risk. *Am J Radiol.* 1984;142:247-253.

38. Dion JE, Gates PC, Fox AJ, et al. Clinical events following neuroangiography: a prospective study. *Stroke.* 1987;18:997-1004.

39. Theodotu BC, Whaley R, Mahaley MS. Complications following transfemoral cerebral angiography for cerebral ischemia: report of 159 angiograms and correlation with surgical risk. *Surg Neurol.* 1987;28:90-92.

40. Wittbrodt ET, Splinter SA. Prevention of anaphilactoid reactions in high-risk patients receiving radiographic contrast media. *Ann Pharmacother.* 1994;28:236.

41. Steinberg EP, Moore RD, Powe NR, et al. Safety and cost effectiveness of high-osmolality as compared with low-osmolality contrast material in patients undergoing cardiac angiography. *N Engl J Med.* 1992;326:425.

42. Rudnick MR, Goldfarb S, Wexler L, et al. Nephrotoxicity of ionic and non-ionic contrast media in 1196 patients—a randomized trial (the Iohexol Cooperative Study). *Kidney Int.* 1995;47:254.

43. Solomon R, Werner C, Mann D, et al. Effects of saline, mannitol, and furosemide on acute decreases in renal function induced by radiocontrast agents. *N Engl J Med.* 1994;331:1416.

44. Stevens MA, McCullough PA, Tobin KJ, et al. A prospective randomized trial of prevention measures in patients with high risk for contrast nephropathy. *J Am Coll Cardiol.* 1999;33:403.

45. Stone GW, McCullough PA, Tumlin JA, et al. Fenoldopam mesylate for the prevention of contrast-induced nephropathy: a randomized controlled trial. *JAMA.* 2003;290:2284-2291.

46. Tepel M, van der Giet M, Schwarzfeld C, et al. Prevention of radiographic-contrast-agent-induced reductions in renal function by N-acetylcysteine. *N Engl J Med.* 2000;343:180-184.

47. Nallamothu BK, Shojania KG, Saint S, et al. Is acetylcysteine effective in preventing contrast-related nephropathy? A meta-analysis. *Am J Med.* 2004;117:938-947.

48. Merten GJ, Burgess WP, Gray LV, et al. Prevention of contrast-induced nephropathy with sodium bicarbonate. A randomized controlled trial. *JAMA.* 2004;291:2328-2334.

49. Barrett BJ, Parfrey PS. Preventing nephropathy induced by contrast medium. *N Engl J Med.* 2006;354:379-386.

Part 3

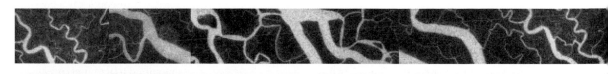

Aortic Arch
and Supraclavicular Artery Disease

4

Subclavian and Upper-Extremity Artery Disease

Jeffrey A. Goldstein, Raghu Kolluri, and Krishna Rocha-Singh

Peripheral artery disease (PAD) involving the lower extremities is mostly manifested in the form of atherosclerosis; however, this is less common in upper extremities. While atherosclerosis may involve the arch vessels, including the subclavian and brachiocephalic arteries, it rarely affects axillary and brachial arteries. The structural or functional difference between the atherosclerosis-prone and -spared areas of the arch vessels and upper extremities is unclear. One hypothesis suggests the difference may be related to the different shear forces and tensile strengths of the upper-extremity blood vessels.[1] The embryonic dissimilarity between the upper- and lower-extremity vasculature is also thought to be a potential cause of this difference.[2]

Unlike lower extremities, abundant collateral vessels in the shoulder and elbow regions prevent severe ischemic symptoms even when main arteries are occluded. As such, upper-limb ischemia is a rather uncommon condition and accounts for approximately 10% to 15% of the endovascular procedures performed.[3,4]

Brachiocephalic and Subclavian Artery Disease

Atherosclerosis remains the most common cause of disease in the brachiocephalic and subclavian arteries and may result in upper-extremity or cerebrovascular symptoms depending on its location and the potential site of atheromatous embolization. The risk factors for the development of disease in these 2 vascular beds include smoking, dyslipidemia, and diabetes. Underlying etiologies that cause brachiocephalic and subclavian artery disease are listed in Table 4.1.

Atherosclerosis
Takayasu's arteritis
Radiation-Induced arteritis
Aneurysmal dilation
Trauma
Fibromuscular dysplasia
Ehlers-Danlos syndrome
Thoracic outlet syndrome

Table 4.1 Diseases of the Brachiocephalic and Subclavian Arteries

Vascular Disease: Diagnostic and Therapeutic Approaches. © 2011 Michael R. Jaff and Christopher J. White, editors. Cardiotext Publishing, ISBN: 978-1-935395-16-4.

Thoracic Outlet Syndrome

Thoracic outlet syndrome (TOS) is a group of clinical entities that affect the shoulder, neck, and upper extremity manifesting in both vascular and neurological symptoms due to compression of the neurovascular bundle as it exits the thoracic outlet. TOS is broadly divided into neurogenic, arterial, and venous forms depending on the involved structure, that is, brachial plexus, subclavian artery, and subclavian vein, respectively.

Arterial TOS is the least common but most serious form of TOS and can present with limb-threatening ischemia or gangrene of the digits. Underlying bony abnormalities such as cervical rib and callus formation due to the fractured first rib or clavicle are primarily responsible for arterial TOS, however, congenital bands or scar tissue formation after shoulder surgery may also predispose to arterial TOS. These anatomical abnormalities compress the subclavian artery, which leads to increased flow velocity at the compression site and poststenotic turbulence. This turbulence increases the shear stress on the arterial wall, exposing the intima, leading to platelet activation and formation of a poststenotic aneurysm. Turbulence increases further with aneurysmal dilation of the poststenotic area resulting in generation of platelet thrombi, which may embolize causing digital ischemia and gangrene.

Axillary/Brachial Artery Disease

Atherosclerosis infrequently affects the axillary artery and rarely affects the brachial artery. More commonly, the pathophysiology of these lesions involves arteritis, radiation injury, trauma, or thromboembolism. In a prospective 20-year study of a 172 patients Deguara et al noted that thromboembolism was the most common etiology (35%) of upper-extremity ischemia.[5] Two-thirds of these patients had underlying atrial fibrillation, and the brachial artery was the site of the embolic event in 85% of the cases.

Fibromuscular dysplasia (FMD) predominantly affects the renal and carotid arteries and, to a lesser extent, the intracerebral arteries; however, it has been reported in the brachial arteries.[6]

Other disease conditions affecting the axillary and brachial arteries include neurofibromatosis-related vascular lesions, Takayasu's disease, connective tissue disorders, and collagen vascular disorders, such as Ehlers-Danlos syndrome and heparin-induced thrombocytopenia.[7] Pheochromocytoma can present with a similar angiographic finding owing to increased catecholamines, leading to functional stenosis.[8] Rare causes of brachial artery occlusion are hypereosinophilic syndrome[9] and HIV-associated arterial thrombosis.[10]

Radial and Ulnar Disease

Disease in the radial and ulnar arterial segments results in digital ischemia and vasospastic phenomenon. This is described in detail in Chapter 19, "Vasospastic Diseases."

Signs and Symptoms

The symptoms of brachiocephalic and subclavian artery occlusive disease occur due to embolism or to ischemia. Brachiocephalic stenosis can cause subclavian-carotid steal, resulting in anterior cerebral hypoperfusion; whereas a subclavian stenosis can cause subclavian-vertebral steal, resulting in posterior cerebral hypoperfusion. These lesions may also cause arm and hand claudication. Stenoses in multiple arch vessels may result in vertebrobasilar insufficiency. Aneurysmal diseases, dissections, and poststenotic dilation due to arterial TOS or FMD result in an embolic phenomenon to the cerebral hemispheres or to the ipsilateral upper extremity.

Patients with history of coronary artery bypass graph (CABG) surgery employing a left internal mammary artery (IMA) or right IMA bypass graft may present with recurrent angina due to subclavian coronary steal, however, the incidence is low at 0.4%.[11]

The signs and symptoms of axillary and brachial artery disease depend on the chronicity and site of the stenosis or occlusion. In chronic stenosis or occlusion, such as in vasculitis, the presenting complaint may be vasospastic phenomenon. It may also present with arm/hand claudication. However, acute digital ischemia and gangrene can occur from embolic occlusions (Figure 4.1). This is described in depth in Chapter 19.

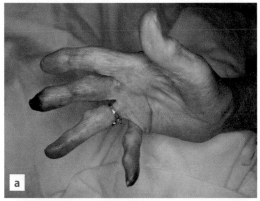

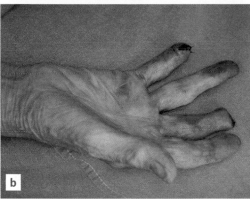

Figure 4.1 (a) Digital gangrene in a patient with acute embolic event to the ulnar artery. (b) Postdigital amputation of gangrenous portions.

Subclavian Steal Phenomenon

In *subclavian steal phenomenon*, a significant proximal subclavian or brachiocephalic stenosis results in the affected arm becoming dependent on blood flow from the posterior cerebral circulation. Retrograde vertebral flow in the ipsilateral arm "steals" blood flow from the posterior circulation resulting in symptoms that are listed in Table 4.2 (Figure 4.2). Acute subclavian steal is seen in patients with trauma or dissection, or it is due to vascular surgery complications and may result in catastrophic vertebrobasilar insuf-

ficiency or infarction. However, in patients with atherosclerosis-related chronic subclavian steal, symptoms may be seen in those with disease involving multiple arch vessels or abnormalities of the Circle of Willis.

Vertigo/dizziness
Diplopia
Dysarthria
Tinnitus
Syncope and near-syncope
Ataxia
Homonymous hemianopsia
Nonhemispheric sensory deficit
Nausea
Vomiting
Upper-extremity claudication

Table 4.2 Subclavian Steal Symptoms

Pathophysiology

Reivich et al[12] first reported subclavian steal syndrome in 2 patients who presented with cerebral ischemia due to retrograde left vertebral flow in the setting of ipsilateral subclavian stenosis proximal to the vertebral artery. The blood pressure distal to the stenosis or occlusion is reduced, resulting in the reversal of flow within the ipsilateral vertebral to maintain the blood flow to the arm.[13]

Although there is reversal of flow in the ipsilateral vertebral artery, sufficient arterial flow from the contralateral vertebral artery via the basilar artery may not affect flow within the Circle of Willis,[14-18] therefore, most patients with chronic subclavian steal phenomenon remain asymptomatic.[16]

Alternatively, in subclavian coronary steal in coronary artery disease patients after CABG surgery, proximal subclavian stenosis or brachiocephalic stenosis may result in retrograde flow through the IMA graft as the upper extremity "steals" blood flow from the coronary circulation (Figure 4.3). This can lead to myocardial ischemia, which may manifest as angina pectoris or even ischemic cardiomyopathy.

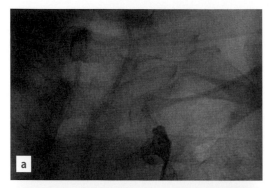

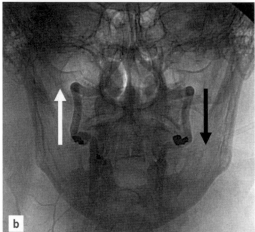

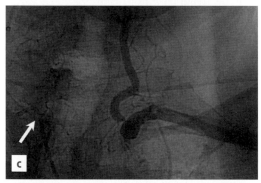

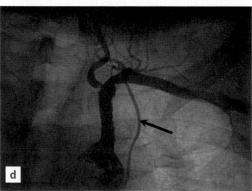

Figure 4.2 (left column) (a) Occluded left subclavian artery in a patient requiring CABG surgery. (b) Right vertebral artery angiography demonstrates antegrade right vertebral (white arrow) and retrograde left vertebral arterial flow (black arrow). (c) Retrograde flow through a stenotic right vertebral artery supplies blood to the left arm. Note the diagnostic catheter in the right subclavian artery (white arrow). (d) The left subclavian artery after PTA and stent placement. The patient underwent CABG surgery the following day utilizing a left IMA (arrow) graft to the left anterior descending coronary artery.

Physical exam

The physical examination should include a thorough palpation of all the pulses. Supraclavicular areas should be palpated for the presence of a cervical rib. Provocative positions that compress the neurovascular bundle, such as the Adson's test and the exaggerated military position of attention and the hyperabduction maneuver, may reproduce these symptoms, however, these tests may be positive even in asymptomatic patients.[19] Roos[20] suggests the use of the *elevated arm stress test (EAST),* which involves the slow opening and closing of the hands for 3 minutes, with the patient in the "surrender position" (90° arm abduction at the shoulder joint and a 90° flexion at the elbow joint) (Figure 4.4). The hand may show pallor and rapid development of claudication pain causing the patient to drop the affected hand onto his or her lap. The Allen test may be positive for occlusion of ulnar or radial arteries.

Laboratory Testing

Laboratory tests, such as CBC, blood sugar, erythrocyte sedimentation rate, electrolytes, and thyroid function, must be ordered to exclude systemic disease and inflammation. Cervical spine films should be obtained to rule out the presence of cervical rib or elongated transverse process of the seventh cervical vertebra.

Noninvasive Testing

Brachiocephalic disease and subclavian disease may be identified clinically by differential arm

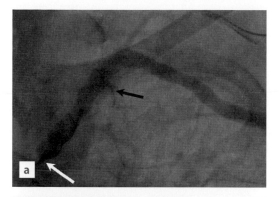

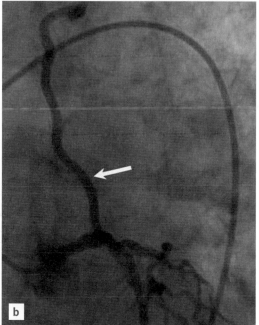

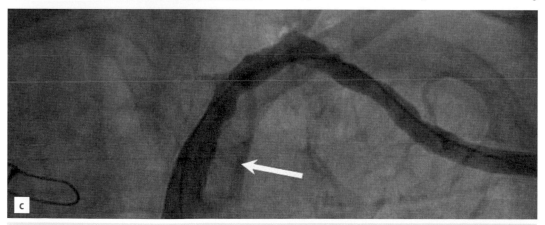

pressures (> 20 mm Hg), diminished radial or ulnar pulses, supraclavicular bruit (ipsilateral), or carotid bruit during physical examination. Although a difference between arm blood pressures is a good screening tool, it is not sensitive in detecting symptomatic subclavian steal. Tan et al[21] reported blood pressure difference only in 55% of patients with subclavian steal phenomenon. Systolic blood pressure difference was also significantly higher in patients with severe subclavian steal with complete reversal of ipsilateral vertebral.

Although noninvasive duplex ultrasonography of the subclavian and brachiocephalic vessels should be the first imaging modality of choice, it is challenging due to the anatomy, the overlying bony structures (sternum and clavicles), and the insonation angle required for complete visualization. However, this test can be performed by trained vascular technologists and is included within the carotid duplex protocol in most labs (Figure 4.5). The limitation of the insonation angle can be overcome with continuous-wave Doppler (Figure 4.6); the proximal portions of the arch vessels can be interrogated from the supraclavicular notch utilizing continuous-wave Doppler probe. Indirect evidence of subclavian steal phenomenon can be obtained from the vertebral waveforms as well. Klierwer et al[22] describes 5 types of vertebral flow patterns found along

Figure 4.3 (a) Selective left subclavian angiogram demonstrating a critical ostial stenosis (white arrow) and absence of antegrade flow in the left IMA (black arrow). (b) Selective left main coronary artery injection demonstrating retrograde flow in the left IMA graft (arrow). (c) Selective left subclavian angiography after PTA and stent placement demonstrating restoration of antegrade left IMA flow (arrow).

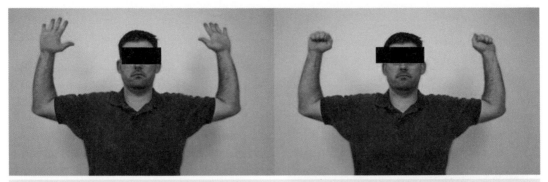

Figure 4.4 The elevated arm stress test (EAST) is used to diagnose TOS. Note alternate opening and closing of the fists.

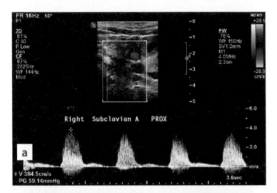

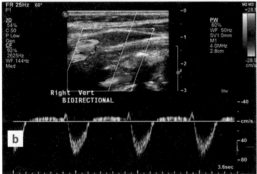

Figure 4.5 (a) Elevated subclavian artery velocity noted in routine carotid duplex study. (b) Ipsilateral vertebral artery partial reversal (bidirectional flow) noted in the same study.

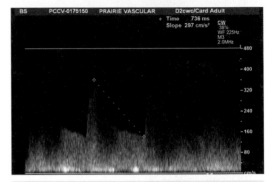

Figure 4.6 Continuous-wave Doppler used to detect elevated velocities within the proximal left common carotid artery.

Gadolinium-enhanced magnetic resonance angiography (MRA) is an excellent technique for visualization of suspected disease involving the brachiocephalic and subclavian vessels. This technique is particularly useful in detecting large vessel vasculitis (Figure 4.10), scar tissue, or congenital bands that may result in thoracic outlet syndrome. The technique is limited by its availability and inability to be used in patients with metallic implants. Computed tomography angiography (CTA) is another noninvasive modality. The drawbacks include radiation and dye-induced nephropathy.

with subclavian stenosis (Figure 4.7). Proximal brachiocephalic or left common carotid stenosis may be suspected when *parvus et tardus* waveforms are noted in the distal branches (ie, common, internal, and external carotid arteries) (Figure 4.8). Subclavian stenosis may also be incidentally identified in patients undergoing routine surveillance duplex ultrasonography of an axillofemoral bypass graft (Figure 4.9).

Indications for Angiography

Angiography of the upper extremities should be performed when the etiology of upper-extremity ischemia remains unclear despite noninvasive evaluation. Indications for upper-

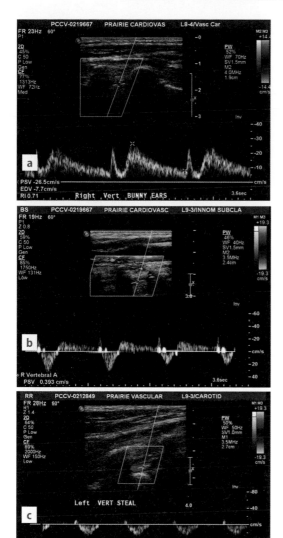

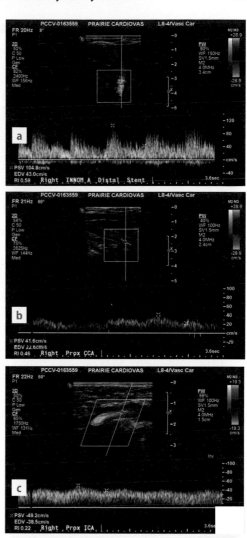

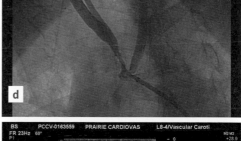

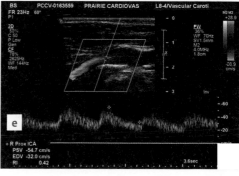

Figure 4.7 (above) (a) Note 2 systolic peaks within this vertebral artery waveform with a deep cleft in between the peaks. The first peak is steep and taller than the second peak. The end diastolic flow is above the baseline. The flow is antegrade. This is an early sign of vertebral steal phenomenon. (b) Same patient after 6 months follow-up shows bidirectional flow (partial reversal) within the vertebral artery. Note the systolic peak and reversal. Flow is antegrade in diastole. (c) Complete reversal within the vertebral artery 1 year after the initial presentation.

Figure 4.8 (right column) (a) Spectral broadening in Innominate artery on routine carotid duplex study. (b) Note parvus et tardus waveforms within the proximal common carotid artery. (c) Note parvus et tardus waveforms within the proximal internal carotid artery. (d) Note stenosis within the innominate stent. (e) Note restoration of proximal ICA waveform after angioplasty of the brachiocephalic stenosis.

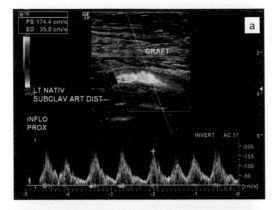

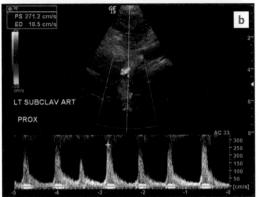

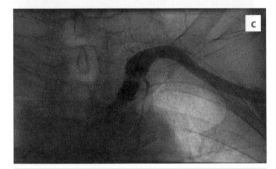

Figure 4.9 (a) Low resistive signal noted in the axillofemoral graft, on routine surveillance graft. (b) Elevated velocities noted in the left proximal subclavian artery suggestive of significant stenosis. (c) Note kink in the subclavian artery causing the elevation in velocities on duplex ultrasonography.

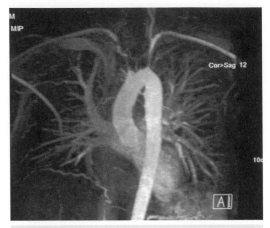

Figure 4.10 MRA of a patient with bilateral arm claudication and Takayasu's arteritis. Note stenoses involving the arch vessels.

extremity angiography include arm claudication, digital ischemia, or trauma with signs of vascular injury.

Prior to selective angiography of the upper extremity an arch aortogram should be performed in the LAO view. This allows for

detection of anomalies and anatomic features that influence the choice of equipment. Even if symptoms are unilateral, bilateral angiography is generally recommended. This will help to distinguish bilateral small-vessel obstructive disease from unilateral small-artery embolic obstruction.

Selective engagement of the subclavian and brachiocephalic arteries is usually achieved with a Judkins Right 4 catheter. Alternatively a Vitek, Simmons, Cobra, or Headhunter catheter may be used. The bifurcation of the brachiocephalic and right subclavian arteries is best delineated in the RAO-caudal projection. The vertebral and IMA arteries are best delineated in the contralateral oblique projection.

Selective axillary or brachial angiography is performed with the diagnostic catheter in the distal subclavian artery. Axillary artery angiography is performed in the neutral position, and brachial artery angiography is performed with the arm abducted with the forearm supine.

Forearm and hand angiography is performed with the diagnostic catheter in the mid to distal brachial artery. Vasodilators should be used to improve visualization of the digital arteries. Alternatively, the hands can be wrapped in warm cloths to promote vasodilation.

Anatomy

The arterial system of the arms and hands consists of the inflow arteries (brachiocephalic and subclavian), the intrinsic arteries (axillary, brachial, antecubital, radial, ulnar, palmar, and digital), and the arterioles, which terminate in sphincters that control flow into the capillaries.[23] The collateral circulation around the shoulder, axilla, and elbow are well developed. In the forearm, hand, and fingers, the radial and ulnar arteries, the deep and superficial palmar arches, and the paired digital arteries provide parallel circulation, which can provide circulation independent of the other (Figure 4.11).

The brachiocephalic artery is the first great vessel arising from the aortic arch. The subclavian arteries arise from the bifurcation of the brachiocephalic artery on the right and the aortic arch on the left. The branches of the subclavian artery are the vertebral and internal mammary arteries and the thyrocervical and costocervical trunks.

The subclavian artery passes through the thoracic outlet before it ends in the axillary artery. The superior surface of the first rib or a cervical rib and the inferior surface of the clavicle form the base and the roof of the thoracic outlet, respectively. The subclavian vein is the most anterior structure of the neurovascular bundle and is surrounded by subclavius muscle, anteriorly and superiorly, and scalenus anterior muscle, posteriorly. The subclavian artery and the brachial plexus lie between the scalenus anterior muscle, anteriorly, and the scalenus medius and the scalenus posterior muscles, posteriorly.

The axillary artery begins at the lateral margin of the first rib and ends at the lower margin of the teres major muscle, where it becomes the brachial artery. The first portion of the axillary artery lies above the pectoris minor muscle and is enclosed in the brachial sheath along with the axillary vein and brachial plexus. The second and third portions of the vessel lie behind and below the pectoralis minor muscle, respectively. The branches of the axillary artery are the superior thoracic, thoracoacromial, lateral thoracic, subscapular, posterior humeral circumflex, and anterior humeral circumflex arteries.

At the lower margin of the tendon of the teres major muscle, the brachial artery begins and ends below the elbow, where it bifurcates into the radial and ulnar arteries. The artery is superficial throughout its course beginning medial to the humerus and, finally, coursing between the epicondyles of the humerus. The branches of the brachial artery are the profunda brachii, superior ulnar collateral, and inferior ulnar collateral, as well as nutrient and muscular arteries.

The ulnar artery is the larger of the 2 terminal branches of the brachial artery. In its proximal portion, it gives rise to the recurrent interosseous artery, which provides collateral flow to the elbow and the anterior and posterior interosseous arteries. Distally the ulnar artery

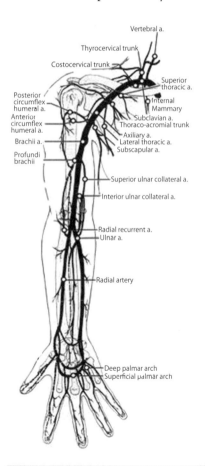

Vertebral a.

Thyrocervical trunk

Costocervical trunk

Superior thoracic a.

Posterior circumflex humeral a.

Anterior circumflex humeral a.

Internal Mammary

Subclavian a.

Thoraco-acromial trunk

Brachii a.

Axiliary a.

Lateral thoracic a.

Subscapular a.

Profundi brachii

Superior ulnar collateral a.

Interior ulnar collateral a.

Radial recurrent a.

Ulnar a.

Radial artery

Deep palmar arch

Superficial palmar arch

Figure 4.11 Arterial anatomy of the upper extremity.

divides to enter the deep and superficial palmar arches.

The branches of the radial artery in the forearm are the radial recurrent, muscular, volar carpal, and superficial volar arteries; at the wrist, it gives rise to the superficial palmar branch. Distally the radial artery unites with the deep palmar branch of the ulnar artery to form the deep palmar arch (Figure 4.12).

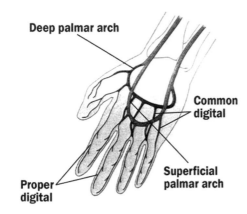

Figure 4.12 Arterial anatomy of the hand.

The ulnar artery supplies the superficial palmar arch and the radial supplies the deep palmar arch. The superficial arch is usually dominant and lies distal to the deep arch. The princeps pollicis and radialis indicis arteries arise from the radial artery and supply the thumb and index finger. The superficial palmar arch gives off common palmar digital arteries, which divide into proper digital arteries that supply apposing surfaces of the fingers.

Common Variations

Congenital variations of the arterial anatomy of the upper extremity occur relatively frequently. An understanding of these anomalies is important for proper interpretation of upper-extremity angiograms. The right subclavian artery may arise separately from the aortic arch. In 0.5% of cases, it arises as the final great vessel off of the aortic arch. Occasionally, the left subclavian and left common carotid arteries share a common origin. The left common carotid and brachiocephalic arteries have a common origin 15% of

the time. A bovine origin of the left common carotid artery occurs in 10% of the population. The course of both the left and right subclavian arteries is variable. In 1% to 5% of patients, the left vertebral artery originates directly from the aortic arch.

Multiple arterial variations of the arm have been described (Table 4.3).[24] Knowledge of these variations is important. For example, a brachioradial artery may be mistakenly interpreted as an occluded radial artery.

Superficial brachial artery
Accessory brachial artery
Superficial brachioulnar artery
Brachioulnar artery
Brachioradial artery
Superficial brachioradial artery
Brachiointerosseous artery
Superficial brachiomedian artery
Superficial brachioulnoradial artery
Superficial radial artery
Absence of the radial artery
Absence of the ulnar artery

Table 4.3 Variations of the Arteries of the Forearm

The arterial anatomy of the hand is highly variable. The superficial palmar arch can be classified as either complete (80%) or incomplete (20%). Patients with a complete arch are described by the anastomotic patterns with the ulnar artery. Those with an incomplete arch are classified by the vessels contributing to the arch. The deep arch is also classified by whether it is complete (97%) or incomplete (3%). The complete deep arch has 4 variations while the incomplete has 2.

Surgical Therapy

Since the 1980s and 1990s, the use of percutaneous angioplasty has increased. Angioplasty with or without stenting has proven to be a satisfactory alternative to surgery due to the high success rates, low periprocedural complications, and a shorter hospital stay. As such, endovascular therapy has been advocated as the primary modality of treatment for subclavian and brachiocephalic disease.[25]

Surgical procedures include *transthoracic* and *extrathoracic surgeries*. Extrathoracic surgical repairs are preferred due to the lower perioperative mortality and morbidity with comparable efficacy and durability.[26,27] The common extrathoracic surgical revascularization procedures include carotid-subclavian, carotid-axillary, and axilloaxillary bypass. Another extrathoracic technique, subclavian-carotid transposition, is also used in some centers.

Primary surgical anastomosis is possible in most cases of brachial artery disease due to its tortuous course. If the resected artery is more than 2 cm long, interposition with a vein graft should be done.[28]

Management of arterial TOS depends on the severity of the symptoms and the severity of the occlusion on the angiograms. The management ranges from thrombectomy to complete vascular reconstruction along with decompression of thoracic outlet, if the arteriogram reveals an external compression. The vascular reconstruction involves graft anastomosis from the supraclavicular subclavian artery to the brachial artery. An extra pleural thoracic sympathectomy can be performed if the patient has significant vasospasm.[19] This may help in decreasing the peripheral resistance and dilating the collaterals.

The most important aspect in the management of hand ischemia is pain management, vasodilator therapy, and supportive care as outlined in Chapter 19. However, in patients with acute hand ischemia due to occupational vascular problems, such as hypothenar hammer syndrome, therapy may involve intra-arterial thrombolytic therapy if ischemia onset is less than 2 weeks. Otherwise, resection of the thrombosed artery and end-to-end transposition with the vein graft harvested from the dorsum of the foot is an accepted therapy for acute hand ischemia (Figure 4.13).[29] Patients with irreversible digital gangrene may require amputation (see Figure 4.1b).

Endovascular Therapy

Most patients with subclavian or brachiocephalic stenosis are asymptomatic due to the abundant collateral circulation and lower metabolic requirements of the arm. In general, arterial revascularization of the upper extremity is reserved for symptomatic patients. Subclavian or brachiocephalic revascularization may be performed to protect inflow into axilloaxillary, axillofemoral, subclavian-carotid, or IMA-coronary graft. Subclavian stenosis may be a cause for failure of hemodialysis fistulas, and subclavian intervention may be indicated for patients undergoing or anticipating hemodialysis. Similarly, intervention is indicated in patients with a significant subclavian stenosis, who are in need of IMA coronary artery bypass grafting (see Figure 4.2). Alternatively, a free IMA graft may be considered.[30]

Although brachiocephalic stenosis is uncommon, the associated symptoms may be severe. A brachiocephalic stenosis may place both the anterior and posterior cerebral circulations at risk (Figure 4.14). An important contraindication to subclavian or brachiocephalic intervention is the presence of thrombus. Intervention in this setting would seemingly increase the risk of embolization to the distal extremity or the anterior or posterior cerebral circulations.

Unfortunately, there are no randomized controlled trials comparing the outcomes of surgical and endovascular management of upper-extremity arterial disease. The success, efficacy, and restenosis rates are derived from available retrospective case series. The restenosis rate after subclavian and brachiocephalic artery percutaneous transluminal angioplasty (PTA) and/or stenting has been reported as 6% to 21% (Table 4.4). Thrombosis or occlusion is exceptionally rare.[30] In a review of the experience of surgical and endovascular revascularization of brachiocephalic and subclavian arteries, the technical success, complication,

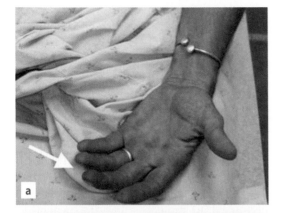

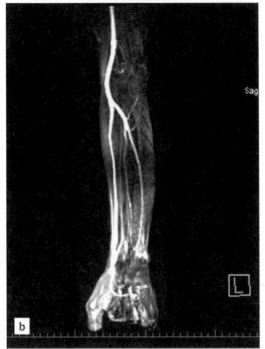

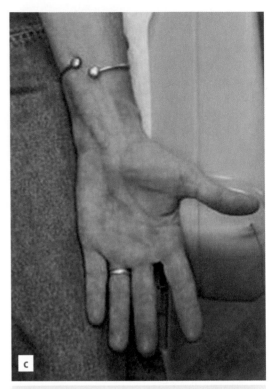

Figure 4.13 (a) Acute digital ischemia and vasospasm due to hypothenar hammer syndrome in a hog farmer. (b) MRA of the upper extremity. Note normal-appearing brachial, radial, and interosseus arteries. Ulnar artery is occluded at the wrist. (c) Postulnar to superficial and deep palmar arch reverse vein graft with restoration of flow to the hand.

and restenosis rate is superior with endovascular techniques (Table 4.5).[30] In the contemporary era, the technical success for endovascular treatment of subclavian and brachiocephalic artery stenosis approaches 100%.[31]

The technical success rate for occlusions is somewhat lower than stenosis. It has been reported as 83% to 90%.[39,40] Restenosis rates for subclavian occlusions with PTA alone has been reported as high as 50% at 1 year.[40] However, with stenting, the restenosis rate, even for occlusions, is probably less than 20%.

Fibromuscular dysplasia (FMD) is amenable to angioplasty without stenting (Figure 4.15; see page 67).

Subclavian Artery Intervention

Atherosclerotic subclavian artery stenosis usually involves the proximal portion of the vessel proximal to the vertebral artery. Occlusions may extend from the ostium to the origin of the vertebral artery. The relationship of the lesion must be defined in relation to the vertebral artery and IMA, and in the right subclavian, the brachiocephalic and right common carotid arteries, before intervention can be planned.

The preferred access site for stenosis is the common femoral artery (CFA). An antegrade approach allows good visualization of the ostium of the vessel. It may be beneficial to obtain

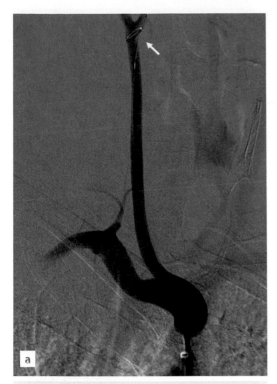

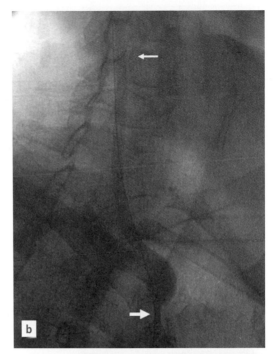

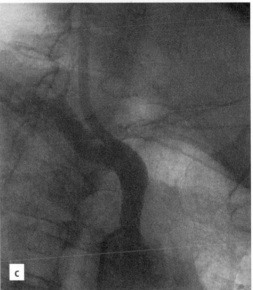

Figure 4.14 (a) High-grade symptomatic brachio-cephalic stenosis. A filter wire embolic protection device, as well as a buddy wire, is seen in the distal right common carotid artery (arrow). (b) Placement of the intravascular stent (large arrow) over the filter wire (small arrow) prior to removal of the buddy wire. (c) Final result after brachiocephalic PTA and stent placement.

both CFA and brachial artery access when intervening on occlusions. It may be necessary to cross an occlusion in a retrograde fashion. The lesion can then be dilated and stented in an antegrade fashion after snaring and externalizing the brachial wire.

Patients should be started on aspirin (81–325 mg daily) prior to subclavian or brachiocephalic intervention. Although not supported by published data, it is our practice to treat these patients with clopidogrel for a minimum of 1 month after stenting. For patients who are undergoing revascularization prior to CABG, usually, clopidogrel is started after the CABG. The choice of anticoagulant during the intervention is dependent on the operator. Most procedures are performed using unfractionated heparin with a goal activated clotting time (ACT) of

250–300 seconds. Although there are no data to support its use for this indication, many interventionalists utilize the direct thrombin inhibitor bivalirudin, due to its ease of use.

The intervention may be performed from the CFA utilizing either a guide or sheath-based platform. When using a sheath, the subclavian artery is usually cannulated with an appropriate

Author, Year	Patients (n)	PTA/Stent	Restenosis Rate	Mean Follow-up
De Vries et al[31]	102	102/0	11%	34 months
Bates et al[32]	89	0/89	10.7%	36 months
Angle et al[33]	21	14/7	21%	27 months
Westerband et al[34]	13	2/11	15.3%	29 months
Al-Mubarak et al[35]	35	0/35	6%	20 months
Henry et al[36]	103	57/46	13%	52 months
Sullivan et al[25]	66	0/66	16%	35 months
Martinez et al[37]	17	0/17	19%	19 months

Table 4.4 Restenosis Rates for Subclavian and Brachiocephalic PTA and Stenting

	Endovascular (n = 108)	Surgery (n = 2496)
Technical Success	97%	96%
Stroke	0%	3%
Death	0%	2%
Complications	6%	16%
Recurrence	3%	16%

Table 4.5 Comparison of Endovascular and Surgical Revascularization of Brachiocephalic and Subclavian Arteries

diagnostic catheter. The lesion may be crossed with a 0.035-in wire and the diagnostic catheter may be exchanged for the appropriate sheath. With more complex lesions, it may be necessary to cross with a hydrophilic or smaller-diameter wire, advance the diagnostic catheter distal to the lesion, and exchange for a supportive 0.035-in wire. In general, a 0.035-in wire is required to provide adequate support for exchanging the sheath. Alternatively, the dilator may be removed from the sheath and a long diagnostic catheter may be telescoped through the sheath. After cannulating the artery and advancing the wire distal to the lesion, the sheath may be advanced over the diagnostic catheter.

The advantage of a guide-based platform is that it may provide for more support and di-rectionality. This may be of greater importance when treating ostial lesions. A long diagnostic catheter may be telescoped through the guide. After engaging the origin of the vessel and crossing the lesion with a supportive wire, the guide may be advanced over the diagnostic catheter.

In general, a 6-Fr or 7-Fr sheath or an 8-Fr or 9-Fr guide catheter is used. One must anticipate the diameter of the balloons and stents to complete the intervention and ensure compatibility with the sheath or guide preprocedure. This will obviate the need to exchange the sheath or guide during the procedure to accommodate a larger device.

In general, balloon angioplasty is performed prior to stent placement. This allows for evaluation of the lesion characteristics and ves-

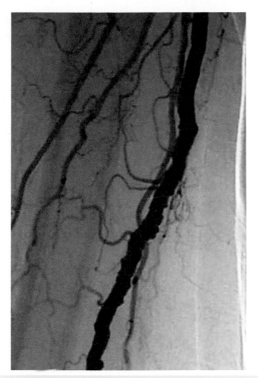 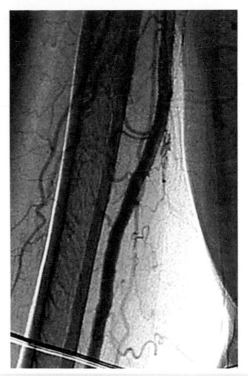

Figure 4.15 Note "string of pearls" appearance in the brachial artery that resolved with angioplasty. (Reproduced from Kolluri R, Ansel G. Fibromuscular dysplasia of bilateral brachial arteries—a case report and literature review. *Angiology*. 2004;55(6):685-689. Reprinted by permission of SAGE Publications.)

sel diameter. Due to the superior patency with stents, balloon angioplasty alone should not be performed in subclavian arteries. In general, predilation is performed with 5- to 7-mm diameter balloon (Table 4.6).

Vessel	Diameter (mm)
Brachiocephalic	8–11
Subclavian	6–8
Axillary	5–7
Brachial	5–7
Radial	3–4
Ulnar	3–4

Table 4.6 Typical Diameters of the Arteries of the Arm

Subclavian stenoses proximal to the vertebral artery are treated with balloon expandable stents due to the need for precise placement and radial force. Most patients will require a 6- to 9-mm diameter stent (Table 4.6). Ostial lesions require special attention to ensure that the ostium is completely covered and 1 to 2 mm of stent is extended into the aorta. This is confirmed with an ipsilateral oblique view. It is important to avoid compromise of the IMA or vertebral artery with the stent. This is achieved with a contralateral oblique view. When the lesion is within close proximity of the vertebral artery or IMA, it may be prudent to protect access to this vessel by placing a 0.014-in wire in the vessel via the brachial artery. This technique is particularly important in patients with an occluded contralateral vertebral artery, as inadvertent occlusion of a solitary vertebral artery may be catastrophic. It is advisable to deploy the stent and postdeploy the stent at higher pressure after slight retraction of the balloon proximally.

This technique may help avoid distal dissection caused by an overhanging balloon. For lesions distal to the vertebral artery, self-expanding stents are generally recommended to accommodate the tapering vessel as well as the flexion of this portion of the vessel.

Ostial subclavian occlusions may require recanalization in a retrograde fashion. This is accomplished using a 6-Fr brachial artery sheath. Generally, crossing these lesions will require the combination of a stiff-angled glide wire supported by a catheter. It is helpful to have a diagnostic catheter placed in the proximal stump of the vessel to guide the wire toward the true lumen (see Figure 4.2c). Once the lesion is crossed the brachial wire should be snared and externalized through the CFA sheath. Once this is accomplished, the appropriate sheath or guide must be exchanged over this wire and the intervention can be completed from the CFA.

Operators must remember the potential for embolization to the posterior circulation via the vertebral artery while performing subclavian interventions. Ringlestein and Zeumer[41] reported that despite successful recanalization of the subclavian stenosis or occlusion, it may take 20 seconds to several minutes before the vertebral flow is corrected from retrograde to antegrade. It is hypothesized that this may impart a protective mechanism against distal embolization to the vertebral artery. The risk of cerebral embolization increases in patients with antegrade vertebral artery flow. As such, it is important to assess the direction of flow within the ipsilateral and contralateral vertebral artery either by duplex ultrasonography or angiography prior to subclavian intervention. In patients with antegrade vertebral flow, the risk of embolization to the posterior cerebral circulation may be lowered by utilizing embolic protection. This may be accomplished from the ipsilateral brachial artery using a filter device. In patients with antegrade vertebral artery flow, retrograde flow may be induced by hyperemia. This can be accomplished by inflation of a blood pressure cuff above systolic pressure for several minutes followed by deflation immediately before balloon inflation and/

or stent deployment. Alternatively, hyperemia may be produced with an intra-arterial vasodilator, such as papaverine.

Brachiocephalic Artery Intervention

Brachiocephalic artery interventions are technically more complicated because of the potential for embolization to the anterior circulation. Distal protection should be used to minimize the risk of embolization to the anterior cerebral circulation via the internal carotid artery. This may be performed by obtaining 6-Fr ipsilateral brachial artery access. A 6-Fr IMA guide catheter may then be used to cannulate the common carotid artery. Through this catheter, a distal protection filter is advanced into either the distal common or proximal internal carotid artery depending on the diameters of the vessels. Owing to the acute angle between the subclavian and common carotid arteries, stiffer, fixed-wire distal protection devices may have a tendency to prolapse into the brachiocephalic artery. For this reason, it is advisable to use a wire-independent device such as the Spider Rx. Once the distal protection device is in place, a sheath or guide catheter may be manipulated from the CFA into proper position as described in the previous section. In general, the wire over which the intervention is performed is advanced into the external carotid artery.

Even with newer embolic protection devices, it may be impossible to safely advance the device from brachial artery into the carotid artery. In this situation, the embolic protection device is advanced from the CFA (see Figure 4.14). A guide catheter is used to ensure coaxial alignment and a supportive buddy wire is used to provide support during positioning of the balloon and stent. Prior to deployment of the stent, the buddy wire is retracted into the guide catheter.

Balloon expandable stents should be utilized in this location. Care must be taken to ensure that neither the ostium of the common carotid nor subclavian artery is compromised by the stent. The bifurcation of these vessels is best viewed in the RAO caudal view.

Axillary and Brachial Artery Intervention

Axillary and brachial arterial stenoses are rare compared to stenoses in more proximal arterial segments. The pathophysiology of these lesions differs markedly from atherosclerotic occlusive disease. These lesions are approached similarly to subclavian lesions. However, angioplasty alone is preferred in locations such as the subclavian-axillary junction, where there is bending and compression. When these lesions do not respond to angioplasty alone, self-expanding stents are used.

Complications

Fortunately, the complication rate with subclavian and brachiocephalic endovascular interventions is as low as 2%.[42] The major risk of these interventions is distal embolization. The risk of distal embolization is less than 1%.[43] Distal embolization to the arm and hand vessels may result in digital ischemia, while embolization to the posterior or anterior circulation can result in transient ischemic attack (TIA) or cerebrovascular accident (CVA). Distal embolization within the arm may require thrombectomy, thrombolysis, or further angioplasty and stenting. Neurovascular rescue must be considered, if available locally, for cerebral embolization, otherwise treatment involves anticoagulation and supportive care.

The most common complications with subclavian and brachiocephalic interventions are associated with the access site and occur in up to 7% of the cases.[39] These include hematoma, bleeding, infection, pseudoaneurysm formation, arteriovenous fistula formation, and retroperitoneal hematoma. Use of the brachial artery increases the risk of access site complications.

The proximal subclavian artery is an intrathoracic structure. Perforation or rupture of this vessel is associated with significant morbidity and mortality. Calcified lesions may increase the risk of this complication. These lesions should be conservatively predilated. Conservative stent sizing is prudent. The stent may be postdilated if necessary (see Table 4.4). A perforation or rupture is treated with balloon tamponade, reversal of anticoagulation, and placement of a covered stent. If a perforation cannot be sealed with a covered stent without occluding a vertebral artery, IMA bypass graft or right common carotid artery emergent operative repair must be considered. However, an occluded vertebral artery may be well tolerated in the setting of a patent contralateral vertebral artery.

Dissections within the brachiocephalic or subclavian arteries are generally treated with intravascular stenting, similar to dissections in other vessels. However, in these vessels careful attention needs to be paid to the right common carotid artery, vertebral arteries, and IMA bypass grafts. Dissections that compromise these vessels may require further stenting to maintain patency.

Hyperperfusion syndrome and hyperemia are described in other vascular territories after revascularization, particularly after carotid endarterectomy. Hyperperfusion syndrome, resulting in cerebral hemorrhage, after subclavian artery stenting, has been described.[44] Management of this complication is supportive and the mortality is high. Hyperperfusion of the hand and deltoid muscle have also been described after endovascular revascularization of the subclavian artery.[45,46] These cases were treated conservatively and with fasciotomy, respectively. Hyperperfusion syndrome must be differentiated from embolization as the treatment differs.

Summary

Compared to lower-extremity disease, upper-extremity vascular disease is uncommon. While atherosclerosis may affect the brachiocephalic and subclavian arteries, it is rare in the more distal vessels of the upper extremities. It is potentially disabling due to its effects on arm and hand function and possible involvement of the cerebral or coronary circulation. Upper-extremity vascular disease may carry a worse prognosis than lower-extremity disease if it is secondary to a systemic disorder.

The evaluation of patients with symptoms of upper-extremity ischemia begins with segmental pressures. This can differentiate between large- and small-vessel disease. Further evaluation of large-vessel disease may involve duplex ultrasonography, MRA, CTA, or angiography. Small-vessel disease is further evaluated with digital pressures and waveforms, lab testing for connective tissue disease, and possibly also angiography.

Endovascular techniques are preferred when brachiocephalic or subclavian revascularization is required. Upper-extremity endovascular revascularization has a high technical success rate, low complication rate, and excellent patency.

References

1. Glagov S, Zarins C, Giddens DP, Ku DN. Hemodynamics and atherosclerosis. Insights and perspectives gained from studies of human arteries. *Arch Pathol Lab Med*. 1988;112(10):1018-1031.

2. Lippert H, Pabst R. *Arterial Variations in Man*. Munich: Verlag; 1985, 107-124.

3. Quraishy MS, Cawthorn SJ, Giddings AE. Critical ischaemia of the upper limb. *J R Soc Med*. 1992;85(5):269-273.

4. Pentti J, Salenius JP, Kuukasjarvi P, Tarkka M. Outcome of surgical treatment in acute upper limb ischaemia. *Ann Chir Gynaecol*. 1995;84(1):25-28.

5. Dequara J, Ali T, Modarai B, Burnand KG. Upper limb ischemia: 20 years experience from a single center. *Vascular*. 2005;13(2):84-91.

6. Kolluri R, Ansel G. Fibromuscular dysplasia of bilateral brachial arteries—a case report and literature review. *Angiology*. 2004;55(6):685-689.

7. Kreidy R, Hatem J. Acute limb ischemia secondary to heparin-induced thrombocytopenia after cardiac surgery. *J Med Liban*. 2004;52(3):175-181.

8. de Mendonca WC, Espat PA. Pheochromocytoma associated with arterial fibromuscular dysplasia. *Am J Clin Pathol*. 1981;75(5):749-754.

9. Ponsky TA, Brody F, Giordano J, Garcia R, Kardon D, Schwartz A. Brachial artery occlusion secondary to hypereosinophilic syndrome. *J Vasc Surg*. 2005;42(4):796-799.

10. Mulaudzi TV, Robbs JV, Pillay W, et al. Thrombectomy in HIV related peripheral arterial thrombosis: a preliminary report. *Eur J Vasc Endovasc Surg*. 2005;30(1):102-106.

11. Belz M, Marshall JJ, Cowley MJ, Vetrovec GW. Subclavian balloon angioplasty in the management of the coronary-subclavian steal syndrome. *Cathet Cardiovasc Diagn*. 1992;25(2):161-163.

12. Reivich M, Holling HE, Roberts B, Toole JF. Reversal of blood flow through the vertebral artery and its effect on cerebral circulation. *N Engl J Med*. 1961;265:878-885.

13. Fields WS, Lemak NA. Joint study of extracranial arterial occlusion. VII. Subclavian steal—a review of 168 cases. *JAMA*. 1972;222(9):1139-1143.

14. Webster MW, Downs L, Yonas H, Makaroun MS, Steed DL. The effect of arm exercise on regional cerebral blood flow in the subclavian steal syndrome. *Am J Surg*. 1994;168(2):91-93.

15. Amar AP, Levy ML, Giannotta SL. Iatrogenic vertebrobasilar insufficiency after surgery of the subclavian or brachial artery: review of three cases. *Neurosurgery*. 1998;43(6):1450-1457; discussion 1457-1458.

16. Berni A, Tromba L, Cavaiola S, Tombesi T, Castellani L. Classification of the subclavian steal syndrome with transcranial Doppler. *J Cardiovasc Surg*. (Torino) 1997;38(2):141-145.

17. Bornstein NM, Krajewski A, Norris JW. Basilar artery blood flow in subclavian steal. *Can J Neurol Sci*. 1988;15(4):417-419.

18. Gosselin C, Walker PM. Subclavian steal syndrome: existence, clinical features, diagnosis and management. *Semin Vasc Surg*. 1996;9(2):93-97.

19. Gilroy J, Meyer JS. Compression of the subclavian artery as a cause of ischaemic brachial neuropathy. *Brain*. 1963;86:733-746.

20. Roos DB. *Overview of Thoracic Outlet Syndromes*. New York: Futura Publishing Company; 1989, 91-106.

21. Tan TY, Schminke U, Lien LM, Tegeler CH. Subclavian steal syndrome: can the blood pressure difference between arms predict the severity of steal? *J Neuroimaging*. 2002;12(2):131-135.

22. Kliewer MA, Hertzberg BS, Kim DH, Bowie JD, Courneya DL, Carroll BA. Vertebral artery Doppler waveform changes indicating subclavian steal physiology. *AJR Am J Roentgenol*. 2000;174(3):815-819.

23. Longo GM, Pearce, WH, Sumner, DS, eds. *Evaluation of the Upper Extremity*. 6th ed. Philadelphia: Elsevier Saunders; 2005, 1274-1293.

24. Rodriguez-Niedenfuhr M, Vazquez T, Nearn L, Ferreira B, Parkin I, Sanudo JR. Variations of the arterial pattern in the upper limb revisited: a morphological and statistical study, with a review of the literature. *J Anat*. 2001;199(Pt 5):547-566.

25. Sullivan TM, Gray BH, Bacharach JM, et al. Angioplasty and primary stenting of the subclavian, innominate, and common carotid arteries in 83 patients. *J Vasc Surg*. 1998;28(6):1059-1065.

26. Edwards WH Jr, Tapper SS, Edwards WH Sr., Mulherin JL Jr., Martin RS III, Jenkins JM. Subclavian revascularization. A quarter century experience. *Ann Surg*. 1994;219(6):673-677; discussion 677-678.

27. Vitti MJ, Thompson BW, Read RC, et al. Carotid-subclavian bypass: a twenty-two-year experience. *J Vasc Surg*. 1994;20(3):411-417; discussion 417-418.

28. Shindo S, Kojima A, Ishimoto T, Iyori K, Kobayashi M, Tada Y. Arterial reconstruction in the upper extremities. *Vascular*. 2004;12(1):57-61.

29. Vayssairat M, Debure C, Cormier JM, Bruneval P, Laurian C, Juillet Y. Hypothenar hammer syndrome: seventeen cases with long-term follow-up. *J Vasc Surg*. 1987;5(6):838-843.

30. Rogers J, Calhoun, RF II. Diagnosis and management of subclavian artery stenosis prior to coronary artery bypass grafting in the current era. *J Cardiac Surg*. 2007;22(1)20-25.

31. De Vries JP, Jager LC, Van den Berg JC, et al. Durability of percutaneous transluminal angioplasty for obstructive lesions of proximal subclavian artery: long-term results. *J Vasc Surg*. 2005;41(1):19-23.

32. Bates MC, Broce M, Lavigne PS, Stone P. Subclavian artery stenting: factors influencing long-term outcome. *Catheter Cardiovasc Interv*. 2004;61(1):5-11.

33. Angle JF, Matsumoto AH, McGraw JK, et al. Percutaneous angioplasty and stenting of left subclavian artery stenosis in patients with left internal mammary-coronary bypass grafts: clinical experience and long-term follow-up. *Vasc Endovascular Surg*. 2003;37(2): 89-97.

34. Westerband A, Rodriguez JA, Ramaiah VG, Diethrich EB. Endovascular therapy in prevention and management of coronary-subclavian steal *J Vasc Surg*. 2003;38(4):699-703; discussion 704.

35. Al-Mubarak N, Liu MW, Dean LS, et al. Immediate and late outcomes of subclavian artery stenting. *Catheter Cardiovasc Interv*. 1999;46(2):169-172.

36. Henry M, Amor M, Henry I, Ethevenot G, Tzvetanov K, Chati Z. Percutaneous transluminal angioplasty of the subclavian arteries. *J Endovasc Surg*. 1999;6(1):33-41.

37. Martinez R, Rodriguez-Lopez J, Torruella L, Ray L, Lopez-Galarza L, Diethrich EB. Stenting for occlusion of the subclavian arteries. Technical aspects and follow-up results. *Texas Heart Inst J*. 1997;24(1):23-27.

38. Hadjipetrou P, Cox S, Piemonte T, Eisenhauer A. Percutaneous revascularization of atherosclerotic obstruction of aortic arch vessels. *J Am Coll Cardiol*. 1999;33(5):1238-1245.

39. Cho L, Casserly IP, Wholey MH, eds. *Manual of Peripheral Vascular Intervention*. Philadelphia, PA: Lippincott Williams & Wilkins; 2005, 120-139.

40. Motarjeme A. Percutaneous transluminal angioplasty of supra-aortic vessels. *J Endovasc Surg*. 1996;3(2):171-181.

41. Ringelstein EB, Zeumer H. Delayed reversal of vertebral artery blood flow following

percutaneous transluminal angioplasty for subclavian steal syndrome. *Neuroradiology.* 1984;26(3):189-198.

42. Wholey MH. The supraaortic and vertebral endovascular interventions. *Tech Vasc Interv Radiol.* 2004;7(4):215-225.

43. Queral LA, Criado FJ. Endovascular treatment of aortic arch occlusive disease. *Semin Vasc Surg.* 1996;9(2):156-163.

44. Salerno JL, Vitek J. Fatal cerebral hemorrhage early after subclavian artery endovascular therapy. *AJNR Am J Neuroradiol.* 2005;26(1):183-185.

45. Klocker J, Chemelli A, Bodner G, et al. Hyperperfusion syndrome of the deltoid muscle after subclavian artery angioplasty and stenting. *J Endovasc Ther.* 2003;10(4): 833-837.

46. Chemelli AP, Bodner G, Perkmann R, Hourmont K, Waldenberger P, Jaschke W. Hyperperfusion syndrome of the left hand after percutaneous transluminal angioplasty and stent placement in a subclavian artery stenosis. *J Vasc Interv Radiol.* 2001;12(3): 388-390.

5

Extracranial Carotid Artery Disease

Christopher J. White and Michael R. Jaff

Stroke is the third leading cause of death in the United States and the second leading cause worldwide. Over 20% of patients die from the acute stroke, and the mortality is as high as 50% at 5 years.[1] Control of several modifiable stroke risk factors, in particular hypertension, diabetes mellitus, dyslipidemia, and tobacco abuse, is integral to stroke prevention.

Extracranial Carotid Artery Stenosis and Stroke Risk

The risk of stroke increases as the severity of the carotid stenosis increases. The stroke rate in patients with carotid stenosis of 75% or less is 1.3% per year, and 10.5% per year if the stenosis is greater than 75%.[2] In symptomatic patients with 70% to 99% carotid stenosis followed medically for 2 years, North American Symptomatic Carotid Endarterectomy Trial (NASCET) investigators demonstrated a 26% risk of ipsilateral stroke and 28% risk of any stroke.[3] It appears, however, that the initial cerebrovascular symptom conveys differing risks of subsequent stroke.

A retinal *transient ischemic attack (TIA),* such as amaurosis fugax, led to an annual stroke rate of 2%. Over 7 years of follow-up, the cumulative rate of cerebral infarction was 14% in patients with amaurosis fugax, compared with 27% in patients with hemispheric TIA as the initial cerebrovascular symptom. The NASCET investigators demonstrated a 2-year risk of fatal and nonfatal stroke of 17% after transient monocular blindness, and 42% after hemispheric TIA.

Regardless of their anatomic location, carotid plaque increases the risk of stroke. The pathogenesis of stroke in extracranial carotid stenosis results from reduced vessel diameter, superimposed thrombosis, and embolization of thrombotic material. This has been demonstrated on transcranial Doppler ultrasonography in patients with transient monocular blindness.[4] Alterations in plaque morphology that may lead to clinical symptoms have been postulated. As in the coronary circulation with acute coronary syndromes, plaque rupture has been postulated to result in acute stroke.

Atherosclerotic carotid artery stenoses most often cause symptoms secondary to emboli (plaque rupture, ulceration), with a minority of symptoms caused by thrombotic

Vascular Disease: Diagnostic and Therapeutic Approaches. © 2011 Michael R. Jaff and Christopher J. White, editors. Cardiotext Publishing, ISBN: 978-1-935395-16-4.

occlusion or hemodynamic impairment, which is in contrast to the pathophysiology of acute coronary syndromes.

Progression of Carotid Stenosis

Carotid artery stenosis demonstrates disease progression in approximately 20% to 40% of cases. In one prospective natural history study of 232 patients with mild (< 50%) and moderate (50%–79%) carotid stenosis followed with annual carotid duplex ultrasonography for a mean of 7 years, 23% demonstrated disease progression. One-half of these patients progressed to severe stenosis (80%–99%) or occlusion. Risk of progression to either 80% to 99% stenosis or occlusion was more likely in patients whose initial stenosis was categorized as 50% to 79% rather than < 50%.[5]

Subsequent data in 425 asymptomatic patients with 50% to 79% carotid stenosis followed for a mean of 38 months demonstrated progression of stenosis in 17% of 282 arteries with at least 2 serial carotid duplex ultrasonography examinations. There was a low incidence of ipsilateral stroke despite this rate of disease progression (0.85% at 1 year, 3.6% at 3 years, 5.4% at 5 years).[6] All natural history studies agree that more severe stenoses carry increasing risks of disease progression and subsequent stroke. Of 242 asymptomatic patients presenting with variable degrees of carotid stenosis, 35 patients suffered stroke or TIA. However, patients with 80% to 99% carotid stenosis demonstrated an annual neurologic event rate of 20.6%.[7]

The risk of stroke with internal carotid artery occlusion is somewhat unpredictable. In a retrospective review of 167 patients with carotid occlusion followed for a mean of 39 months, 27% had no symptoms, 43% suffered stroke, and 17% had a TIA. Over the course of follow-up, 18% had a stroke, and 67% were ipsilateral to the occlusion. The contralateral stroke event rate was 33%, with a lower 5-year stroke-free event rate in patients with stenoses of 50% to 99% (77%) compared with < 50% (94%) (P = 0.08).[8]

Plaque ulceration clearly increases the risk of subsequent stroke. Plaque ulceration over 2 years of follow-up in the medically treated NASCET patients increased the risk of ipsilateral stroke from 26.3% to 73.2% as the degree of stenosis progressed from 75% to 99%. In patients without plaque ulceration, the 2-year stroke risk was 21.3% regardless of the degree of stenosis.[9]

The History and Physical Examination

Perhaps the most important aspect of the evaluation of patients with extracranial carotid artery disease is determining the symptomatic status of the patient in relation to the carotid artery stenosis. Treatment options, and the outcomes of these treatment options, vary greatly depending on the symptomatic nature of the carotid artery stenosis.

Symptoms suggestive of cerebral ischemia are categorized by the location and amount of the brain affected, by the duration of symptoms, and the reversibility of the symptoms. For example, transient retinal ischemia, classically referred to as amaurosis fugax, is described as a "dark shade" resulting in temporary loss of vision in one visual field. Amaurosis fugax classically resolves within minutes. This is a TIA. Other symptoms may involve the dominant hemisphere, resulting in contralateral hemiparesis and aphasia. Nondominant hemispheric ischemia will result in the patients' lack of awareness of symptoms, or anosognosia. Posterior circulation ischemia, or vertebrobasilar insufficiency (VBI), will result in symptoms of dysarthria, diplopia, vertigo, drop attacks, and/or transient confusion.

Recently, the American Stroke Association proposed a revision of the definition of TIA to include imaging findings with the clinical presentation. As defined, a TIA is defined as

- "Transient episode of neurologic dysfunction caused by focal brain, spinal cord, or retinal ischemia without acute infarction."
- "…[These patients' risk] can be stratified by clinical scale, vessel imaging,

and diffusion magnetic resonance imaging."[10]

A stroke (cerebrovascular accident, or CVA) is a more permanent manifestation of cerebral ischemia, with symptoms lasting more than 24 hours.

Palpation of the carotid artery upstroke is a nonspecific physical finding. A diminished carotid upstroke may suggest cardiac valvular pathology or a global reduction in left ventricular systolic function. In fact, occlusion of the internal carotid artery is often accompanied by a normal carotid upstroke, as the location of the internal carotid artery is cephalad to the angle of the mandible. However, the finding of a cervical bruit has significant implications.

Evaluation of the Carotid Bruit

A carotid bruit is the audible and sometimes palpable result of turbulent blood flow. Many physicians view the cervical bruit as the only true indication for further investigation of the carotid bifurcation. A cervical bruit occurs in approximately 1% of healthy adults,[11] and it increases in frequency with age, from 2.3% in subjects aged 45 to 54 years to 8.2% in subjects older than 75 years.[12] Carotid atherosclerosis is a common cause of cervical bruits; however, thyrotoxicosis, anemia, and arteriovenous fistulae can result in a similar physical finding. A recent meta-analysis of 22 studies evaluating the impact of carotid bruits on cardiovascular events and mortality included 17,295 patients.[13] This analysis demonstrated the rate of myocardial infarction as 3.69 per 100 patient-years for those patients with a carotid bruit compared with 1.86 per 100 patient-years for patients without carotid bruits. Annual cardiovascular mortality rates were significantly greater among patients with carotid bruits (2.85 per 100 patient-years vs. 1.11 per 100 patient-years for those without bruits).

The natural history of patients with carotid bruits is not significantly different from patients without a bruit. In one study of 241 nursing home residents over the age of 75, 12% had carotid bruits. The 3-year cumulative incidence of cerebrovascular events was similar in this group

(10%) to those patients without bruits (9%).[14] Loss of the baseline bruit occurred in 60% of patients and was not associated with adverse clinical events.

The low predictive accuracy of carotid bruits for significant carotid stenosis is in part due to the low prevalence of significant carotid atherosclerosis in the population. In the Framingham Heart Study, in individuals between 66 and 93 years of age, the actual prevalence of significant carotid atherosclerosis was only 8%.[15] The positive predictive value of a carotid bruit resulting in 50% or greater internal carotid artery stenosis is less than 40%.

Differential Diagnosis of Cerebral Ischemia, Stroke, and Carotid Artery Disease

There are many causes of stroke other than atherosclerotic carotid artery disease. The most common etiology is an embolic event, most often from a cardiac source. When considering the cardiac pathology, nonvalvular atrial fibrillation, rheumatic mitral valve disease, and cardiac chamber thrombi (prior myocardial infarction) are identified by electrocardiography and echocardiography. More recently, a common source of cerebral emboli is aortic arch atherosclerosis, identified with transesophageal echocardiography. Paradoxical emboli must be considered and thoroughly investigated with transesophageal echocardiography, especially in light of new percutaneous approaches to closure of occult patent foramen ovale. Other uncommon causes of stroke include intracranial tumors, intracerebral hemorrhage (rupture of an aneurysm), central nervous system vasculitis, and intracranial arteriovenous malformations.

Risk Factors for Stroke and Carotid Artery Disease

Control of several modifiable stroke risk factors, in particular hypertension, diabetes mellitus, hyperlipidemia, and tobacco abuse, is integral to stroke prevention. For example, patients with diabetes mellitus have twice the stroke risk of nondiabetics. Similarly, those who smoke are at increased risk of all stroke subtypes, with a relative risk of 2.58 compared to those patients who have never smoked. Both low levels of high-density lipoprotein (HDL) cholesterol and a high total to HDL cholesterol (TC:HDL) ratio are risk factors for carotid atherosclerosis; however, hypercholesterolemia is not a strong independent risk factor for stroke.

As many as 60% of all strokes are attributable to hypertension, the most important risk factor for ischemic stroke, and both the incidence and mortality increase as the blood pressure rises above 110/75 mm Hg. It is estimated that two-thirds of the population's stroke risk is attributable to hypertension. Trials of antihypertensive therapy have demonstrated that even a modest reduction in blood pressure reduces the incidence of stroke. Many prospective trials suggest a linear relationship between blood pressure and stroke risk, with a lower incidence of stroke regardless of how low the blood pressure. However, other largely cohort studies have suggested a "J-shaped" phenomenon, with increased stroke rates at both very high and very low blood pressure levels. An evaluation of 7 meta-analyses of randomized trials suggests that the relationship is a linear one, with a 31% risk reduction associated with every 10 mm Hg drop in systolic blood pressure.

Atherosclerosis of the extracranial carotid arteries is a leading cause of stroke. Hypertension promotes the development of atherosclerosis at the bifurcation of the common carotid into the internal and external carotid arteries. Carotid atherosclerosis is generally found to be most severe within 2 cm of the common carotid artery bifurcation, and often involves the posterior wall of the vessel.

The presence of hypertension appears to be as important as plaque morphology and severity in predicting neurological events. A prospective study of serial carotid duplex ultrasonography suggested that hypertension, in addition to plaque echolucency and lesion progression, predicted patient symptoms.

Patients with diabetes mellitus are twice as likely to suffer a stroke in their lifetime. Tobacco use is a risk factor for cerebrovascular ischemia. Oral contraceptives, resulting in hypercoagulability in association with active tobacco use, are an important risk factor.

The impact and magnitude of risk factors for stroke have been highlighted in a study evaluating patients presenting in 22 countries.[16] Investigators completed a standardized questionnaire, physical examination, and laboratory tests. In the first 3000 patients, 78% of whom suffered an ischemic stroke, the most important risk factors were hypertension (odds ratio [OR] 2.64), tobacco use (odds ratio 2.09), and waist to hip ratio (OR 1.65).

Diagnostic Testing in Carotid Artery Disease

The gold standard to evaluate the presence and severity of carotid stenosis is intra-arterial digital subtraction angiography (Figure 5.1). Although serious complications are associated with cerebral arteriography, in skilled centers, these risks approach 1.0% morbidity and 0.1% mortality. However, this is an impractical test to establish the presence of carotid artery stenosis, as it is invasive and cost prohibitive.

If the patient has ischemic symptoms, a computed tomography (CT) scan of the brain should be performed initially. The CT demonstrates hemorrhagic infarction, subarachnoid hemorrhage, tumor, intracranial aneurysms, and arteriovenous malformations (Figure 5.2). Magnetic resonance imaging (MRI) of the brain offers a more sensitive indicator of small and hyperacute infarcts and necrosis related to the ischemia.

Several noninvasive tests are available to evaluate for the presence of carotid disease in patients with a cervical bruit or in patients at high risk for carotid stenosis. Carotid duplex ultrasonography (CDUS), magnetic resonance

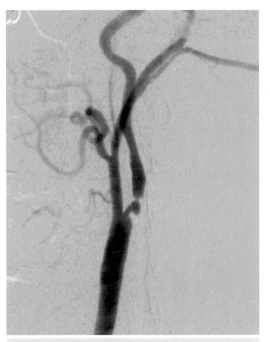

Figure 5.1 Digital subtraction arteriogram demonstrating severe internal carotid artery stenosis.

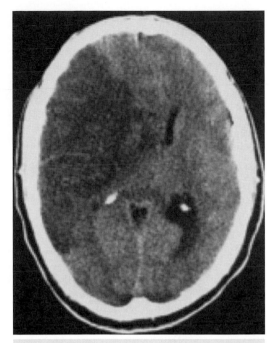

Figure 5.2 Unenhanced computerized tomographic scan of brain demonstrating right hemispheric infarct.

angiography (MRA), and computed tomography angiography (CTA) are now the reliable and noninvasive tests available.

Carotid Duplex Ultrasonography

Carotid duplex ultrasonography (CDUS) combines gray-scale, B-mode, and Doppler ultrasonography to detect focal increases in systolic and end-diastolic velocities, ranges of which indicate moderate and severe extracranial carotid artery stenosis.[17]

The gray-scale image provides information on the location of the extracranial carotid arteries (common carotid, internal carotid, external carotid, and vertebral arteries). In addition, it provides an assessment of plaque location and composition (heterogeneous, or fibrotic plaque; homogeneous, or "fatty plaque"), along with plaque ulceration. The color image facilitates rapid identification of arterial stenosis, but it is the Doppler evaluation that defines the presence and severity of carotid artery stenosis. CDUS is the ideal modality for evaluating the adequacy of revascularization over time.

The peak systolic velocity is most frequently used to gauge stenosis severity, but end-diastolic velocity, and the peak systolic velocity ratio of the internal carotid and distal common carotid artery, provides greater information (Figure 5.3). Color Doppler improves efficiency, but not necessarily diagnostic accuracy. Doppler ultrasonography may also provide information about plaque composition, and intraplaque hemorrhage, which can impact prognosis.

Some centers utilize transcranial Doppler in conjunction with CDUS to determine the collateral pathways in the intracranial circulation. In addition, cerebral vasospasm is well visualized with this technique.

The utility of CDUS to evaluate carotid artery stenting (CAS) remains controversial. Early reports suggested that CDUS was less accurate for determining stent patency as the stent may alter the Doppler-derived velocities.[18-20] Although the exact mechanism for alteration in these velocities is unclear, some investigators have suggested that alterations in compliance of the internal carotid artery after CAS results in elevations in peak systolic velocities. This may

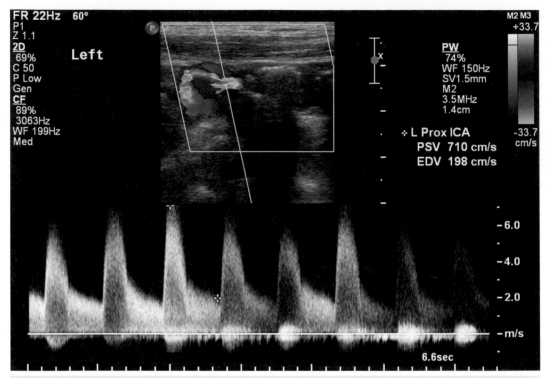

Figure 5.3 Carotid duplex ultrasound consistent with severe (80-99%) stenosis of the left internal carotid artery. (PSV=Peak systolic velocity; EDV=End diastolic velocity)

thereby require new criteria for the stented internal carotid artery.[21] However, more recent data demonstrating restenosis rates after CAS utilized Doppler velocity criteria unchanged from native internal carotid arteries.[22]

Independent analysis of CDUS images as part of large-scale multicenter trials of CAS has demonstrated excellent reduction in Doppler velocities after stent deployment with durable preservation of these Doppler measurements to 1 year of follow-up.[23]

Magnetic Resonance Angiography

Magnetic resonance angiography (MRA) utilizes the energy generated by controlled shifts of protons in an electromagnetic field to produce a 3D image of the carotid bifurcation in order to detect carotid stenoses. High-quality MRA requires the administration of a magnetic resonance contrast agent, commonly gadolinium, via a peripheral venous catheter. MRA requires

less operator skill than CDUS. However, interpretation of the source images and image postprocessing are important. The reformatted images are not sufficient to provide an accurate determination of stenosis severity. In fact, without the administration of gadolinium, the 2-dimensional time-of-flight images commonly overestimate moderate stenoses as severe, and severe stenoses as occluded. In addition, there are several scenarios in which MRA cannot be performed, including in severely ill or morbidly obese patients, in patients with claustrophobia, and in those patients with an implantable cardioverter, defibrillator, or pacemaker.

CDUS and MRA have similar reported sensitivities (83%–86%) and specificities (89%–94%). A meta-analysis of these 2 imaging modalities demonstrated that both are reliable to detect carotid artery occlusion and > 70% stenosis. Current algorithms commonly deploy the results of 2 imaging modalities to determine the anatomic options for carotid revascularization.

Multidetector Computed Tomography Angiography

More recently, multidetector *computed tomography angiography (CTA)* has been utilized to identify patients with carotid artery stenosis. Early experience with first-generation devices has demonstrated sensitivity to detect 70% to 99% stenosis when compared to angiography of 85%, with specificity of 93%. Calcification at the area of significant stenosis impairs the image interpretation. In addition, CTA is not practical for serial surveillance of a carotid stenosis, as the test requires significant external beam radiation and administration of iodinated contrast media.

Invasive Arteriography

Angiography is considered the gold standard for cerebrovascular arteriography. Given the progressive improvement in noninvasive imaging, cerebrovascular arteriography as a diagnostic test is infrequently required. The major drawback for invasive angiography has been the risk of adverse events associated with the procedure. In the Asymptomatic Carotid Artery Surgery (ACAS) trial, there was a 1.2% risk of stroke related to angiography. If 2 noninvasive tests performed by expert laboratories are discordant, an arteriogram is indicated.

The gold standard to evaluate carotid stenosis is cervical angiography, but this is a relatively expensive and invasive procedure associated with 1.0% morbidity and 0.1% mortality. Similarly, MRA produces a reproducible 3D image of the carotid bifurcation in order to detect high-grade stenoses. MRA is less operator dependent than Doppler ultrasonography but has limitations when patients are critically ill, are unable to lie supine, or have ferromagnetic implants.

Carotid duplex ultrasonography and MRA have similar reported sensitivities (83%–86%) and specificities (89%–94%). Both of these imaging modalities, however, have misclassification rates ranging from 28% compared to catheter angiography for duplex ultrasonography, to 18% compared to angiography with MRA. Many believe that such noninvasive tests should not be the sole determinant for assessing the need for carotid revascularization.

Recently, CTA has been used to confirm findings of carotid artery stenosis (see Figure 5.4). Early experience with single-slice CTA has demonstrated sensitivity to detect 70% to 99% stenosis when compared to angiography of 85%, with specificity of 93%. All 3 noninvasive modalities (CDUS, MRA, and CTA), offer significant advantages and improved patient acceptance over invasive arteriography.[24]

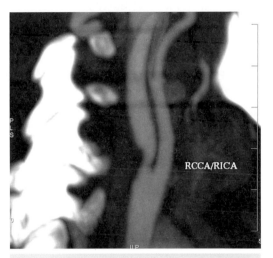

Figure 5.4 Contrast-enhanced Computerized Tomographic Arteriogram demonstrates moderate right internal carotid artery stenosis.

Therapeutic Alternatives

Medical Therapy

Effective primary and secondary stroke prevention requires aggressive risk factor modification, specifically blood pressure control and smoking cessation. Aspirin therapy (75–325 mg daily) results in a 25% relative risk reduction compared to placebo.[25,26] There is consensus that doses of aspirin higher than 325 mg per day are not more effective for stroke prevention.[27] The Clopidogrel Versus Aspirin in Patients at Risk of Ischaemic Events (CAPRIE) trial demonstrated a significant benefit for clopidogrel for the combined end point of isch-emic stroke, myocardial infarction, or vascular death, but it did not show a reduction in stroke risk with clopidogrel compared to aspirin alone.[28] The Management of a Therothrombosis with Clopidogrel in High-risk Patients (MATCH) trial showed no stroke reduction benefit for aspirin and clopidogrel compared to clopidogrel alone, although the bleeding risk was increased with the combination therapy.[26] Despite isolated data from a single trial regarding secondary prevention, the preponderance of evidence is that the addition of dipyridamole to aspirin alone for primary or secondary stroke prevention is of marginal benefit.[25,26,29] Warfarin is only useful for stroke prevention in patients with atrial fibrillation.[30]

Despite the absence of epidemiological data to link elevated cholesterol levels with stroke, large studies of several statins have demonstrated stroke reduction with this class of drugs.[31] Both the 4S Trial (simvastatin) and the Cholesterol and Recurrent Events (CARE) trial (pravastatin) demonstrated a 30% relative risk reduction for stroke compared to placebo.[32,33] Interestingly, the stroke benefit was delayed and did not appear until after 3 years of therapy.

Surgical Therapy

Carotid endarterectomy (CEA) was established in the late twentieth century as superior to medical therapy for stroke prevention in pa-tients with symptomatic ≥ 50% carotid steno-ses and asymptomatic ≥ 60%. There are no data comparing revascularization therapy to more modern potent blood pressure medications (angiotensin-converting enzyme inhibitors), antiplatelet agents (dipyridamole, clopidogrel, or prasugrel), or antiatherosclerotic agents, that is, statins, with CEA for stroke prevention.

For symptomatic patients, the landmark trials of the 1990s compared aspirin alone to aspirin with CEA for prevention of stroke and death in symptomatic patients. The NASCET, the Veterans Affairs Trial (VA309), and the European Carotid Surgery Trial (ECST) demonstrated superiority for CEA using a selected group of experienced surgeons and patients who had ≥ 50% carotid stenoses causing hemispheric or ocular symptoms (Figure 5.5).[34-39] In NASCET patients, for severe lesions (70%–99%) the *number needed to treat (NNT)* with CEA to prevent one stroke was 8, while for more modest lesions (50%–69%), the NNT was 15. For symptomatic patients, with moderate to severe (50%–69%) carotid stenosis, males had a significant benefit, whereas females did not.[37]

There is expert consensus that the 30-day perioperative risk of stroke and death from CEA should not exceed 6% for symptomatic patients.[40,41] Unfortunately, none of the randomized surgical trials for symptomatic patients met this threshold, with a combined incidence of 30-day perioperative stroke and death rate of 7.1% (ECST 7.5%, 6.3–8.8; NASCET 6.5%, 5.3–

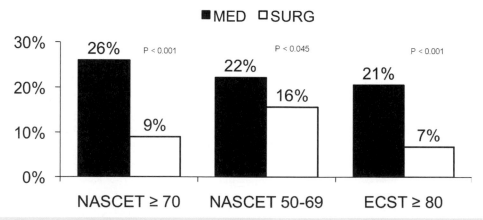

Figure 5.5 Data demonstrating statistically significant reduction in stroke and death over 2 years in symptomatic patients with CEA compared to medical therapy (MED) in major randomized trials.[35,37-39]

7.9; VA 7.7%, 3.1–15.2).[42] In a meta-analysis of CEA in symptomatic patients (n = 51 studies), the strongest predictor of stroke or death was the authorship of the manuscript.[43] That is, when a neurologist was lead author the risk of stroke and death was 7.7% (95% CI, 5.0–10.2), however, when a single-author surgeon was the author, the risk was reported as 2.3% (95% CI, 1.8–7.0). The authors suggested 3 possible reasons for this apparent bias, including (1) scientific fraud, with surgeons underreporting complications, (2) a negative publication bias as surgeons are less likely to publish poor results, and (3) a diagnostic bias as surgeons may fail to identify a minor, subtle, or unusual presentation of a stroke. Whichever explanation is used, one of the reasons for confusion and debate about CEA outcomes is that the literature for CEA is heterogeneous, making nonrandomized comparisons to other therapies difficult.

For asymptomatic patients there is expert consensus that the 30-day perioperative risk of stroke and death from CEA should not exceed 3%.[40,41] Three large, randomized controlled trials have been completed to determine the benefit of CEA plus aspirin compared to aspirin therapy alone to prevent stroke in asymptomatic patients with carotid artery disease. The Veterans Affairs Cooperative Study (VACS) included 444 men who were followed for 4 years.[44] Best medical care consisted of 650 mg of aspirin twice a day, although 43% of the patients were unable to take any aspirin at all, or took a smaller dose. The risk of stroke as a result of diagnostic angiography was 0.4%. There was no difference between the groups for stroke and death. The combined end point of all ipsilateral neurological events (TIA, transient monocular blindness, and stroke) was reduced from 20.6% in the medical therapy (MED) group to 8% in the CEA arm ($P < 0.001$). The 30-day perioperative risk of stroke and death was 4.7%.

The Asymptomatic Carotid Atherosclerosis Study (ACAS) was a randomized trial that screened over 42000 patients, to randomize 1662 asymptomatic patients with ≥ 60% stenosis (by ultrasonography) ages 40 to 79 years, to CEA plus medical therapy (n = 825) or medical therapy alone (n = 834).[45] Medical therapy

consisted of 325 mg of aspirin daily with attention to risk factor management including hypertension, lipids, diabetes control, and smoking discontinuation advice. Angiography was required in the CEA group and was associated with 1.2% risk of stroke. The 30-day perioperative stroke or death rate was 2.7%. CEA achieved a 5-year risk reduction among asymptomatic patients of 53% (95% CI, 22%–72%; P = 0.004) for ipsilateral stroke or a perioperative stroke or death (11% for MED vs. 5.1% for CEA) (Figure 5.6). The NNT with CEA to prevent one ipsilateral stroke at 5 years was 19. For men, CEA yielded a 66% risk reduction for ipsilateral stroke over 5 years, compared with only 17% for women. Women trended toward a higher perioperative complication rate than men (3.6% vs. 1.7%, $P = 0.12$). At 5-years follow-up there was no difference for the rates of all stroke and death between MED (31.9%) or CEA (25.6%, $P = 0.08$).

The Asymptomatic Carotid Surgery Trial (ACST) randomized 3,120 asymptomatic patients with ≥ 70% carotid artery stenosis by ultrasonography ages 40 to 91 years.[46] Medical therapy included antiplatelet therapy (80% at randomization and > 90% at the last follow-up visit), antihypertensive therapy (60% at randomization and 81% at the last follow-up visit), and lipid-lowering therapy (17% at randomization and 70% at the last follow-up visit). By intention to treat, there was a 3.1% risk of stroke or death within 30 days of operation. The 5-year risk of any stroke or perioperative death was 11.8% with medical therapy compared with 6.4% with CEA ($P < 0.0001$) (Figure 5.6). CEA for those with moderate stenoses (60%–80%) demonstrated equal benefit compared with those with severe stenoses (80%–99%). The perioperative risk was slightly, but not significantly, higher in women at 3.8% compared with 2.7% in men. The number of nonperioperative carotid territory strokes over 5 years was reduced by CEA in both men (CEA = 18 vs. MED = 77, $P < 0.0001$) and women (CEA = 8 vs. MED = 28, $P < 0.001$). Similar to ACAS, the overall risk of any stroke or death over 5 years was not different between MED (31.2) and CEA (28.9%, $P = 0.172$).

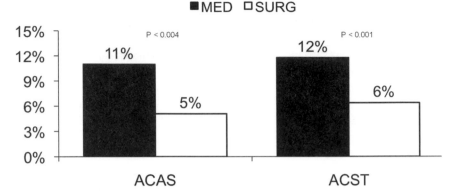

Figure 5.6 Data demonstrating statistically significant reduction in stroke and death over 5 years in asymptomatic patients with CEA compared to medical therapy (MED) in major randomized trials.[45,46]

Endovascular Therapy

Percutaneous revascularization techniques have dramatically altered the management of both coronary and peripheral vascular disease. Many conditions, such as iliac, subclavian, and renal artery lesions; and angioplasty with or without stent placement, have virtually replaced open surgical approaches. As the durability and safety of percutaneous methods have improved, applications in other vascular distributions have become accepted alternatives to surgical procedures.

The major advantage of these percutaneous methods is that they are less invasive than open surgical procedures, offering revascularization without the risk of general anesthesia, less risk of procedural morbidity and mortality, shorter hospital stay, and lower cost. In patients with serious comorbidities who are at increased risk of surgical complications, percutaneous revascularization techniques become more attractive. The most recent extension of percutaneous revascularization procedures has been to explore their safety and efficacy in stenotic extracranial carotid arteries for stroke prevention (Figure 5.7).

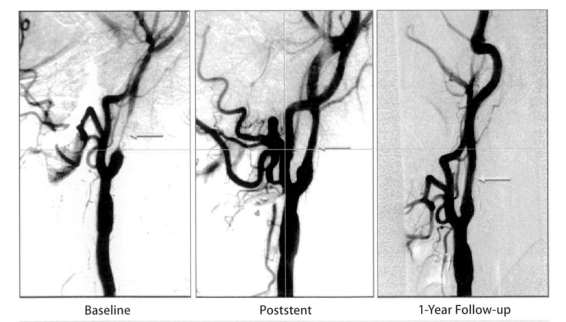

Baseline   Poststent   1-Year Follow-up

Figure 5.7 Carotid artery stent placement with 1-year follow-up.

Indication

The current indication for carotid artery stenting (CAS) is for stroke prevention in patients at increased risk for CEA (Table 5.1). Current Medicare reimbursement is limited to carotid stenosis ≥ 70% in a symptomatic, high-surgical-risk patient. Medicare will also reimburse carotid stenosis ≥ 50% in symptomatic patients and ≥ 80% in asymptomatic patients enrolled in FDA-sponsored investigational trials.

Contraindications

There are well-recognized patient- and lesion-related features that increase the risk of stent complications (Table 5.2).[47] The more severely elongated the aortic arch, the more difficult will be access from the femoral artery (Figures 5.8

and 5.9).[48] Other contraindications to CAS include patients with large disabling strokes, severe dementia, and life-threatening reactions to iodinated contrast material.

CAS outcomes—high surgical risk

Patients with high-surgical-risk features (see Table 5.1) for CEA are proven to have outcomes similar to CEA in a randomized controlled trial (Figure 5.10).[49] Three-year outcomes have confirmed the durable and beneficial results obtained in the only randomized controlled trial in this high-risk subset of patients.[50] Additional supporting peer-reviewed and published evidence include a meta analysis,[51] and multiple premarket[52-61] and postmarket[62-66] surveillance trials (Figure 5.11). A multispecialty document

Anatomic Features	Medical Comorbidities
High cervical or intrathoracic lesion	Age ≥ 80 years
Prior neck surgery or radiation therapy	Class III/IV congestive heart failure
Contralateral carotid artery occlusion	Class III/IV angina pectoris
Prior ipsilateral CEA	Left main or severe multivessel coronary disease
Contralateral laryngeal nerve palsy	Need for open heart surgery
Tracheostoma	Ejection fraction ≤ 30%
Immobilized neck due to arthritis	Recent (6 weeks) myocardial infarction
	Severe chronic obstructive lung disease

Table 5.1 Increased Risk for Carotid Artery Surgery

Clinical Features	Angiographic Features
Age ≥ 75/80	≥ 2 acute (90º) bends
Dementia	Circumferential calcification
Bleeding disorder	Cerebral microangiopathy
Multiple lacunar strokes	Intravascular filling defect (thrombus)
Renal failure	No or difficult vascular access

Table 5.2 Increased Risk for Carotid Stent

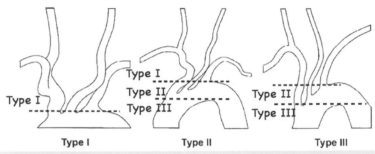

Figure 5.8 Three types of aortic arch morphology are shown. The type I aortic arch is characterized by origin of all 3 great vessels in the same horizontal plane as the outer curvature of the aortic arch. In a type II aortic arch, the innominate artery originates between the horizontal planes of the outer and inner curvatures of the aortic arch. For the type III aortic arch, the innominate artery originates below the horizontal plane of the inner curvature of the aortic arch.[48]

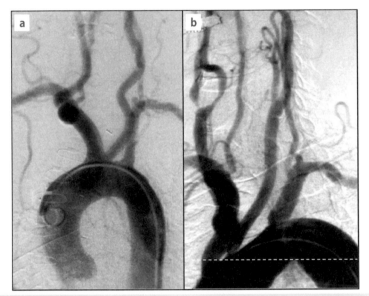

Figure 5.9 (a) Bovine arch with the left common carotid artery arising from the innominate artery. (b) A type III aortic arch, with the innominate artery arising below the horizontal plane of the inner curvature of the aortic arch.

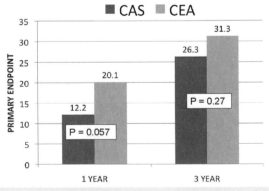

Figure 5.10 One-year follow-up of SAPPHIRE trial with data analyzed by treatment received.[49]

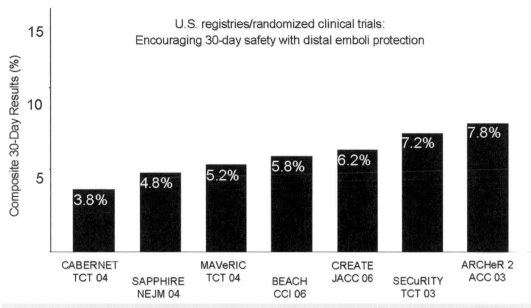

Figure 5.11 US clinical trials of CAS 30-day results in high-surgical-risk patients.[52-61]

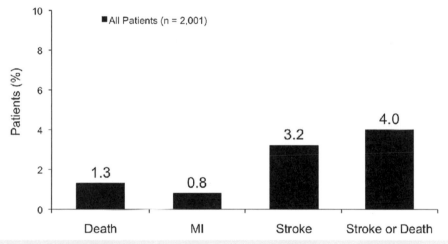

Figure 5.12 SAPPHIRE Worldwide postmarket surveillance registry.[63]

from the American College of Cardiology also supports the benefit of CAS in high-surgical-risk (anatomic and comorbid features) symptomatic (> 50% stenosis) and asymptomatic (> 80% stenosis) patients.[67]

Three large, postmarket surveillance trials evaluating CAS in a "real-world" environment, with independent neurologic assessment, have been published. The Stenting and Angioplasty with Protection in Patients at High Risk for Endarterectomy (SAPPHIRE Worldwide)

postmarket approval registry evaluated 30-day safety and efficacy outcomes after CAS was performed in 2001 symptomatic and asymptomatic high-surgical-risk patients with CAS operators of varying experience.[63] The 30-day stroke and death rate was 4% (Figure 5.12).

Two FDA-mandated, postmarket surveillance trials (EXACT, n = 2145; CAPTURE-2, n = 4175) with independent neurologic assessment reported on more than 6,000 high-surgical-risk patients treated by CAS operators with varying levels of experience.[66] The 30-day stroke and death was 4.1% for 2145 EXACT patients and 3.4% for the 4175 CAPTURE-2 patients. In patients comparable to those included in the 2006 American Heart Association (AHA) published guidelines (< 80 years),[68] the 30-day stroke and death rate for symptomatic patients (≥ 50% stenosis) was 5.3% (benchmark for CEA ≤ 6%) and for asymptomatic patients (≥ 80% stenosis) it was 2.9% (benchmark for CEA ≤ 3%) (Figure 5.13).[66] These postmarket surveillance trials, in more than 8,000 patients, strongly support clinical equipoise between CAS and CEA for high-surgical-risk patients.

The very elderly (≥ 75–80 years of age) are at increased risk of periprocedural complications not only from CEA[69-71] but also from CAS.[47,53,66,72] However, 3 peer-reviewed articles report on CAS with embolic protection in 389 high-surgical-risk patients ≥ 80 years of age.[73-75] The overall 30-day stroke and death rate with independent neurological assessment in patients ≥ 80 years of age was 3.3%, 2.7%, and 0.8%. The authors emphasized the importance of operator experience and case selection to avoid CAS high-risk features such as difficult aortic arch access, excessive lesion tortuosity, and heavy calcification.[47] These excellent results in octogenarians have been confirmed in a multicenter report of 418 patients who were treated at 4 high-volume centers, with independent neurological assessment with a very favorable 30-day stroke and death rate combined among asymptomatic and symptomatic patients of 2.8% (Figure 5.14).[76]

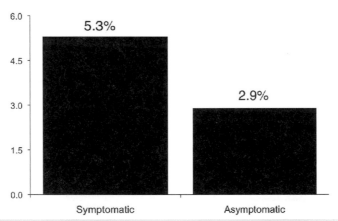

Figure 5.13 Thirty-day stroke and death results from CAPTURE-2 and EXACT trials.

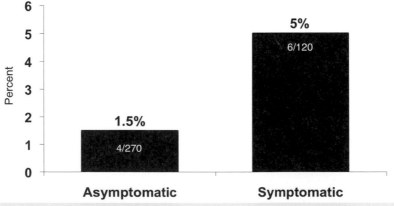

Figure 5.14 Thirty-day stroke and death results from CAS in octogenarians.[76]

CAS outcomes—average surgical risk

The only trial dedicated to average-surgical-risk asymptomatic patients is the Asymptomatic Carotid Trial (ACT 1). ACT 1 is an ongoing trial randomizing asymptomatic patients with carotid stenoses ≥ 70% and ≤ 99% in patients < 80 years of age (Table 5.3). The randomization is 3:1 for CAS to CEA. So far, the initial results in 145 CAS patients have demonstrated a 1.4% risk of stroke, no deaths, and no heart attacks. Follow-up at 1 year in 106 patients has shown no ipsilateral strokes. The goal is to randomize over 1800 patients among 50 centers.

A total of 4 reasonably large, randomized controlled trials in average-surgical-risk symptomatic (one trial included asymptomatic patients as well) patients have been completed. The seriously flawed Endarterectomy Versus Angioplasty in Patients with Severe Symptomatic Carotid Stenosis (EVA-3S) trial randomized 527 symptomatic (≥ 60%), average-risk patients to CAS or CEA.[77] The 30-day incidence of stroke or death for CEA was 3.9% and 9.6% for CAS. Early in the trial, use of an *embolic protection device (EPD)* was not required, which resulted in a stroke rate of 25% (5 of 20). This caused the trial to be stopped and restarted with EPD use required. These very inexperienced interven-tionalists, some trainees who required tutoring while placing carotid stents, were a significant limitation of this study. The patients in EVA-3S had similar risk profiles as the Carotid Revascularization Endarterectomy Versus Stenting Trial (CREST) roll-in patients, but CREST required at least 20 cases of carotid stent experience with audited results and mandated the use of an EPD. EVA-3S appears to have been a trial designed for CAS to fail.

The Stent-Supported Percutaneous Angioplasty of the Carotid Artery Versus Endarterectomy (SPACE) trial showed no difference between CEA and CAS in average-surgical-risk symptomatic patients with optional use of EPDs.[78] The 30-day stroke and death rate for CAS was 6.8% and for CEA was 6.3%, not clinically or statistically different.[79] A major flaw of the SPACE trial was the lack of EPD use in 73% of the study subjects. After 2 years of follow-up, there continued to be no difference in outcomes between CEA and CAS, however, for patients who were < 68 years at randomization there were significantly fewer events (30-day stroke and death and ipsilateral stroke for 2 years) with CAS (4.8%) compared with CEA (8.0%, $P < 0.005$) (Figure 5.15).[79,80]

The more recent publication of the multi-

Event	30 Days, N = 145
Death, stroke, and myocardial infarction	1. 4%
All stroke and death	1.4%
Major stroke and death	0.0%
Death	0.0%
All stroke	1.4%
Major stroke	0.0%
Minor stroke	1.4%
Myocardial infarction	0.0%
31–365 days, N = 106	
Ipsilateral stroke	0.0%

Table 5.3 Lead-in Patients from the ACT 1 Study

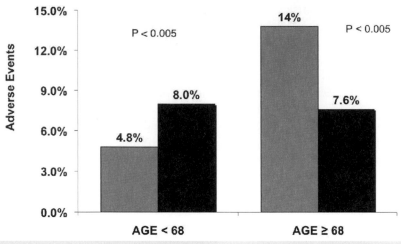

Figure 5.15 Two-year outcomes for the SPACE trial.[80]

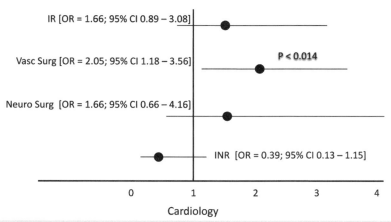

Figure 5.16 CREST lead-in results by operator specialty.[83]

center International Carotid Stenting Study (ICSS) suggests no difference for the primary end point of disabling stroke or death (CAS 4.0% vs. CEA 3.2%, $P = 0.34$).[81] For this interim report researchers did find an excess of minor strokes (Rankin score < 3, and/or resolved by 30 days) in the CAS group. Once again, there was a significant imbalance in the experience level of the investigators performing CEA compared to those performing CAS. Investigators were permitted to enroll patients while being tutored in the procedure, and EPDs were not required. Two inexperienced sites produced 5 of the total 17 major strokes observed in the trial while treating only 11 patients.

The CREST lead-in phase reported on 1246 patients with a 30-day stroke and death rate of 3.9% (95% CI, 2.9%–5.2%) with 5.6% (95% CI, 3.3%–8.7%) being for symptomatic patients and 3.4% (95% CI, 2.3%–4.9%) for asymptomatic patients.[82] Data on variations among operators by specialty was recently published (Figure 5.16).[83] The authors reported that subspecialties training in catheter-based techniques (ie, cardiology, radiology, and neuroradiology) had a statistically lower complication rate than did the non-catheter-based specialty of vascular surgery. Vascular surgeons had a statistically significant 2-fold increase in rate of stroke and death compared to the other groups.

CREST enrolled 2502 average-surgical-risk symptomatic (53%) and asymptomatic

(47%) patients.[84] For the primary end point (any stroke, myocardial infarction [MI], or death with the periprocedural period, plus any ipsilateral stroke thereafter), there was no difference between CAS and CEA (Figure 5.17). Four-year follow-up revealed no difference between CAS (7.2%) and CEA (6.8%) with a hazard ratio of 1.11 (95% CI, 0.81–1.51; $P = 0.51$). There was an excess of minor strokes with CAS but there was no difference for major strokes (CAS 0.9% vs. CEA 0.7%). The CEA group had twice as many MIs (2.3%) compared with CAS (1.1%). Cranial nerve palsy occurred in 4.8% of the CEA patients. There was an age effect, with younger patients (< 69 years) doing better with CAS and older patients doing better with CEA.

For both ICSS and CREST there were no differences between CEA and CAS for major stroke and death. Both trials demonstrated more minor strokes in the CAS group and more heart attacks in the CEA group. CREST required more experience for CAS operators than did ICSS. The ICSS surgeons reported far fewer periprocedural MIs (0.5%) than the CREST sur-geons (2.3%), suggesting a potential problem with underreporting surgical complications.[81,84]

Technical and Procedure Issues

It is likely that equipment and device evolution will impact the incidence of periprocedural complications for carotid stenting. Operators are making choices ranging from the most appropriate guiding catheter versus a sheath, to closed-cell versus open-cell stents, to which embolic protection device is best. From the femoral artery access, the consensus is that type III aortic arch should be avoided and these patients should be offered CEA. Another option is to approach a patient with complex aortic arch from a radial or brachial artery access. When approaching a complex aortic arch from the femoral artery, it is best to use an 8-Fr guiding catheter (eg, Hockey stick, Amplatz, or Simmons shapes) and to not deeply intubate the common carotid artery to avoid trauma to the arch.

Several clinical trials have noted increased complications with the use of open-cell stents (Figure 5.18, Table 5.4). There were almost

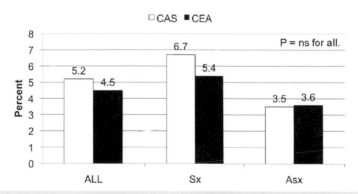

Figure 5.17 Periprocedural all stroke, death, and MI in CREST. Sx = symptomatic; Asx = asymptomatic

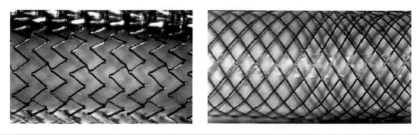

Figure 5.18 Open-cell compared (left) to closed-cell stents (right).

Closed-Cell Stent	Open-Cell Stent
Wallstent (Boston Scientific)	Precise (Cordis)
X-act (Abbott)	Acculink (Abbott)
NexStent (EndoTex)	Zilver (Cook)
	Protege (ev3)
	Memotherm (Bard)

Table 5.4 Design Differences for Stents

twice as many adverse events with open-cell versus closed-cell stents in the SPACE trial, which included symptomatic, average-surgical-risk patients (Figure 5.19).[85] In another trial of symptomatic patients, the risk of 30-day adverse events was increased almost 4-fold in open-cell stents (11.1%) compared with closed-cell stents (3.0%).[86] A third study correlated free-cell area in stents with events and found that symptomatic patients had more events with greater free-cell area.[87] Finally, diffusion-weighted imaging (DWI), an imaging tool used to identify new embolic lesions after CAS, demonstrated a lower incidence of new DWI lesions with closed-cell stents (31%) than for open-cell stents (51%, $P < 0.01$).[88] However, one large CAS study did not show any relationship between the stent type (open- vs. closed-cell) and complications.[89] The authors pointed out that a randomized control trial is necessary to neutralize confounders, such as lesion morphology, which drives stent choice, and may account for the observed outcomes.

Embolic protection devices

Three methods of embolic protection have been developed to reduce cerebral embolization associated with CAS, and these include distal occlusion balloons, distal filter devices, and proximal protection devices with and without flow reversal (Figure 5.20). No randomized trials have been completed to demonstrate the safety and efficacy of any of these devices. Many have received FDA approval as a "bundled" device with a carotid stent and approved for use as a "system." Although an early meta-analysis concluded that EPDs did reduce the risk of stroke,[90] this was a collection of heterogeneous data on early generation devices. The lack of proven efficacy for EPDs has been somewhat problematic because complications related to their use have been documented.[91,92]

Most DWI studies agree with transcranial Doppler studies showing that there are fewer new lesions after CEA compared to CAS,[93] although when nonischemic cerebral com-

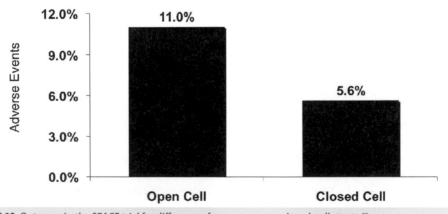

Figure 5.19 Outcome in the SPACE trial for differences for open- versus closed-cell stents.[85]

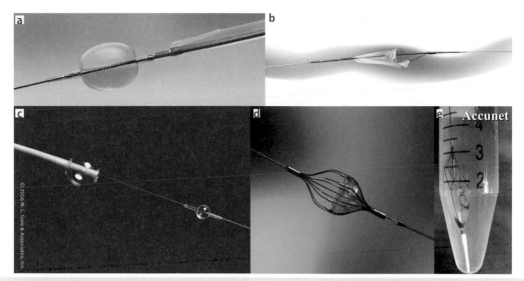

Figure 5.20 Several of the available EPDs. **a.** Medtronic GuardWire. Courtesy of Medtronic. **b. Boston Scientific FilterWire EZ.** Courtesy of Boston Scientific. **c. GORE® Flow Reversal System.** Courtesy of W.L. Gore & Associates. **d. Cordis Angioguard.** © Cordis Corporation 2010. **e. Abbott Accunet.** Image courtesy of Abbott Vascular. © 2010 Abbott Laboratories. All Rights Reserved.

plications are included, there is no difference between CEA or CAS.[94,88] The majority of DWI lesions are asymptomatic and about half of them will disappear over several months, making their clinical importance uncertain.[95] When a filter device is used versus no EPD, there was a reduction in new lesions seen by DWI.[88] Kim and colleagues[96] compared a distal occlusion balloon to a filter using DWI. There was no difference in the number of new cerebral lesions between the filter group and distal balloon occlusion group.

The source of embolic events associated with CAS appears to be more related to the aortic arch anatomy than the carotid artery lesion.[97] When DWI imaging is done after cerebral diagnostic angiography, there is a correlation with new brain lesions consistent with embolic events and difficult to cannulate arteries, more contrast usage, and longer fluoroscopic times.[98] New brain lesions by DWI during CAS correlate with aortic arch characteristics such as difficult arch morphology (type III) and complex atherosclerotic arch lesions by transesophageal echocardiography (complex > 5 mm or mobile debris).[99] Even more compelling than these emboli that are released with catheter manip-

ulation in the aortic arch is that new embolic lesions may be seen on the contralateral hemisphere or posterior circulation and not ipsilateral to the CAS procedure.[100]

The distal occlusion balloon (PercuSurge GuardWire [now Medtronic GuardWire, Medtronic]) was the first clinically used protection device with CAS and had problems related to intolerance (~ 5%) of ischemia related to interruption of cerebral blood flow (Figure 5.20). Occlusion of blood flow also meant the operator could not visualize the lesion with contrast injections while deploying the stent. Even with distal carotid occlusion, emboli could still reach the brain via collaterals or by incomplete aspiration at the completion of the procedure.[101,102]

Filter devices rapidly replaced the distal occlusion balloon because they were much easier to use (Figure 5.20).[103,104] Filter EPDs were well tolerated by patients because they did not require interruption of blood flow to the brain. Filters allowed contrast injections throughout the procedure, enabling the interventionalist to visualize the lesions during stent deployment. Filters are guide-wire-like devices that are compatible with conventional CAS equipment including stents and 6-Fr delivery sheaths or 8-Fr guiding catheters. The weakness of filter EPDs is that by definition, they are "partially" occlusive, allowing particles smaller than their pore sizes to pass through the filter, to the brain. There are complications associated with filter use. Sometimes retrieval of a filter EPD can be difficult. A tortuous internal carotid artery can make entry with the retrieval catheter difficult.[105,106] If the filter catches on the edge of a deployed stent, it can be damaged or torn, potentially "dumping" its contents. Rarely, the filter is so full of debris that it must be aspirated prior to its removal so that it doesn't spill its contents.

Proximal endovascular occlusion (PEO) devices have many advantages but have not been readily adopted by clinicians because they are more difficult to use than filter-based EPDs. PEO devices are more complex, requiring occlusion of the external carotid artery, which is not required with filters. One of the devices (Parodi, W.L. Gore) uses active flow reversal and requires a venous access sheath (Figure 5.20)[107] and one (MoMa, Invatec, Medtronic) does not. PEO devices require aspiration steps at the completion of the procedure that are not necessary with filter devices. The guiding catheters are larger than usual, making vascular access complications a concern. Finally, because there is occlusion of antegrade flow, PEO devices share many of the difficulties of the distal occlusion balloon. Approximately 1 patient in 20 (5%) has some level of intolerance to interruption of blood flow to the brain during the procedure, and the operator cannot inject contrast to visualize the target lesion to guide stent deployment. The emergence of PEO devices as clinically available devices appear to have lowered postprocedural CAS complication rates.[108] These devices have an advantage of cerebral protection before the lesion is crossed with a wire, and for the entire procedure no antegrade flow occurs, thus protecting the patient against procedure-related emboli. A recent trial reported a 1.4%, 30-day stroke and death rate with a PEO in 1288 consecutive patients.[109] The risk of 30-day stroke and death in the trial was < 1% for asymptomatic patients and near 3% in symptomatic patients.

Transcranial Doppler was used to compare filter-type EPDs and the PEO with active flow reversal. There was continuing embolization with the filter EPD while there were no embolic signals with the PEO with the flow reversal system.[110] However, embolic signals were detected during placement of the PEO and again during removal of the device.

A report from Italy describes a single-center registry of 1300 CAS patients treated with a PEO with a 30-day stroke and death rate of 1.4%, supported by independent neurological assessment.[109] Consistent with prior CAS studies, there was higher risk of 30-day stroke and death in symptomatic versus asymptomatic patients (3.0% vs. 0.8%, $P < 0.05$), and for patients at high surgical risk compared to average-surgical-risk patients (1.9% vs. 1.1%, $P < 0.05$). Older patients experienced no increase in complications of CAS, with the 30-day stroke and death for octogenarians not significantly different than for younger patients. A small number (n = 4, 0.3%) of patients could not complete the CAS procedure due to intolerance. Interestingly, 12.5% of the treated patients had a critical stenosis or occlusion of their contralateral internal carotid artery, which did not prevent PEO success. The only factors that independently predicted adverse outcome was lack of CAS experience, the presence of a symptomatic lesion, and the absence of clinical hypertension.

Proximal protection, in experienced hands, is associated with a dramatic reduction in the expected 30-day stroke and death rate compared to other CAS registry reports.[67] This low event rate, supported by independent neurological assessment, was obtained despite the PEO device not being able to prevent cerebral emboli during its insertion or removal, or contralateral emboli related to aortic arch pathology. In these experienced interventionalists' hands, the incidence of femoral access complications was quite low for this 8-Fr and 10-Fr system, and the rapidity with which they were able to complete the CAS procedure resulted in < 1% of all patients unable to tolerate proximal occlusion.

Summary

Data obtained in multiple population risk strata is now available to be evaluated for CAS supporting the beneficial, useful, and effectiveness of CAS (ACC/AHA Class I; Level of Evidence A). Importantly, in high-surgical-risk patients, there is clinical equipoise between CAS and CEA for both symptomatic and asymptomatic patients with anatomic or comorbid features that place them at increased risk for CEA. The current recommendation for patients at increased risk for surgery who require carotid revascularization for prevention of stroke, is that CAS should be considered a reasonable alternative.

There is no consensus regarding the relative outcomes of CAS versus CEA in average-surgical-risk patients. Recent clinical trials in this patient population have ranged from EVA-3S, which strongly favored CEA, to the most recently reported PEO experience with extremely low stroke and death rates in both symptomatic and asymptomatic patients. The SPACE trial split the difference, showing a benefit for CAS for patients < 69 years old and a benefit for CEA in older patients. CREST, a large randomized controlled trial with distal emboli protection, has recently been published and demonstrated equivalent safety and efficacy of CAS and CEA among standard risk symptomatic and asymptomatic patients. Patients undergoing CAS had an increased risk of minor stroke, whereas patients randomized to CEA suffered a greater incidence of myocardial infarction.[111]

References

1. Lloyd-Jones D, Adams RJ, Brown TM, et al. Heart disease and stroke statistics—2010 update: A report from the American Heart Association. *Circulation*. 2010;121:e46-e215.

2. Norris JW, Zhu CZ, Bornstein NM, et al. Vascular risks of asymptomatic carotid stenosis. *Stroke*. 1991;22:1485-1490.

3. North American Symptomatic Carotid Endarterectomy Trial Collaborators. Beneficial effect of carotid endarterectomy in symptomatic patients with high-grade carotid stenosis. *N Engl J Med*. 1991;325:445-453.

4. The Amaurosis Fugax Study Group. Current management of amaurosis fugax. *Stroke*. 1990;21:201-208.

5. Johnson BF, Verlato F, Bergelin RO, et al. Clinical outcome in patients with mild and moderate carotid artery stenosis. *J Vasc Surg*. 1995;21:120-126.

6. Rockman CB, Riles TS, Lamparello PJ, et al. Natural history and management of the asymptomatic, moderately stenotic internal carotid artery. *J Vasc Surg*. 1997;25:423-431.

7. Bock RW, Gray-Weale AC, Mock PA, et al. The natural history of asymptomatic carotid artery disease. *J Vasc Surg*. 1993;17:160-171.

8. Faught WE, van Bemmelen PS, Mattos MA, et al. Presentation and natural history of internal carotid artery occlusion. *J Vasc Surg*. 1993;18:512-524.

9. Carr S, Farb A, Pearce WH, et al. Atherosclerotic plaque rupture in symptomatic carotid artery stenosis. *J Vasc Surg*. 1996;23:755-766.

10. Easton JD, Saver SL, Albers GJ, et al. Definition and evaluation of transient ischemic attack. A scientific statement from the American Heart Association/American Stroke Association Stroke Council: Council on Cardiovascular Surgery and Anesthesia; Council on Cardiovascular Radiology and Intervention; Council on Cardiovascular Nursing; and the Interdisciplinary Council on Peripheral Vascular Disease. *Stroke*. 2009;40:2276-2293.

11. Wadia NH, Monckton G. Intracranial bruits in health and disease. *Brain*. 1957;80:492-509.

12. Heyman A, Wilkinson WE, Heyden S, et al. Risk of stroke in asymptomatic persons with cervical arterial bruits: a population study in Evans County, Georgia. *N Engl J Med*. 1980;302:838-841.

13. Pickett CA, Jackson JL, Hemann BA, Atwood JE. Carotid bruits as a prognostic indicator of cardiovascular death and myocardial infarction: a meta-analysis. *Lancet*. 2008;371:1587-1594.

14. Van Ruiswyk J, Noble H, Sigmann P. The natural history of carotid bruits in elderly persons. *Ann Intern Med.* 1990;112:340-343.

15. Wolf PA, Kannel WB, Sorlie P, McNamara P. Asymptomatic carotid bruit and risk of stroke: the Framingham Study. *JAMA.* 1981;245:1442-1445.

16. O'Donnell MJ, Xavier D, Liu L, et al. Risk factors for ischaemic and intracerebral haemorrhagic stroke in 22 countries (the Interstroke Study): a case-control study. *Lancet.* 2010;376:112-123.

17. Jahromi AS, Cina CS, Liu Y, Clase CM. Sensitivity and specificity of color duplex ultrasound measurement in the estimation of internal carotid artery stenosis: a systematic review and meta-analysis. *J Vasc Surg.* 2005;41:962-972.

18. Ringer AJ, German JW, Guterman LR, Hopkins LN. Follow-up of stented carotid arteries by Doppler ultrasound. *Neurosurgery.* 2002;51:639-643.

19. Robbin ML, Lockhart ME, Weber TM, et al. Carotid artery stents: early and intermediate follow-up with Doppler US. *Radiology.* 1997;205:749-756.

20. Willfort-Ehringer A, Ahmadi R, Gscwandtner ME, et al. Healing of carotid stents: a prospective duplex ultrasound study. *J Endovasc Ther.* 2003;10:636-642.

21. Lal BK, Hobson RW, Goldstein J, Chakhtoura EY, Duran WN. Carotid artery stenting: is there a need to revise the ultrasound velocity criteria? *J Vasc Surg.* 2004;39(1):220-226.

22. McCabe DJH, Pereira AC, Clifton A, Bland JM, Brown MM. Restenosis after carotid angioplasty, stenting, or endarterectomy in the Carotid and Vertebral Artery Transluminal Angioplasty Study (CAVATAS). *Stroke.* 2005;36:281-286.

23. Fleming SE, Bluth EI, Milburn J. Role of sonography in the evaluation of carotid artery stents. *J Clin Ultrasound.* 2005;33:321-328.

24. Patel SG, Collie DA, Wardlaw JM, et al. Outcome, observer reliability, and patient preferences if CTA, MRA, or Doppler ultrasound were used, individually or together, instead of digital subtraction angiography before carotid endarterectomy.[see comment]. *J Neurol, Neurosurg & Psychiatry.* 2002;73(1):21-28.

25. MRC/BHF Heart Protection Study of cholesterol lowering with simvastatin in 20 536 high-risk individuals: a randomised placebo-controlled trial. *Lancet.* 2002;360:7-22.

26. Albers GW, Amarenco P, Easton JD, Sacco RL, Teal P. Antithrombotic and thrombolytic therapy for ischemic stroke: the Seventh ACCP Conference on Antithrombotic and Thrombolytic Therapy. *Chest.* 2004;126:483S-512S.

27. Taylor DW, Barnett HJ, Haynes RB, et al. Low-dose and high-dose acetylsalicylic acid for patients undergoing carotid endarterectomy: a randomised controlled trial. ASA and Carotid Endarterectomy (ACE) Trial Collaborators. *Lancet.* 1999;353:2179-2184.

28. CAPRIE Steering Committee. A randomised, blinded, trial of clopidogrel versus aspirin in patients at risk of ischaemic events (CAPRIE). *Lancet.* 1996;348:1329-1339.

29. Diener HC, Cunha L, Forbes C, Sivenius J, Smets P, Lowenthal A. European Stroke Prevention Study. 2. Dipyridamole and acetylsalicylic acid in the secondary prevention of stroke. *J Neurol Sci.* 1996;143:1-13.

30. Mohr JP, Thompson JL, Lazar RM, et al. A comparison of warfarin and aspirin for the prevention of recurrent ischemic stroke. *N Engl J Med.* 2001;345:1444-1451.

31. Law MR, Wald NJ, Rudnicka AR. Quantifying effect of statins on low density lipoprotein cholesterol, ischaemic heart disease, and stroke: systematic review and meta-analysis. *BMJ.* 2003;326:1423.

32. Randomised trial of cholesterol lowering in 4444 patients with coronary heart disease: the Scandinavian Simvastatin Survival Study (4S). *Lancet.* 1994;344:1383-1389.

33. Sacks FM, Pfeffer MA, Moye LA, et al. The effect of pravastatin on coronary events after myocardial infarction in patients with average cholesterol levels. Cholesterol and Recurrent Events Trial investigators. *N Engl J Med.* 1996;335:1001-1009.

34. European Carotid Surgery Trialists' Collaborative Group. Randomised trial of endarterectomy for recently symptomatic carotid stenosis:

final results of the MRC European Carotid Surgery Trial (ECST). *Lancet*. 1998;351:1379-1387.

35. North American Symptomatic Carotid Endarterectomy Trial Collaborators. Beneficial effect of carotid endarterectomy in symptomatic patients with high-grade carotid stenosis. *N Engl J Med*. 1991;325:445-453.

36. Mayberg MR, Wilson SE, Yatsu F, et al. Carotid endarterectomy and prevention of cerebral ischemia in symptomatic carotid stenosis. Veterans Affairs Cooperative Studies Program 309 Trialist Group. *JAMA*. 1991;266:3289-3294.

37. Barnett HJ, Taylor DW, Eliasziw M, et al. Benefit of carotid endarterectomy in patients with symptomatic moderate or severe stenosis. North American Symptomatic Carotid Endarterectomy Trial Collaborators. *N Engl J Med*. 1998;339:1415-1425.

38. Rothwell PM, Gutnikov SA, Warlow CP. Reanalysis of the final results of the European Carotid Surgery Trial. *Stroke*. 2003;34:514-523.

39. Ferguson GG, Eliasziw M, Barr HW, et al. The North American Symptomatic Carotid Endarterectomy Trial: surgical results in 1415 patients. *Stroke*. 1999;30:1751-1758.

40. Beebe HG, Clagett GP, DeWeese JA, et al. Assessing risk associated with carotid endarterectomy. A statement for health professionals by an Ad Hoc Committee on Carotid Surgery Standards of the Stroke Council, American Heart Association. *Circulation*. 1989;79:472-473.

41. Biller J, Feinberg WM, Castaldo JE, et al. Guidelines for carotid endarterectomy: a statement for healthcare professionals from a special writing group of the Stroke Council, American Heart Association. *Stroke*. 1998;29:554-562.

42. Rothwell PM, Eliasziw M, Gutnikov SA, et al. Analysis of pooled data from the randomised controlled trials of endarterectomy for symptomatic carotid stenosis. *Lancet*. 2003;361:107-116.

43. Rothwell PM, Slattery J, Warlow CP. A systematic review of the risks of stroke and death due to endarterectomy for symptomatic carotid stenosis. *Stroke*. 1996;27:260-265.

44. Hobson RW II, Weiss DG, Fields WS, et al. Efficacy of carotid endarterectomy for asymptomatic carotid stenosis. The Veterans Affairs Cooperative Study Group. *N Engl J Med*. 1993;328:221-227.

45. Executive Committee for the Asymptomatic Carotid Atherosclerosis Study (ACAS). Endarterectomy for asymptomatic carotid artery stenosis. *JAMA*. 1995;273:1421-1428.

46. Halliday A, Mansfield A, Marro J, et al. Prevention of disabling and fatal strokes by successful carotid endarterectomy in patients without recent neurological symptoms: randomised controlled trial. *Lancet*. 2004;363:1491-1502.

47. Roubin GS, Iyer S, Halkin A, Vitek J, Brennan C. Realizing the potential of carotid artery stenting: proposed paradigms for patient selection and procedural technique. *Circulation*. 2006;113:2021-2030.

48. Casserly I, Yadav J. Carotid intervention. In: Casserly I, Sachar R, Yadav J, eds. *Manual of Peripheral Vascular Intervention*. Philadelphia: Lippincott; 2005:83-109.

49. Yadav JS, Wholey MH, Kuntz RE, et al. Protected carotid-artery stenting versus endarterectomy in high-risk patients. *N Engl J Med*. 2004;351:1493-1501.

50. Gurm HS, Yadav JS, Fayad P, et al. Long-term results of carotid stenting versus endarterectomy in high-risk patients. *N Engl J Med*. 2008;358:1572-1579.

51. Gurm HS, Nallamothu BK, Yadav J. Safety of carotid artery stenting for symptomatic carotid artery disease: a meta-analysis. *Eur Heart J*. 2008;29:113-119.

52. SECURITY Investigators. United States Food and Drug Administration, Center for Devices and Radiological Health: Abbott Xact® Carotid Stent System, summary of the safety and effectiveness data, 2005. Accessed at http://www.fda.gov/ohrms/dockets/dockets/05m0381/05m-0381-aav0001-03-PMA-02-SSED-vol1.pdf.

53. Iyer SS, White CJ, Hopkins LN, et al. Carotid artery revascularization in high-surgical-risk patients using the Carotid WALLSTENT and FilterWire EX/EZ: 1-year outcomes in the BEACH Pivotal Group. *J Am Coll Cardiol*. 2008;51:427-434.

54. Gray W. Two-year composite endpoint results for the Archer Trials: Acculink for revascular-

ization of carotids in high risk patients. *Am J Cardiol.* 2004;94:62E.

55. Safian RD, Bresnahan JF, Jaff MR, et al. Protected carotid stenting in high-risk patients with severe carotid artery stenosis. *J Am Coll Cardiol.* 2006;47:2384-2389.

56. Whitlow P. Security: more good data for protected carotid stenting in high-risk surgical patients. 2003. (Accessed at http://www.medscape.com/viewarticle/461721_print.) [electronic reference]

57. White CJ, Iyer SS, Hopkins LN, Katzen BT, Russell ME. Carotid stenting with distal protection in high surgical risk patients: the BEACH trial 30 day results. *Catheter Cardiovasc Interv.* 2006;67:503-512.

58. White CJ, for the Beach Investigators. BEACH Trial: 30 day outcomes of carotid wallstent and filterwire EX/EZ distal protectioin system placement for treatment of high surgical risk patients. *J Am Coll Cardiol.* 2005;45:28A.

59. Ramee S, Higashida R. Evaluation of the Medtronic self-expanding carotid stent system with distal protection in the treatment of carotid artery stenosis (Abstract). *Am J Cardiol.* 2004;94:61E.

60. Hopkins LN, Myla S, Grube E, et al. Carotid artery revascularization in high surgical risk patients with the NexStent and the Filterwire EX/EZ: 1-year results in the CABERNET trial. *Catheter Cardiovasc Interv.* 2008;71:950-960.

61. Gray WA, Hopkins LN, Yadav S, et al. Protected carotid stenting in high-surgical-risk patients: the ARCHeR results. *J Vasc Surg.* 2006;44:258-268.

62. Gray WA, Yadav JS, Verta P, et al. The CAPTURE registry: results of carotid stenting with embolic protection in the post approval setting. *Catheter Cardiovasc Interv.* 2007;69:341-348.

63. Massop D, Dave R, Metzger C, et al. Stenting and Angioplasty with Protection in Patients at High-Risk for Endarterectomy: SAPPHIRE Worldwide Registry First 2,001 Patients. *Catheter Cardiovasc Interv.* 2008:DOI 10.1002/ccd.21844.

64. Gray WA, Yadav JS, Verta P, et al. The CAPTURE registry: predictors of outcomes in carotid artery stenting with embolic protection for high surgical risk patients in the early post-approval setting. *Catheter Cardiovasc Interv.* 2007;70:1025-1033.

65. Katzen BT, Criado FJ, Ramee SR, et al. Carotid artery stenting with emboli protection surveillance study: thirty-day results of the CASES-PMS study. *Catheter Cardiovasc Interv.* 2007;70:316-323.

66. Gray WA, Chaturvedi S, Verta P. Thirty-day outcomes for carotid artery stenting in 6320 patients from 2 prospective, multicenter, high-surgical-risk registries. *Circ Cardiovasc Interv.* 2009;2:159-166.

67. Bates ER, Babb JD, Casey DE Jr, et al. ACCF/SCAI/SVMB/SIR/ASITN 2007 clinical expert consensus document on carotid stenting: a report of the American College of Cardiology Foundation Task Force on Clinical Expert Consensus Documents (ACCF/SCAI/SVMB/SIR/ASITN Clinical Expert Consensus Document Committee on Carotid Stenting). *J Am Coll Cardiol.* 2007;49:126-170.

68. Sacco RL, Adams R, Albers G, et al. Guidelines for prevention of stroke in patients with ischemic stroke or transient ischemic attack: a statement for healthcare professionals from the American Heart Association/American Stroke Association Council on Stroke: co-sponsored by the Council on Cardiovascular Radiology and Intervention: the American Academy of Neurology affirms the value of this guideline. *Stroke.* 2006;37:577-617.

69. Wennberg D, Lucas F, Birkmeyer J, Bredenberg C, Fisher E. Variation in carotid endarterectomy mortality in the Medicare population. *JAMA.* 1998;279:1278-1281.

70. Kazmers A, Perkins AJ, Huber TS, Jacobs LA. Carotid surgery in octogenarians in Veterans Affairs medical centers. *J Surg Res.* 1999;81:87-90.

71. Miller MT, Comerota AJ, Tzilinis A, Daoud Y, Hammerling J. Carotid endarterectomy in octogenarians: does increased age indicate "high risk?" *J Vasc Surg.* 2005;41:231-237.

72. Hobson RW II, Howard VJ, Roubin GS, et al. Carotid artery stenting is associated with increased complications in octogenarians:

30-day stroke and death rates in the CREST lead-in phase. *J Vasc Surg.* 2004;40:1106-1111.

73. Chiam P, Roubin G, Iyer S, et al. Carotid artery stenting in elderly patients: importance of case selection. *Catheter Cardiovasc Interv.* 2008;72:318-324.

74. Henry M, Henry I, Polydorou A, Hugel M. Carotid angioplasty and stenting in octogenarians: is it safe? *Catheter Cardiovasc Interv.* 2008;72:309-317.

75. Velez CA, White CJ, Reilly JP, et al. Carotid artery stent placement is safe in the very elderly (> or =80 years). *Catheter Cardiovasc Interv.* 2008;72:303-308.

76. Grant A, White C, Ansel G, Bacharach M, Metzger C, Velez C. Safety and efficacy of carotid stenting in the very elderly. *Catheter Cardiovasc Interv.* 2009;9999:NA.

77. Mas JL, Chatellier G, Beyssen B, et al. Endarterectomy versus stenting in patients with symptomatic severe carotid stenosis. *N Engl J Med.* 2006;355:1660-1671.

78. Ringleb PA, Allenberg J, Bruckmann H, et al. 30 day results from the SPACE trial of stent-protected angioplasty versus carotid endarterectomy in symptomatic patients: a randomised non-inferiority trial. *Lancet.* 2006;368:1239-1247.

79. Stingele R, Berger J, Alfke K, et al. Clinical and angiographic risk factors for stroke and death within 30 days after carotid endarterectomy and stent-protected angioplasty: a subanalysis of the SPACE study. *Lancet Neurol.* 2008;7:216-222.

80. Eckstein HH, Ringleb P, Allenberg JR, et al. Results of the Stent-Protected Angioplasty versus Carotid Endarterectomy (SPACE) study to treat symptomatic stenoses at 2 years: a multinational, prospective, randomised trial. *Lancet Neurol.* 2008;7:893-902.

81. International Carotid Stenting Study Investigators. Carotid artery stenting compared with endarterectomy in patients with symptomatic carotid stenosis (International Carotid Stenting Study): an interim analysis of a randomised controlled trial. *Lancet Neurol.* 2010:10.1016/S0140-6736(10)60239-5.

82. Roubin G, Clark W, Chakhtoura E, et al. Low complication rates for carotid artery stenting in the credentialling phase of the carotid revascularization endarterectomy versus stenting trial (Abstract). *Stroke.* 2006;37:620.

83. Hopkins LN, Roubin GS, Chakhtoura EY, et al. The Carotid Revascularization Endarterectomy versus Stenting Trial: credentialing of interventionalists and final results of lead-in phase. *J Stroke Cerebrovasc Dis.* 2010;19:153-162.

84. Clark WM, for the Crest Investigators. *Carotid Revascularizaton and Endarterectomy versus Stenting Trial.* San Antonio, TX: American Stroke Association; 2010.

85. Jansen O, Fiehler J, Hartmann M, Bruckmann H. Protection or nonprotection in carotid stent angioplasty: the influence of interventional techniques on outcome data from the SPACE Trial. *Stroke.* 2009;40:841-846.

86. Hart JP, Peeters P, Verbist J, Deloose K, Bosiers M. Do device characteristics impact outcome in carotid artery stenting? *J Vasc Surg.* 2006;44:725-730; discussion 730-731.

87. Bosiers M, de Donato G, Deloose K, et al. Does free cell area influence the outcome in carotid artery stenting? *Eur J Vasc Endovasc Surg.* 2007;33:135-141; discussion 142-143.

88. Schnaudigel S, Groschel K, Pilgram SM, Kastrup A. New brain lesions after carotid stenting versus carotid endarterectomy: a systematic review of the literature. *Stroke.* 2008;39:1911-1919.

89. Schillinger M, Gschwendtner M, Reimers B, et al. Does carotid stent cell design matter? *Stroke.* 2008;39:905-909.

90. Kastrup A, Groschel K, Krapf H, Brehm BR, Dichgans J, Schulz JB. Early outcome of carotid angioplasty and stenting with and without cerebral protection devices: a systematic review of the literature. *Stroke.* 2003;34:813-819.

91. Barbato JE, Dillavou E, Horowitz MB, et al. A randomized trial of carotid artery stenting with and without cerebral protection. *J Vasc Surg.* 2008;47:760-765.

92. Cloft HJ. Distal protection: maybe less than you think. *AJNR Am J Neuroradiol.* 2008;29:407-408.

93. Poppert H, Wolf O, Resch M, et al. Differences in number, size and location of intracranial microembolic lesions after surgical versus endovascular treatment without protection

device of carotid artery stenosis. *J Neurol.* 2004;251:1198-1203.

94. Roh HG, Byun HS, Ryoo JW, et al. Prospective analysis of cerebral infarction after carotid endarterectomy and carotid artery stent placement by using diffusion-weighted imaging. *AJNR Am J Neuroradiol.* 2005;26:376-384.

95. Palombo G, Faraglia V, Stella N, Giugni E, Bozzao A, Taurino M. Late evaluation of silent cerebral ischemia detected by diffusion-weighted MR imaging after filter-protected carotid artery stenting. *AJNR Am J Neuroradiol.* 2008;29:1340-1343.

96. Kim SJ, Roh HG, Jeon P, et al. Cerebral ischemia detected with diffusion-weighted MR imaging after protected carotid artery stenting: comparison of distal balloon and filter device. *Korean J Radiol.* 2007;8:276-885.

97. Hammer FD, Lacroix V, Duprez T, et al. Cerebral microembolization after protected carotid artery stenting in surgical high-risk patients: results of a 2-year prospective study. *J Vasc Surg.* 2005;42:847-853; discussion 853.

98. Bendszus M, Koltzenburg M, Burger R, Warmuth-Metz M, Hofmann E, Solymosi L. Silent embolism in diagnostic cerebral angiography and neurointerventional procedures: a prospective study. *Lancet.* 1999;354:1594-1597.

99. Faggioli G, Ferri M, Rapezzi C, Tonon C, Manzoli L, Stella A. Atherosclerotic aortic lesions increase the risk of cerebral embolism during carotid stenting in patients with complex aortic arch anatomy. *J Vasc Surg.* 2009;49:80-85.

100. Schluter M, Tubler T, Steffens JC, Mathey DG, Schofer J. Focal ischemia of the brain after neuroprotected carotid artery stenting. *J Am Coll Cardiol.* 2003;42:1007-1013.

101. Schluter M, Tubler T, Mathey DG, Schofer J. Feasibility and efficacy of balloon-based neuroprotection during carotid artery stenting in a single-center setting. *J Am Coll Cardiol.* 2002;40:890-895.

102. Henry M, Polydorou A, Henry I, Hugel M. Carotid angioplasty under cerebral protection with the PercuSurge GuardWire System. *Catheter Cardiovasc Interv.* 2004;61:293-305.

103. Reimers B, Corvaja N, Moshiri S, et al. Cerebral protection with filter devices during carotid artery stenting. *Circulation.* 2001;104:12-15.

104. Henry M, Polydorou A, Henry I, et al. New distal embolic protection device the FiberNet 3 dimensional filter: first carotid human study. *Catheter Cardiovasc Interv.* 2007;69:1026-1035.

105. Shilling K, Uretsky BF, Hunter GC. Entrapment of a cerebral embolic protection device—a case report. *Vasc Endovascular Surg.* 2006;40:229-233.

106. Ganim RP, Muench A, Giesler GM, Smalling RW. Difficult retrieval of the EPI Filterwire with a 5 French FR4 coronary catheter following carotid stenting. *Catheter Cardiovasc Interv.* 2006;67:309-311.

107. Parodi JC, Ferreira LM, Sicard G, La Mura R, Fernandez S. Cerebral protection during carotid stenting using flow reversal. *J Vasc Surg.* 2005;41:416-422.

108. Kelso R, Clair DG. Flow reversal for cerebral protection in carotid artery stenting: a review. *Perspect Vasc Surg Endovasc Ther.* 2008;20:282-290.

109. Stabile E, Salemme L, Sorrropago G, et al. Proximal endovascular occlusion for carotid artery stenting: results from a prospective registry of 1300 patients. *J Am Coll Cardiol.* 2010:55:1661-1667.

110. Garami ZF, Bismuth J, Charlton-Ouw KM, Davies MG, Peden EK, Lumsden AB. Feasibility of simultaneous pre- and postfilter transcranial Doppler monitoring during carotid artery stenting. *J Vasc Surg.* 2009;49:340-344, 345 e1-2; discussion 345.

111. Brott TG, Hobson RW, Howard G, et al. Stenting versus endarterectomy for treatment of carotid-artery stenosis. *N Engl J Med* 2010;363:11-23.

6

Vertebrobasilar Insufficiency

J. Stephen Jenkins and Tyrone J. Collins

Introduction

The incidence of vertebral artery stenosis in a population of patients with positive markers for atherosclerosis is not insignificant. Patients with documented peripheral vascular disease have a 40% incidence of vertebral artery stenosis.[1] The Joint Study of Extracranial Arterial Occlusion examined 3800 patients who presented for angiography due to symptomatic cerebral vascular disease. In this population of patients there was a 40% incidence of vertebral artery stenosis and a 10% incidence of complete occlusion of one vertebral artery.[2] Stenosis of the extracranial vertebral artery affects 25% to 40% of the patient population with documented atherosclerotic disease of the brachiocephalic vessels.[3-5] The vertebral basilar system is responsible for 25% of ischemic cerebral vascular events. Transient ischemic attacks due to extracranial posterior circulation disease are associated with a 5-year stroke rate of 30%.[3-5] The natural history of intracranial, symptomatic vertebral basilar disease that is managed medically has a poor prognosis. In a retrospective cohort of 102 patients with symptomatic intracranial vertebral stenosis, the 1-year and 5-year mortality rates were 21% and 52%, respectively, if the patients were managed medically.[6] Posterior circulation strokes have a mortality rate of 20% to 30%, much higher than anterior circulation strokes.[7,8]

The pathogenesis of posterior circulation symptoms is somewhat confusing for several reasons. It is well known in the surgical literature that ligature of one of the vertebral arteries is well tolerated in humans.[9] Occlusion of one vertebral artery should be insignificant if the contralateral vertebral artery is intact provided no other significant aortic arch disease exists. This scenario is rarely the case in a population of diffusely atherosclerotic patients with vertebral vascular disease. There is also collateral blood supply from the carotid artery and thyrocervical trunk that develops in the presence of proximal vertebral artery ischemic disease.[10,11] Although artery-to-artery emboli represent a potential cause of ischemic stroke in the posterior circulation, this pathophysiology occurs more commonly in the anterior circulation due to the plaque composition of carotid artery atherosclerosis. The majority of vertebral artery atherosclerotic plaques are ostial, hard, smooth, and not as prone to ulceration as carotid plaques, making them an ideal candidate

Vascular Disease: Diagnostic and Therapeutic Approaches. © 2011 Michael R. Jaff and Christopher J. White, editors. Cardiotext Publishing, ISBN: 978-1-935395-16-4.

for percutaneous treatment. Angioplasty of the vertebral artery ostium represents the majority of cases reported in the literature (Figure 6.1).[11-13]

Diagnostic Evaluation

History and Physical

Accepted ischemic symptoms of the posterior circulation include diplopia, dizziness, drop attacks, gait disturbances, dysphasia, and bilateral homonymous hemianopia. Less-common symptoms include confusion, global amnesia, syncope, occipital headaches, nausea, vomiting, nystagmus, bilateral facial numbness, cortical blindness, and altered mental status. Although symptoms of *vertebrobasilar insufficiency (VBI)* is most commonly due to bilateral vertebral artery disease, other possible combinations of innominate, carotid, and subclavian disease as well as intracranial disease have to be considered in this atherosclerotic population of patients. All patients presenting with VBI symptoms should undergo a complete neurological history and physical examination by an independent neurologist who does not participate in the revascularization procedure.

Noninvasive Evaluation

Noninvasive imaging of the ostial and proximal vertebral artery (V_1), the most frequent site of vertebral atherosclerotic obstructive disease, is often difficult and incomplete due to its location. Duplex ultrasonography at best can visualize antegrade or retrograde flow necessitating digital angiography, which is the gold standard for identifying vertebral disease. More recently, magnetic resonance angiography (MRA) and computed tomography angiography (CTA) have been used to evaluate proximal vertebral artery

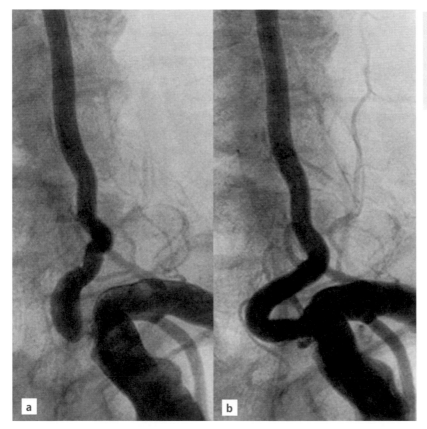

Figure 6.1 (a) Ostial left vertebral artery stenosis 95%. (b) Ostial left vertebral artery postangioplasty with a 4x12-mm balloon expandable stent.

disease, but data confirming their ability to reliably detect vertebral disease is not available.[14]

Invasive Evaluation

Contrast angiography using digital subtraction techniques is the gold standard to identify vertebral basilar atherosclerotic disease. Angiographic evaluation includes an aortic arch and 4-vessel study with selective angiography of bilateral carotid and vertebral arteries, including intracranial imaging. The intracranial distribution of the anterior and posterior circulation and the Circle of Willis should also be defined in several views, making certain to identify any collateral blood supply.

Normal Anatomy/ Variations/Collaterals

The vertebral arteries arise at a 90° angle as the first branch of the subclavian artery. The anatomic course is divided into 4 segments defined by bony landmarks. The ostium of the vertebral artery is the most frequent location of disease in this vessel. The 4 segments are designated V_1 to V_4 and are illustrated in Figure 6.2. The V_1 segment begins at the vertebral artery origin from the subclavian artery and travels cephalad until entering the transverse foramina of either the fifth or sixth cervical vertebrae. The V_2 segment is encased in the protective bony canal of the transverse foramina from C2 to C6. The V_3 segment begins as the artery exits the bony canal of transverse foramina at C2 and ends as the vessel penetrates the dura mater and becomes an intracranial vessel. This extremely tortuous portion of the vertebral artery passes posterior to the arch of C1 and between the atlas and occiput. This segment requires excessive redundancy to allow mobility of the atlanto-occipital and atlanto-axial joints. Collateral flow from both the occipital branch of the external carotid artery or the thyrocervical trunk is capable of supplying the V_3 segment in the presence of proximal vertebral artery disease. The V_4 segment is the most distal portion of the vertebral artery and runs along the inferior portion of the pons until joining the contralateral vertebral artery to form the basilar artery. Important branches of the V_4 segment include the posterior inferior cerebellar arteries (PICA) and the anterior spinal artery formed from branches of the V_4 segment, which join in the midline and supply the anterior two-thirds of the spinal cord. It is because of these branches that angioplasty of the V_4 segment is extremely risky and is rarely attempted except for acute stroke intervention or severe symptoms unresponsive to medical treatment. One vertebral artery is hypoplastic in 6% of the population and makes no contribution to the formation of the basilar artery. The hypoplastic vertebral artery in these cases terminates at the

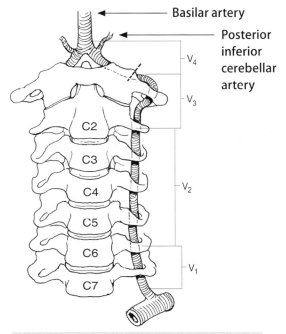

Figure 6.2 Anatomy of the vertebral artery. The V1 segment originates from subclavian artery and ends at the transverse formina of C5 or C6. V2 is encased in transverse foramina from C5 or C6 and ends at C2. V3 begins at the transverse foramina of C2 and ends as the vessel penetrates the dura mater at the foramen magnum. V4 begins at the foramen magnum and ends at the basilar artery. (Reproduced with permission from Elsevier: Silva JA, White CJ. Peripheral vascular intervention. In: Kern MJ. *The Interventional Cardiac Catheterization Handbook.* 2nd ed. Philadelphia: Mosby; 2004:386-440.)

V_4 segment immediately distal to the posterior inferior cerebellar artery. Anomalous origin of the left vertebral artery from the aortic arch just proximal to the left subclavian artery or from the proximal subclavian artery occurs in 5% to 10% of the patient population.[15]

Therapeutic Options

Medical Therapy

Although medical therapy for the management of posterior circulation ischemia includes Coumadin anticoagulation and antiplatelet therapy, there is lack of evidence-driven data comparing these drugs in the management of extracranial vertebral artery disease. The Warfarin–Aspirin Symptomatic Intracranial Disease (WASID) trial randomized patients with stroke or TIA caused by angiographically verified 50% to 99% intracranial stenosis to receive Coumadin (target international normalized ratio [INR] 2–3) or high-dose aspirin (1300 mg/day) in a double-blind, multicenter trial.[16] The stenotic artery was located in the intracranial posterior circulation in 26% of this cohort of patients. Using ischemic stroke, brain hemorrhage, or death from vascular causes other than stroke, warfarin provided no benefit over aspirin (22.8% vs. 22.1% $P = 0.83$) and was associated with significantly higher rates of adverse events than the aspirin group. The MATCH trial[17] randomized 7599 high-risk patients with recent ischemic stroke or TIA and at least one additional vascular risk factor who were already receiving clopidogrel 75 mg to either aspirin 75 mg per day or placebo. The primary composite end point was ischemic stroke, myocardial infarction, vascular death, or rehospitalization for vascular events. Although the addition of aspirin to clopidogrel was associated with nonsignificant reduction in vascular events (15.7% vs. 16.7%), the risk of life-threatening or major bleeding was increased by the addition of aspirin.

The INR should be maintained between 2 and 3 when using Coumadin to treat VBI symptoms. Antiplatelet agents including both aspirin and the adenosine diphosphate inhibitors can also be used to treat posterior circulation ische-mic symptoms. Aspirin 81 to 325 mg per day and clopidogrel 75 mg per day are commonly utilized to reduce the risk of recurrent ischemic events in patients with VBI. Ticlopidine 250 mg per day is an acceptable alternative for patients with side effects or intolerance to clopidogrel.[18-21]

Surgical Revascularization

Three surgical revascularization techniques have been described in the literature to treat one vertebral artery in patients with bilateral vertebral artery stenosis. As with some of the early percutaneous revascularization series, most of the surgical literature does not include solely vertebral artery reconstruction but combines subclavian, innominate, and vertebral arteries into one treatment group.

Surgical revascularization of vertebral disease is not without significant morbidity. In one series by Berguer et al,[22] 174 patients undergoing proximal vertebral artery reconstruction had no in-hospital deaths, and reported complications were as follows: recurrent laryngeal nerve palsy, 2%; Horner's syndrome, 15%; lymphocele, 4%; chylothorax, 0.5%; and acute thrombosis, 1%. Secondary patency rates were 95% and 91% at 5 and 10 years, respectively. Seventy-five patients in this study who had reconstruction of the distal vertebral artery experienced a mortality rate of 4% and an immediate graft thrombosis rate of 8%. Secondary patency rates for distal vertebral artery reconstruction were 87% and 82% at 5 and 10 years, respectively.

Another series by Thevenet and Ruotolo[23] reported a mortality rate of 0.6%, with a high rate of postoperative Horner's syndrome (28%). Postoperative angiograms were obtained in one-third of the patients demonstrating a 5% occlusion rate. Sixty-eight percent of patients were asymptomatic at 5-year follow-up. This series of 290 patients included 86 isolated vertebral lesions and 204 carotid and/or subclavian lesions.

Koskas et al[24] reported a series of 92 vertebral artery reconstructions of the V_3 segment via a direct transposition of the vertebral artery to the internal carotid artery. There was no mortality in this series and the primary patency rate at 5 years was 89%. Nine percent of the transposed vertebral arteries were occluded at early follow-up, and 2% of patients had transient ischemic attacks.

Mortality rates for the surgical treatment of this disease are acceptable, however, excessive postoperative morbidity limits this technique for widespread use in the treatment of vertebral artery disease.

Endovascular Therapy

Indications/contraindications

The initial management of VBI symptoms with anticoagulant and antiplatelet agents was just discussed. Indications for vertebral artery angioplasty are severe obstructive stenoses of the proximal vertebral artery causing VBI symptoms or posterior circulation strokes despite medical treatment with one or more of these agents. Additional indications include instances where vertebral angioplasty would increase total cerebral blood flow to patients with diffuse atherosclerotic disease involving occlusions of both carotid arteries. Vertebral angioplasty should not be attempted once the vessel is totally occluded. Although some percentage of total occlusions could technically be angioplastied, the distal embolic debris would be clinically devastating to the V_4 segment and the basilar artery causing cerebellar, midbrain, pons, medullary, or brainstem infarctions. Total occlusion of the vertebral artery is a contraindication to endovascular treatment.

Balloon angioplasty

The first reported successful treatment of a vertebral artery stenosis by Sundt et al[25] in 1980 was performed using intraoperative transluminal angioplasty. Since his initial report, multiple case reports and series have been reported describing the successful use of percutaneous transluminal angioplasty (PTA) to treat posteri-

or circulation atherosclerotic disease. In a series of 121 patients treated with PTA for supra-aortic stenoses, Motarjeme[26] attempted 39 vertebral revascularizations. Balloon angioplasty alone was successful in 36 (92%) of these cases. Three ostial lesions could not be treated due to excessive tortuosity of the proximal subclavian arteries. One patient undergoing bilateral vertebral artery PTA experienced transient blindness believed to be due to cortical blindness associated with contrast toxicity and subsequent cerebral edema. Higashida et al[27] treated 42 lesions of the vertebral and basilar arteries with PTA for critical symptomatic stenosis. Thirty-four lesions involved the proximal vertebral artery, 5 lesions were located in the distal vertebral artery, and 3 were located in the basilar artery. Complications included 4 transient ischemic attacks, one vessel rupture, one vessel occlusion, and one stroke. One patient with vessel occlusion died within 48 hours of the procedure. Follow-up angiography in the 34 proximal vertebral artery lesions demonstrated an 8.8% incidence of restenosis. Vertebral artery lesions in the V_2 and V_3 segment or the basilar artery proved to be more risky as well as a more difficult to treat. Only 3 transient ischemic attacks occurred in the 34 patients with proximal (V_1 segment) vertebral artery lesions treated. These were intraprocedural events thought to be due to spasm that resolved with intra-arterial nitroglycerine.

The vertebral artery stenosis subgroup of the Carotid and Vertebral Artery Transluminal Angioplasty Study (CAVATAS) trial is the only randomized data to date involving the vertebral artery.[8] In this trial, 16 patients were equally randomized to either vertebral artery angioplasty or medical treatment. As the CAVATAS group began randomizing in 1992, before stents were available, 6 patients in the interventional arm received balloon angioplasty alone with the last 2 receiving stents. Endovascular treatment was successful in all patients with 2 procedurally related TIA that did not require additional treatment or prolonged admission. With regard to the primary outcome, there were no strokes or death in either arm at the 30-day end point.

Stenting

There have been 4 case series of stenting for extracranial vertebral artery stenosis reported in the literature that have at least 30 arteries treated (Table 6.1).

Chastain et al[28] performed vertebral artery stenting in 50 patients with ischemic VBI symptoms and reported their 30-day and 2-year results. Technical success was 98% with no procedural-related complications. One patient died of nonneurological causes and one patient suffered a stroke due to a complicated coronary intervention within the 30-day postprocedural period. Clinical follow-up at 25 ± 10 months revealed 2 patients (4%) with recurrent VBI symptoms. Angiographic follow-up in 90% of the eligible patients demonstrated a binary restenosis rate of 10%.

Yen-Hung Lin et al[29] reported their experience with endovascular treatment of 58 patients with symptomatic ostial vertebral artery stenoses. Technical success was 100% and periprocedural stroke occurred in 3 patients (5%). At a mean follow-up of 31 ± 17.1 months there was one death after coronary artery bypass surgery and one patient with recurrent VBI symptoms. Angiographic evaluation of 32 (48%) lesions revealed restenosis in 8 (25%) vessels.

Jenkins et al[30] evaluated the safety and long-term outcome of endovascular therapy for the treatment of symptomatic VBI in 38 vessels of 32 patients. Technical success without periprocedural stroke or death was achieved in all 38 vessels. One patient experienced a TIA 1 hour after the procedure. At follow-up (mean 10.6 months) all patients were alive and 31 (97%)

were asymptomatic. One patient (3.5%) had in-stent restenosis at 3.5 months and was successfully treated with balloon angioplasty.

Albuquerque et al[12] assessed the rate of restenosis after ostial vertebral artery stenting in 33 patients. Thirty of these patients presented with TIA or strokes and 31 manifested other brachiocephalic stenoses, including 27 patients with occlusion, hypoplasia, or stenosis of the contralateral vertebral artery. Angiographic follow-up (mean 16.2 months) was obtained in 30 patients. Two deaths unrelated to vertebral artery stenting occurred during the follow-up period and one patient refused follow-up angiogram. Although the technical success rate was high (97%) in this population of diffusely atherosclerotic patients, most having concomitant brachiocephalic stenoses elsewhere, in-stent restenosis > 50% occurred in 13 patients (43.3%).

The most recent series of vertebral artery stenting by Jenkins et al[31] represented 105 cases in a single center between 1995 and 2006. The procedure was technically successful in 100% of cases, with nearly 80% of patients remaining asymptomatic at 1 year of follow-up.

Complications and future devices

Procedural complications of vertebral artery stenting include major and minor stroke, TIA, and all other complications that accompany percutaneous procedures including death, access site bleeding, and renal failure. The FDA approval of distal embolic protection devices (EPDs) for the coronary vasculature has allowed availability for off-label use of these devices in the vertebral artery. Although EPDs

Authors	n	Technical Success Rate	Procedural Complications	Improvement in Symptoms	Mean Follow-up	Late Stroke	Restenosis
Albuquerque[12]	33	97%	CVA (1)	27/33	16.2 mo	1/33	43%
Chastain[28]	50	98%	None	48/50	25.0 mo	1/50	10%
Yen-Hung Lin[29]	58	100%	CVA (3)	56/58	31.3 mo	0/58	25%
Jenkins[30]	32	100%	TIA (1)	31/32	10.6 mo	0/32	3%

Table 6.1 Studies of Vertebral Artery Stenting

were not intended or approved for the vertebral artery, this artery is one the most ideal vessels for use of this device in humans. Cerebral tissue is the most sensitive tissue in humans to embolic debris. The size (3–5 mm) of the vertebral artery and the usually long, straight V_1 and V_2 segments, which extend from the subclavian artery to the C2 vertebral body, are a combination rarely found elsewhere in the human vasculature, where endovascular treatment is performed. This creates a long landing zone if the vertebral stenosis occurs in the ostial and V_1 segment, the most common location of vertebral artery atherosclerosis (Figure 6.3). Placement of EPDs should be attempted in all vertebral angioplasty procedures if the stenotic segment allows passage of an EPD.

Technical Procedural Issues

Adjunctive pharmacotherapy

Low-dose, weight-adjusted heparin is utilized for vertebral angioplasty procedures to maintain an activated clotting time > 200 seconds. Bivalirudin is an acceptable alternative in pa-tients with heparin-induced thrombocyto-penia. All patients should be pretreated with aspirin (325 mg/day) and Plavix (75 mg/day) 1 day prior to the procedure. Plavix should be continued for 1 month postprocedure and as-pirin should be continued indefinitely. If drug-eluting stents are used, dual antiplatelet therapy should be continued at least 3 months with sirolimus and 6 months with paclitaxel at a minimum. It is not unreasonable to continue dual antiplatelet therapy indefinitely with the use of drug-eluting stents to prevent the occur-rence of late stint thrombosis.

Equipment choices and tips

A 5-Fr Berenstein is the diagnostic catheter of choice to perform selective angiography of the vertebral artery. A 4-Fr, 5 Fr, or 6-Fr Judkins right, internal mammary, or Vitek curved cath-eters are acceptable; multipurpose curves are useful when procedures are performed using the brachial access. A 0.035-in hydrophilic wire or J-wire should be used to place the diagnos-tic catheter in the subclavian artery distal to the vertebral artery ostium. A manifold is connect-ed and continuous pressure monitored while

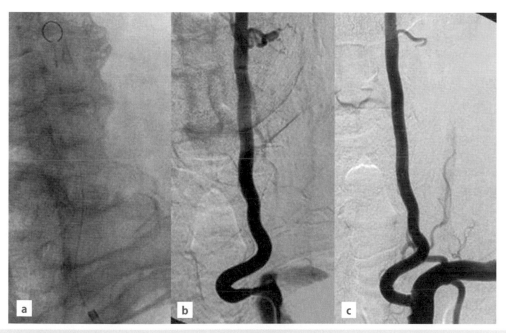

Figure 6.3 (a) An EPD placed in the V2 segment. (b) An 80% ostial stenosis in the V1 segment of the vertebral artery. (c) Final result after placement of a 3.5x12.0-mm balloon expandable stent.

engaging the vertebral artery ostium. A 0.014-in soft guide wire or filter wire is recommended for use with a rapid exchange or monorail balloon to predilate the stenotic lesion. Embolic protection devices are not FDA approved for use in the vertebral artery; however, it should be strongly considered if there is a comfortable landing zone distal to the index lesion. The predilation balloon should be 0.5 mm less than the reference vessel diameter. The physician must be very diligent to keep the tip of the guide wire within view at all times during the procedure as guide-wire perforation can cause fatal intracranial hemorrhage. This can happen with any guide wire but is of particular concern when a hydrophilic guide wire is used. Balloon-expandable coronary or peripheral stents on a 0.014-in platform work well in the vertebral artery ostium. The proximal stent should be extended 1 to 2 mm into the subclavian artery to ensure coverage of the vertebral artery ostium. Both balloon-expandable and self-expanding stents are acceptable in the V_1 and V_2 segments of the vertebral artery.

Summary

Endovascular treatment of the ostial and proximal portions of the vertebral artery can be performed with very high technical success rates, and appears to be safe and effective for alleviating symptoms and improving cerebral blood flow to the posterior circulation. The procedure is also durable as evidenced by low restenosis rates in multiple large series reported in the literature with both balloon angioplasty alone and endovascular stent placement. The restenosis rate of 43% reported by Albuquerque et al[12] is the highest ever reported in any vertebral artery angioplasty series. The causes are likely multifactorial but certainly a population of patients, 95% of whom had significant concomitant brachiocephalic atherosclerosis, contributed to this finding. Because considerable elastic recoil often accompanies PTA alone and historically, ostial lesions have a poor response to PTA

alone, primary stent placement is an attractive treatment option for atherosclerotic vertebral ostial disease. Finally, clinical follow-up should be performed at 3, 6, and 12 months and yearly thereafter, if clinical relief of symptoms occurs. Patients with recurrent symptoms should undergo repeat angiography to identify restenosis or progression of atherosclerotic disease.

References

1. Phatouros CC, Higashida RT, Malek AM, et al. Endovascular treatment of noncarotid extracranial cerebrovascular disease. *Neurosurg Clin N Am*. 2000;11:331-350.

2. Fields WS, North RR, Hass WK, et al. Joint study of extracranial arterial occlusion as a cause of stroke. I. Organization of study and survey of patient population. *JAMA*.1968;203:955-960.

3. Crawley F, Brown MM. Percutaneous transluminal angioplasty and stenting for vertebral artery stenosis. *Cochrane Database Syst Rev*. 2000:CD000516.

4. Imparato AM. Vertebral arterial reconstruction: a nineteen-year experience. *J Vasc Surg*. 1985;2:626-634.

5. Spetzler RF, Hadley MN, Martin NA, Hopkins LN, Carter LP, Budny J. Vertebrobasilar insufficiency. Part 1: Microsurgical treatment of extracranial vertebrobasilar disease. *J Neurosurg*. 1987;66:648-661.

6. Qureshi AI, Ziai WC, Yahia AM, et al. Stroke-free survival and its determinants in patients with symptomatic vertebrobasilar stenosis: a multicenter study. *Neurosurgery*. 2003;52:1033-1039; discussion 1039-1040.

7. Higashida RT, Hieshima GB, Tsai FY, Halbach VV, Norman D, Newton TH. Transluminal angioplasty of the vertebral and basilar artery. *Am J Neuroradiol*. 1987;8:745-749.

8. Coward LJ, Featherstone RL, Brown MM. Percutaneous transluminal angioplasty and stenting for vertebral artery stenosis. *Cochrane Database Syst Rev*. 2005:CD000516.

9. Alexander W. The treatment of epilepsy by

ligature of the vertebral artery. *Brain.* 1942; 5:170-180.

10. Wityk RJ, Chang HM, Rosengart A, et al. Proximal extracranial vertebral artery disease in the New England Medical Center Posterior Circulation Registry. *Arch Neurol.* 1998;55:470-478.

11. Caplan LR, Amarenco P, Rosengart A, et al. Embolism from vertebral artery origin occlusive disease. *Neurology.* 1992;42:1505-1512.

12. Albuquerque FC, Fiorella D, Han P, Spetzler RF, McDougall CG. A reappraisal of angioplasty and stenting for the treatment of vertebral origin stenosis. *Neurosurgery.* 2003;53:607-614; discussion 614-606.

13. Moufarrij NA, Little JR, Furlan AJ, Williams G, Marzewski DJ. Vertebral artery stenosis: long-term follow-up. *Stroke.* 1984;15:260-263.

14. Rocha-Singh K. Vertebral artery stenting: ready for prime time? *Catheter Cardiovasc Interv.* 2001;54:6-7.

15. Wholey MH, Wholey MH. The supraaortic and vertebral endovascular interventions. *Tech Vasc Interv Radiol.* 2004;7:215-225.

16. Chimowitz MI, Lynn MJ, Howlett-Smith H, et al. Comparison of warfarin and aspirin for symptomatic intracranial arterial stenosis. *N Engl J Med.* 2005;352:1305-1316.

17. Diener HC, Bogousslavsky J, Brass LM, et al. Aspirin and clopidogrel compared with clopidogrel alone after recent ischaemic stroke or transient ischaemic attack in high-risk patients (MATCH): randomised, double-blind, placebo-controlled trial. *Lancet.* 2004;364:331-337.

18. Whisnant JP, Cartlidge NE, Elveback LR. Carotid and vertebral-basilar transient ischemic attacks: effect of anticoagulants, hypertension, and cardiac disorders on survival and stroke occurrence—a population study. *Ann Neurol.* 1978;3:107-115.

19. Sivenius J, Rickkinen PJ, Smets P, Laakso M, Lowenthal A. The European Stroke Prevention Study (ESPS): results by arterial distribution. *Ann Neurol.* 1991;29:596-600.

20. Gent M, Blakely JA, Easton JD, et al. The Canadian American Ticlopidine Study (CATS) in thromboembolic stroke. *Lancet.* 1989;1:1215-1220.

21. Hass WK, Easton JD, Adams HP Jr, et al. A randomized trial comparing ticlopidine hydrochloride with aspirin for the prevention of stroke in high-risk patients. Ticlopidine Aspirin Stroke Study Group. *N Engl J Med.* 1989;321:501-507.

22. Berguer R, ed. Long-term results of reconstructions in the vertebral artery. In Yao J, Pierce W, *Long-Term Results in Vascular Surgery.* Norwalk, CT: Appleton & Lange; 1993.

23. Thevenet A, Ruotolo C. Surgical repair of vertebral artery stenoses. *J Cardiovasc Surg.* (Torino) 1984;25:101-110.

24. Koskas F, Kieffer E, Rancurel G, Bahnini A, Ruotolo C, Illuminati G. Direct transposition of the distal cervical vertebral artery into the internal carotid artery. *Ann Vasc Surg.* 1995;9:515-524.

25. Sundt TM Jr, Smith HC, Campbell JK, Vlietstra RE, Cucchiara RF, Stanson A. Transluminal angioplasty for basilar artery stenosis. *Mayo Clin Proc.* 1980;55:673-680.

26. Motarjeme A. Percutaneous transluminal angioplasty of supra-aortic vessels. *J Endovasc Surg.* 1996;3:171-181.

27. Higashida RT, Tsai FY, Halbach VV, et al. Transluminal angioplasty for atherosclerotic disease of the vertebral and basilar arteries. *J Neurosurg.* 1993;78:192-198.

28. Chastain HD II, Campbell MS, Iyer S, et al. Extracranial vertebral artery stent placement: in-hospital and follow-up results. *J Neurosurg.* 1999;91:547-552.

29. Lin YH, Juang JM, Jeng JS, Yip PK, Kao HL. Symptomatic ostial vertebral artery stenosis treated with tubular coronary stents: clinical results and restenosis analysis. *J Endovasc Ther.* 2004;11:719-726.

30. Jenkins JS, White CJ, Ramee SR, et al. Vertebral artery stenting. *Catheter Cardiovasc Interv.* 2001;54:1-5.

31. Jenkins JS, Patel SN, White CJ, et al. Endovascular stenting for vertebral artery stenosis. *J Am Coll Cardiol.* 2010;55:538-42.

7

Hemodialysis Access Intervention

John A. Bittl

The rising number of patients with end stage renal disease (ESRD) has increased the need for hemodialysis access. The creation of dialysis fistulas and grafts has become the most common type of vascular surgery performed in the United States and accounts for 40% to 50% of the operative volume in some programs.[1] The patency of hemodialysis fistulas and grafts, however, remains disappointingly low.

During the past decade, the management of failing hemodialysis accesses has shifted from surgical repair to catheter-based approaches.[2] The National Kidney Foundation-Dialysis Outcomes Quality Initiative (NKF KDOQI) document[3] has endorsed endovascular approaches in centers with local expertise to avoid placing temporary hemodialysis catheters, to preserve venous segments for future access, and to prolong total survival time on hemodialysis. Catheter-based therapies now fill a prominent role in the lives of hemodialysis patients, who consider their dialysis accesses to be a lifeline.

This chapter defines the pathophysiology of dialysis access failure, reviews the success rates for endovascular treatments, and illustrates the catheter-based approaches for treating failing and thrombosed fistulas and grafts.

Epidemiology and Prevalence

The number of patients enrolled in the US Medicare programs for ESRD was 2400 in 1972, rose 10-fold to 27,000 in 1977, and rose another 10-fold to 260,000 in 1997. With a prevalence of more than 1 in 1000 persons, the number of patients with ESRD requiring *renal replacement therapy (RRT)* exceeded 340,000 in 2006.[4] More than 80% of patients requiring RRT in the United States undergo hemodialysis. The US hemodialysis program now makes up more than 6% of the entire Medicare budget.[4]

Survival statistics for patients on hemodialysis remain sobering. The overall annual mortality rate on hemodialysis exceeds 20%.[5] The mortality rate during the first year after initiation of dialysis for elderly, debilitated adults is 58%.[6] Almost 40% of patients with ESRD have concomitant coronary artery disease, and 10% of dialysis patients experience a myocardial infarction every year.[7] In the hemodialysis population, the 1-year mortality rate after myocardial infarction is 59%.[8]

The number of patients undergoing hemodialysis has been growing at 6% per year and will thus double in 12 years. By the year 2020,

Vascular Disease: Diagnostic and Therapeutic Approaches. © 2011 Michael R. Jaff and Christopher J. White, editors. Cardiotext Publishing, ISBN: 978-1-935395-16-4.

the number of patients with ESRD may be as high as 750,000.[4] The rising prevalence of ESRD can be attributed primarily to changing demographics and the undertreatment of hypertension, diabetes, and chronic kidney disease (CKD) in the general population.

Access Anatomy and Pathophysiology of Access Failure

The selection of a particular type of arteriovenous conduit for hemodialysis is based on evidence favoring the creation of an autogenous fistula whenever possible before using a *polytetrafluoroethylene (PTFE) graft*—an approach commonly called "fistula first."[9-11] The selection of a particular site for permanent access creation is based on the suitability of venous (Figure 7.1) and arterial anatomy (Figure 7.2). The selection of a specific location is based on the recommended sequence of using the nondominant arm before the dominant arm, the forearm before the upper arm, and the upper extremity before the lower extremity.[9]

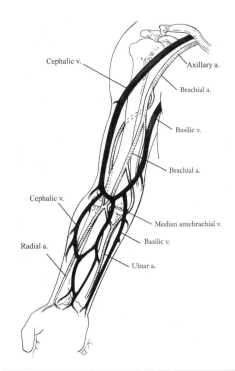

Figure 7.2 Pertinent arterial and venous anatomy of the upper extremity. a = artery, v = vein.

An autogenous arteriovenous access is surgically created by directly anastomosing a native inflow artery to a native outflow vein. A common type is the Brescia-Cimino radial-cephalic fistula constructed at the wrist between the radial artery and the cephalic vein (Figure 7.3), usually in the form of an end-to-side anastomosis. In the upper arm, the creation of a transposed brachial-basilic fistula requires mobilization and tunneling of the basilic vein laterally and superficially for easy cannulation.

A prosthetic arteriovenous access is constructed by surgically interposing a segment of PTFE between a native artery and a native vein in either a straight or looped configuration. Common patterns include the brachial-cephalic configuration in the forearm or the brachial-basilic configuration in the upper arm (Figure 7.3). Other configurations include the prosthetic femoral-saphenous vein inguinal loop access, in which a loop of PTFE is connected end-to-side with the superficial femoral artery and end-to-end with the greater saphenous vein (Figure 7.4).

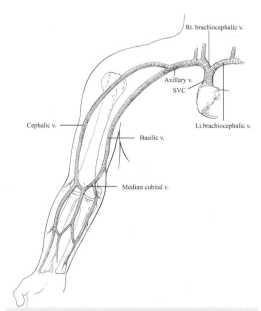

Figure 7.1 Venous anatomy of the upper extremity. Rt = right, SVC = superior vena cava, v = vein.

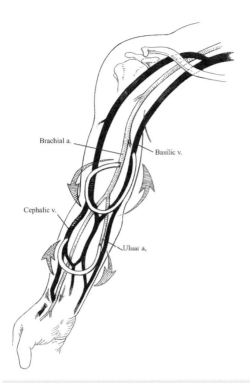

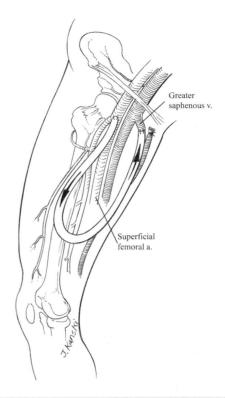

Figure 7.3 Access anatomy of the upper extremity. A radial-cephalic fistula (small distal flow arrows) is created by an end-to-side anastomosis between the cephalic vein and the radial artery, with ligation of the distal stump of the cephalic vein. A brachial-cephalic graft in the forearm (large arrows) requires the surgical interposition of a polytetrafluoroethylene (PTFE) loop using end-to-side connections. A brachial-basilic graft in the upper arm (larger arrows) requires the surgical insertion of a PTFE loop using end-to-side connections. a = artery, v = vein.

Figure 7.4 Access anatomy of the thigh. Creation of a thigh graft involves the surgical placement of a polytetrafluoroethylene (PTFE) loop connected end-to-side with superficial femoral artery and end-to-end with the greater saphenous vein. a = artery, v = vein.

Additional details about access nomenclature are available in dedicated reports.[12] For the purposes of this chapter, however, autogenous arteriovenous accesses will be referred to as *fistulas,* prosthetic arteriovenous accesses as *grafts,* and when mentioned together, both types will be generically referred to as *accesses.* All hemodialysis accesses are short circuits, in which blood is diverted via an inflow artery into an outflow vein and thence into the central venous circulation.

Two modes of failure (Figure 7.5) commonly affect fistulas and grafts, and both types of failure are amenable to interventional treatment (Table 7.1). In newly placed fistulas, the development of an arteriovenous anastomotic stenosis restricts inflow and prevents hypertrophy and adequate maturation.[13-15] In chronically used fistulas and grafts, high pressures and flow in the thin-walled outflow vein raise shear stress and trigger fibromuscular hyperplasia.[16,17] When the hyperplasia is exuberant, a severe stenosis appears, reduces flow, and precipitates thrombosis.

About 50% of malfunctioning accesses contain thrombus,[18] but thrombosis is not the primary cause of failure. Instead, a culprit stenosis in the access circuit initiates the pathophysiologic cascade of events leading to thrombosis (Figure 7.5). The success of catheter-based treatments of access thrombosis requires delineating and treating the stenosis that initiated the pathologic process of stasis and thrombosis. Stenoses can occur anywhere in the dialysis access, but the most common site in 47% to 65% of cases involves the anastomosis between the

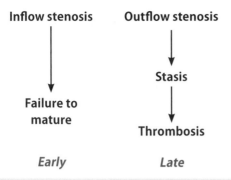

Inflow stenosis   Outflow stenosis

Failure to mature   Stasis

    Thrombosis

Early   *Late*

Figure 7.5 Pathogenesis of dialysis access failure. The early appearance of an inflow (anastomotic) stenosis may lead to failure of fistula maturation. The late development of a stenosis in the outflow segment of a fistula or graft is the cause of stasis and access thrombosis.

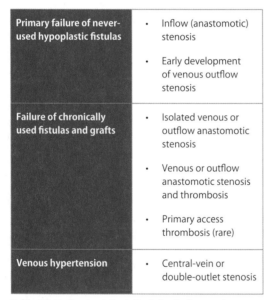

Primary failure of never-used hypoplastic fistulas	• Inflow (anastomotic) stenosis • Early development of venous outflow stenosis
Failure of chronically used fistulas and grafts	• Isolated venous or outflow anastomotic stenosis • Venous or outflow anastomotic stenosis and thrombosis • Primary access thrombosis (rare)
Venous hypertension	• Central-vein or double-outlet stenosis

Table 7.1 Pathophysiologic Basis for Endovascular Intervention

prosthetic graft and the outflow vein.[19-21] Other sites for stenosis formation include a nonanastomotic location within a peripheral outflow vein in 37% to 53%, the graft itself in 38% to 50%, central veins in 3% to 20%, and multiple sites in 31% to 59%.[19-21] Fistulas contain no outflow anastomosis, but like grafts, they are nonetheless susceptible to stenosis formation in the "arterialized" outflow vein.

The bulk of the thrombus that occurs secondarily within a clotted access is typically red thrombus, which is rich in fibrin and red cells and easily extracted with rheolytic methods or pulse-spray thrombolysis. The platelet-rich white clot at the arterial inflow anastomosis is usually resistant to rheolytic or thrombolytic methods and may require mechanical removal with Fogarty thrombectomy.[22]

After surgical creation, fewer than 50% of fistulas are able to provide reliable hemodialysis.[23-27] The disappointing primary unassisted patency rates may improve slightly after successful intervention or surgical salvage, so that secondary patency rates at 1 year are 10% to 20% higher.[2,24] The failure of autogenous fistulas to mature is a more common problem in patients with diabetes and in the elderly. The patency of upper-arm brachial-cephalic and transposed basilic vein fistulas in patients with diabetes at 18 months (78%) may be significantly better than that of forearm fistulas (33%).[28]

When fistulas have been used for hemodialysis, they fail after a median of 3 to 7 years.[29-31] An autogenous fistula has a greater chance for long-term patency than a prosthetic arteriovenous graft, but the primary patency of fistulas remains low because of the lack of suitable anatomy in many cases and the inability to achieve adequate hypertrophy.

Patients who are not candidates for fistulas can have prosthetic grafts constructed from PTFE. Although the primary patency of a prosthetic grafts exceeds 80%,[1] grafts fail after a median lifetime of only 12 to 18 months.[29-32]

Diagnostic Evaluation

The National Kidney Foundation-Dialysis Outcomes Quality Initiative (NKF KDOQI) document[3] recommends establishing an organized nephrology program to identify failing fistulas and grafts. *Monitoring* is carried out with regular physical examinations and assessment of dialysis adequacy. *Surveillance* refers to the performance of noninvasive testing to gather further information about access structure and function. *Diagnostic testing* refers to the performance of invasive procedures to define access anatomy and hemodynamics.

A successful endovascular intervention is the ability to complete at least one dialysis session via the treated access. The definition of *patency duration* is the time from intervention to referral for repeat intervention, vascular surgery, or placement of a temporary dialysis catheter because of a failing or thrombosed access. A significant stenosis refers to at least a 50% diameter stenosis, as detected by angiography and associated with increased bleeding, thrombus formation, or abnormally elevated or low access pressures.

History and Physical Examination (Monitoring)

The history and physical examination may reveal evidence of an inflow or outflow stenosis. A history of increased postdialysis bleeding suggests the development of an outflow stenosis. This may be accompanied by the presence of a focal and short high-pitched bruit. In contrast, a well-functioning fistula or graft should have a continuous medium-pitched bruit similar to the continuous murmur of a patent ductus arteriosus, associated with a prominent thrill along an easily palpable and ballotable course in the subcutaneous tissue. A soft bruit and inconspicuous thrill over recently created, slowly maturing, hypoplastic radial-cephalic fistula may indicate the presence of an anastomotic inflow stenosis. On the other hand, prominent access pulsation is abnormal and usually signifies elevated pressure caused by an outflow stenosis. Multiple aneurysmal segments in the distribution of a large, serpiginous access used for many years may indicate impaired hemostasis secondary to chronic access hypertension.

Access assessment should be carried out weekly by the dialysis nephrologist and should include inspection and palpation for a pulse and a thrill at the arterial, midportion, and venous sections. Marked arm edema, sometimes producing *peau d'orange,* usually indicates dual venous obstruction (cephalic and basilic) or a subclavian vein stenosis or occlusion.

Symptoms and signs of infection may be blunted in uremic patients. Although mild isolated erythema without tenderness or edema is usually not a sign of infection, it is important to recognize that fever and leukocytosis as signs of infection may be masked in uremic patients. Constitutional symptoms suggestive of infection include anorexia, weight loss, and myalgias. Signs of infection include cellulitis, fluctuance, skin breakdown, or purulent discharge. Access infection is a contraindication to interventional treatment because sepsis may ensue when infected thrombus is agitated.

Noninvasive Evaluation (Surveillance)

Nephrologists, who can measure intra-access flow and static venous dialysis pressures, assess hemodialysis adequacy regularly. The finding of rising pressures of more than 150 mm Hg at a constant flow of 200 mL/min on dialysis may indicate the presence of an outflow stenosis. Estimating the recirculation fraction using urea concentrations or clinical parameters such as body weight, volume status, or serum potassium concentration may indicate incomplete dialysis. These are probably relatively late predictors of hemodialysis access failure and become abnormal at the time of impending thrombosis.

Repeat ultrasonographic studies may identify early stenosis formation before physical signs are apparent,[33] but the cost of noninvasive methods and the uncertain benefits of preemptive graft intervention are factors that have tempered enthusiasm for noninvasive surveillance.[3]

Invasive Evaluation and Hemodynamics (Diagnostic Testing)

Hemodynamic measurements made during catheter-based intervention can be critical to assessing procedural success. An inflow stenosis may reduce access pressures to less than 15 mm Hg and prevent adequate filling. An outflow stenosis may increase access pressures to arterial levels. The ideal systolic pressure of an access should be less than 50 mm Hg, and the optimal ratio of systolic pressure in the access to systolic systemic pressure should be 0.30 to 0.40.[19,34] Modest elevations of venous pressures to 60 mm Hg caused by central-vein stenoses or occlusions can cause limb edema. If treatment (Figure 7.6) normalizes pressures (Figure 7.7), edema may improve within 1 to 2 days.

Indications for angiography (diagnostic testing)

The generic term *fistulogram* refers to the angiographic study of either an autogenous arteriovenous fistula or a prosthetic arteriovenous graft. A fistulogram is indicated when hemo-

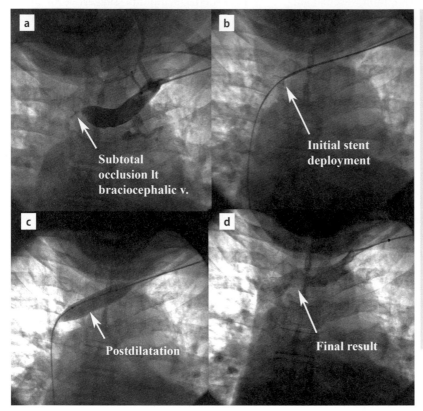

Figure 7.6 Stenting of a subtotal occlusion in the left brachiocephalic vein. Arm edema appeared after creation of an ipsilateral autogenous brachial-basilic access. Venography disclosed the presence of subtotal occlusion of the left brachiocephalic vein (a). Placement of a 14-mm nitinol stent is confirmed with contrast injection and traction applied to the initially deployed stent to avoid slippage (b). Postdilatation angioplasty is performed with a 14-mm balloon (c). The final angiogram shows brisk flow and complete stent expansion (d). lt = left, v = vein.

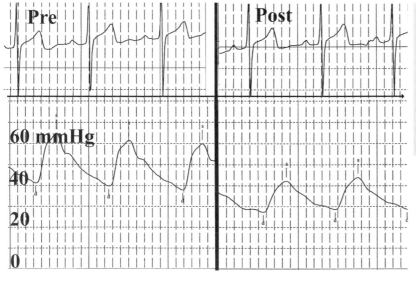

Figure 7.7 Hemodynamic improvement after treatment of subtotal occlusion of the left brachiocephalic vein. After stent placement and balloon angioplasty, as shown in Figure 7.6, fistula pressure fell from 62 to 42 mm Hg and arm edema improved.

dialysis cannot be successfully carried out or when there is evidence from monitoring or surveillance to suggest that thrombosis is imminent or has already occurred (Table 7.2).

Indications for Invasive Evaluation of Failing or Thrombosed Dialysis Accesses
Absence or decrease in thrill
Absence of bruit or pulse
Change from medium-pitched continuous bruit to high-pitched short bruit
New prominent pulsation over access
Increased postdialysis bleeding
Pseudoaneurysm formation
Recurrent thrombosis of dialysis access needle
Repeated difficulty accessing fistula or graft
Decreased dialysis efficiency
Increased dialysis time
Increasing pressure in return line at constant flow
Peripheral edema in graft extremity
Increased recirculation fraction to > 20%
Delayed maturation of hypoplastic fistula

Table 7.2 Indications for Invasive Evaluation of Failing or Thrombosed Dialysis Accesses

Normal anatomy (inflow and outflow)

An access in the arm may have either a looped or straight configuration. In the forearm, the radial-cephalic autogenous fistula is a commonly encountered form (see Figure 7.3), usually with venous outflow carried by the cephalic vein. If the cephalic vein is atretic or occluded, the antecubital vein may carry venous return to the basilic vein. In the forearm, the most common graft configuration is the brachial-cephalic graft (see Figure 7.3), which follows a medial-to-lateral course and continues to the central circulation via the cephalic vein along the lateral aspect of the arm, traverses the pectoral groove, and anastomoses with the axillary vein where it becomes the subclavian vein. In the upper arm, the most common graft configuration is the brachial-basilic graft, which follows a lateral-

to-medial course and continues in a straight line into the axillary vein, subclavian vein, and thence into the central circulation (see Figure 7.3). In the thigh, the most common configuration follows a lateral-to-medial course that connects the superficial femoral artery with the greater saphenous vein (see Figure 7.4).

Important collateral circulation

Venous collaterals are diagnostic of a critical venous stenosis or occlusion. In the peripheral circulation, critical stenoses can be suggested by the presence of either bridging collaterals or large collateral networks connecting the cephalic and basilic veins. In the central circulation, critical stenoses or occlusions of the subclavian vein can be diagnosed when filling of the large axillary vein terminates abruptly and is associated with a medusa-like network of collaterals draining into the internal jugular vein (Figure 7.8). After successful treatment, collaterals will no longer be apparent on angiography (see Figure 7.6). In the central circulation, critical stenoses or total occlusions are usually associated with tunneled catheters or leads from a pacemaker or defibrillator.

Common variations to know

Few anatomic variations of hemodialysis accesses are commonly encountered. Alternative patterns for prosthetic grafts in the forearm include the lateral-to-medial course of the brachial-

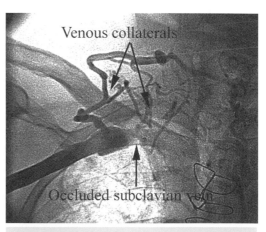

Figure 7.8 Occluded right subclavian vein associated with venous collaterals.

basilic graft or, in the upper arm, the medial-to-lateral course of brachial-cephalic graft. In both sites, loop grafts are more common than straight grafts because they potentially increase the accessible length of the graft for needle entry.

Another configuration in the forearm consists of the proximal radial artery anastomosed in a side-to-side manner with the median antebrachial vein, producing a double-outlet configuration coursing proximally and distally from the arteriovenous anastomosis.[35] Another type of "double-outlet" access is the Brescia-Cimino fistula at the wrist, which empties into both the cephalic and basilic veins, a desirable variation that theoretically avoids fistula thrombosis if one limb develops an outflow stenosis.

Therapeutic Options for Hemodialysis Access Failure

Medical Therapy
Although several randomized trials of antiplatelet agents have been reported, none has shown clear success in preventing access thrombosis.[36-38] In a randomized trial of 877 patients,[25] clopidogrel was no better than placebo in allowing autogenous arteriovenous fistulas to mature adequately after surgical creation for successful hemodialysis (38% vs. 40%). In a separate randomized trial of 649 patients,[26] dipyridamole was modestly better than placebo in achieved primary unassisted patency of autogenous arteriovenous fistulas at 1 year (28% vs. 23%).

Primary thrombosis of chronically used hemodialysis accesses occurs rarely. It may occur unpredictably and unavoidably after major surgery, myocardial infarction, or sepsis associated with hypotension or hyperfibrinogenemia. Other causes of primary access thrombosis are excessive postdialysis access compression, hyperviscosity from hemoconcentration, polycythemia, or hypovolemia. When primary thrombosis of an access occurs without an identifiable pathogenic stenosis or in the setting of a

hypercoagulable state such as Factor V Leiden or the antiphospholipid syndrome,[39] chronic anticoagulation with warfarin is recommended.

No medical therapy has been identified that prevents the development of a venous outflow stenosis or an arterial inflow stenosis.

Surgical Therapy
Percutaneous methods have replaced surgical procedures in many centers to treat acutely failing grafts, but surgical approaches remain important for many indications. In newly placed but hypoplastic fistulas, surgical ligation of tributaries, superficialization, and revision of anastomoses can salvage some autogenous accesses.[40] When fistulas or grafts have recurrent venous outflow stenoses that require frequent balloon angioplasty procedures, surgical excision with end-to-end repair may be recommended.

Endovascular Therapy
A 4-step procedure is applicable for thrombosed fistulas and grafts (Table 7.3). This is based on the understanding of the pathophysiology of access failure (see Figure 7.5). The most common primary cause of access failure is the development of an outflow stenosis, which was observed in every case in a recent series.[19] Access thrombosis occurred at least once in 109 of 179 patients (61%) in a contemporary prospective series (Tables 7.4 and 7.5).

Four-Step Approach for Endovascular Treatment of Failing or Thrombosed Hemodialysis Accesses
1. Thrombectomy of outflow and inflow segments
2. Percutaneous transluminal angioplasty of venous outflow stenosis
3. Fogarty thrombectomy of adherent clot at the arterial inflow anastomosis
4. Angiography of central veins

Table 7.3 Four-Step Approach for Endovascular Treatment of Failing or Thrombosed Hemodialysis Accesses

	Overall	Patients with Fistulas	Patients with Grafts	P
N	179	88 (49)	91 (51)	
Age (mean + SEM, years)	64 ± 15	63 ± 16	64 ± 15	0.334
Sex				< 0.001
Male	102 (57%)	63 (71.6)	39 (42.9)	
Female	77 (43%)	25 (28.4)	52 (57.1)	
Etiology				0.096
Diabetes	80 (44.7)	44 (50.0)	36 (39.6)	
Hypertension	55 (30.7)	25 (28.4)	30 (33.0)	
Interstitial nephritis	10 (5.6)	9 (10.2)	1 (1.1)	
Renal cell carcinoma	8 (4.5)	2 (2.3)	6 (6.6)	
Atheroemboli	5 (2.8)	2 (2.3)	3 (3.3)	
Glomerulonephritis	5 (2.8)	1 (1.1)	4 (4.4)	
Polycystic kidney disease	5 (2.8)	1 (1.1)	4 (4.4)	
Lupus nephritis	5 (2.8)	2 (2.3)	3 (3.3)	
IgA nephropathy	2 (1.1)	2 (2.3)	0 (0.0)	
Bright's disease	1 (0.6)	0 (0.0)	1 (1.1)	
Multiple myeloma	1 (0.6)	0 (0.0)	1 (1.1)	
Pyelonephritis	1 (0.6)	0 (0.0)	1 (1.1)	
Wegener's granulomatosis	1 (0.6)	0 (0.0)	1 (1.1)	
Race				0.148
White	116 (64.8)	62 (70.5)	54 (59.3)	
Black	62 (34.6)	25 (28.4)	37 (40.7)	
Asian	1 (0.06)	1 (0.8)	0 (0.0)	
Current smoker	3 (1.7)	1 (1.1)	2 (2.2)	0.567

Table 7.4 Patient Characteristics. Baseline characteristics and outcomes were compared between fistula and graft patients with the use of independent-sample t-tests, chi-square, and Wilcoxon rank-sum tests. (Adapted from Bittl and Feldman.[19])

The procedures outlined here define an approach that can be performed by interventional cardiologists, nephrologists, or radiologists with predictably high success.[18,41]

1. Indications and contraindications

Emergency indications for catheter-based treatment include hyperkalemia, volume overload, or refractory hypertension associated with a failing or thrombosed access. Another emergency indication for interventional therapy is the inability to achieve hemostasis after dialysis.

An urgent indication for endovascular treatment is access thrombosis. Endovascular treatment for access thrombosis should be per-

formed within 24 hours of diagnosis and within 48 hours of the most recent dialysis session, because further delays may increase the risks of life-threatening complications or the need for temporary catheter placement.

A semiurgent indication for angiography is the finding of a malfunctioning but nonthrombosed dialysis access (see Table 7.2), which should be referred within 48 hours of discovery because thrombosis may be imminent. Indications for endovascular treatment include the presence of more than 50% stenosis associated with evidence of access malfunction.

Contraindications to percutaneous treatment include graft infection, a central right-to-

	All Accesses	Fistulas	Grafts	P
N	294	128 (43.5)	166 (56.5)	
Graft age (days, median, IQR)	516 (184, 1009)	331 (121, 933)	569 (322, 1101)	0.001
No malfunction identified (%)	6 (2.0)	3 (2.3)	3 (1.8)	0.747
Inflow anastomotic stenosis (%)	24 (8.2)	21 (16.4)	3 (1.8)	< 0.001
Resistant inflow thrombus (%)	128 (43.5)	31 (24.2)	97 (58.4)	< 0.001
Outflow anastomotic stenosis (%)	107 (36.4)	—	107 (64.5)	< 0.001
Peripheral venous stenosis (%)	157 (53.4)	104 (81.3)	53 (31.9)	< 0.001
Central venous occlusion (%)	61 (20.7)	31 (24.2)	30 (18.1)	0.198
Totally thrombosed (%)	144 (49.0)	39 (30.5)	105 (63.3)	< 0.001
Prior PTA (%)	139 (47.3)	38 (29.7)	101 (60.8)	< 0.001
Prior stent (%)	17 (5.8)	5 (3.9)	12 (7.2)	0.226
New PTA (%)	247 (84.0)	94 (73.4)	153 (92.3)	< 0.001
New PTA and stent (%)	27 (9.2)	9 (7.0)	18 (10.8)	0.262
Cutting balloon atherotomy (%)	4 (1.7)	4 (3.1)	0 (0.0)	0.022
Largest balloon used (mm, %)				< 0.001
None	6 (2.0)	3 (2.3)	3 (1.8)	
4	10 (3.4)	10 (7.8)	0 (0.0)	
5	2 (0.6)	2 (1.6)	0 (0.0)	
6	40 (13.6)	32 (25.0)	8 (4.8)	
7	108 (36.7)	40 (31.3)	68 (41.0)	
8	97 (33.0)	25 (19.5)	72 (43.4)	
9	27 (9.2)	16 (12.5)	11 (6.6)	
10	4 (1.4)	0 (0.0)	4 (2.4)	
Fogarty used (%)	128 (43.5)	31 (24.2)	97 (58.4)	< 0.001
Pretreatment				
% stenosis		71 ± 3	84 ± 2	< 0.001
Pressure (mm Hg)		76 ± 4	102 ± 2	< 0.001
Posttreatment				
% stenosis		22 ± 2	19 ± 2	0.120
Pressure (mm Hg)		50 ± 3	43 ± 2	< 0.001
Pressure ratio		0.33 ± 3.1	0.36 ± 3.7	0.066
Overall success (%)	281 (95.6)	120 (93.8)	161 (97.0)	0.181
Success in 144 thrombosed				
Accesses (%)	134 (93.0)	34 (87.2)	100 (95.2)	0.091
Complications (%)				0.526
Foreign body extraction	1 (0.03)	1 (0.08)	0 (0.0)	
Dissection	2 (0.07)	1 (0.08)	1 (0.06)	
Grade I hematoma	4 (1.4)	2 (1.6)	2 (1.2)	
Grade II hematoma	0 (0.0)	0 (0.00)	0 (0.0)	
Grade III hematoma	1 (0.3)	0 (0.0)	1 (0.06)	
Arterial embolization	0 (0.0)	0 (0.0)	0 (0.0)	
Oxygen desaturation	0 (0.0)	0 (0.0)	0 (0.0)	

Table 7.5 Graft Characteristics and Procedural Findings. Baseline characteristics and outcomes were compared between fistula and graft patients with the use of independent-sample t-tests, chi-square, and Wilcoxon rank-sum tests. (Adapted from Bittl and Feldman.[19]) IQR = interquartile range, PTA = percutaneous transluminal angioplasty

left shunt, or pulmonary hypertension (Table 7.6). A relative contraindication to catheter-based therapy is thrombosis of a new fistula or graft within 30 days of creation or surgical revision. In this situation, thrombosis has likely arisen from a technical problem or unfavorable biology not amenable to catheter-based therapy.

Contraindications to Endovascular Treatment of Thrombosed Dialysis Accesses
Right-to-left intracardiac shunt
Pulmonary hypertension
Infected access
Surgical revision < 30 days earlier (relative contraindication)

Table 7.6 Contraindications to Endovascular Treatment of Thrombosed Dialysis Accesses

The routine referral of functioning fistulas and grafts for angiography and preemptive angioplasty remains controversial (see section 4.a. "Preemptive angioplasty" following). The Vascular Access Work Group has concluded that as a preventive strategy, "There is considerable debate concerning whether PTA interventions improve long-term outcomes."[42]

2. Outcomes and clinical success

The acute success rate for endovascular treatment depends on access type and failure mode. The published success rates for fistulas range from 78% to 87%[18,19,41] and the success rates for grafts range from 93% to 96%.[18,19,41] In a recent report involving 1437 consecutive procedures,[18] catheter-based interventions resulted in successful hemodialysis for at least 30 days without repeat angiography or surgical intervention in 1317 procedures (91.7%). The angiographic success rates were lower for thrombosed fistulas than for thrombosed grafts (80% vs. 94%). A high proportion of unsuccessful procedures involved 87 hypoplastic fistulas that failed to mature, of which only 44 (51%) were able to undergo hemodialysis.

Long-term patency after endovascular treatment also depends on access type and the presence of thrombosis. Six-month patency rates after endovascular treatment range from 61% to 66%, and the 1-year patency rates range from 38% to 41%.[19,43] Fistulas have longer median patencies than grafts[19,44] unless thrombosis has occurred. Thrombosed accesses have shorter patency durations after percutaneous intervention than malfunctioning but non-thrombosed accesses (136 vs. 238 days, $P < 0.001$),[19] perhaps reflecting lead-time bias. The final pressure achieved in the access is inversely related to the duration of patency,[19,34] and along with postprocedural residual stenosis, may be one of the strongest predictors of patency duration.[34]

3. Complications

Complications from endovascular treatment of dialysis access failure are rare but usually mild and controllable. Hematomas have been categorized by severity.[45] Grade I hematomas are minor and non–flow limiting (Figure 7.9), whereas grade II hematomas are large and flow limiting. Grade III hematomas are massive, associated with pulsatile extravasation or free perforation (Figure 7.10). Free-flowing rupture usually requires firm compression and placement of a VIABAHN Endoprosthesis (W.L. Gore and Associates), Fluency Plus Tracheobronchial Stent Graft (Bard Peripheral Vascular), or polyethylene teryltolate-covered stent (Wallgraft, Boston Scientific) after upsizing to an 11-Fr sheath. Pinhole perforations can usually be controlled by manual compression alone or with suture placement.

Several studies have reported the risk of major complications during catheter-based treatment of malfunctioning hemodialysis accesses. In one series,[46] venous rupture occurred in 40 of 2414 procedures (1.7%). Wallstents (Boston Scientific) were successful in 28 of 37 cases, but a leak was still visible at the end of the intervention in 11 cases. A covered Cragg Endopro stent (MinTec) was needed in one case, and surgical drainage was required for one patient. In another series,[47] venous rupture occurred in 12 of 579 procedures (2.1%). Stents were successful in 10 of 12 patients. In another

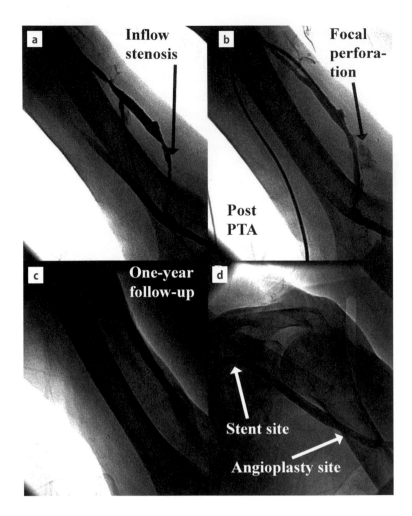

Inflow stenosis

Focal perforation

Post PTA

One-year follow-up

Stent site

Angioplasty site

Figure 7.9 Hematoma development in an immature fistula. Balloon dilatation of the inflow stenosis of a new immature fistula (a) was followed by formation of a non–flow limiting hematoma (b). One year later, the fistula had matured (c) and had been used regularly for hemodialysis 3 times weekly, but a stenosis in the midportion of the cephalic vein required angioplasty and the confluence between the cephalic and axillary veins required stenting (d).

series of 23 patients with venous rupture,[48] the use of Wallstents led to a patency rate of 26% at 180 days.

In one series of 1242 procedures,[49] venous rupture or perforation occurred in 11 (0.9%). No patient with a rupture or perforation died or required emergency or urgent surgical repair. Two of 11 patients (18.2%) required transfusions, 8 of 11 patients (72.7%) required stenting, and 6 of 8 (75.0%) who needed stenting received covered stents to achieve hemostasis. Rupture led to access thrombosis within 30 days in 9 of 11 cases (82%). Multivariable logistical regression analysis suggested that using a balloon catheter more than 2 mm larger than the diameter of the hemodialysis access or using peripheral cutting balloons increased the risk of rupture or perforation.[49]

Other complications include catheter or device breakage requiring retrieval with snares. Arterial embolization requires Fogarty thrombectomy or surgical treatment. Pulmonary embolism is rare after endovascular treatment of thrombosed accesses. No scintigraphic evidence of pulmonary embolism was seen in a systematic evaluation after various catheter-based approaches to treat thrombosed dialysis accesses.[50]

4. Clinical trials and registries
a. Preemptive angioplasty

Several studies have evaluated the ability of preemptive angioplasty to prevent access thrombosis, but results have been mixed. Positive reports include a small study[51] of 21 patients with prosthetic arteriovenous accesses that had not previ-

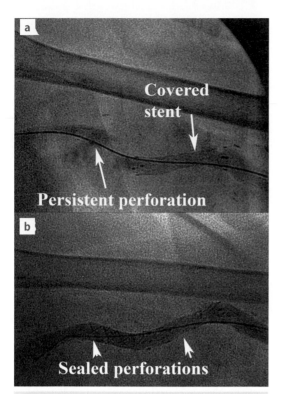

Figure 7.10 Rupture of dialysis fistula. A free-flowing perforation was refractory to compression and persisted after placement of a single covered stent (a). This was successfully sealed after placement of several covered stents (b).

ously clotted or required intervention, in which preemptive angioplasty reduced the risk of thrombosis from 44% to 10% per 100 patients-years (*P* = 0.01). Another small study[52] reported that prophylactic angioplasty (N = 32) was superior to the standard treatment of fistulas (N = 30) in reducing thrombosis rate from 25% to 16% per 100 patient-years. Tessitore and colleagues[53] evaluated the cost effectiveness of access blood-flow measurements and preemptive angioplasty in 159 patients and observed that a 3-fold increase in the number of angiographic procedures offset a 77% reduction in thrombosis events and a 65% reduction in fistula loss, thus defining an "economically dominant therapy" (ie, cost-saving).

Several randomized studies have suggested that preemptive angioplasty fails to prevent access thrombosis. A prospective randomized trial of 64 patients monitored with monthly static venous-to-systolic blood pressure ratios compared prophylactic angioplasty with the strategy of delayed invasive management at the time of thrombosis and observed similar rates of thrombosis rates and access loss.[54] Another randomized trial[55] of 112 patients compared monthly access blood-flow measurements with standard surveillance and reported that the greater number of interventions that were performed in the surveillance group than in the control group did not reduced the rate of access thrombosis (41% vs. 51% per 100 patient-years, *P* = NS).

A recent economic analysis suggested that preemptive percutaneous transluminal angioplasty (PTA) produced a decline in access thrombosis from 27.6 to 22.0 events per 100 patient-years (*P* < 0.029) at a net cost of $34,586 per 100 patient-years and an incremental cost-effectiveness ratio of $6177 per thrombosis event avoided.[56] This appeared to be less economically appealing than increasing the proportion of fistulas in the hemodialysis population.

b. Preemptive use of stent grafts
Haskal and colleagues[57] randomized 190 hemodialysis patients with venous anastomotic stenoses to undergo either balloon angioplasty alone or placement of a nitinol PTFE stent graft (Flair, Bard Peripheral Vascular). At 6 months, the primary end points of target lesion patency (51% vs. 23%, *P* < 0.001) and access patency (38% vs. 20%, *P* = 0.008) were greater in the stent-graft group than in the balloon-angioplasty group. A potential drawback of the study was the 81% higher likelihood of access thrombosis in the stent-graft group than in the balloon-angioplasty group (odds ratio [OR], 1.81; 95% confidence interval [CI], 0.93 – 3.51), which did not reach statistical significance but raised the question of a type II statistical error and a safety signal. Access thrombosis, though treatable, compromises outcomes by reducing long-term access patency from 136 versus 238 days (*P* < 0.001)[19] and costs more per procedure than malfunctioning but nonthrombosed accesses ($3336 vs. $1939, *P* < 0.05).[56] Another potential drawback of widespread adoption of

the stent grafting involves cost. The retail cost of each Flair stent graft ranges from $2065 to $2495 (Bard Peripheral Vascular), whereas the entire cost of supplies and personnel for balloon angioplasty of malfunctioning but nonthrombosed dialysis accesses treated with balloon angioplasty has been reported to be $1939 (95% CI, $1880–$1999).[56] The cost of the insertion of 1 stent graft could double the cost of the entire procedure, and inserting 2 or 3 stent grafts would triple or quadruple the cost of each treatment. No formal cost analysis of preemptive stent graft insertion has been reported.

c. Registry results

In a prospective analysis, successful outcomes were obtained in 275 of 294 malfunctioning hemodialysis accesses (96%) treated with catheter-based methods.[19] Successful results were achieved in 134 of 144 completely thrombosed accesses (93%). Successful procedures were less likely in thrombosed fistulas than in thrombosed grafts (87% vs. 95%). The median patency after intervention was 206 days (interquartile range, 79–457 days), the 6-month patency rate was 66%, and the 1-year patency rate was 41% (Figure 7.11). Several factors, including access

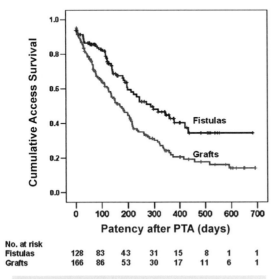

No. at risk								
Fistulas	128	83	43	31	15	8	1	1
Grafts	166	86	53	30	17	11	6	1

Figure 7.11 Kaplan-Meier survival curves for 294 fistulas and grafts after percutaneous intervention. PTA = percutaneous transluminal angioplasty. (Adapted from Bittl and Feldman.[19])

types and the presence of thrombosis, influenced long-term patency (Table 7.7). Fistulas were associated with longer median patency durations after intervention than grafts (286 vs. 170 days, $P < 0.001$). Nonthrombosed accesses had longer patency durations than thrombosed accesses (238 vs. 136 days, $P < 0.001$).

The presence of thrombosis reduced the long-term patency for all accesses and eliminated the fistula advantage (Figure 7.12); thrombosed fistulas had similar patency durations as thrombosed grafts (140 vs. 136 days). The presence of diabetes had no impact on long-term patency (199 days for diabetics vs. 212 days for nondiabetics, $P = 0.767$). In-stent restenosis tended to reduce long-term patency (206 days for unstented vs. 150 days for previously stented accesses, $P = 0.091$). Bailout stenting, which was used for failed balloon procedures, produced a trend toward reduced patency (210 days for unstented vs. 196 days for stented accesses, $P = 0.290$). The presence of a central occlusion produced higher access pressures (63 ± 4 vs. 42 ± 2 mm Hg, $P < 0.001$) and produced a trend toward reduced patency (135 vs. 215 days, $P = 0.183$). Restenotic lesions had shorter patency than *de novo* lesions (181 vs. 286 days, $P = 0.002$). Postprocedural graft pressure and postprocedural pressure ratio were inversely related to long-term patency. In a multivariate Cox proportional hazards model (Figure 7.13), several factors emerged as significant independent correlates of long-term graft survival.[19]

In a more recent series,[18] catheter-based interventions resulted in successful hemodialysis for at least 30 days without repeat angiography or surgical intervention in 1317 of 1437 procedures (92%). The angiographic success rate was lower for thrombosed fistulas than for thrombosed grafts (80% vs. 94%, $P = 0.001$). In another series, Beathard[43] reported 6-month patency rates of 61% and a 1-year patency rate of 38% after a variety of catheter interventions by interventional nephrologists. Several studies have confirmed that autogenous arteriovenous fistulas tend to have longer median patency durations than prosthetic grafts after catheter-based intervention.[44,56]

Characteristic	Patency (days [IQ range])	Univariable P	Multivariable P
Overall	206 (79, 457)		
Access type		< 0.001	0.071
Autogenous (fistula)	286 (124, 600)		
Nonthrombosed	378 (196, 600)		
Thrombosed	140 (30, 308)		
Prosthetic (graft)	170 (63, 340)		
Nonthrombosed	205 (77, 359)		
Thrombosed	136 (33, 340)		
Etiology		0.767	0.705
Diabetes	199 (103, 433)		
No diabetes	212 (176, 457)		
New stent		0.290	0.213
Present	196 (111, 321)		
Absent	210 (77, 420)		
Central occlusion		0.183	0.232
Present	136 (35, 378)		
Absent	215 (89, 457)		
Lesion		0.002	0.001
Restenotic	181 (67, 319)		
De novo	286 (98, 344)		
Balloon size (mm)		0.208	
Postprocedural access pressure		0.038	0.001
> 50 mm Hg	198 (68, 420)		
≤ 50 mm Hg	343 (168, 407)		
Access age		0.029	

Table 7.7 Univariable and Multivariable Proportional Hazards Model for Patency Durations After Catheter-Based Intervention (Adapted from Bittl and Feldman[19]) IQ = interquartile

5. Future devices and approaches

Several experimental methods are under investigation to enhance the long-term patency of arteriovenous grafts by targeting intimal hyperplasia in the venous outflow. External beam radiation has been tried, but in a small series of patients this was unable to reduce the likelihood of repeat restenosis.[58] The concept of endothelial cell seeding of PTFE grafts was based on the concept that these cells form a biologically active lining to reduce the release from flowing blood of mitogens for vascular smooth muscle cells. Lining of PTFE grafts with anti-CD34 antibodies, which can bind bone marrow–derived CD34(+) endothelial progenitor cells that proliferate and differenti-

ate into mature endothelial cells in an experimental model, resulted in almost complete endothelialization of the grafts but paradoxically increased neointimal hyperplasia at the graft-vein anastomosis.[59]

The routine use of nitinol stents has uncertain benefits in treating malfunctioning dialysis accesses,[60,61] but other potential developments include the use of drug-eluting stents for dialysis accesses. The promising initial results with stent grafts[61] await independent confirmation.

6. Technical and procedural issues
a. Preparation of the patient

Information should be gathered about the etiology of ESRD, concurrent illnesses, access

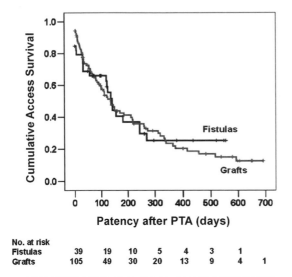

No. at risk							
Fistulas	39	19	10	5	4	3	1
Grafts	105	49	30	20	13	9	4	1

Figure 7.12 Kaplan-Meier survival curves for 144 thrombosed fistulas and grafts after percutaneous intervention. PTA = percutaneous transluminal angioplasty. (Adapted from Bittl and Feldman.[19])

history, and indications (see Table 7.2) or contraindications (see Table 7.6). Physical examination should focus on the presence of volume overload and adequacy of circulation in the access extremity (eg, Allen test). The measurement of the serum potassium level should be made if a dialysis session has been missed. In hemodialysis patients treated chronically with oral anticoagulants, warfarin or other vitamin K antagonists do not need to be withheld before performing a fistulogram. Intravenous lines should not be placed in any potential venous site for future access creation, but hand veins ipsilateral to an access site are permissible sites.[3]

The process of informed consent should include a discussion of the indications for endovascular treatment, the alternatives of watchful waiting or surgery, the use of conscious sedation, and the low risk of bleeding, thrombosis, or pulmonary embolism.

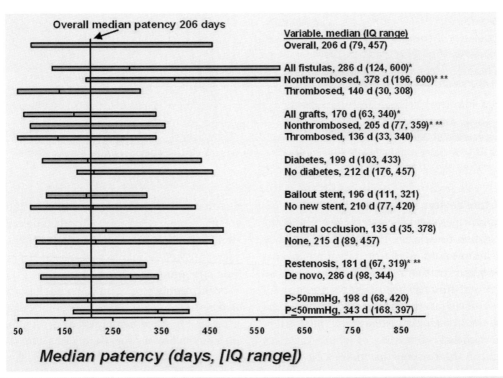

Figure 7.13 Cox proportional hazards analysis for access patency after percutaneous intervention. Median duration of access patency with interquartile (IQ) ranges in days are presented and grouped according to baseline demographic and procedural variables. A multivariable Cox proportional hazards analysis was conducted to determine whether the interaction between fistulas and accesses was independent of other clinical factors. Patency durations are presented as median and interquartile ranges (days). d = days, P = access pressure, * < .05 by univariable analysis, ** < .05 by multivariable analysis. (Adapted from Bittl and Feldman.[19])

b. Adjunctive pharmacotherapy

Aspirin 325 mg is often given orally before the procedure but can be omitted or replaced with clopidogrel in allergic patients. For thrombosed accesses, heparin is usually given intravenously in a dose of 5000 U during the procedure. Lower doses of heparin can be considered or heparin can be omitted altogether if the risk of bleeding or perforation is increased, as in recently created thin-walled fistulas. Antibiotic prophylaxis with cephalothin 1 g intravenously is commonly recommended. If an allergy to cephalosporins exists, vancomycin 1 g intravenously can be substituted and given over 1 hour. Warfarin is recommended if no stenosis is found.

c. Equipment choices and options
i. Thrombosed accesses

Before angiography, flow direction within an access may be disclosed either by the patient, the vascular surgeon, or the operative report; but foreknowledge of flow direction is not mandatory. Placing 2 sheaths in a thrombosed access ensures that the inflow and outflow segments will both be adequately evaluated and treated.

Percutaneous 18-gauge needles are inserted into the occluded fistula or graft near the usual entry sites, which are marked by needle tracks and induration. An alternative approach is to begin with a 4-Fr micropuncture set (Cook). In either case, a "pop" may be felt as the needle penetrates the dura. It is important to avoid puncturing the back wall of the graft, because an extrinsic hematoma may compress the access. Because no flashback is seen and no blood can be aspirated from a thrombosed access, intra-access entry is confirmed by smooth guide wire advancement under fluoroscopy.

Two 6-Fr sheaths are placed within the access, one in the direction of the venous outflow and one in the direction of the arterial inflow (Figure 7.14). Although the method is called the "cross-sheath" technique,[62] the tips of the sheaths face each other but do not actually overlap. Two 150-cm, 0.018-in V-18 hydrophilic control wires (Boston Scientific Medi-Tech) are advanced through the sheaths under fluoroscopic guidance without contrast injections, one in the

outflow direction and one in the inflow direction. If it is difficult to identify or advance the wire beyond the outflow stenosis or to enter the inflow artery, a 65-cm 5-Fr multipurpose A1 catheter (Cordis) can be inserted for additional maneuverability. The resistant stenosis can usually be penetrated with a 0.035-in hydrophilic curved wire and subsequently replaced with the 0.018-in guide wire for thrombectomy. Brisk contrast injections in a thrombosed access are prohibited, because thrombus may dislodge and embolize.

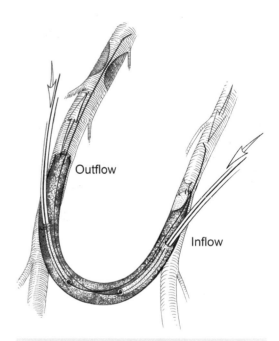

Figure 7.14 Cross-sheath method. A 6-Fr sheath is inserted into the access near the arterial-inflow anastomosis and directed into the direction of the outflow, and a 6-Fr sheath is inserted into the access near the venous-outflow in the direction of the inflow. Guide wires are advanced in the direction of the inflow and outflow under fluoroscopic guidance. No contrast is injected into a thrombosed access.

The first step is to de-clot the access, and several thrombectomy devices are available, including the dedicated AngioJet AVX rheolytic thrombectomy catheter (MEDRAD), pulse-spray infusion catheters (Cook), pulse-spray side-slit catheters (AngioDynamics), the Amplatz Thrombectomy Device (Microvena), the Arrow-Trerotola Percutaneous Thrombolytic

Device (Arrow International), and the Gelbfish EndoVac device (Neovascular Technology).

Thrombectomy is carried out first in the outflow direction (Figure 7.15), and then in the inflow direction (Figure 7.16). After flow is achieved, the access sheaths are flushed with heparinized saline, and angiography is performed to identify the outflow stenosis.

The second step involves venous angioplasty of the culprit outflow stenosis with 4-mm to 10-mm balloons (Figure 7.17). The venous stenoses tend to be fibrotic, are resistant to dilatation, and occasionally require pressures greater than 20 atmospheres (atm). High-pressure, noncompliant balloons (Conquest or Dorado, Bard Peripheral Vascular) with rated burst pressures of 20 to 24 atm can be used. Cutting Balloons (Boston Scientific) can be used when high-pressure balloons are unsuccessful,[63-65] but the use of peripheral cutting balloons in one study was associated with an increased risk of rupture.[49] Stents are usually reserved for severe recoil, venous perforations, or stenoses in surgically inaccessible veins, but the use of stent grafts will likely increase in an effort to reduce restenosis.[57]

The third step involves Fogarty thrombectomy using an over-the-wire 4-Fr Thru-Lumen Embolectomy Catheter (Edwards Lifesciences) to extract resistant thrombus at the arterial inflow (Figures 7.18 and 7.19).

The fourth step entails venography of the entire venous outflow and central veins (Figure

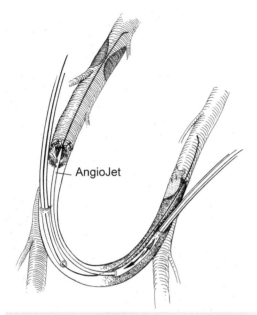

Figure 7.15 Rheolytic thrombectomy of venous outflow.

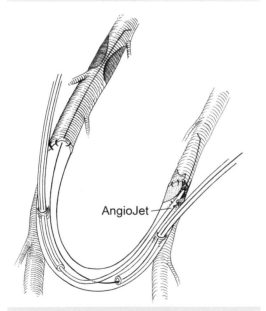

Figure 7.16 Rheolytic thrombectomy of arterial inflow.

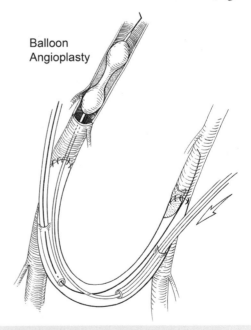

Figure 7.17 Balloon dilatation of outflow stenosis. The outflow stenosis is commonly found at or near the venous outflow anastomosis but can be encountered anywhere in the peripheral vein.

central-vein stenoses remains controversial. Levit et al[66] evaluated the success of preemptive angioplasty or stenting for central venous stenoses ipsilateral to hemodialysis accesses in 35 patients who underwent 86 angiograms over a 6-year period. Angioplasty or stenting of asymptomatic stenoses was associated with more rapid stenosis progression and escalation of lesions than the strategy of watchful waiting.

A successful procedure is characterized by angiographic evidence of widely patent access with excellent flow (Figure 7.20), minimal residual thrombus, and systolic pressure in the access approximately 30% to 40% that of systemic. Intradermal Z-sutures are used for immediate hemostasis without compression after sheath withdrawal. Sutures are removed in 1 to 2 days.

ii. Nonthrombosed accesses

Nonthrombosed fistulas and grafts respond to an abbreviated endovascular approach. A diagnostic fistulogram can usually be obtained through a 4-Fr micropuncture catheter placed in either direction. The catheter should be directed toward the inflow if the fistula is hypoplastic. The catheter should be directed toward the outflow if the access has been chronically used for hemodialysis and demonstrates signs of increased pressure.

When a stenosis is identified, angioplasty can be carried out through the 4-Fr micropuncture sheath using a coronary balloon (Maverick, Boston Scientific) or through 4-Fr or 5-Fr sheaths using peripheral monorail balloons (Sterling, Boston Scientific Medi-Tech). If ultra-high-pressure balloons are needed, however, larger sheaths may be required.

d. Tips and tricks

Needle entry of a thrombosed fistula may occasionally be challenging when accesses have failed to mature or are located deep in the subcutaneous tissue under lichenified skin. If an access cannot be entered, the transradial approach may be useful for a diagnostic fistulogram but it is less ideal than a transvenous approach for endovascular treatment. Once an access can be entered, a guide wire can be advanced and used

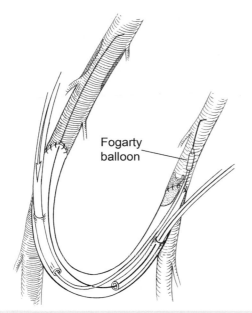

Figure 7.18 Fogarty embolectomy catheter advancement beyond the resistant inflow thrombus.

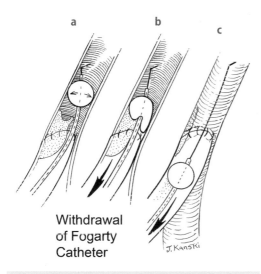

Figure 7.19 Fogarty embolectomy. The balloon catheter is inflated (a), pulled back to the thrombus (b), and forcefully withdrawn to mechanically dislodge the resistant inflow stenosis (c).

7.20). This is necessary to rule out the presence of a central stenosis. If treatment of a central-vein stenosis is recommended, it requires large-diameter devices such the XXL balloon (Boston Scientific Medi-Tech), Atlas balloon (Bard), or SMART Control stent (Cordis) up to 14 mm in diameter. However, treatment of incidental

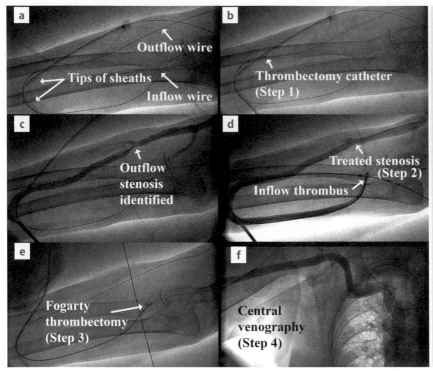

a
Outflow wire
Tips of sheaths
Inflow wire

b
Thrombectomy catheter
(Step 1)

c
Outflow
stenosis
identified

d
Treated stenosis
(Step 2)
Inflow thrombus

e
Fogarty
thrombectomy
(Step 3)

f
Central
venography
(Step 4)

Figure 7.20 Four-step technique for right forearm brachiocephalic graft. Step 1 involves placement of 2 sheaths, guide wires (a), and rheolytic thrombectomy of outflow (b) and inflow. Step 2 requires identification and treatment of the outflow stenosis (c and d). Step 3 entails identification and Fogarty thrombectomy of the resistant inflow thrombus (e). Step 4 involves completion central venous angiography to reveal a widely patent venous outflow, peripheral vein, and central venous circulation (f).

as a fluoroscopic target for needle entry (Figure 7.21). When a catheter is placed in the direction of the outflow, a diagnostic angiogram of the inflow can still be obtained using the technique of compression angiography (Figure 7.22).

Advancement of rheolytic thrombectomy catheters may occasionally snag the blunt, leading edge of a facing sheath. When this occurs, transient insertion of the sheath dilator presents a smoother transition for passage of the thrombectomy catheter.

Persistent thrombosis is most successfully treated with repeat Fogarty thrombectomy of the inflow. The catheter must be withdrawn forcefully to dislodge the resistant thrombus. If this fails and the access continues to have low

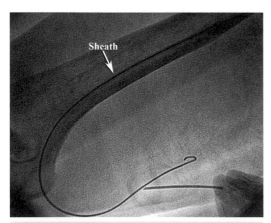

Sheath

Figure 7.21 Difficult entry of a thrombosed fistula. A guide wire inserted through one sheath can be used as fluoroscopic target for insertion of a second sheath.

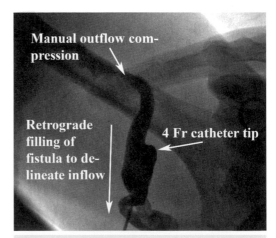

Manual outflow compression

Retrograde filling of fistula to delineate inflow

4 Fr catheter tip

Figure 7.22 Compression angiogram for retrograde delineation of arterial inflow.

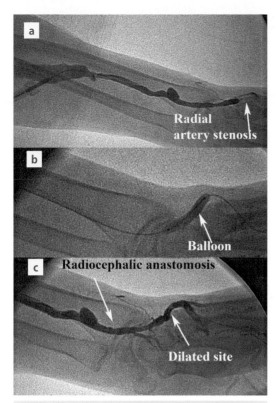

Figure 7.23 Radial artery angioplasty. Underfilling of radial-cephalic fistula is caused by the occlusion of the radial artery and significant stenosis in the palmar arch (arrow, a). Balloon dilatation (b) resulted in improved inflow (c).

pressure, balloon angioplasty of the arterial inflow anastomosis with a 6-mm dilatation catheter can be tried. An approach of last resort is to perform balloon angioplasty along the entire length of the access.

An uncommon cause of low fistula or graft pressure is a stenosis within the native inflow artery. When a patient has an occluded radial artery and has a fistula perfused via the ulnar artery and palmar arch, retrograde advancement of a coronary angioplasty balloon may be required (Figure 7.23).

e. Postcare
Almost all procedures are carried out on an outpatient basis. After a successful procedure a prominent thrill and a continuous medium-pitched bruit should be present. No bleeding or hematoma should be detected. The distal circu-

lation should be intact. Patients can be referred immediately for hemodialysis or discharged to home within 30 minutes of completion of the procedure. Sutures placed for hemostasis should be removed in 24 to 48 hours.

Summary

Catheter-based therapies for thrombosed and failing dialysis fistulas and grafts achieve success in more than 80% of cases. The Hobson's choice of placing a temporary catheter or consuming precious venous conduit has been supplanted by catheter-based approaches that prolong the function of fistulas and grafts for the growing and vulnerable population of patients with ESRD who undergo hemodialysis.

Optimal Diagnostic Algorithm
Hemodialysis fistulas and grafts have limited long-term patency. When thrombosis appears to be imminent or has already occurred or physical evidence suggests the presence of an inflow or outflow stenosis, prompt referral for a fistulogram is warranted to avoid interruption in hemodialysis and to enhance the long-term patency of accesses (Figure 7.24).

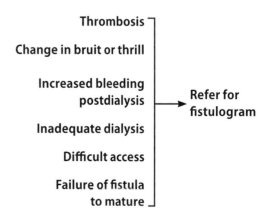

Figure 7.24 Optimal diagnostic algorithm. The causes of hemodialysis access failure are thrombosis, outflow stenosis, or inflow stenosis.

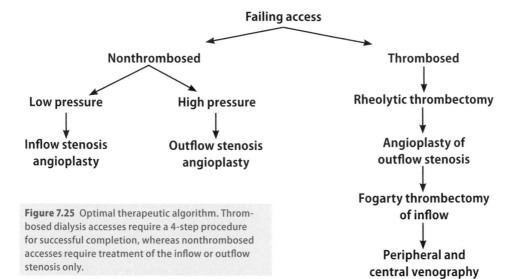

Figure 7.25 Optimal therapeutic algorithm. Thrombosed dialysis accesses require a 4-step procedure for successful completion, whereas nonthrombosed accesses require treatment of the inflow or outflow stenosis only.

Optimal Therapeutic Algorithm

The therapeutic approach to thrombosed dialysis fistulas and grafts entails a 4-step procedure (Figure 7.25). The approach to nonthrombosed dialysis fistulas and grafts entails an abbreviated form of the 4-step approach and focuses on the treatment of the underlying inflow or outflow stenosis.

References

1. Weiswasser JM, Sidawy AN. Strategies of arteriovenous dialysis access. In: Rutherford RB, ed. *Vascular Surgery*. Philadelphia: Elsevier Saunders; 2005:1669-1676.

2. Hodges TC, Fillinger MF, Zwolak RM, Walsh DB, Bech F, Cronenwett JL. Longitudinal comparison of dialysis graft access methods: risk factors for failure. *J Vasc Surg.* 1997;26:1009-1019.

3. Anonymous. NKF-K/DOQI clinical practice guidelines for vascular access: update 2000. *Am J Kidney Dis.* 2001;37:S137-S181.

4. Collins AJ, Foley RN, Herzog C, et al. Excerpts from the United States Renal Data System 2007 annual data report. *Am J Kidney Dis.* 2008;51(Suppl 1):S1-S320.

5. US Renal Data System. USRDS 2004 Annual Data Report: atlas of end-stage renal disease in the United States. *Am J Kidney Dis.* 2005;45(Suppl 1):S1-S280.

6. Kurella TM, Covinsky KE, Chertow GM, Yaffe K, Landefeld CS, McCulloch CE. Functional status of elderly adults before and after initiation of dialysis. *N Engl J Med.* 2009;361:1539-1547.

7. Chueng AK, Sarnak MJ, Yan G, et al. Cardiac diseases in maintenance hemodialysis patients: results of the HEMO Study. *Kidney Int.* 2004;65:2380-2389.

8. Herzog CA, Ma JZ, Collins AJ. Poor long-term survival after acute myocardial infarction among patients on long-term dialysis. *N Engl J Med.* 1998;339:799-805.

9. Vascular Access 2006 Work Group. NKF-DOQI clinical practice guidelines for vascular access, update 2006. *Am J Kidney Dis.* 2006;48(Suppl 1):S176-S306.

10. Jindal K, Chan CT, Deziel C, et al. Hemodialysis clinical practice guidelines for the Canadian Society of Nephrology. *J Am Soc Nephrol.* 2006;17:S1-S27.

11. Ohira S, Naito H, Amono I, et al. 2005 Japanese Society for Dialysis Therapy guidelines for vascular access construction and repair for chronic hemodialysis. *Ther Apher Dial.* 2006;10:449-62.

12. Sidawy AN, Gray R, Besarab A, et al. Recommended standards for reports dealing with

arteriovenous hemodialysis accesses. *J Vasc Surg*. 2002;35:603-610.

13. Beathard GA, Arnold P, Jackson J, Litchfield T. Aggressive treatment of early fistula failure. *Kidney Int*. 2003;64:1487-1484.

14. Achkar K, Nassar GM. Salvage of a severely dysfunctional arteriovenous fistula with a strictured and occluded outflow tract. *Semin Dial*. 2005;18:336-342.

15. Bittl JA, von Mering GO, Feldman RL. Adaptive remodeling of hypoplastic hemodialysis fistulas salvaged with angioplasty. *Catheter Cardiovasc Interv*. 2009;73:974-978.

16. Swedberg SH, Brown BG, Sigley R, Wight TN, Gordon D, Nicholls SC. Intimal fibromuscular hyperplasia at the venous anastomosis of PTFE grafts in hemodialysis patients. Clinical, immunocytochemical, light and electron microscopic assessment. *Circulation*. 1989;80:1726-1736.

17. Roy-Chaudhury P, Kelly BS, Miller MA, et al. Venous neointimal hyperplasia in polytetrafluoroethylene dialysis grafts. *Kidney Int*. 2001;59:2325-2334.

18. Bittl JA. Catheter interventions for hemodialysis fistulas and grafts. *J Am Coll Cardiol Interv*. 2010;3:1-11.

19. Bittl JA, Feldman RL. Prospective assessment of hemodialysis access patency after percutaneous intervention: Cox proportional hazards analysis. *Catheter Cardiovasc Interv*. 2005;66:309-315.

20. Kanterman RY, Vesely TM, Pilgram TK, Guy BW, Windus DW, Picus D. Dialysis access grafts: anatomic location of venous stenosis and results of angioplasty. *Radiology*. 1995;195(1):135-139.

21. Beathard GA. Angioplasty for arteriovenous grafts and fistulae. *Semin Nephrol*. 2002;22:202-210.

22. Valji K. Transcatheter treatment of thrombosed hemodialysis access grafts. *AJR Am J Roentgenol*. 1995;164:823-829.

23. Asif A, Gadalean FN, Merrill D, et al. Inflow stenosis in arteriovenous fistulas and grafts: a multicenter, prospective study. *Kidney Int*. 2005;67:1986-1992.

24. Berman SS, Gentile AT. Impact of secondary procedures in autogenous arteriovenous fistula maturation and maintenance. *J Vasc Surg*. 2002;34:866-771.

25. Dember LM, Beck GJ, Allon M, et al. Effect of clopidogrel on early failure of arteriovenous fistulas for hemodialysis: a randomized controlled trial. *JAMA*. 2008;299:2164-2171.

26. Dixon BS, Beck GJ, Vazquez MA, et al. Effect of dipyridamole plus aspirin on hemodialysis graft patency. *N Engl J Med*. 2009;360:2191-2201.

27. Patel ST, Hughes J, Mills JL Sr. Failure of arteriovenous fistula maturation: an unintended consequence of exceeding Dialysis Outcome Quality Initiative guidelines for hemodialysis access. *J Vasc Surg*. 2003;38:439-445.

28. Hakaim A, Nalbandian M, Scott T. Superior maturation and patency of primary brachiocephalic and transposed basilic vein arteriovenous fistulae in patients with diabetes. *J Vasc Surg*. 1998;27:154-157.

29. Huber MS, Mooney JF, Madison J, Mooney MR. Use of a morphologic classification to predict clinical outcome after dissection from coronary angioplasty. *Am J Cardiol*. 1991;68:467-471.

30. Perera GB, Mueller MP, Kubaska SM, Wilson SE, Lawrence PF, Fujitani RM. Superiority of autogenous arteriovenous hemodialysis access: maintenance of function with fewer secondary interventions. *Ann Vasc Surg*. 2004;18:66-73.

31. Schwartz C, McBrayer C, Sloan J, Meneses P, Ennis W. Thrombosed dialysis grafts: comparison of treatment with transluminal angioplasty and surgical revision. *Radiology*. 1995;194:337-341.

32. Schwab SJ. Vascular access for hemodialysis. *Kidney Int*. 1999;55:2078-2090.

33. Malik J, Slavikova M, Svobodova J, Tuka V. Regular ultrasonographic screening significantly prolongs patency of PTFE grafts. *Kidney Int*. 2005;67:1554-1558.

34. Lilly RZ, Carlton D, Barker J, et al. Predictors of arteriovenous graft patency after radiologic intervention in hemodialysis patients. *Am J Kidney Dis*. 2001;37:945-953.

35. Bruns SD, Jennings WC. Proximal radial artery as inflow site for native arteriovenous fistula. *J Am Coll Surg*. 2003;197:58-63.

36. Domoto DT, Bauman JE, Joist JH. Combined aspirin and sulfinpyrazone in the prevention of recurrent hemodialysis vascular access thrombosis. *Thromb Res.* 1991;62:737-743.

37. Kaufman JS, O'Connor TZ, Zhang JH, et al. Randomized controlled trial of clopidogrel plus aspirin to prevent hemodialysis access graft thrombosis. *J Am Soc Nephrol.* 2003;14:2313-2321.

38. Sreedhara R, Himmelfarb J, Lazarus JM, Hakim RM. Anti-platelet therapy in graft thrombosis: results of a prospective, randomized double-blind study. *Kidney Int.* 1994;45:1477-1483.

39. Knoll GA, Wells PS, Young D, et al. Thrombophilia and the risk for hemodialysis vascular access thrombosis. *J Am Soc Nephrol.* 2005;16:1108-1114.

40. Gelabert HA, Freischlag JA. Angioaccess. In: Rutherford RB, ed. *Vascular Surgery.* 4th ed. Philadelphia: W.B. Saunders, 2000:1466-1477.

41. Beathard GA, Litchfield T. Effectiveness and safety of dialysis vascular access procedures performed by interventional nephrologists. *Kidney Int.* 2004;66:1622-1632.

42. Vascular Access 2006 Work Group. NKF-DOQI clinical practice guidelines for vascular access, update 2006: Clinical practice recommendations for guideline 4: detection of access dysfunction: monitoring, surveillance, and diagnostic testing. *Am J Kidney Dis.* 2006;48 (Suppl 1):S269-S270.

43. Beathard GA. Percutaneous transvenous angioplasty in the treatment of vascular access stenosis. *Kidney Int.* 1992;42:1390-1397.

44. Woods JD, Turenne MN, Strawderman RL, et al. Vascular access survival among incident hemodialysis patients in the United States. *Am J Kidney Dis.* 1997;30:50-57.

45. Beathard GA. Management of complications of endovascular dialysis access procedures. *Semin Dial.* 2003;16:309-313.

46. Raynaud AC, Angel CY, Sapoval MR, Beyssen B, Pagny JY, Auguste M. Treatment of hemodialysis access rupture during PTA with Wallstent implantation. *J Vasc Interv Radiol.* 1998;9:437-442.

47. Sofocleous CT, Schur I, Koh E, et al. Percutaneous treatment of complications occurring during hemodialysis graft recanalization. *Eur J Radiol.* 2003;47:237-246.

48. Funaki B, Szymski GX, Leef JA, Rosenblum JD, Burke R, Hackworth CA. Wallstent deployment to salvage dialysis graft thrombolysis complicated by venous rupture: early and intermediate results. *AJR Am J Roentgenol.* 1997;169:1435-1437.

49. Bittl JA. Venous rupture during percutaneous treatment of hemodialysis fistulas and grafts. *Catheter Cardiovasc Interv.* 2009;74:1097-1101.

50. Petronis JD, Regan F, Briefel G, Simpson PM, Hess JM, Contoreggi CS. Ventilation-perfusion scintigraphic evaluation of pulmonary clot burden after percutaneous thrombolysis of clotted hemodialysis access grafts. *Am J Kidney Dis.* 1999;34:207-211.

51. Martin LG, MacDonald MJ, Kikeri D, Cotsonis GA, Harker LA, Lumsden AB. Prophylactic angioplasty reduces thrombosis in virgin ePTFE arteriovenous dialysis grafts with greater than 50% stenosis: subset analysis of a prospectively randomized study. *J Vasc Interv Radiol.* 1999;10:389-396.

52. Schwab SJ, Oliver MJ, Suhocki P, McCann R. Hemodialysis arteriovenous access: detection of stenosis and response to treatment by vascular access blood flow. *Kidney Int.* 2001;59:358-362.

53. Tessitore N, Bedogna V, Poli A, et al. Adding access blood flow surveillance to clinical monitoring reduces thrombosis rates and costs, and improves fistula patency in the short term: a controlled cohort study. *Nephrol Dial Transplant.* 2008;23:3578-3584.

54. Dember LM, Holmberg EF, Kaufman JS. Randomized controlled trial of prophylactic repair of hemodialysis arteriovenous graft stenosis. *Kidney Int.* 2004;66:390-398.

55. Moist LM, Churchill DN, House AA, et al. Regular monitoring of access flow compared with monitoring of venous pressure fails to improve graft survival. *J Am Soc Nephrol.* 2003;14:2645-2653.

56. Bittl JA, Cohen DJ, Seek MM, Feldman RL. Economic analysis of angiography and pre-

emptive angioplasty to prevent hemodialysis-access thrombosis. *Cathet Cardiovasc Interv.* 2010;75:14-21.

57. Haskal ZJ, Trerotola S, Dolmatch B, et al. Stent graft versus balloon angioplasty for failing dialysis-access grafts. *N Engl J Med.* 2010;362:494-503.

58. Parikh S, Nori D, Rogers D, et al. External beam radiation therapy to prevent postangioplasty dialysis access restenosis: a feasibility study. *Cardiovasc Radiat Med.* 1999;1:36-41.

59. Rotmans JI, Heyliger JMM, Verhagen HJM, et al. In vivo seeding using anti-CD34 antibodies successfully accelerates endothelialization but stimulates intimal hyperplasia in porcine arteriovenous expanded polytetrafluoroethylene grafts. *Circulation.* 2005;112:12-18.

60. Vogel PM, Parise C. SMART stent for salvage of hemodialysis access grafts. *J Vasc Interv Radiol.* 2004;15:1051-1060.

61. Sreenarasimhaiah VP, Margassery SK, Martin KJ, Bander SJ. Salvage of thrombosed dialysis access grafts with venous anastomosis stents. *Kidney Int.* 2005;67:678-684.

62. Aruny JE. Dialysis access shunt and fistula recanalization. In: Kandarpa K, Aruny JE, eds. *Handbook of Interventional and Radiologic Procedures.* Boston: Little, Brown; 1996:115-124.

63. Bittl JA, Feldman RL. Cutting balloon angioplasty for undilatable venous stenoses causing dialysis graft failure. *Catheter Cardiovasc Interv.* 2003;58:524-526.

64. Vesely TM, Siegel JB. Use of the peripheral cutting balloon to treat hemodialysis-related stenoses. *J Vasc Interv Radiol.* 2005;16:1593-1603.

65. Wu CC, Sen SC. Cutting balloon angioplasty for resistant venous stenoses of dialysis access: immediate and patency results. *Cathet Cardiovasc Interv.* 2008;71:250-254.

66. Levit RD, Cohen RM, Kwak A, et al. Asymptomatic central venous stenosis in hemodialysis patients. *Radiology.* 2006;238:1051-1056.

Part 4

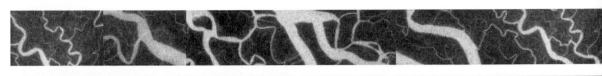

Aortic, Visceral, and Renal Artery Disease

8

Diseases of the Thoracic Aorta

Mark F. Conrad and Richard P. Cambria

Unlike the abdominal aorta, wherein degenerative aneurysm and some element of aortoiliac occlusive disease are the pathologies of concern, the thoracic aorta is potentially involved with a spectrum of pathologies whose management involves the full expertise of cardiovascular specialists. Certain of these pathologies, such as uncomplicated type B aortic dissections and giant cell arteritis, are typically managed primarily or exclusively with medical therapies. Alternatively, entities such as traumatic aortic tear are circumstances in which acute interventions are typically required. Additional considerations make a thorough understanding of natural history and clinical decision-making prescient. To wit, conventional surgical treatment of thoracic aortic pathologies is accompanied by significant morbidity and mortality when compared, for example, to repair of abdominal aortic aneurysm. Finally, the recent emergence of stent-graft repair in the thoracic aorta (which is likely the most important advance in the treatment of thoracic aortic pathology in our lifetime) has the potential to substantially diminish the morbidity of surgical repair, and even alter long-standing treatment paradigms.

In this chapter, we review the spectrum of thoracic aortic pathologies, emphasizing natural history data and clinical decision making rather than technical nuances of interventions. Recognizing that the ultimate role of stent-graft repair in a number of pathologies is yet to be defined, an update on the indications and results of open surgical and/or endovascular repair is presented.

The Thoracic Aorta

From the standpoint of implications for interventional therapies, the *thoracic aorta* can be divided into 3 segments: the *ascending aorta*, the *aortic arch*, and the *descending aorta* extending to the diaphragmatic hiatus; beyond same is the *visceral aortic segment* wherein the renal and visceral vessels arise. Often, various lengths of the descending aorta have in continuity pathology with the visceral and/or abdominal aorta; such lesions are referred to as "thoracoabdominal" in extent (Figure 8.1). The ascending aorta arises from the heart at the level of the aortic valve and follows an anterior course in the

Vascular Disease: Diagnostic and Therapeutic Approaches. © 2011 Michael R. Jaff and Christopher J. White, editors. Cardiotext Publishing, ISBN: 978-1-935395-16-4.

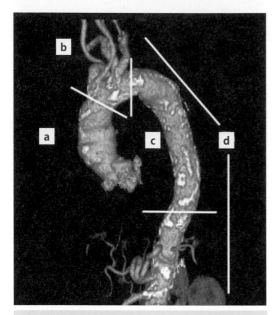

Figure 8.1 Helical CT 3D reconstruction of the aorta. The ascending aorta begins at the aortic root and extends to the innominate artery (a). The aortic arch includes the great vessels (b). The descending thoracic aorta begins at the left subclavian artery and extends to the diaphragm (c). The thoracoabdominal aorta includes the descending aorta and the infra-diaphragmatic aorta to the iliac bifurcation (d).

right chest toward the mediastinum, ending at the innominate artery. The aortic arch begins with the innominate artery and traverses the mediastinum along a posterior course to the left chest. The arch gives rise to the great vessels, including the innominate artery, the left carotid artery, and the left subclavian artery. The descending thoracic aorta begins beyond the transverse arch, distal to the left subclavian artery and traverses the left chest to the level of the diaphragm.

Degenerative Aneurysms of the Thoracic and Thoracoabdominal Aorta

There are 2 morphologic classifications of true aneurysms (ie, composed of native aortic wall):

fusiform, defined as a circumferential expansion of the aorta, and *saccular,* which is characterized by an asymmetric bulge in the involved arterial segment. A false aneurysm, or pseudoaneurysm, is defined as being bound by inflammatory or fibrotic tissue rather than the aortic wall per se, representing a contained rupture of the aorta.

Classification of Thoracic Aneurysms

The ascending aorta can be divided into 2 portions: the *sinus portion* proximally and the *tubular portion* distally. The sinus portion is also know as the aortic root and encompasses the aortic valve, the sinus of Valsalva, and the origins of the coronary arteries. The sinus and tubular portions join at the most superior aspect of the valve commissures at a point appropriately termed the *sinotubular junction.* The tubular portion begins at the sinotubular junction and extends to the innominate artery distally.

Descending thoracic aortic aneurysms are classified as confined to the thoracic aorta or involving the thoracic and abdominal aortae. The latter, termed *thoracoabdominal aortic aneurysms,* are classified according to the scheme originally devised by Crawford that in the most basic terms considers whether the lesion is primarily a caudal extension of a descending thoracic aneurysm, or a cephalad extension of a total abdominal aortic aneurysm (Figure 8.2). This classification is especially useful in patients requiring operative repair, since it has direct implications for both the technical conduct of operation and the incidence of operative complications; in particular, ischemic spinal cord injury. However, the classification scheme outlined in Figure 8.2 does not consider the patient with a contiguous aneurysm involving parts or all of the ascending aorta and aortic arch. While synchronous proximal aneurysms are noted in 6% to 13% of degenerative thoracic aortic aneurysm patients, contiguous arch and thoracoabdominal aneurysms are rare, typically occurring only in patients with a prior ascending aortic dissection and/or those with Marfan's syndrome.[1]

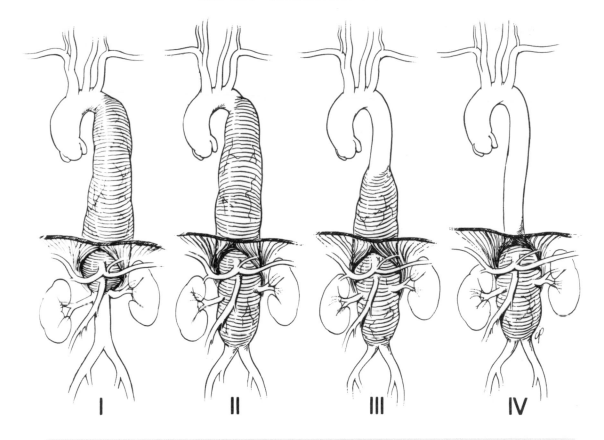

Figure 8.2 Crawford classification of thoracoabdominal aneurysms.

Etiology and Pathogenesis

The ascending thoracic aorta and arch derive their embryonic origin from the aortic sac, while the descending thoracic aorta is formed by the fusion of the paired dorsal aortae.[2] As a result, the ascending thoracic aorta differs from the descending thoracoabdominal aorta in structure and cell biology. In the ascending aorta, the intima is thin and the media is thick when compared to the descending thoracic aorta, in which the opposite is true. In addition, the thoracic aorta (compared to the abdominal aorta) has a higher content of collagen and elastin but a lower collagen to elastin ratio.[3,4] Finally, the vascular smooth muscle cells of the ascending aorta are derived from the neural crest, while those of the descending aorta originate from mesodermal and endothelial cells.[5,6] Nearly 60% of thoracic aortic aneurysms involve the ascending aorta or the aortic root, while the remaining 40% affect the descending aorta. There is over-lap of aortic segments in many cases, with 10% of thoracic aneurysms involving the aortic arch and 10% involving the thoracoabdominal aorta. The etiology, pathogenesis, natural history, and therapeutic principles differ with each segment.

Descending thoracic aorta

Aneurysms of the descending thoracic aorta develop through a complex process involving a combination of genetic and environmental factors. The majority of thoracic aortic aneurysms are degenerative in nature, and indistinguishable on either gross or microscopic pathology from the more typically encountered *abdominal aortic aneurysm (AAA)*. However, genetic predisposition remains an important etiologic factor as 20% to 30% of aortic aneurysm patients have a first-order relative with the disease.[7,8] While there continues to be debate over whether aneurysmal degeneration is a sequela of atherosclerosis or a primary connective tissue weakness,[7,9] recent studies have shown that although there is significant overlap between the 2 populations, the propensity to develop weakening of the adventitia and media seen with aneurysmal disease is certainly different from the intimal proliferative process associated with atherosclerosis. Indeed, both processes can diminish aortic compliance and wall tensile strength, resulting in aneurysm formation such that the terms "atherosclerotic" and "degenerative" are used interchangeably when applied to aortic aneurysms.

The second most common etiology of descending thoracic aortic aneurysms is as the sequela of chronic aortic dissection.[10-14] Of patients experiencing acute aortic dissection, 25% to 40% will develop chronic aneurysmal dilatation of the outer wall of the false lumen, which renders them susceptible to late aneurysm rupture and death.[15-19] Other causes are less common. Aneurysms secondary to the sequelae of giant cell arteritis are typically seen in women and can result from either Takayasu's arteritis or the nonspecific variety of giant cell aortitis. In addition, there may be no known prior diagnosis of aortitis or other associated collagen vascular disease. Such aneurysms can be either focal or diffuse along the thoracoabdominal aorta, and are frequently associated with other known sequelae of inflammatory aortitis, namely, visceral aneurysms, and renal artery occlusive disease.

Patients with Marfan's syndrome may have true cystic medial necrosis, a rare pathology that predisposes the thoracic aorta to aneurysmal degeneration and dissection. Marfan's syndrome is an autosomal dominant, inherited mutation of the *fibrillin-1* gene, a structural protein that is the major component of the microfibrils that form elastin. Such mutations lead to a decrease in the amount of elastin in the aortic wall and the deposition of disarrayed microfibrillar connective tissue precipitating subsequent aortic degeneration. Aortic root aneurysms that predispose patients to acute dissection represent the single most common vascular manifestation of Marfan's, followed by aortic dissection.[20]

Thoracic aortic aneurysms secondary to an infectious process present challenging management issues because the dual goals of eradication of sepsis and arterial reconstruction typically demand an in situ type of reconstruction, that is, placement of a prosthetic graft in a contaminated field. The term *mycotic aneurysm* continues to be applied to these lesions, although this term more precisely relates to aneurysms that develop secondary to embolization from infected cardiac vegetations. In contemporary practice, the pathogenesis of these lesions is usually hematogenous seeding of atherosclerotic plaque that leads to the development of focal aortitis and dissolution of the aortic wall resulting in the formation of a false aneurysm. All such aneurysms are, in fact, contained aortic ruptures.

Our data are consistent with published reviews regarding the distribution of the various etiologies of thoracic aneurysms, namely, some 80% are degenerative, 15% to 20% the sequelae of chronic dissection (including 5% of patients with Marfan's syndrome), 2% are related to infection, and 1% to 2% are the sequelae of previous aortitis.[11,21]

Ascending aorta

Unlike those of the descending aorta, cystic medial degeneration, characterized by a loss of vascular smooth muscle cells and elastic fiber destruction, is the most common etiology of ascending aortic aneurysms. This process is a normal consequence of aging to some extent but has been found to be greatly accelerated in patients who are hypertensive[22] and those who develop aneurysmal dilatation of the ascending aorta.[4] Aneurysms that involve the aortic root are termed *annulo-aortic ectasia* and are often associated with well-defined connective tissue disorders such as Marfan's syndrome, Ehler-Danlos syndrome, or a bicuspid aortic valve.[23]

Other causes of ascending aortic aneurysms are less common. Bacterial infection is a rare etiology that is usually secondary to endocarditis or seeding of laminar clot within an existing aneurysm. The most common causal organisms include *Staphylococcus aureus* and epidermidis, salmonella, and *Streptococcus* species.[23] Although syphilis was once the most common cause of ascending aortic aneurysms, aggressive early treatment with appropriate antibiotics has made luetic aneurysms rare. Aortitis is another rare cause of ascending aortic aneurysms. Takayasu's arteritis is a chronic inflammatory disease that typically causes obliterative luminal changes but is associated with a 15% incidence of aortic dilation, which ultimately results in aneurysm formation.[13] Giant cell arteritis typically affects the temporal or cranial arteries but it can also produce aneurysms of the ascending aorta. Finally, *pseudoaneurysms* can occur secondary to trauma, infection, or iatrogenically at the site of a previous aortic cannulation.

Natural History

The expected natural history of thoracic aortic aneurysms is progressive enlargement and eventual rupture regardless of etiology or location. Since thoracic aneurysms are uncommon when compared to AAA, fewer natural history studies are available. Furthermore, natural history studies of degenerative thoracic aneurysms often include aortic dissections that may skew results as many of these patients succumb during the acute phase of the disease.[24,25] Finally, women make up half of thoracic aneurysm patients as opposed to 10% to 20% of those with AAA making size criteria for operation in thoracic aneurysms less clearly defined than for AAA.

A recent longitudinal study found that the mean rate of growth for all thoracic aneurysms is 0.1 cm per year. Aneurysm growth is greater for descending thoracic aneurysms (0.19 cm/year) than for the ascending aorta (0.07 cm/year) and it is also accelerated in patients with dissections and connective tissue disorders such as Marfan's syndrome.[26] The size of the aorta at initial diagnosis has been shown to be an important predictor of future dilation, but there still remains substantial variation in individual aneurysm growth rates making prediction of future aortic size difficult.[13]

Population-based studies, since they are exempt from the inherent bias of referral center series, offer the best insight. Two studies performed 20 years ago form the foundation of descending thoracic aneurysm epidemiology. These studies reported an incidence of 5.9 descending thoracic aortic aneurysms per 100,000 patient-years over a 30-year period.[24] When left untreated, the actuarial 3-year survival was 35% and the 5-year survival was a mere 13%, with aneurysm rupture identified as the cause of death in nearly 75% of patients (> 50% of these patients were not known to have an aneurysm prior to their death).[24,27] Johansson et al[25] reported that the incidence of rupture of all thoracic aortic aneurysm during 2 separate time intervals (1980 and 1989) was 5 per 100,000 patients and remained stable over the decade examined. Rupture was nearly uniformly fatal, and approximately half of all ruptures occurred in the ascending aorta. These investigators also found that there was an equal gender distribution with respect to ruptured thoracic aortic aneurysm; however, these data are clearly complicated by the inclusion of acute proximal aortic dissections.

Recently, Clouse and associates[28] reevaluated the prognosis of degenerative thoracic aortic aneurysms found in Olmsted County, Minnesota, between 1980 and 1994. The descending aorta was the principal segment affected in 60% of patients. This study was notable in that while the overall 5-year rupture risk was 20%, and 24% of patients required surgery, significantly more (nearly 80%) ruptures occurred in women, and female gender was identified as an independent variable predicting rupture (relative risk [RR] 6.8; 95% CI, 2.3–19.9; $P = 0.01$). In a prospective evaluation of the natural history of thoracic aneurysms, Juvonen et al[29] also identified patient age, the presence of pain (even atypical), and a history of chronic obstructive pulmonary disease as patient-specific independent risk factors for rupture. Aneurysm-specific variables also strongly correlating with rupture included symptoms attributable to the aneurysm and dissection developing within the degenerative aneurysm, further establishing their importance in surgical decision making as emphasized by others.[29,30] Finally, increasing aneurysm size led to higher rupture risk, where aneurysms that were > 6cm had a 30% 5-year rupture rate while those that were < 4cm had a rupture rate of essentially 0, and, rupture accounted for 30% of all deaths, occurring with an incidence of 3.5 per 100,000 patient-years.[31]

The size criteria recommendations for operative repair of descending thoracic aortic aneurysms were inferred from a series of 117 patients treated for rupture. Crawford and associates[32] noted that 80% of all ruptures occurred in aneurysms less than 10 cm, dispelling the previously held myth that only exceedingly large thoracic aneurysms ruptured. Rupture occurred with smaller-sized aneurysms when

acute dissection was the causative pathology, and indeed, 13% of all ruptures occurred at a site where the aneurysm was less than 6 cm. In addition, rupture was observed in 10% of patients with aneurysms less than 6 cm in diameter and the authors recommended elective operation when a 5-cm diameter threshold was exceeded. More recent referral center reports have advanced insight into the expected natural history and rupture risk of patients considered for descending thoracic and thoracoabdominal aneurysm resection. These valuable data have delineated both patient-specific and aneurysm-specific factors that influence prognosis (Table 8.1). Descending thoracic aneurysms appear to expand at more rapid rates as they become

Prognostic Factors (End Point)		
Reference	Aneurysm-Specific	Patient-Specific
Cambria et al[33]	Size ≥ 5 cm (rupture)	COPD (expansion, rupture trend) Chronic renal failure (rupture trend)
Dapunt et al[34]	Size ≥ 5 cm (expansion, survival)	Smoking (expansion)
Perko et al[35]	Dissection (rupture) Size ≥ 6 cm (rupture, survival)	Hypertension (survival) Respiratory insufficiency (survival) Renal failure (rupture, survival)
Masuda et al[36]	Size (expansion) Abdominal aneurysmal disease (expansion)	Diastolic hypertension (expansion) Renal failure (expansion)
Griepp et al[37]	Dissection (rupture, survival) Smaller max size (dissection rupture) Increasing extent (rupture)	Age (rupture) Hypertension (dissection rupture) COPD (rupture) Pain-even atypical (rupture)
Coady et al[38,39]	Size ≥ 6 cm (rupture or dissection)	None
Bonser et al[40]	Intraluminal thrombus (expansion) Mid descending aorta (expansion)	Smoking (expansion) Prior stroke (expansion) Peripheral vascular disease (expansion)
Juvonen et al[29,41]	Size ≥ 5 cm (smaller max for dissection rupture)	Age (rupture) COPD (rupture) Pain-even atypical (rupture) Hypertension (dissection rupture)
Lobato et al[42]	Size ≥ 5 cm (rupture) Expansion (rupture)	None
Davies et al[26]	Size ≥ 5 cm (rupture) Size ≥ 6 cm (rupture or acute dissection) Descending aorta (survival) Elective repair (survival) Expansion (rupture trend)	Female gender (rupture or acute dissection) Prior stroke (rupture or acute dissection) Marfan's syndrome (rupture or acute dissection)

Table 8.1 Reports from Referral Centers Describing Thoracic/Thoracoabdominal Aortic Aneurysm Prognosis. (Note: Prognostic factors are stratified by aneurysm- and patient-specific factors and the end points of individual studies are depicted in parentheses.)

larger, and several investigators have correlated increased expansion rates with rupture.[36,42,43] Further, these studies indicate rupture risk is negligible in aneurysms less than 5 cm, is equivalent to the risk of surgical morbidity in the 5- to 6-cm range, and increases substantially at aneurysm diameters larger than 6 cm and/or growth rates of ≥ 10 mm per year. To wit, 6 cm is the surgical threshold to consider intervention in patients with degenerative aneurysms of the descending thoracic aorta.

Ascending aortic aneurysms grow at an average rate of 1 to 4 mm per year, and major event risk (ie, rupture or dissection) varies with location and primary cause.[23] Joyce et al[44] evaluated the natural history of ascending aortic aneurysms and found that the 5-year survival of patients with aneurysmal diameters > 6 cm was 38%, while those with aneurysms < 6 cm had a 5-year survival of 61%. In addition, Coady et al[38] noted that the incidence of dissection and rupture increased with aneurysm size and identified 6 cm as the median size at the time of dissection and rupture for ascending aortic aneurysms. Factors contributing to risk of expansion and rupture include the presence of a chronic dissection, the size of the aneurysm at the time of diagnosis, and the etiology. Marfan's syndrome deserves special mention because 90% of deaths from Marfan's syndrome are associated with complications related to the ascending aorta.[45] As these aortic root aneurysms grow beyond 6 cm, the potential for dissection, rupture, and aortic regurgitation increases so that most authors recommend elective repair at 5.0 cm in these patients.[38,46]

These natural history observations have led to the acceptance of 6 cm as a generally appropriate size threshold for recommendation of surgical intervention for degenerative ascending and descending thoracic aneurysms and 5.0 to 5.5 cm for aneurysms involving the abdominal aorta. Increasing expansion rate is used as an indicator of heightened rupture risk as is the presence of aortic tenderness, and, in such cases, consideration is given to earlier operation. In the cases of chronic dissection and Marfan's syndrome, a 5-cm size threshold is maintained due to rupture tendency at smaller sizes.[37,39,41]

Clinical Presentation

Although patients commonly present in an asymptomatic fashion with incidental detection during radiologic surveillance for other causes, symptoms referable to thoracic aneurysms do occur and should be evaluated in a timely manner. In addition to the acute onset of severe pain, which may be associated with aneurysm expansion, rupture, and/or acute dissection, large thoracic aneurysms may produce symptoms of back, epigastric, or flank pain related either to compression of local structures or to chronic inflammatory changes of the mediastinal pleura. Unlike AAA, where back pain usually indicates an acute event, the pain associated with thoracic aneurysms may be atypical or chronic in nature. Juvonen et al[29,41] noted that the presence of even uncharacteristic pain is an independent risk factor of rupture and stated that the dismissal of such complaints (even if they are chronic) in patients with a history of thoracic aneurysms is inappropriate and can have morbid consequences. Frequently, pain is localized to the left lower hemithorax or, when the aneurysm is largest in the region of the aortic hiatus, pain is experienced in the midback and epigastrium. When the aneurysm erodes into the thoracolumbar spine or chest wall, complaints of chest and back pain can be prominent and again, may be present for weeks or even months. In severe cases, such complaints are often related to a chronic state of contained aneurysm rupture. In the ascending thoracic aorta, compression of the overlying sternum can result in chronic anterior chest pain, which has been reported by 25% to 75% of these patients.[23]

Depending on the topography of the aneurysm, other symptoms may be referable to a variety of compression and/or erosion phenomena. The new onset of hoarseness can be related to a left recurrent laryngeal nerve palsy, while compression or erosion of the tracheobronchial tree or pulmonary parenchyma will produce a chronic cough, hemoptysis, or dyspnea, and, dysphasia lusoria is a possible but uncommon symptomatic manifestation of thoracic aneurysms.[47] Similar to AAA, distal embolization of atheromatous debris has been observed, but it has constituted a rare indication for operation in our experience.

Perhaps related to reluctance to recommend operation because of the threat of surgical morbidity, up to 40% of thoracic aortic aneurysm patients will present with symptoms.[11,14] This explains the higher incidence of patients treated for rupture when compared to AAA operations. Our results are consistent with those available from a review of the literature indicating that some 25% of patients will be treated under urgent or emergent circumstances, with approximately half of these presenting with a frank rupture.[11,14,48-50] Unfortunately, we and others have demonstrated that such nonelective operations are associated with a significant increase in morbidity.[51,52]

Associated Diseases

Associated vascular diseases and comorbid conditions are commonplace in patients presenting for treatment of thoracic aneurysms. Synchronous aneurysms typically involving the ascending aorta or arch have been observed in some 10% of patients being evaluated for descending thoracic aneurysm repair, and a familial aneurysm history has been identified in 7.5% of our thoracic and thoracoabdominal aneurysm patients. Prior operation for aortic aneurysm disease is seen in one-third of patients and as noted, the most common of these is a previous infrarenal aneurysm repair. In addition, Coselli et al[53] detailed experience in 123 patients undergoing thoracic aneurysm resection after a prior infrarenal AAA repair. These patients were likely to present with symptoms at a mean interval of 8.2 ± 5.4 years after the initial AAA resection.

Since the majority of patients seen in consideration for descending thoracic aneurysm resection are those with degenerative aneurysms, demographic and clinical features typical of a patient population with diffuse atherosclerosis

are the rule. Patients treated for degenerative aneurysm average 70 years in age, and a history of hypertension is nearly universal. Cigarette smoking and/or significant *chronic obstructive pulmonary disease (COPD)* are frequently encountered. Pulmonary function studies have been routinely performed prior to operation, and 25% of patients will have significant COPD as manifested by an FEV1 of less than 50% predicted. Cerebrovascular disease, prior stroke, and symptomatic manifestations of lower-extremity arterial occlusive disease occur in 15% of patients.

Associated visceral and renovascular occlusive disease to some degree has been reported in 30% of patients.[54] Indeed, in our experience, 15% of patients had significant renal insufficiency as manifested by a preoperative serum creatinine of $\geq$ 1.8 mg/dL.[11] The coexistence of renovascular disease and some degree of renal insufficiency is especially commonplace in patients with thoracoabdominal aneurysms and has important implications for accurate assessment of perioperative risk and long-term preservation of renal function. Because, the majority of thoracoabdominal aneurysms present with involvement of the entire visceral aortic segment, occlusive lesions of the mesenteric and renal arteries or total ostial occlusion of one or more of these vessels frequently accompanies aneurysmal dilation of this region of the aorta. Accordingly, we believe extreme levels of preoperative azotemia (serum creatinine greater than 2.5 cm/dL) constitute a relative contraindication to elective operation unless preoperative studies indicate some potential for salvage or retrieval of renal function with renal artery reconstruction. In many series, the presence of an abnormal preoperative serum creatinine is at least a univariate correlate of perioperative mortality.[11,14,48,55-57] Indeed, assessment of renal function and associated renovascular disease is an important component of patient evaluation and choice of therapy.

Many patients with ascending aortic aneurysms are found to have an underlying stenotic congenitally bicuspid aortic valve. Although this relationship has long been attributed to a poststenotic dilatation of the ascending aorta, a recent study by Nistri et al[58] identified aortic dilation in 52% of young patients with normally functioning bicuspid aortic valves. Indeed, other studies have demonstrated that aortic dilation associated with a bicuspid valve occurs independently of the functional status of the valve.[13] Although the exact mechanism behind this relationship remains unclear, it is important that patients with a known bicuspid aortic valve should have their ascending aorta imaged regularly.

Diagnostic Imaging

Plain x-ray
Several characteristic findings of thoracic aneurysmal disease seen with a chest x-ray include widening of the mediastinal silhouette, enlargement of the aortic knob, and tracheal deviation. Although thoracic aortic aneurysms are often evident on chest x-ray, it is difficult to differentiate between normal thoracic aortic tortuosity

associated with advancing age (usually identified as an "ectatic aorta" by radiologists) and actual aneurysmal dilatation. Consequently, it is important to have a low threshold for obtaining more detailed imaging when findings associated with aortic pathology are encountered on plain film.

Computed tomography
In contemporary practice, a dynamic, fine-cut, contrast-enhanced *computed tomography (CT) scan* with or without helical reconstruction (Figure 8.3) provides the physician with the following information:

- accurate assessment of aneurysm size and extent;
- a baseline study to which future images may be compared;
- determination of anatomic suitability for endovascular repair;
- if open surgery is required, the anatomic extent of resection and risk of subsequent spinal cord ischemia.

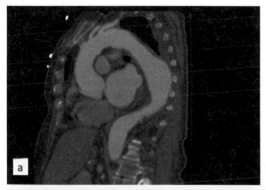

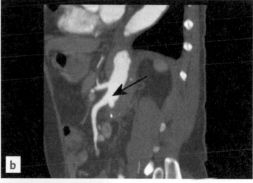

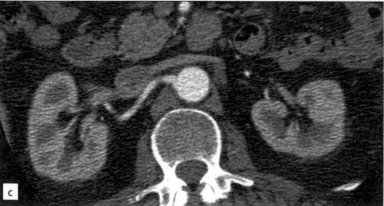

Figure 8.3 Helical CT with reconstruction is the only imaging study required in the majority of cases. It provides evaluation of (a) aortic quality, luminal thrombus, (b) aortic and branch topography (arrow pointing to patent SMA), and (c) renovisceral patency, as well as aortic cross-clamp site or proximal and distal seal zones depending on the planned method of repair.

Accurate assessment of the size of thoracic aortic aneurysms is contingent upon measurement in the appropriate perpendicular plane. When imaging a tortuous aorta or evaluating sections through the aortic arch or lower descending aorta, it is important to understand that individual axial images may section the aorta in a plane that is off axis (Figure 8.4). Such measurements result in an erroneous overestimation of aortic diameter and underscore the importance of personally viewing CT scans prior to initiation of therapy. One way to avoid this error is through 3D reconstruction of the thoracic aorta with determination of the centerline of axis, which ensures that any cross-sectional measurement will be perpendicular to the aortic axis. The quality of current CT scanners with 3D reconstruction is exceptional and in our practice, this has become the image modality of choice for the evaluation and treatment of thoracic aortic aneurysms.

Magnetic resonance imaging

CT scanning of the aortic root is not as accurate as with the rest of the thoracic aorta as motion artifacts related to aortic root pulsation are recognized in nearly 60% of patients.[59] As a result, *magnetic resonance imaging (MRI)* is the preferred imaging modality of this location. Contrast-enhanced MRI and 3D MRI techniques can be used to accurately assess the aorta and have become the imaging investigation of choice for patients with stable aortic disease and a contraindication to contrast such as renal insufficiency or contrast allergy. In general, MRI is susceptible to scatter effects from metal

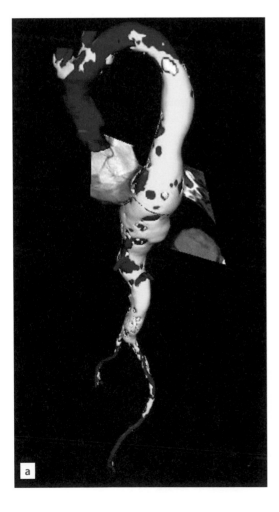

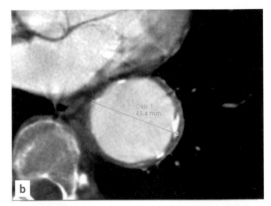

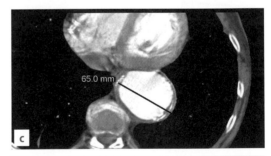

Figure 8.4 Helical CT with reconstruction showing the variation of aortic measurement with changes in axial plane. (a) 3D reconstruction showing adjusted axial plane to ensure diameter measurement along the centerline axis. (b) Axial image along same plane yields diameter of 4.9 cm. (c) Axial image at same level with traditional CT plane overestimates aortic diameter by 1.6 cm.

in stent grafts, making it a less robust option for most postoperative graft surveillance.

Contrast arteriography

Catheter-based aortic angiography was once the diagnostic modality of choice for both open and endovascular repair. However, in contemporary practice, it is rarely used as a purely diagnostic procedure, rather, it is utilized at the time of endovascular repair to ensure accurate placement of stent grafts.

Echocardiography

Transthoracic echocardiography (TTE) is an excellent method of imaging the aortic root. Its benefits include availability, minimal invasiveness, and lack of nephrotoxicity. In skilled hands, TTE can be used to visualize and evaluate the aortic root and segments of the arch with a high degree of accuracy. However, TTE can be limited in sicker patients who require mechanical ventilation or are unable to maintain appropriate positioning.[59] In contrast, the accuracy of *transesophageal echocardiography (TEE)* can be similar to that of quality axial imaging studies in identifying ascending aortic dissections, evaluating root complications, and determining accurate dimensions of the ascending aorta. In addition, TEE can evaluate the structure and function of the aortic and mitral valves yielding information that will help direct therapy in patients with ascending aortic aneurysms. One limitation of TEE is an inability to accurately visualize the aorta at and beyond the level of the diaphragm, and TEE is not used for aortic surveillance because of the invasive nature of the test.

Principles of Therapy

Medical management

Few medical therapies are known to retard the growth of thoracic aortic aneurysms or reduce the risk of the dreaded complications of dissection and rupture. However, blood pressure control with beta-blocker therapy has been shown to decrease the rate of aortic dilation and reduce

aneurysm-related mortality in patients with Marfan's syndrome.[60] Whether it is appropriate to apply these results to patients with degenerative aneurysms of the descending thoracic aorta or ascending aneurysms associated a bicuspid aortic valve is unknown. However, it is intuitive that blood pressure control would be beneficial for all patients with thoracic aneurysms, and most authors recommend beta-blockers as initial therapy for this patient population. The goal of antihypertensive therapy is to keep the systolic pressure at a low-normal range of 105 to 120 mm Hg, and this often requires additional medications to maintain.[13]

Patients should be informed of the typical symptoms of the acute aortic syndrome that could represent aortic expansion, the development of an aortic dissection, or early, contained aortic rupture. These symptoms include significant back, neck, or abdominal pain that occurs abruptly; their presence should prompt the patient to seek medical attention immediately. Risk factor modification is another important aspect of patient education regarding thoracic aneurysms. Patients should be counseled regarding smoking cessation and given appropriate support to achieve this goal.

It should be noted that there is a significant association of cardiovascular disease with thoracic aortic aneurysms, and these should be aggressively identified and controlled. In addition, up to one-quarter of patients with thoracic aortic disease have concomitant AAA, and all patients should undergo baseline imaging of the abdominal and pelvic aorta at the time of initial diagnosis.[13] Finally, because several etiologies of thoracic aortic aneurysms, including Marfan's syndrome and bicuspid aortic valve, are familial, it is important to identify and screen first-degree relatives of patients with these entities.

Open surgical repair of descending thoracic and thoracoabdominal aneurysms

The choice of surgical technique depends upon the anatomy of the aneurysm, including aortic location and distal extent of aortic involvement. In contemporary practice, several schemes of open repair of descending thoracic and thoracoabdominal aneurysms are utilized (Figure 8.5). The 2 general approaches involve a clamp-and-sew technique, often supplemented by adjuncts to minimize complications related to spinal cord, renal, and visceral ischemia versus the use of distal aortic perfusion through an atriofemoral artery bypass circuit. The rationale for distal aortic perfusion is the reduction of ischemic times to the intercostal, visceral, and renal vessels since these vascular beds are perfused during creation of the proximal anastomosis; distal perfusion has been favored for repair of isolated thoracic aneurysms.[61] Clearly, comparable results have been achieved in contemporary practice using both clamp-and-sew and distal perfusion techniques.[11,48,54,62,63] In addition, atriofemoral bypass will provide easily titratable mechanical unloading of the left ventricle, which may be desirable in patients with antecedent aortic valvular dysfunction or significant degrees of left ventricular dysfunction.

An accurate assessment of associated comorbid conditions is mandatory to guide appropriate decision making with respect to recommending open surgical repair. All patients should be evaluated with dipyridamole thallium scanning or the equivalent thereof to assess perioperative myocardial ischemic potential. In addition, patients with a history of symptoms suggestive of heart failure should have an assessment of left ventricular function. While patients with significant impairments of pulmonary reserve can usually be detected on a historical basis alone, we routinely obtain preoperative pulmonary function studies. Advanced age is an important component only in as much as it is accompanied by overall fragility and impaired functional status. We routinely hospitalize patients for at least 12 hours prior to surgery for intravenous fluid hydration, intravenous dopamine infusions if any degree of renal insufficiency is present, and a mechanical and antibiotic bowel prep. The latter is based on evidence indicating that bacterial translocation during the course of supraceliac clamping may contribute to disorders of blood coagulation during the conduct of operation.[64]

Although the technical conduct of specific procedures is beyond the scope of this discussion, there are several principles of therapy aimed at reducing complications that apply to all patients. Postoperative paraplegia secondary to interruption of potential blood supply to the spinal cord is by far the most feared nonfatal complication of descending thoracic aneurysm repair. In an effort to minimize this risk, we developed and applied a technique for the provision of regional hypothermic protection to that segment of the spinal cord typically at risk for ischemic injury during descending thoracic and thoracoabdominal aneurysm repair that involves an epidural infusion of iced saline during aortic cross-clamping.[65,66] Other adjuncts aimed at reducing the risk of paraplegia include cerebrospinal fluid drainage, reimplantation of patent critical intercostal arteries, the use of evoked-potential monitoring, and atriofemoral bypass to maintain distal aortic perfusion. Spinal cord ischemia remains an unsolved problem despite considerable improvements in the overall incidence of this complication. As detailed in Table 8.2, contemporary results from centers of excellence show that although paraplegia rates have improved, spinal cord ischemia remains a significant risk of open thoracic and thoracoabdominal aortic aneurysm repair. Renal protection is achieved through the direct installation of renal preservation fluid (4°C lactated Ringers with 25 g of Mannitol per liter and 1 g Methyl Prednisolone per liter) into the renal artery ostia after the aorta is opened causing a rapid decline of renal core temperature. This is important because of the significant impact of postoperative renal failure (defined as a doubling of baseline creatinine or absolute level > 3.0 mg/dL) on operative mortality. Indeed, in our series, patients who sustained significant postoperative renal failure had an 8-fold increase in their mortality risk (OR 7.8; 95% CI, 3.4–17.9; $P < 0.0001$).[51] The final adjunct in our overall approach involves in-line mesenteric shunting. As displayed in Figure 8.5, immediately after performance of the proximal anastomosis, pro-grade pulsatile perfusion can be established into either the celiac axis or superior

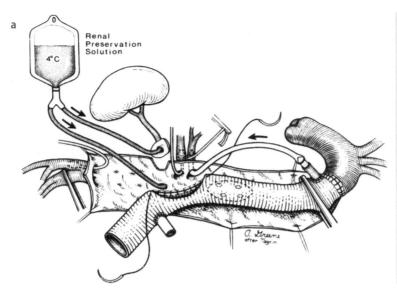

Figure 8.5 Approaches to operative conduct of thoracoabdominal aneurysm repair. (a) Our clamp-and-sew technique with associated adjuncts of mesenteric shunting, renal cold perfusion, and epidural cooling (not shown). (b) Distal perfusion (left heart bypass) using the heparin-impregnated Bio-Medicus pump where perfusion distal to the proximal cross-clamp is initially maintained via the femoral artery and then by multiple perfusion catheters once reconstruction proceeds distally.

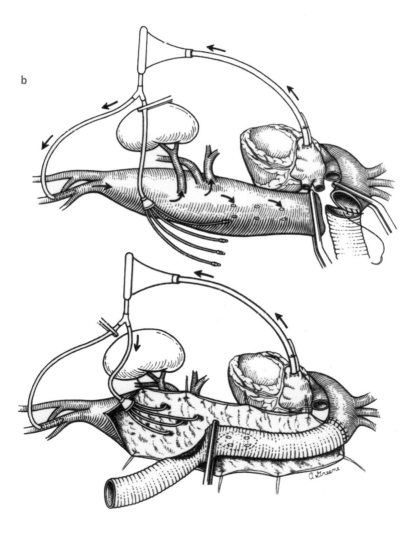

mesenteric artery to minimize visceral ischemic time and its potential contribution to coagulopathic bleeding.[71]

In the majority of clinical series, postoperative respiratory failure is the single most common complication after thoracoabdominal aneurysm resection, occurring in 25% to 45% of patients.[14,49,51,65,72] There may be confusion as to how this is defined, since the term "prolonged" ventilatory support (which is the most common problem) may be variably interpreted. A slow wean from ventilatory support, often planned to proceed over several days, is appropriate management in certain patients after extensive descending thoracic aortic resection, particularly those with baseline pulmonary insufficiency. Despite varying definitions, postoperative respiratory insufficiency occurs commonly, and the variables predictive of his complication include active cigarette smoking; baseline COPD, especially in those with significant reductions in forced expiratory volume in the first second of expiration (FEV_1); and cardiac, renal, or bleeding complications.[65,73,74] In the circumstance of elective operation, risk factor modification with smoking cessation and bronchodilator therapy for patients with COPD are vital for acceptable outcomes. However, institution of preoperative steroid therapy with the intent of improving respiratory function is contraindicated since we

have observed this maneuver to precipitate aneurysm rupture.

Despite the widespread use of the preceding adjunctive techniques, representative large clinical series, including the most recent publications, indicate that the mortality of descending thoracic and thoracoabdominal aneurysm repair remains in the 10% range (Table 8.2).[14] A consideration of variables predictive of operative mortality reveals consistent themes. In the recent update of our experience, operative mortality was 6.8% for elective operations and it increased to 12.9% in nonelective situations ($P = 0.06$).[51]

Another negative predictor reported in the literature is advanced age, although we find overall functional status is more important than chronological age per se.[12,14,48,49] The presence of increasing numbers of comorbid conditions can naturally be expected to increase overall operative risk. Individual series variously demonstrate increased operative risks with patients with antecedent coronary artery disease, significant COPD, and in particular preoperative renal insufficiency.[11,14,48,49,51,52,55,56] Significant antecedent dysfunction in these respective organ systems increases the risks of organ-specific complications after operation, and patients who sustain major neurologic deficits, postoperative renal failure, and cardiopulmonary complica-

Reference	Year Published	# Patients	Op. Mortality n (%)	Paraplegia/ Paraparesis n (%)	Comment
Svensson et al[14]	1993	1509	155 (10)	234 (16)	
Coselli et al[49]	2000	1220	93 (7.5)	56 (4.6)	
Schepens et al[57]	1996	172	18 (10.5)	24 (14.7)	
Grabitz et al[67]	1996	260	37 (14.2)	39 (15)	
Acher et al[48]	1998	217	21 (9.7)	17 (7.8)	desc TA included
Estrera et al[68]	2001	654	106 (16)	33 (5)	desc TA included
Jacobs et al[69]	2002	184	20 (10.8)	5 (2.7)	Types I–III TAA
van Dongen et al[70]	2002	118	4 (3.4)	5 (4.2)	desc TA included elective cases only
Conrad et al[51]	2006	455	39 (8.2)	43 (9.5)	
Totals		4789	493 (10)	456 (9.5)	

Table 8.2 Contemporary Clinical Series of Descending Thoracic and Thoracoabdominal Aneurysm Repair
Abbreviations: Desc TA= descending thoracic aortic aneurysm; TAA= thoracoabdominal aortic aneurysm

tions have a significantly increased risk of operative mortality.[11,12,14,48,51,75]

Open surgical repair of ascending aortic aneurysms

Repair of the ascending thoracic aorta requires the institution of cardiopulmonary bypass and, depending on the location, is generally achieved with an appropriately sized supracoronary tube graft. When the aneurysm involves the aortic root, it can be repaired by replacing the aortic root while either replacing or sparing the aortic valve. Aortic valve replacement is usually reserved for patients with associated significant aortic regurgitation secondary to dysfunction of the valvular leaflets. A valve-sparing root replacement usually involves excising the sinuses of Valsalva while sparing the aortic leaflets and reimplanting the valve leaflets within the graft to restore the normal anatomic configuration.[76]

Operative mortality after open repair of the ascending thoracic aorta varies depending upon the acuity of the operation and function of the left ventricle. The mortality of elective repair ranges from 3% to 10%, and the early re-exploration rate for bleeding is 8% to 15%.[13,77] In contrast, in the acute setting, the operative risk increases substantially with mortality rates approaching 25%.[77]

Endovascular reconstruction

Endoluminal treatment of isolated thoracic aortic aneurysm with stent grafting was introduced in 1994, by Dake et al.[78] Since then, pivotal and comparative (vs. open repair) trial data are emerging for the spectrum of thoracic aortic pathology.[79-82] However, descending thoracic aortic aneurysms occur less frequently than their abdominal counterparts such that from a regulatory standpoint, the development of thoracic endograft technology has proceeded much more slowly than that of technology for treating abdominal aortic aneurysms. Despite a lack of late results from clinical trials and a paucity of level I data from randomized controlled trials, the recent advent of a FDA-approved, commercially available device has caused the treatment paradigm for a variety of thoracic aortic pathologies to evolve toward stent-grafting strategies.

Endovascular repair of thoracic aortic aneurysms offers the benefit of aneurysm exclusion without the physiologic insult associated with thoracotomy and clamping of the proximal aorta. The procedure is conceptually simple, involving the insertion of a presized covered stent graft that is deployed under fluoroscopic guidance (Figure 8.6). However, there are several anatomic factors including aortic or iliac artery tortuosity, proximity of the aneurysm to the brachiocephalic or visceral vessels, and occlusive disease of the iliac vessels that can make device delivery a challenge. Indeed, the success of endovascular thoracic aneurysm repair is predicated upon obtaining quality aortic imaging, careful patient selection, and appropriate preprocedural planning. There are several anatomic barriers to thoracic stent grafting. The first is the size and length of the aortic neck. The neck is the area of normal aorta that will be used to seal the stent graft both proximally and distally. In addition, the proximal and distal seal zones should be at least 2 cm in length to ensure an adequate fixation and seal. Finally, the delivery systems for thoracic endografts are larger than their abdominal counterparts, with the largest devices requiring an iliac diameter of 9 mm to pass. In the presence of extensively calcified or narrow iliac arteries, a prosthetic conduit sewn to the common iliac artery may be required for successful device delivery and should be planned in advance.

Several large series have evaluated the effectiveness of endovascular stent grafting for the repair of descending thoracic aneurysms. The PIVITOL trial is a prospective, nonrandomized multicenter trial that compared 140 patients treated with thoracic endografts to 94 patients treated with open repair during the same time period. This resulted in lower perioperative mortality in the endovascular group (2.1% vs. 11.7%, $P < 0.001$) as well as lower rates of spinal cord ischemia (3% vs. 14%), respiratory failure (4% vs. 20%), and renal insufficiency (1% vs. 13%). However, there was no difference in all-cause mortality between the

2 groups at 2-year follow-up.[79] A recent evaluation of the European EUROSTAR and the United Kingdom Thoracic Endograft registries (prospectively gathered databases of aortic pathology) identified 249 patients who underwent endovascular repair for degenerative thoracic aneurysms. They reported a 30-day mortality of 5.3% and paraplegia rate of 4% with an 80% 1-year survival.[81]

We have previously reported our experience with 105 patients undergoing thoracic aortic stent grafting and compared the results to 93 patients treated with open surgery during the same time period. Despite borderline statistical significance, the operative mortality was halved in the stent-graft group when compared with the open (7.6% vs. 15.1%, $P = 0.09$).[83] While a 7.6% mortality lies in the lower end of reported rates for thoracic endografts, which have been up to 20%,[84,85] it is substantially higher than that of our updated experience with 873 infrarenal AAA endovascular repairs (1.8%)[86] or the PIVI-

TOL trial[79] and may be related to the fact that 30% of the endograft patients were not considered open surgical candidates.[83] The spinal cord ischemia rate was 6.7% in our stent-graft population, with 2 patients experiencing transient paraparesis that resolved prior to discharge.[83] These results are similar to those of 2 published multicenter trials that both reported spinal cord ischemia rates of 3%.[79,82] In addition, available reviews suggest that 8% to 43% of landing sites in descending aortic aneurysms will not allow an appropriate 2-cm length for secure proximal fixation.[84,85,87] Indeed, in 20% of our patients, the left subclavian artery was intentionally covered (11.5% underwent preprocedural subclavian artery bypass).[83] The 4-year survival for this group was 54% and freedom from reintervention rate was 81%.[83]

The anatomic constraints of the 2-cm proximal and distal seal zones will eliminate many patients from endovascular consideration. As descending thoracic aneurysms extend to the

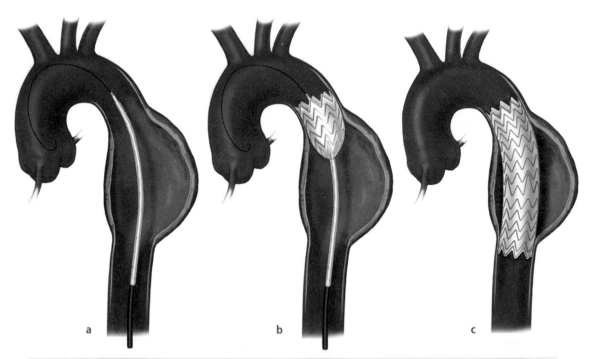

a   b   c

Figure 8.6 Cartoon depiction of endovascular repair of descending thoracic aortic aneurysm. (a) Descending thoracic aneurysm with adequate proximal and distal seal zones. A stiff wire has been advanced to the level of the aortic valve and the device is positioned under fluoroscopic guidance. (b) Initiation of device deployment. (c) The completed endovascular repair.

thoracoabdominal aorta, the extent of surgery with consequent risks of paraplegia, renal insufficiency, and death increases. Although, in our experience, the perioperative mortality after thoracoabdominal aneurysm repair is around 8%,[51] a recent review of the National Inpatient Sample (a stratified discharge database of a representative 20% of US hospitals) reported an overall "real-world" mortality of 22.3%.[88] To wit, extension of stent-graft repair to patients with thoracic aneurysms that involve the sub-

clavian artery or visceral abdominal aorta with a so-called "hybrid" operation has the potential to afford genuine benefit to these "high-risk" patients. In this instance, the proximal or distal seal zone can be extended by first bypassing the offending vessels with grafts from the ascending thoracic aorta for proximal vessels and the infrarenal aorta for visceral vessels. This hybrid approach has been advocated by some with early success (Figure 8.7). Black et al[89] reported data on 25 high-risk patients treated with hybrid procedures (80% had type II or III thoracoabdominal aneurysms). They identified an elective mortality of 17% and no paraplegia with the procedure.

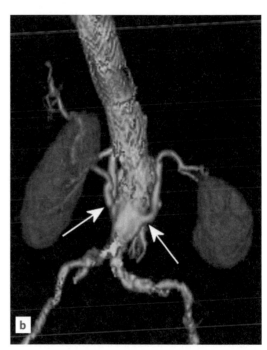

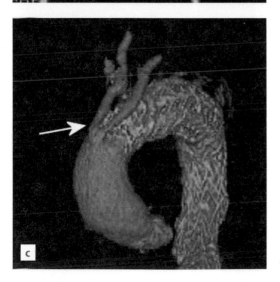

Figure 8.7 Helical CT 3D reconstruction of hybrid procedure of the visceral vessels. (a) Debranching of visceral vessels with infrarenal aortic replacement. The aorto–left renal bypass originates from the infrarenal graft (thin arrow) while a bifurcated graft (also originating from the infrarenal graft) was used to bypass the celiac and SMA (fat arrow). (b) Posterior view of hybrid procedure with arrows pointing to aortorenal grafts originating from the infrarenal graft. (c) Debranching of the great vessels to extend endovascular treatment of thoracic aneurysm. A bifurcated graft originating from the ascending aorta was used to bypass the innominate and left carotid arteries (arrow).

Acute Aortic Dissection

Acute aortic dissection is the most common catastrophe affecting the aorta, with an incidence exceeding that of ruptured abdominal aortic aneurysm (AAA) and a mortality rate approaching 1% per hour in the absence of treatment during the acute phase.[90] Early studies reported that the mortality reached 75% within the first 2 weeks after the onset of symptoms if no therapy was instituted.[91] Despite advances in the diagnosis and management of aortic dissection, the morbidity and mortality remain significant, being 27% in the initial report of the International Registry of Acute Aortic Dissection (IRAD).[92] The treatment paradigm for certain types of acute aortic dissection is likely to change as trials of endovascular stent-graft repair for type B dissections emerge. A thorough understanding of the clinical presentation, classification, and pathologic anatomy of aortic dissection is a necessary prerequisite for clinical decision making.

General Features

The pathognomonic lesion of aortic dissection begins with a tear in the intimomedia, allowing the surging blood column to enter the aortic intramural space. Histopathology within this area of aortic wall may reveal deterioration of medial collagen and elastin fibers, although it is important to emphasize that aortic dissection can occur in a histologically normal aorta. The typical tear is transverse, not circumferential, and the intimomedial layer is cleaved both longitudinally and circumferentially for a variable distance.[93] The blood flow is usually antegrade within the aortic wall, although retrograde flow and dissection may occur. The so-called false lumen, which is adventitially bound, represents the blood-filled space between the dissected layers of the aortic wall. Depending on the circumference involved, dilation and pressurization of the false channel may diminish both size and flow capacity of the true lumen. Fenestrations (connections between the true and false lumens) occur within the intimal flap downstream, usually at branch vessel ostia, which are cleaved by the dissection process; these serve as sites of reentry

of blood flow into the true lumen, thus maintaining false lumen patency. The most common pattern of dissection in the thoracoabdominal aorta is along the left posterolateral aspect of the aorta with the celiac, superior mesenteric, and right renal arteries typically originating from the true lumen, while the left renal artery is fed from the false lumen; however, variations from this pattern are frequently encountered (Figure 8.8).[91,94]

Classification

Aortic dissection is classified both temporally and by anatomy, the latter having major implications for treatment. An acute aortic dissection is

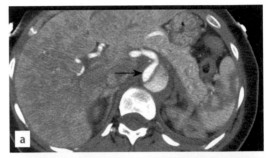

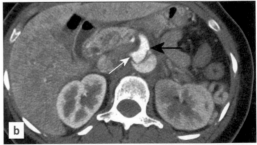

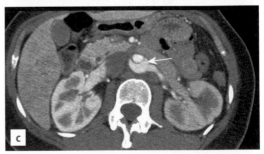

Figure 8.8 CT scan imaging of typical configuration of visceral aortic segment involvement of aortic dissection. The true lumen is smaller than the false lumen. (a) The celiac axis (thin black arrow); (b) SMA (thick black arrow) and right renal artery (white arrow) originate from the true lumen. (c) The left renal artery (white arrow) originates from the false lumen.

diagnosed within 2 weeks of the onset of symptoms, while chronic occurs beyond this time point. This designation, while arbitrary, is logical since the majority of lethal complications associated with aortic dissection will occur during the initial 2-week interval. Anatomically, 3 classification schemes have been described based on site of entry and direction of tear. Sixty-five percent of intimal tears occur in the ascending aorta, 20% in the descending aorta, 10% in the aortic arch, and 5% in the abdominal aorta.[92] The DeBakey classification is most commonly used and specifically delineates the extent of the descending aortic dissection (Figure 8.9).[95]

- Type I: dissection originates in the ascending aorta, extends through the aortic arch and into the descending aorta and/or abdominal aorta for a varying distance.
- Type II: dissection originates in and is confined to the ascending aorta and/or the aortic arch.

- Type III: dissection originates in the descending aorta and is limited to it in type IIIa; type IIIb involves descending and variable extents of the abdominal aorta.

The second anatomic classification scheme, proposed by Daily and colleagues,[96] simplifies aortic dissection into Stanford type A and B. Stanford type A includes dissections that involve the ascending aorta (DeBakey type I and II), irrespective of the site of origin. Stanford type B includes dissections that originate in and are confined to the descending aorta. The most recent classification scheme further simplifies aortic dissection into the anatomic categories "proximal" and "distal," equivalent to Stanford type A and B. Based upon this classification, the IRAD data revealed that approximately 60% of patients presented with Stanford type A and 40% have type B dissections.

The most important initial step in diagnosis of aortic dissection is determination of the

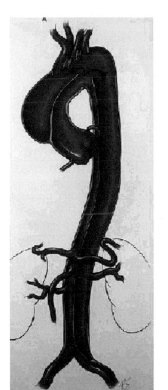
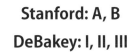
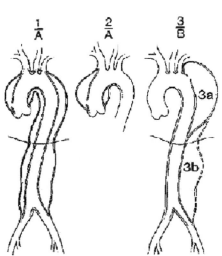
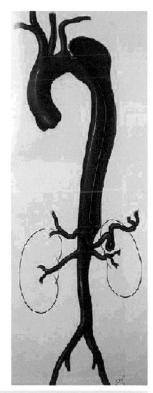

Stanford: A, B
DeBakey: I, II, III

Figure 8.9 DeBakey and Stanford classification schemes for acute aortic dissection. The principal distinction between proximal and distal dissections is the involvement of the ascending aorta.

location of the aortic entry tear and/or involvement of the ascending aorta, as this predicts the likelihood of proximal cardioaortic complications and directs early therapy. Typically, if the dissection involves the ascending aorta, the entry tear is located in the proximal ascending aorta, yet retrograde dissection from a more distal entry tear can occur. Early diagnosis and rapid classification are essential for appropriate initial management, as proximal dissections usually require emergent graft replacement of the ascending aorta due to the high risk of cardioaortic complications, including aortic rupture, cardiac tamponade, acute aortic insufficiency, or coronary artery ostial occlusion. Distal dissections currently are managed medically unless specific complications, such as malperfusion syndrome, complicate the dissection.

Incidence and Epidemiology

Although epidemiological information regarding acute aortic dissection is sparse, a recent study by Clouse et al[31] reported its incidence to be 3.5 per 100,000 persons. Men are more frequently afflicted, with a male to female ratio of 5:1.[91,97] The average age at presentation is 50 to 60 years for proximal dissections and 60 to 70 years for distal dissections.[92] Two-thirds of acute aortic dissections are proximal (DeBakey I, II; Stanford A) with the remaining third distal dissections (Figure 8.10).[98]

The most common associated risk factors for the development of aortic dissection include hypertension and advanced age, in particular for distal dissection (Figure 8.10). Aortic wall structural abnormalities and the presence of a bicuspid aortic valve (even in the absence of aortic root dilatation) are also established risk factors. Patients with connective tissue disorders, such as Ehlers-Danlos and Marfan's syndromes, are prone to develop cystic medial degeneration of the aortic wall. Marfan's syndrome accounts for 5% of all aortic dissections, making it the leading cause of dissection in patients under the age of 40.[99] Indeed, aortic root repair in patients with Marfan's syndrome is usually performed

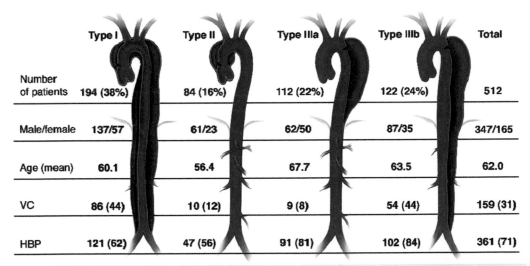

	Type I	Type II	Type IIIa	Type IIIb	Total
Number of patients	194 (38%)	84 (16%)	112 (22%)	122 (24%)	512
Male/female	137/57	61/23	62/50	87/35	347/165
Age (mean)	60.1	56.4	67.7	63.5	62.0
VC	86 (44)	10 (12)	9 (8)	54 (44)	159 (31)
HBP	121 (62)	47 (56)	91 (81)	102 (84)	361 (71)

Figure 8.10 Demographic and clinical features of 512 patients with acute aortic dissection classified by the DeBakey system treated at the Massachusetts General Hospital between 1965 and 1999. The distribution of dissection extent, demographic features, and incidence of peripheral vascular complications were similar over the 35-year period during which these patients were treated. Patients with type III dissections tend to be older and almost universally hypertensive. As anticipated, vascular complications (ie, aortic branch compromise) tend to cluster among the more extensive type I and IIIb dissections. HBP = high blood pressure; VC = vascular complications. (Adapted from: Lauterbach SR, Cambria RP, Brewster DC, et al. Contemporary management of aortic branch compromise resulting from acute aortic dissection. *J Vasc Surg.* 2001;33(6):1185-1192. Cambria RP, Brewster DC, Gertler J, et al. Vascular complications associated with spontaneous aortic dissection. *J Vasc Surg.* 1988;7(2):199-209.)

with the intention of preventing aortic dissection rather than rupture. Cocaine ingestion and pregnancy associated with hypertension and preeclampsia are rare causes of acute aortic dissection in otherwise healthy individuals.[93]

Natural History

Started in 1996, the International Registry of Aortic Dissection (IRAD) database is an ongoing, multinational, academic medical center registry of consecutive patients with acute aortic dissection. The IRAD study reported an overall mortality of 27.4% for all types of aortic dissection, including 26.0% for surgical treatment of proximal dissection and 58.0% for medical management alone, although it may be inferred that patients in the latter group were not surgical candidates due to advanced age, comorbidities, or refusal of treatment. In distal aortic dissection, mortality was 10.7% with medical therapy but rose to 31.0% in the presence of complications requiring intervention;[92] clearly, patients in these 2 treatment groups were not comparable. Branch vessel involvement, termed *malperfusion syndrome* when ischemic complications arise, is a frequent indication for surgery in aortic dissection and occurs in 30% to 42% of patients.[18,100,101] False lumen thrombosis occurs in 2% to 3% of medically treated patients and only 15% to 30% of surgically treated patients. Continued false lumen patency is a risk factor for recurrent dissection and/or aneurysmal degeneration irrespective of surgical repair.[102] Progression to aneurysm formation within 4 years of initial diagnosis occurs in 30% to 50% of patients with distal dissection initially treated with medical therapy.[103,104]

Our cumulative experience affords a perspective over a 35-year period involving 512 patients with acute aortic dissection.[98] The overall mortality during the interval 1990 to 1999 was significantly lower when compared to an earlier report from 1965 to 1986 (18% vs. 37%, $P < 0.006$).[100] Nearly one-third of the patients had evidence of branch occlusion, with 32% of these patients requiring directed peripheral vascular intervention to restore circulation. In discerning the factors associated with improved results over time, several variables were important: (1) aortic rupture occurred in just 6% of patients versus 18% in the prior interval. Presumably, patients were being diagnosed and referred more promptly. (2) The impact of branch occlusion on mortality was no longer significant, implying that early recognition and treatment of malperfusion syndromes had improved overall results. (3) Overall mortality in surgical repair of proximal dissection had improved from 33% to 15% due to advances in cardiac surgical techniques. (4) The presence of mesenteric ischemia receives treatment priority in virtually all patients and constitutes an exception to prompt central aortic repair of type A dissection. The later management change is based upon work by Deeb et al,[105] which showed that delaying central aortic repair until the patient has recovered from the effects of mesenteric ischemia and reperfusion improved mortality from 87% to 37%.

Clinical Presentation

The most common presenting symptom is pain (located in the back, abdomen, or chest), reported in over 93% of patients, with 85% specifying an abrupt onset.[92,106] While the pain is typically described as anterior in location in type A dissections, for type B dissections the pain was more often experienced in the back.[92] Although the classic description of pain associated with aortic dissection is ripping or tearing (50%), patients more frequently complain of sharp, stabbing pain (68%) and less often experience migratory symptoms (19%). Typically, the pain is severe, causing the patient to seek medical attention within minutes to hours of onset. The localization of pain to the abdomen was reported by 21% of patients with type A and 43% of patients with type B dissections.[92] In such patients, a high index of suspicion for mesenteric vascular compromise is warranted. The control of pain by antihypertensive therapy is considered to be of paramount importance in the early management of acute aortic dissection, and the recurrence of pain implies failure of medical therapy and warrants repeat imaging to direct therapy. In the absence of clinical or radiographic signs of pathoanatomic changes, medical therapy remains the appropriate management of patients with early recurrent pain after type B dissection.[107]

Syncope may complicate the presentation of acute aortic dissection in 5% to 10% of patients, and its presence often indicates the development of cardiac tamponade or involvement of the brachiocephalic vessels.[108] Overall, patients in the IRAD study presenting with syncope were more likely have a type A dissection than type B dissection (19% vs. 3%, $P < 0.001$) and more likely to have cardiac tamponade (28% vs. 8%, $P < 0.001$).[92] Similarly, they were more likely to have a stroke (18% vs. 4%, $P < 0.001$) and more likely to die in the hospital (34% vs. 23%, $P = 0.01$). Although patients presenting with syncope had a higher rate of severe complications (tamponade, stroke, death), in almost half, these were not the cause of their loss of consciousness.[108]

Spinal cord ischemia from the interruption of intercostal vessels is clearly more common with type B aortic dissections; occurring in 2% to 3% of patients. On initial physical examination, hypertension is present in 70% of type B dissections, but only in 25% to 35% of type A dissections (Figure 8.10). The presence of hypotension complicating a type B dissection is rare (< 5% of patients). In contrast, hypotension may be present in 25% of dissections that involve the ascending aorta, potentially as a result of aortic valve disruption or cardiac tamponade.[92] The malperfusion of brachiocephalic vessels involved with the dissection may falsely depress brachial cuff pressures. Hypertension that is refractory to medical management is common in type B dissections, occurring in 64% of patients with involvement of the descending aorta.[109] However, such refractory hypertension is usually not associated with renal artery compromise or aortic dilatation.

Pulse deficits are common and occur in 30% to 50% patients in whom the aortic arch and/or the thoracoabdominal aorta is involved.[18,100,101] In examination of the IRAD population, the involvement of the brachiocephalic trunk was noted in 14.5% of all patients, left common carotid artery in 6.0%, left subclavian in 14.5%, and femoral arteries in 13.0% to 14.0%.[110] Patients presenting with pulse deficits more often have neurologic deficits, coma, and hypotension. Carotid pulse deficits, not surprisingly, are strongly correlated with fatal stroke, consistent with prior observations.[98] The number of pulse deficits is clearly associated with increased mortality. Within 24 hours of presentation, 9.4% of patients with no deficits died, 15.8% of patients with 1 or 2 deficits died, and 35.3% of patients with 3 or more deficits died.[110] Interestingly, it is uncommon for isolated lower-extremity pulse deficits to cause mortality as a result of lower-extremity ischemia or its sequelae.[100] Regardless, leg ischemia is an indication of extensive dissection and is often accompanied by compromise of other vascular territories. Indeed, the clinical course of lower-extremity ischemia can be quite variable as up to one-third of this group demonstrates spontaneous return of pulses.[100]

Related Conditions of the Thoracic Aorta

Intramural hematoma (IMH) and *penetrating atheromatous ulcer (PAU)* are 2 closely related (possibly the same) aortic conditions that commonly cause diagnostic confusion with classic aortic dissection. However, PAU is often noted as a radiographic curiosity on CT scans obtained for evaluation of the thoracic aorta whereas IMH is a dissecting process and patients can present with symptoms typical of the acute aortic syndrome that include the abrupt onset of severe pain in the chest, neck, back, and/or abdomen. Paradoxically, both are manifestations of degenerative aortic pathology, typically occurring in older patients with significant hypertension and often with diffuse degenerative disease of the thoracic aorta. IMH of the thoracic aorta has been characterized as a distinct clinical entity whose distinguishing radiographic features are the absence of a definable intimal flap (as seen with classic aortic dissection) or penetrating ulceration.[111,112] The extent of this IMH is variable both in terms of length of the aorta involved, circumference, and direction of propagation. The etiology of IMH was initially thought to involve spontaneous rupture of the vasa vasorum within the medial layers of the aortic wall. More consistent with our own observations, a penetrating atheromatous ulcer phenomenon is usually the origin of IMH and whether or not the ulcerlike projection is radiographically demonstrated is merely serendipity.[113] PAU is used to describe these lesions when a caplike projection of contrast is seen (on CT scan) beyond the usual luminal aortic boundary.

The natural history of IMH and PAU has been reported to include progression to aortic dissection, false aneurysm formation, rupture, or spontaneous regression.[113] The IRAD database examined 1010 patients who presented with symptoms of the acute aortic syndrome and identified a 5.7% incidence of IMH. This affected the descending aorta in 60% of cases, whereas classic aortic dissection more commonly affected the ascending aorta (65% of cases). The overall mortality of IMH was similar to that of classic aortic dissection, 20.7% versus 23.9%, both for proximal (39.1% vs. 29.9%) and distal (8.3% vs. 13.1%) locations. Among the 51 patients whose initial diagnostic study revealed IMH, 8 (16%) progressed to aortic dissection on a second imaging study. A normal aortic diameter in the acute phase was the best predictor of IMH regression without complications.

The IRAD investigators recommended prompt surgical therapy for IMH involvement of the ascending aorta. Intense medical therapy alone (goal of systolic blood pressure < 120/80, heart rate < 60) was recommended for involvement of the arch and descending aorta.[114]

A recent report of 35 patients with IMH detailed a significant correlation between disease progression and initial aortic diameter and/or hematoma thickness. Those patients with an initial aortic diameter > 40 mm had a 30-fold increased risk of progression to either aneurysm formation or rupture. In addition, hematoma thickness of > 1 cm, was associated with a 9-fold increased risk of progression. This suggests that the degree of separation of the aortic wall layers may contribute to chronic aneurysmal degeneration.[115]

Although such focal pathology may be ideally suited for stent-graft repair (Figure 8.11), the majority of patients with IMH or PAU of the descending aorta are currently managed with medical therapy. Indications for intervention include aortic diameter > 6 cm, rupture, impending rupture, or major progression in size despite medical therapy. Those patients with involvement of the ascending aorta are usually treated surgically due to the high risk of cardioaortic complications. Surveillance imaging of patients with IMH or PAU treated medically should be frequent, especially those with evidence of aneurysmal dilation.

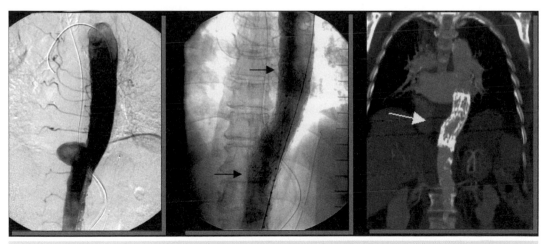

Figure 8.11 Stent-graft treatment of a mid-descending thoracic aorta penetrating atheromatous ulcer.

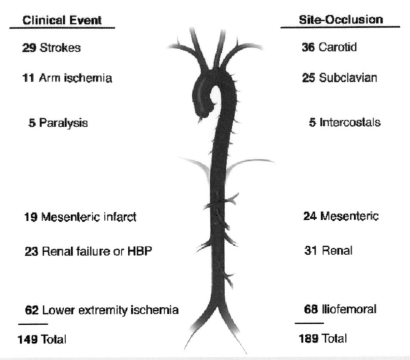

Clinical Event	Site-Occlusion
29 Strokes	36 Carotid
11 Arm ischemia	25 Subclavian
5 Paralysis	5 Intercostals
19 Mesenteric infarct	24 Mesenteric
23 Renal failure or HBP	31 Renal
62 Lower extremity ischemia	68 Iliofemoral
149 Total	189 Total

Figure 8.12 Distribution of peripheral vascular complications in 512 patients over a 35-year period (1965–1999) treated at the Massachusetts General Hospital. Peripheral vascular complications are classified by aortic branch site. Differences between site occlusions and clinical events represent asymptomatic occlusions.

Pathogenesis of Malperfusion Syndromes

Aortic branch compromise, often termed malperfusion syndrome when vascular beds are critically compromised, may occur in aortic dissection through several mechanisms. One or more vascular beds may be simultaneously affected. Branch vessel obstruction is often subtotal, waxing and waning in severity after symptom onset. It should be emphasized that the terms aortic branch compromise and malperfusion syndrome are not equivalent, since (1) obstruction is often subtotal, producing variable degrees of end organ ischemia, and (2) certain affected vessels (eg, subclavian and celiac arteries) may not produce critical ischemia, even with total occlusion, because of collateral circulation. Aortic branch compromise may complicate aortic dissection in up to 31% of patients.[18,100,101] We documented that such aortic branch compromise was associated with increased early mortality.[98] Virtually any aortic branch can be affected and, as intui-

tively suspected, the morbid clinical events will vary as a function of the vascular territory involved. Mesenteric vessel involvement is often associated with intestinal infarction, whereas subclavian and/or lower-extremity occlusive events are often well tolerated (Figure 8.12). Identifying the mechanisms of branch compromise is critical to formulate effective treatment plans. In the minutes after an aortic dissection is initiated, the true lumen collapses to a variable degree and the false lumen expands.[116] The adventitially bound outer wall of the false lumen must expand to a larger diameter to accommodate the same wall tension at any given blood pressure, as governed by the Law of LaPlace. The true lumen, which contains the majority of the elastic components of the aortic wall, undergoes radial elastic collapse.[116] Therefore, the degree to which the true lumen recoils and the false lumen expands (ie, their respective cross-sectional area) is dependent upon the percentage of the total aortic circumference involved with the dissection. When the dissection involves a significant portion of the aortic circumference, the true lumen can be narrowed to the point of near obliteration (Figure 8.13). A compressed true lumen will lead to impaired perfusion of distal structures and should increase the index of suspicion for visceral and renal ischemia.

Two mechanisms for aortic branch vessel compromise have been identified, each of which has specific treatment implications in the management of malperfusion syndromes. In *dynamic obstruction,* the compressed true lumen is unable to provide adequate flow volume, or the dissection flap may prolapse into the vessel ostium, which remains anatomically intact. This is the more common mechanism of branch compromise, being responsible for some 80% of malperfusion syndromes.[117] The severity of true lumen collapse and the degree of the aortic-level ostial vessel occlusion is determined by the circumference of the aorta dissected, blood pressure, heart rate, and peripheral resistance of the outflow vessel. Pulse deficits based on dynamic obstruction may wax and wane over time due to the variability of the aforementioned variables (Figure 8.14).[118,119]

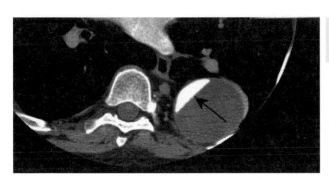

Figure 8.13 Helical CT imaging showing a narrow true lumen that may lead to end organ compromise.

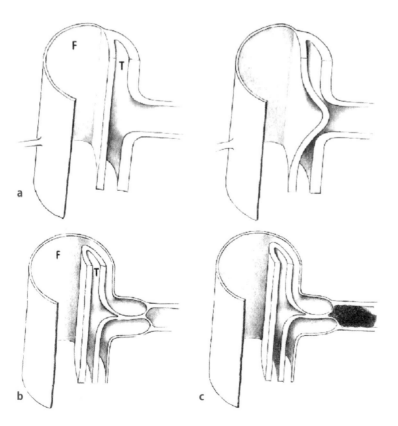

Figures 8.14 Mechanisms of aortic branch obstruction in acute dissection. (a) In dynamic obstruction, the septum may prolapse into the vessel ostium during the cardiac cycle, and the compressed true (T) lumen flow is inadequate to perfuse branch vessel ostia, which remain anatomically intact. (b) Near complete circumferential dissection with static obstruction—the cleavage plane of the dissection extends into the ostium and compromises inflow. Thrombosis beyond the compromised ostia may further worsen perfusion. (c) Spontaneous perfusion of aortic branches perfused from the false (F) lumen occurs if the dissecting process tears the ostia away from the true lumen. Such spontaneous "fenestrations" often account for persistent false lumen flow.

In acute dissection the false lumen is highly thrombogenic as a result of the exposed adventitial and medial layers. Thrombus formation may occur in the blind end of the dissection column. If the blind end or the propagating end of the dissection column enters and constricts the ostia of a branch vessel, organ injury can occur by thrombosis or hypoperfusion of the involved vessel. This mechanism for malperfusion syndrome involves the dissecting process extending into the branch vessel proper, narrowing it to a variable degree—so-called *static obstruction*.[117] This obstruction is unlikely to resolve with restoration of aortic true lumen flow alone, and some manipulation of the vessel itself (ie, stent, bypass graft) will typically be required. More common than static obstruction is the dissection process itself shearing the aortic intimomedia around the vessel ostium; the vessel anatomy remains intact with flow provided by the false lumen (Figure 8.14c). Most branches perfused from the false lumen do not show evidence of ongoing malperfusion as long as there is distal decompression and continued flow.

Diagnostic Studies

In most environments, a contrast-enhanced, fine-cut CT scan of the entire aorta is the preferred diagnostic modality. The findings of aortic dissection on chest radiography are nonspecific and rarely diagnostic. The most common chest x-ray abnormality seen in aortic dissection is widening of the aortic silhouette, appearing in 60% to 90% of cases.[92]

Aortography

Formerly the gold standard for the diagnosis of aortic dissection, with a sensitivity of 88% and a specificity of 94%, aortography has largely yielded, as a diagnostic study, to axial imaging studies.[120,121] False-negative aortograms may occur when thrombosis of the false lumen has occurred, in the presence of an intramural hematoma, or when equal flow into the true and false lumen obscures delineation. The aortographic findings considered supportive of a diagnosis of aortic dissection include distortion of the normal contrast column, flow reversal or stasis into a false channel, failure of major branches to fill, and aortic valvular regurgitation. Contemporary diagnostic algorithms have de-emphasized the role of aortography. Furthermore, pressurized contrast injections into either lumen in the presence of aortic dissection can, in fact, lead to diagnostic confusion with respect to malperfusion syndromes. For example, branch ostiae are anatomically normal in circumstances of dynamic obstruction and the true lumen will typically appear normal with contrast injections. Therefore, in contemporary practice, aortography is unnecessary prior to surgical repair of proximal dissection, and is essentially not used as a diagnostic modality.[122] It is now reserved for situations in which endovascular management is necessary.

Transesophageal echocardiography

The sensitivity of transesophageal echocardiography (TEE) has been reported to be as high as 98%, and the specificity ranges from 63% to 96%.[123] The advantages of TEE include wide availability, ease of use, and bedside capability. In addition, TEE possesses the ability to detect entry tear sites, false lumen flow/thrombus, involvement of the arch or coronary arteries, degrees of aortic valvular regurgitation, and pericardial effusions. The addition of color flow Doppler patterns may decrease false positives by recognizing differential flow velocities in the true and false lumens. The chief limitation of TEE is the anatomic blind spot in the distal ascending aorta and arch secondary to the air-filled trachea and left main stem bronchus, and the inability to document dissection extension beyond the diaphragm. Despite these shortcomings, TEE can be particularly useful in delineating dissection and relevant surgical pathology in the ascending aorta. Moreover, in the unstable patient with a suspected acute dissection in the ascending aorta, TEE may be performed in the operating room to expedite diagnosis and definitive therapy. In the IRAD study, TEE was number 2 in most frequent usage (after CT) in the diagnosis and workup of an acute aortic dissection.[123]

Computed tomography

All patients with suspected acute aortic dissection should be thoroughly evaluated with both chest and abdominal dynamic, contrast-enhanced fine-cut CT scanning. CT scanning has a reported sensitivity of 83% to 95% and a specificity of 87% to 100% for the diagnosis of acute aortic dissection.[124] The chief limitation is the ascending aorta, where the sensitivity may drop to < 80%, but this is readily overcome with the addition of TEE. Three-dimensional CT scan reconstructions can aid in treatment planning, but axial imaging affords the best opportunity to detect topographic relationships of the true and false lumens and potential aortic branch compromise. In most cases, the true lumen may be localized by its continuity with an undissected segment of the aorta. The presence of intraluminal thrombus is a fairly good marker of the false lumen, but in patients with a concomitant degenerative aneurysm, thrombus may be present in the true lumen. The finding of greatest significance was the observation in the descending thoracic aorta of the false lumen being larger than the true lumen in over 90% of cases ($P < 0.05$) and this simple guideline is clinically quite useful.[125] A compressed true lumen is perhaps the key radiographic finding, which should substantially raise the index of suspicion for renal/visceral/lower-extremity malperfusion syndrome (see Figure 8.13). Indeed, it may be appropriate, if open surgical intervention is chosen as the revascularization procedure, to proceed directly to surgery after CT alone in circumstances where the clinical and/or laboratory signs dictate the need for urgent revascularization. Compared to other modalities, CT scanning is the least operator dependent, provides useful anatomic correlates for surgical and endovascular therapy, and most reliably collects information for follow-up analysis and measurement.

Principles of Treatment

Prompt institution of intravenous antihypertensive medications to lower systemic blood pressure and pulse (dP/dT) is a key element of initial therapy for all patients, with the goal of stabilizing the extent of the dissection, reducing intimal flap mobility, relieving dynamic aortic branch obstruction, and decreasing the risk of rupture. Mortality in the acute phase of a proximal dissection may exceed 1% per hour related to the central cardioaortic complications of tamponade, acute aortic valvular insufficiency, and coronary obstruction. Thus, prompt ascending aortic graft replacement plus or minus aortic valve repair/replacement is the treatment of choice for the majority of patients with type A aortic dissection. For patients with type B dissections, the catastrophic complication of rupture is uncommon, except in those patients who present with advanced false lumen dilatation or the equivalent of aneurysm formation at the aortic entry site.[118] Furthermore, in patients with uncomplicated type B dissections, surgical therapy (ie, graft replacement of the aortic entry tear site) has not demonstrated superiority over medical or interventional therapy for stable patients.[106]

Aortic branch compromise by the propagating false lumen and subsequent malperfusion syndrome may complicate the initial presentation of patients with extensive type B dissections. A complication-specific approach involving open surgical and endovascular options to treat such malperfusion syndromes is advocated and reviewed next. The application of stent-graft repair at the entry tear may alter this paradigm in the near future.

Medical Therapy

Medical treatment of aortic dissection was first advocated in the 1960s by Wheat[126] (ironically, a surgeon) as an alternative for those patients too ill to withstand surgical therapy. Currently, medical management in an intensive care unit is now the initial therapy for virtually all patients with the tentative diagnosis of aortic dissection. The immediate management of acute aortic dissection is directed toward reducing the hemodynamic forces that have initiated and propagated the intimal tear and cleavage of the aortic wall. The goal of medical therapy is to eliminate the pain of dissection and reduce systolic blood pressure and dP/dT.[127] By reducing dP/dT, the forces predisposing the dissected aorta to rupture or compromise of branch vessels will be lessened. Intravenous antihypertensive therapy should be started in all patients in whom acute aortic dissection is suspected, with the exception of those with hypotension.[127] For those patients with hypotension in the setting of acute dissection, an expeditious evaluation for tamponade is warranted, but percutaneous pericardiocentesis as a temporizing measure is not advised as it often accelerates bleeding or shock.[128] In contemporary practice, a combination of a beta-blocker and vasodilator is standard medical therapy. In addition, the beta-blocker should be initiated before the direct vasodilator (ie, sodium nitroprusside); otherwise, the reflex sympathetic stimulation from direct vasodilation will stimulate catecholamine release, and resultant increases in dP/dT, opposite of the desired effect. The cornerstones of medical therapy are the reduction of both dP/dT and arterial blood pressure. For the acute reduction of dP/dT, an intravenous beta-blocker is infused in incremental doses until evidence of effective beta-blockade is achieved, usually indicated by a heart rate of 60 to 80 beats per minute. Beta-blockers that achieve both alpha- and beta-adrenergic blockade (such as Labetalol) may achieve both dP/dT reduction in concert with blood pressure lowering. Short-acting beta-blockers (like Esmolol) may be particularly useful as a test of beta-blockade tolerance in patients at risk for bronchospasm or COPD flare. In these patients, a cardioselective beta-blocker such as atenolol or metoprolol may be desirable. For the acute reduction of arterial pressure, the direct vasodilator sodium nitroprusside is very effective and should be used after beta-blockade is achieved.

Patients should be placed in the intensive care unit during the acute period with continuous blood pressure monitoring via an intra-arterial catheter, telemetry monitoring of cardiac rhythms, and hemodynamic surveillance involving a Foley catheter and pulmonary artery catheter if necessary. Once the patient's blood pressure has been controlled to a systolic of 105 to 120 mm Hg (or mean of 60–70 mm Hg) and pain has resolved, the individual can be transitioned to oral antihypertensives. Patients who are managed medically should be followed with serial surveillance imaging studies that should consist of a contrast CTA. The first can be obtained 6 months after discharge and then on a yearly basis if the aorta shows no change from the initial scan.[13]

Surgical Therapy—Graft Replacement of Ascending Aortic Dissection

A complete review of the literature and state-of-the-art surgical management of acute type A dissection is beyond the scope of this review. Urgent surgical repair of acute type A dissection is the treatment of choice for all patients unless major neurologic deficits or peripheral vascular complications of the dissection pose greater overall risk (ie, visceral ischemia) than the threat of proximal rupture (Figure 8.15). The IRAD study group found an overall operative mortality of 25.1% in patients with proximal aortic dissection and noted a significant difference between stable patients and those who were unstable at presentation (16.7% vs. 31.4%, $P < 0.001$).[92,129] Improvements in cardiac surgical techniques, including routine use of profound hypothermic circulatory arrest, improved strategies for cerebral protection, avoidance of routine aortic valve replacement, and avoidance of extensive arch resections, have led to improvements in outcome. Despite the advances in surgical techniques and perioperative care, operative mortality remains significant, between 15% and 30%.[98,129,130]

Graft Replacement of Descending Aortic Dissection

Threatened or actual rupture at the aortic intimal tear in the proximal descending aorta remains, in our view, the only indication for acute graft replacement of the proximal descending aorta in distal dissection. Unless an extensive aneurysm is present, resection should be con-

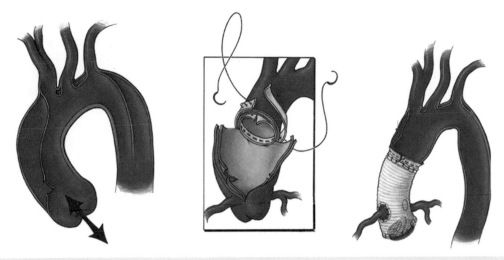

Figure 8.15 Repair of type A dissection with replacement of the ascending aorta. Anatomic goals of replacement include (a) resection of aortic tear, (b) resuspension/repair or replacement of aortic valve as necessary, and (c) routine use of circulatory arrest to perform at least the distal anastomosis, and reconstruction of the aortic layers so as to redirect flow into the true lumen and eliminate false lumen flow (this is successful only 50% of the time).

fined to the proximal descending aorta, as mortality and spinal cord ischemia risk increase dramatically with extensive aortic replacement in the setting of an acute dissection. Even in the circumstances where graft replacement of the proximal descending aorta is indicated for actual or threatened rupture, stent-graft repair will usually be preferred over open surgical correction because of decreased morbidity and mortality. The mortality rate for the open repair of acute type B aortic dissection has ranged from 6% to 69% in several large series (Table 8.3). In a series of nearly 100 type B dissection

patients over the course of a decade, we applied this approach only once.[98] In addition, central aortic grafting may be unsuccessful in alleviating distal malperfusion syndromes depending on the mechanism of obstruction, the anatomic complexity of the dissection, and the successful obliteration of false lumen flow.

Surgical Treatment of Malperfusion Syndromes

Since dynamic obstruction at the aortic level is the most common mechanism of malperfusion

Author	Period	Adjuncts	# Patients	Mortality	Paraplegia/ Paraparesis
Jex[131]	1962–1983	PB (66%)	29	45%	24%
Verdant[132]	1974–1994	NA	52	12%	0%
Glower[133]	1975–1988	PB (44%) GS (39%)	19	18%	NA
Miller[134]	1977–1982	PB (NA%)	26	13%	25%
Neya[17]	1979–1991	PB (NA%)	13	69%	NA
Fann[101]	1983–1992	PB (100%)	17	41%	NA
Svennson[135]	1986–1989	PB (NA%)	67	6%	25%
Coselli[54]	1986–1994	PB (NA%) CSF (NA%)	28	14%	7%

Table 8.3 Results of Open Surgical Graft Replacement of Acute Type B Aortic Dissection. NA: not available; PB: partial bypass; CSF: cerebrospinal fluid drainage; GS: Gott shunt. Adapted from Black JH, Cambria RP. Aortic dissection: perspectives for the vascular/ endovascular surgeon. In: *Rutherford's Textbook of Vascular Surgery.* 6th Ed. Philadelphia: Elsevier Saunders; 2005.

syndromes (see Figure 8.14), surgical fenestration (accomplished by an open or endovascular approach) has been the most commonly applied procedure.[118] The open surgical technique involves wide resection of the dissected septum to relieve aortic obstruction by equalizing flow between the true and false lumenae. A variety of technical and anatomic features will determine whether the fenestration is limited to the infrarenal aorta (Figure 8.16a) or carried widely into the visceral aortic segment. Application of such a "complication-specific" approach to malperfusion syndromes has produced favorable results both in our experience[98] and that of others (Eleftriades et al[136] were able to relieve ischemia in 93% of patients with a 77% 3-year survival). Fenestration has also been performed with endovascular techniques using catheters and balloons to decompress the false lumen in a process that is usually guided by intravascular ultrasonography (Figure 8.16b). The largest reported series of percutaneous balloon fenestration in the setting of acute aortic dissection reported a 93% success rate in restoring blood flow to ischemic territories with a 25% 30-day mortality in this critically ill population.[137]

We reviewed a decade of our experience involving 187 patients with acute aortic dissection treated during the 1990s, and in an attempt to clarify the role of open surgical fenestration and peripheral endovascular intervention in patients with malperfusion syndromes.[98] Nearly a third of the patients had evidence of branch occlusion; 17 of 53 (32%) patients underwent peripheral vascular intervention to restore circulation. Surgical fenestration was used in 9 patients with mesenteric or renal malperfusion syndromes. Restoration of flow was successful in all patients and all patients so treated survived, whereas 2 deaths occurred in patients with mesenteric ischemia managed with percutaneous fenestration. Open aortic fenestration is an excellent method of restoring circulation to vascular territories affected

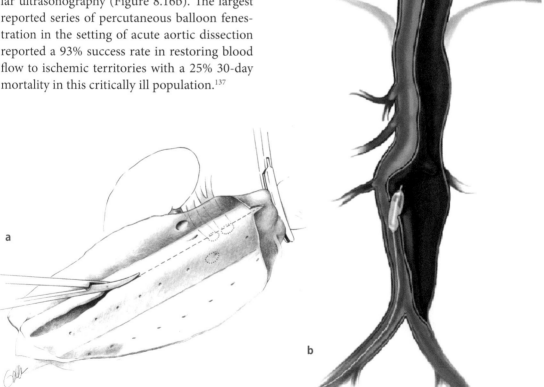

Figure 8.16 Surgical and endovascular fenestration of the infrarenal aorta. (a) With open fenestration, the septum is excised up to the clamp (dashed line), and the visceral vessel ostea are re-created prior to closure of the aorta. (b) With endovascular fenestration, a balloon is used to enlarge natural fenestrations and renovisceral vessels are made to originate from the true lumen (often requires stenting of the orifice).

by malperfusion syndromes, especially when mesenteric and renal beds are involved, and it affords the opportunity to assess bowel viability and plan second-look procedures. However, in current practice, patients who have branch vessel compromise and no evidence of bowel infarction are preferentially managed with stent-graft obliteration of the aortic entry tear. Treatment priority should be assigned to the most life-threatening condition in patients with acute aortic dissection. The presence of mesenteric ischemia assumes such priority in virtually all patients, and constitutes an exception to prompt central aortic repair in those with type A dissections.[98]

Stent-Graft Repair of Aortic Dissection Entry Site

Stent-graft repair at the aortic entry tear may ultimately provide the means to accomplish both the short-term goal of maintenance of end-organ perfusion and the long-term goal of false lumen thrombosis and aortic wall remodeling with the prevention of aneurysmal degeneration, while obviating the substantial morbidity of conventional open surgical repair. In 1999, the endovascular treatment of acute type B dissections with stent-graft technology was described in 2 sentinel reports.[138,139] Such an approach would effectively treat malperfusion syndromes (at least those caused by dynamic obstruction) and at least theoretically reduce late aortic-related complications by minimizing the incidence of aneurysmal degeneration of the outer wall of the false lumen. Yet, from a practical perspective, stent-graft repair of acute dissection in the United States has only been available since April 2005 coincident with initial FDA approval of a commercially available thoracic stent graft. The concept of inducing false lumen thrombosis by sealing the aortic tear with an aortic endograft has the potential to reduce both early and late complications of type B dissection (Figure 8.17).[140] Indeed, Dake et al[138] were able to achieve complete or partial

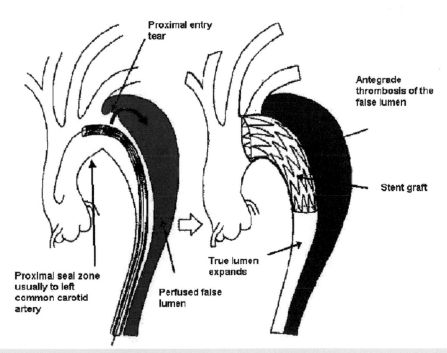

Figure 8.17 Stent-graft deployment to cover the proximal entry tear in the hopes of inducing false lumen thrombosis and true lumen re-expansion. The latter should also alleviate "downstream" branch compromise caused by dynamic obstruction mechanisms. False lumen thrombosis in the thoracic aorta should, in theory, minimize subsequent aneurysmal expansion of the outer wall of the false lumen.

thrombosis of the false lumen in 100% of patients, with relief of corresponding symptoms in 76% of patients and morbidity/mortality rates that compared favorably to open surgery. In the natural history of medically managed type B dissections, continued patency of the false lumen is an independent risk factor for progression of chronic dissections to aneurysmal dilatation.[141] During the first 4 to 7 years after acute aortic dissection managed medically, aneurysmal degeneration of the false lumen in the thoracic aorta may develop in 14% to 40% of patients treated with medical therapy alone.[92]

The Eurostar/UK registry report is the largest compendium of patients treated with thoracic aortic stent grafts to date. In the combined registry, 131 patients with aortic dissection (5% proximal, 81% distal, 14% not classified) were treated with stent grafts; 57% had symptoms of rupture, aortic expansion, or side branch occlusion. Although no meaningful long-term data are available, primary technical success was achieved in 89% and 30-day mortality was 8.4%.[81] Paraplegia occurred in 0.8% of those treated, and survival at 1 year after treatment was reported in 90% of 67 patients who had such follow-up.

A recent meta-analysis of all published series of stent-graft repair for aortic dissection prior to 2005 identified 609 patients with a procedural success of 98.2%. The 30-day mortality was 5.3% and was 3-fold higher in patients with acute dissection, and the neurologic complication rate was 2.9%.[142] A more recent study from China looked at 63 patients with acute dissection who underwent stent-graft placement within 2 weeks of symptoms. These researchers reported a clinical success rate of 95.2% with a 30-day mortality of 3.2%, no paraplegia, and a 1-year false lumen thrombosis rate of 98.4%.[143]

These preliminary data suggest that stent-graft repair may ultimately become the treatment of choice for the majority of patients with distal dissections; the available data consisting largely of registry and/or single-center retrospective reviews permit only the conclusion that stent-graft repair of the aortic entry tear can afford effective treatment of complicated type B dissections with the inherent advantages of a minimally invasive approach. However, the available data are insufficient to make treatment plans, in particular, with reference to patients with uncomplicated distal dissections (those typically treated with medical therapy). Indeed, medical therapy in such patients has typically produced favorable results, perhaps not a surprising finding, as these patients do not have immediately threatening anatomic complications of their dissection.

To potentially clarify (although it has not) the role of stent-graft treatment of type B aortic dissections, the INSTEAD trial was designed as a prospective, randomized, multicenter trial performed in Europe that compared stent grafting to medical therapy for the treatment of chronic, uncomplicated type B aortic dissection. However, it is important to understand that this trial was designed to address all-cause 1-year mortality (its principal end point) in patients with chronic type B dissections. Patients were only randomized to medical versus stent-graft therapy 2 weeks after the onset of symptoms. Thus, patients with early complications (those who would likely benefit from endovascular therapy) were essentially subtracted out of the study cohort. Not surprisingly, the investigators found no difference in 30-day or 1-year mortality between the 2 groups, but the stent-graft group noted false lumen thrombosis in over 90% of patients at 1 year (significantly higher than the medically treated group). Clearly, comparative clinical trials are needed to clarify the role of stent-graft repair in acute distal dissections.

Natural History and Follow-up

The primary late complication of aortic dissection is aneurysmal dilatation of the outer wall of the false lumen; of patients surviving acute dissection, 25% to 40% will progress to have aneurysmal dilation of the dissected aorta despite medical management.[103,104] In most clinical series of thoracoabdominal aneurysms, some 20% of cases are the sequelae of chronic dissection, for which conventional open repair is typically the only treatment option in contemporary practice.[11] Indeed, a variety of technical and anatomic considerations indicate that stent-graft repair of aneurysms of chronic dissection etiology remain a major challenge.[144] Factors that appear to have a significant impact on chronic aneurysm development after dissection include poorly controlled hypertension, maximal aortic diameter of at least 4 cm in the acute phase, and continued patency of the false lumen. Furthermore, some 10% to 20% of those with dissection will subsequently experience late rupture of the aneurysm,[102] and conventional surgical repair of such lesions is considerably more complex than with degenerative aneurysms.

Similar to so-called hybrid procedures for degenerative thoracoabdominal aortic aneurysm repair, elaborate stent-graft repair of such extensive aneurysms has recently been reported. Mossop et al[145] from Australia described their experience in 25 patients with a staged thoracoabdominal and branch vessel endoluminal repair. Initial treatment involved endograft closure of the proximal entry tear and bare metal, self-expanding Z-stenting of the true lumen, thereby supporting the true lumen and stabilizing the dissection flap. At 1-week follow-up, secondary reentry tears were then sealed by a variety of endovascular approaches, including placement of branch vessel covered stents, short segment covered aortic endografts, and coil embolization of the false lumen. In their series over 4 years, they reported no Z stent migration or stent-related intimal trauma resulting in rupture. Induction of false lumen thrombosis was achieved in 85% of patients. Survival at mean follow-up of 2.5 years was 100%.

Aneurysms that are the sequelae of chronic dissection tend to be more extensive and occur in younger patients compared with degenerative aneurysms. Treatment with effective beta-blockade is an essential feature of long-term therapy and follow-up. The rationale of such therapy is based on the recognition that patients with aortic dissection have a systemic illness that places their entire aorta at risk for further dissection, aneurysm, or rupture. Guidelines recommend progressive upward titration of beta-blockade to achieve a blood pressure < 125/80 mm Hg in usual patients and < 120 in those with Marfan's syndrome. In addition, aggressive beta-blockade has been shown to retard the growth of the aortic root in Marfan's syndrome patients and may have a similar effect on the thoracoabdominal aorta.[60] Serial imaging is the cornerstone of long-term follow-up, and axial imaging modalities should encompass the entire aorta. While in the developmental stages at present, branched stent-graft technologies will likely have an important role in the future management of patients with aneurysms of chronic dissection etiology.

Summary

Considerable progress has been demonstrated in the overall results of treatment for diseases of the thoracic aorta. A broad clinical awareness of aortic dissection and aneurysmal disease and improved methods of diagnosis have helped reduce the morbidity and mortality associated with these disease processes. Indeed, clinicians who understand the principles of both medical and surgical management of diseases of the thoracic aorta can effectively separate patients who require surgical intervention from those who can be managed medically with serial imaging studies. Although open surgery has been the standard of care for many years, it is clear that a wide variety of thoracic aortic pathologies are amenable to endovascular therapy. As stent-graft technology continues to evolve, it is clear that this is will become the primary method of thoracic aortic repair in anatomically suitable patients.

References

1. Panneton JM, Hollier LH. Nondissecting thoracoabdominal aortic aneurysms: Part I. *Ann Vasc Surg.* 1995;9(5):503-514.
2. Mann D, Mehta V. Cardiovascular embryology. *Int Anesthesiol Clin.* 2004;42(4):15-28.

3. Ghorpade A, Baxter BT. Biochemistry and molecular regulation of matrix macromolecules in abdominal aortic aneurysms. *Ann N Y Acad Sci.* 1996;800:138-150.

4. Guo DC, Papke CL, He R, Milewicz DM. Pathogenesis of thoracic and abdominal aortic aneurysms. *Ann N Y Acad Sci.* 2006;1085:339-352.

5. Bergwerff M, Verberne ME, DeRuiter MC, et al. Neural crest cell contribution to the developing circulatory system: implications for vascular morphology? *Circ Res.* 1998;82(2):221-231.

6. Gittenberger-de Groot AC, DeRuiter MC, Bergwerff M, Poelmann RE. Smooth muscle cell origin and its relation to heterogeneity in development and disease. *Arterioscler Thromb Vasc Biol.* 1999;19(7):1589-1594.

7. Tilson MD. Aortic aneurysms and atherosclerosis. *Circulation.* 1992;85(1):378-379.

8. Webster MW, Ferrell RE, St Jean PL, et al. Ultrasound screening of first-degree relatives of patients with an abdominal aortic aneurysm. *J Vasc Surg.* 1991;13(1):9-13; discussion 13-14.

9. Reed D, Reed C, Stemmermann G, Hayashi T. Are aortic aneurysms caused by atherosclerosis? *Circulation.* 1992;85(1):205-211.

10. Tsai TT, Fattori R, Trimarchi S, et al. Long-term survival in patients presenting with type B acute aortic dissection: insights from the International Registry of Acute Aortic Dissection. *Circulation.* 2006;114(21):2226-2231.

11. Cambria RP, Davison JK, Zannetti S, et al. Thoracoabdominal aneurysm repair: perspectives over a decade with the clamp-and-sew technique. *Ann Surg.* 1997;226(3):294-303; discussion 303-305.

12. Coselli JS, LeMaire SA, de Figueiredo LP, Kirby RP. Paraplegia after thoracoabdominal aortic aneurysm repair: is dissection a risk factor? *Ann Thorac Surg.* 1997;63(1):28-35; discussion 35-36.

13. Isselbacher EM. Thoracic and abdominal aortic aneurysms. *Circulation.* 2005;111(6):816-828.

14. Svensson LG, Crawford ES, Hess KR, et al. Experience with 1509 patients undergoing thoracoabdominal aortic operations. *J Vasc Surg.* 1993;17(2):357-368; discussion 368-370.

15. Sueyoshi E, Sakamoto I, Hayashi K, et al. Growth rate of aortic diameter in patients with type B aortic dissection during the chronic phase. *Circulation.* 2004;110(11 Suppl 1):II256-261.

16. Kato M, Bai H, Sato K, et al. Determining surgical indications for acute type B dissection based on enlargement of aortic diameter during the chronic phase. *Circulation.* 1995;92(9 Suppl):II107-12.

17. Neya K, Omoto R, Kyo S, et al. Outcome of Stanford type B acute aortic dissection. *Circulation.* 1992;86(5 Suppl):II1-7.

18. DeBakey ME, McCollum CH, Crawford ES, et al. Dissection and dissecting aneurysms of the aorta: twenty-year follow-up of five hundred twenty-seven patients treated surgically. *Surgery.* 1982;92(6):1118-1134.

19. Schor JS, Yerlioglu ME, Galla JD, et al. Selective management of acute type B aortic dissection: long-term follow-up. *Ann Thorac Surg.* 1996;61(5):1339-1341.

20. Kim SY, Martin N, Hsia EC, et al. Management of aortic disease in Marfan Syndrome: a decision analysis. *Arch Intern Med.* 2005;165(7):749-755.

21. Panneton J, Hollier, LM. Basic data underlying clinical decision making: Non-dissecting thoracoabdominal aortic aneurysms: Part I. *Ann Vasc Surg.* 1995;9:503-514.

22. Guo D, Hasham S, Kuang SQ, et al. Familial thoracic aortic aneurysms and dissections: genetic heterogeneity with a major locus mapping to 5q13-14. *Circulation.* 2001;103(20):2461-2468.

23. Nataf P, Lansac E. Dilation of the thoracic aorta: medical and surgical management. *Heart.* 2006;92(9):1345-1352.

24. Bickerstaff LK, Pairolero PC, Hollier LH, et al. Thoracic aortic aneurysms: a population-based study. *Surgery.* 1982;92(6):1103-1108.

25. Johansson G, Markstrom U, Swedenborg J. Ruptured thoracic aortic aneurysms: a study of incidence and mortality rates. *J Vasc Surg.* 1995;21(6):985-988.

26. Davies RR, Goldstein LJ, Coady MA, et al. Yearly rupture or dissection rates for thoracic aortic aneurysms: simple prediction based on

size. *Ann Thorac Surg.* 2002;73(1):17-27; discussion 27-28.

27. Estes JE Jr. Abdominal aortic aneurysm; a study of one hundred and two cases. *Circulation.* 1950;2(2):258-264.

28. Clouse WD, Hallett JW Jr, Schaff HV, et al. Improved prognosis of thoracic aortic aneurysms: a population-based study. *JAMA.* 1998;280(22):1926-1929.

29. Juvonen T, Ergin MA, Galla JD, et al. Prospective study of the natural history of thoracic aortic aneurysms. *Ann Thorac Surg.* 1997;63(6):1533-1545.

30. Cambria RP, Brewster DC, Moncure AC, et al. Spontaneous aortic dissection in the presence of coexistent or previously repaired atherosclerotic aortic aneurysm. *Ann Surg.* 1988;208(5):619-624.

31. Clouse WD, Hallett JW Jr, Schaff HV, et al. Acute aortic dissection: population-based incidence compared with degenerative aortic aneurysm rupture. *Mayo Clin Proc.* 2004;79(2):176-180.

32. Crawford ES, Hess KR, Cohen ES, et al. Ruptured aneurysm of the descending thoracic and thoracoabdominal aorta. Analysis according to size and treatment. *Ann Surg.* 1991;213(5):417-425; discussion 425-426.

33. Cambria RA, Gloviczki P, Stanson AW, et al. Outcome and expansion rate of 57 thoracoabdominal aortic aneurysms managed nonoperatively. *Am J Surg.* 1995;170(2):213-217.

34. Dapunt OE, Galla JD, Sadeghi AM, et al. The natural history of thoracic aortic aneurysms. *J Thorac Cardiovasc Surg.* 1994;107(5):1323-1332; discussion 1332-1333.

35. Perko MJ, Norgaard M, Herzog TM, et al. Unoperated aortic aneurysm: a survey of 170 patients. *Ann Thorac Surg.* 1995;59(5):1204-1209.

36. Masuda Y, Takanashi K, Takasu J, et al. Expansion rate of thoracic aortic aneurysms and influencing factors. *Chest.* 1992;102(2):461-466.

37. Griepp RB, Ergin MA, Galla JD, et al. Natural history of descending thoracic and thoracoabdominal aneurysms. *Ann Thorac Surg.* 1999;67(6):1927-1930; discussion 1953-1958.

38. Coady MA, Rizzo JA, Hammond GL, et al.

What is the appropriate size criterion for resection of thoracic aortic aneurysms? *J Thorac Cardiovasc Surg.* 1997;113(3):476-491; discussion 489-491.

39. Coady MA, Rizzo JA, Hammond GL, et al. Surgical intervention criteria for thoracic aortic aneurysms: a study of growth rates and complications. *Ann Thorac Surg.* 1999; 67(6):1922-1926; discussion 1953-1958.

40. Bonser RS, Pagano D, Lewis ME, et al. Clinical and patho-anatomical factors affecting expansion of thoracic aortic aneurysms. *Heart.* 2000;84(3):277-283.

41. Juvonen T, Ergin MA, Galla JD, et al. Risk factors for rupture of chronic type B dissections. *J Thorac Cardiovasc Surg.* 1999;117(4):776-786.

42. Lobato AC, Puech Leao P. Predictive factors for rupture of thoracoabdominal aortic aneurysm. *J Vasc Surg.* 1998;27(3):446-453.

43. Galla JD, Ergin MA, Lansman SL, et al. Identification of risk factors in patients undergoing thoracoabdominal aneurysm repair. *J Card Surg.* 1997;12(2 Suppl):292-299.

44. Joyce JW, Fairbairn JF II, Kincaid OW, Juergen JL. Aneurysms of the thoracic aorta. A clinical study with special reference to prognosis. *Circulation.* 1964;29:176-181.

45. Fuster V, Andrews P. Medical treatment of the aorta. I. *Cardiol Clin.* 1999;17(4):697-715, viii.

46. Gott VL, Pyeritz RE, Magovern GJ Jr, et al. Surgical treatment of aneurysms of the ascending aorta in the Marfan syndrome. Results of composite-graft repair in 50 patients. *N Engl J Med.* 1986;314(17):1070-1074.

47. Cooke JC, Cambria RP. Simultaneous tracheobronchial and esophageal obstruction caused by a descending thoracic aneurysm. *J Vasc Surg.* 1993;18(1):90-94.

48. Acher CW, Wynn MM, Hoch JR, Kranner PW. Cardiac function is a risk factor for paralysis in thoracoabdominal aortic replacement. *J Vasc Surg.* 1998;27(5):821-828; discussion 829-830.

49. Coselli JS, LeMaire SA, Miller CC III, et al. Mortality and paraplegia after thoracoabdominal aortic aneurysm repair: a risk factor analysis. *Ann Thorac Surg.* 2000;69(2):409-414.

50. Safi HJ, Miller CC III, Carr C, et al. Importance of intercostal artery reattachment during tho-

racoabdominal aortic aneurysm repair. *J Vasc Surg.* 1998;27(1):58-66; discussion 66-68.

51. Conrad MF, Crawford RS, Davison JK, Cambria RP. Thoracoabdominal aneurysm repair: a 20-year perspective. *Ann Thorac Surg.* 2007;83:S856-S861.

52. LeMaire SA, Miller CC III, Conklin LD, et al. Estimating group mortality and paraplegia rates after thoracoabdominal aortic aneurysm repair. *Ann Thorac Surg.* 2003;75(2):508-513.

53. Coselli JS, LeMaire SA, Buket S, Berzin E. Subsequent proximal aortic operations in 123 patients with previous infrarenal abdominal aortic aneurysm surgery. *J Vasc Surg.* 1995;22(1):59-67.

54. Coselli JS. Thoracoabdominal aortic aneurysms: experience with 372 patients. *J Card Surg.* 1994;9(6):638-647.

55. Cox GS, O'Hara PJ, Hertzer NR, et al. Thoracoabdominal aneurysm repair: a representative experience. *J Vasc Surg.* 1992;15(5):780-787; discussion 787-788.

56. Gilling-Smith GL, Worswick L, Knight PF, et al. Surgical repair of thoracoabdominal aortic aneurysm: 10 years' experience. *Br J Surg.* 1995;82(5):624-629.

57. Schepens MA, Dekker E, Hamerlijnck RP, Vermeulen FE. Survival and aortic events after graft replacement for thoracoabdominal aortic aneurysm. *Cardiovasc Surg.* 1996;4(6):713-719.

58. Nistri S, Sorbo MD, Marin M, et al. Aortic root dilatation in young men with normally functioning bicuspid aortic valves. *Heart.* 1999;82(1):19-22.

59. Hartnell GG. Imaging of aortic aneurysms and dissection: CT and MRI. *J Thorac Imaging.* 2001;16(1):35-46.

60. Shores J, Berger KR, Murphy EA, Pyeritz RE. Progression of aortic dilatation and the benefit of long-term beta-adrenergic blockade in Marfan's syndrome. *N Engl J Med.* 1994;330(19):1335-1341.

61. von Oppell UO, Dunne TT, De Groot KM, Zilla P. Spinal cord protection in the absence of collateral circulation: meta-analysis of mortality and paraplegia. *J Card Surg.* 1994;9(6):685-691.

62. Mauney MC, Tribble CG, Cope JT, et al. Is clamp and sew still viable for thoracic aortic

resection? *Ann Surg.* 1996;223(5):534-540; discussion 540-543.

63. Schepens MA, Defauw JJ, Hamerlijnck RP, Vermeulen FE. Use of left heart bypass in the surgical repair of thoracoabdominal aortic aneurysms. *Ann Vasc Surg.* 1995;9(4):327-338.

64. Cohen JR, Angus L, Asher A, et al. Disseminated intravascular coagulation as a result of supraceliac clamping: implications for thoracoabdominal aneurysm repair. *Ann Vasc Surg.* 1987;1(5):552-557.

65. Cambria RP, Davison JK, Zannetti S, et al. Clinical experience with epidural cooling for spinal cord protection during thoracic and thoracoabdominal aneurysm repair. *J Vasc Surg.* 1997;25(2):234-241; discussion 241-243.

66. Davison JK, Cambria RP, Vierra DJ, et al. Epidural cooling for regional spinal cord hypothermia during thoracoabdominal aneurysm repair. *J Vasc Surg.* 1994;20(2):304-310.

67. Grabitz K, Sandmann W, Stuhmeier K, et al. The risk of ischemic spinal cord injury in patients undergoing graft replacement for thoracoabdominal aortic aneurysms. *J Vasc Surg.* 1996;23(2):230-240.

68. Estrera AL, Miller CC III, Huynh TT, et al. Neurologic outcome after thoracic and thoracoabdominal aortic aneurysm repair. *Ann Thorac Surg.* 2001;72(4):1225-1230; discussion 1230-1231.

69. Jacobs MJ, de Mol BA, Elenbaas T, et al. Spinal cord blood supply in patients with thoracoabdominal aortic aneurysms. *J Vasc Surg.* 2002;35(1):30-37.

70. van Dongen EP, Schepens MA, Morshuis WJ, et al. Thoracic and thoracoabdominal aortic aneurysm repair: use of evoked potential monitoring in 118 patients. *J Vasc Surg.* 2001;34(6):1035-1040.

71. Cambria RP, Davison JK, Giglia JS, Gertler JP. Mesenteric shunting decreases visceral ischemia during thoracoabdominal aneurysm repair. *J Vasc Surg.* 1998;27(4):745-749.

72. Hollier LH, Money SR, Naslund TC, et al. Risk of spinal cord dysfunction in patients undergoing thoracoabdominal aortic replacement. *Am J Surg.* 1992;164(3):210-213; discussion 213-214.

73. Money SR, Rice K, Crockett D, et al. Risk

of respiratory failure after repair of thoracoabdominal aortic aneurysms. *Am J Surg*. 1994;168(2):152-155.

74. Svensson LG, Hess KR, Coselli JS, et al. A prospective study of respiratory failure after high-risk surgery on the thoracoabdominal aorta. *J Vasc Surg*. 1991;14(3):271-282.

75. Safi HJ, Campbell MP, Miller CC III, et al. Cerebral spinal fluid drainage and distal aortic perfusion decrease the incidence of neurological deficit: the results of 343 descending and thoracoabdominal aortic aneurysm repairs. *Eur J Vasc Endovasc Surg*. 1997;14(2):118-124.

76. David TE, Ivanov J, Armstrong S, et al. Aortic valve-sparing operations in patients with aneurysms of the aortic root or ascending aorta. *Ann Thorac Surg*. 2002;74(5):S1758-1761; discussion S1792-1799.

77. Yun KL. Ascending aortic aneurysm and aortic root disease. *Coron Artery Dis*. 2002;13(2):79-84.

78. Dake MD, Miller DC, Semba CP, et al. Transluminal placement of endovascular stent-grafts for the treatment of descending thoracic aortic aneurysms. *N Engl J Med*. 1994;331(26):1729-1734.

79. Bavaria JE, Appoo JJ, Makaroun MS, et al. Endovascular stent grafting versus open surgical repair of descending thoracic aortic aneurysms in low-risk patients: a multicenter comparative trial. *J Thorac Cardiovasc Surg*. 2007;133(2):369-377.

80. Cho JS, Haider SE, Makaroun MS. Endovascular therapy of thoracic aneurysms: Gore TAG trial results. *Semin Vasc Surg*. 2006;19(1):18-24.

81. Leurs LJ, Bell R, Degrieck Y, et al. Endovascular treatment of thoracic aortic diseases: combined experience from the EUROSTAR and United Kingdom Thoracic Endograft registries. *J Vasc Surg*. 2004;40(4):670-679; discussion 679-680.

82. Makaroun MS, Dillavou ED, Kee ST, et al. Endovascular treatment of thoracic aortic aneurysms: results of the phase II multicenter trial of the GORE TAG thoracic endoprosthesis. *J Vasc Surg*. 2005;41(1):1-9.

83. Stone DH, Brewster DC, Kwolek CJ, et al. Stent-graft versus open-surgical repair of the thoracic aorta: mid-term results. *J Vasc Surg*. 2006;44(6):1188-1197.

84. Greenberg R, Resch T, Nyman U, et al. Endovascular repair of descending thoracic aortic aneurysms: an early experience with intermediate-term follow-up. *J Vasc Surg*. 2000;31(1 Pt 1):147-156.

85. Mitchell RS, Miller DC, Dake MD, et al. Thoracic aortic aneurysm repair with an endovascular stent graft: the "first generation." *Ann Thorac Surg*. 1999;67(6):1971-1974; discussion 1979-1980.

86. Brewster DC, Jones JE, Chung TK, et al. Long-term outcomes after endovascular abdominal aortic aneurysm repair: the first decade. *Ann Surg*. 2006;244(3):426-438.

87. Grabenwoger M, Hutschala D, Ehrlich MP, et al. Thoracic aortic aneurysms: treatment with endovascular self-expandable stent grafts. *Ann Thorac Surg*. 2000;69(2):441-445.

88. Cowan JA Jr, Dimick JB, Henke PK, et al. Surgical treatment of intact thoracoabdominal aortic aneurysms in the United States: hospital and surgeon volume-related outcomes. *J Vasc Surg*. 2003;37(6):1169-1174.

89. Black SA, Wolfe JH, Clark M, et al. Complex thoracoabdominal aortic aneurysms: endovascular exclusion with visceral revascularization. *J Vasc Surg*. 2006;43(6):1081-1089; discussion 1089.

90. Kouchoukos NT, Dougenis D. Surgery of the thoracic aorta. *N Engl J Med*. 1997;336(26):1876-1888.

91. Hirst AE, Johns VJ, Klime SW. Dissecting aneurysm of the aorta: a review of 505 cases. *Medicine*. 1958;37:217-219.

92. Hagan PG, Nienaber CA, Isselbacher EM, et al. The International Registry of Acute Aortic Dissection (IRAD): new insights into an old disease. *JAMA*. 2000; 283(7):897-903.

93. Khan IA, Nair CK. Clinical, diagnostic, and management perspectives of aortic dissection. *Chest*. 2002;122(1):311-328.

94. Williams D. Pathophysiology of aortic dissection. In: Ernst CB, ed. *Current Therapy in Vascular Surgery*; Mosby, Philadelphia, PA; 1997:211-215.

95. Debakey ME, Henley WS, Cooley DA, et al. Surgical management of dissecting aneurysms of the aorta. *Thorac Cardiovasc Surg*. 1965;49:130-148.

96. Daily PO, Trueblood HW, Stinson EB, et al. Management of acute aortic dissection. *Ann Thorac Surg.* 1970;10:237-246.

97. Auer J, Berent R, Eber B. Aortic dissection: incidence, natural history and impact of surgery. *J Clin Basic Cardiol.* 2002;3:151-154.

98. Lauterbach SR, Cambria RP, Brewster DC, et al. Contemporary management of aortic branch compromise resulting from acute aortic dissection. *J Vasc Surg.* 2001;33(6):1185-1192.

99. Larson EW, Edwards WD. Risk factors for aortic dissection: a necropsy study of 161 cases. *Am J Cardiol.* 1984;53(6):849-855.

100. Cambria RP, Brewster DC, Gertler J, et al. Vascular complications associated with spontaneous aortic dissection. *J Vasc Surg.* 1988;7(2):199-209.

101. Fann JI, Smith JA, Miller DC, et al. Surgical management of aortic dissection during a 30-year period. *Circulation.* 1995;92(9 Suppl):II113-121.

102. Bernard Y, Zimmermann H, Chocron S, et al. False lumen patency as a predictor of late outcome in aortic dissection. *Am J Cardiol.* 2001;87(12):1378-1382.

103. Panneton JM, Hollier LH. Dissecting descending thoracic and thoracoabdominal aortic aneurysms: Part II. *Ann Vasc Surg.* 1995;9(6):596-605.

104. Hollier LH, Symmonds JB, Pairolero PC, Cherry KJ, Hallett JW, Gloviczki P. Thoracoabdominal aortic aneurysm repair. Analysis of postoperative morbidity. *Arch Surg.* 1988;123(7):871-875.

105. Deeb GM, Williams DM, Bolling SF, et al. Surgical delay for acute type A dissection with malperfusion. *Ann Thorac Surg.* 1997;64(6):1669-1675; discussion 1675-1677.

106. Nienaber CA, Eagle KA. Aortic dissection: new frontiers in diagnosis and management: Part II: therapeutic management and follow-up. *Circulation.* 2003;108(6):772-778.

107. Januzzi JL, Movsowitz HD, Choi J, et al. Significance of recurrent pain in acute type B aortic dissection. *Am J Cardiol.* 2001;87(7):930-933.

108. Nallamothu BK, Mehta RH, Saint S, et al. Syncope in acute aortic dissection: diagnostic, prognostic, and clinical implications. *Am J Med.* 2002;113(6):468-471.

109. Januzzi JL, Sabatine MS, Choi JC, et al. Refractory systemic hypertension following type B aortic dissection. *Am J Cardiol.* 2001;88(6):686-688.

110. Bossone E, Rampoldi V, Nienaber CA, et al. Usefulness of pulse deficit to predict in-hospital complications and mortality in patients with acute type A aortic dissection. *Am J Cardiol.* 2002;89(7):851-855.

111. von Kodolitsch Y, Csösz SK, Koschyk DH, et al. Intramural hematoma of the aorta: predictors of progression to dissection and rupture. *Circulation.* 2003;107(8):1158-1163.

112. Nienaber CA, von Kodolitsch Y, Petersen B, et al. Intramural hemorrhage of the thoracic aorta. Diagnostic and therapeutic implications. *Circulation.* 1995;92(6):1465-1472.

113. Muluk SC, Kaufman JA, Torchiana DF, et al. Diagnosis and treatment of thoracic aortic intramural hematoma. *J Vasc Surg.* 1996;24(6):1022-1029.

114. Evangelista A, Mukherjee D, Mehta RH, et al. Acute intramural hematoma of the aorta: a mystery in evolution. *Circulation.* 2005;111(8):1063-1070.

115. Sueyoshi E, Imada T, Sakamoto I, et al. Analysis of predictive factors for progression of type B aortic intramural hematoma with computed tomography. *J Vasc Surg.* 2002;35(6):1179-1183.

116. Williams DM, LePage MA, Lee DY. The dissected aorta: part I. Early anatomic changes in an in vitro model. *Radiology.* 1997;203(1):23-31.

117. Williams DM, Lee DY, Hamilton BH, et al. The dissected aorta: percutaneous treatment of ischemic complications—principles and results. *J Vasc Interv Radiol.* 1997;8(4):605-625.

118. Cambria RP. Surgical treatment of complicated distal aortic dissection. *Semin Vasc Surg.* 2002;15(2):97-107.

119. Young JR, Kramer J, Humphries AW. The ischemic leg: a clue to dissecting aneurysm. *Cardiovasc Clin.* 1975;7(1):201-205.

120. Guthaner DF, Miller DC. Digital subtraction angiography of aortic dissection. *AJR Am J Roentgenol.* 1983;141(1):157-161.

121. Petasnick JP. Radiologic evaluation of aortic dissection. *Radiology*. 1991;180(2):297-305.

122. Rizzo RJ, Aranki SF, Aklog L, et al. Rapid non-invasive diagnosis and surgical repair of acute ascending aortic dissection. Improved survival with less angiography. *J Thorac Cardiovasc Surg*. 1994;108(3):567-574; discussion 574-575.

123. Moore AG, Eagle KA, Bruckman D, et al. Choice of computed tomography, transesophageal echocardiography, magnetic resonance imaging, and aortography in acute aortic dissection: International Registry of Acute Aortic Dissection (IRAD). *Am J Cardiol*. 2002;89(10):1235-1238.

124. Hartnell G, Costello P. The diagnosis of thoracic aortic dissection by noninvasive imaging procedures. *N Engl J Med*. 1993;328(22):1637; author reply 1638.

125. LePage MA, Quint LE, Sonnad SS, et al. Aortic dissection: CT features that distinguish true lumen from false lumen. *AJR Am J Roentgenol*. 2001;177(1):207-211.

126. Wheat M Jr, Palmer, RF. Dissecting aneurysms of the aorta: present status of drug versus surgical therapy. *Prog Cardiovasc Dis*. 1968;11(3):198-210.

127. Isselbacher E. Diseases of the aorta. In: Braunwald E, ed. *Heart Disease*. 2002:1422-1455.

128. Isselbacher E, Cigarroa JE, Eagle KA. Cardiac tamponade complicating proximal aortic dissection: is pericardiocentesis harmful? *Circulation*.1994;90:2375-2379.

129. Trimarchi S, Nienaber CA, Rampoldi V, et al. Contemporary results of surgery in acute type A aortic dissection: the International Registry of Acute Aortic Dissection experience. *J Thorac Cardiovasc Surg*. 2005;129(1):112-122.

130. Lai DT, Robbins RC, Mitchell RS, et al. Does profound hypothermic circulatory arrest improve survival in patients with acute type a aortic dissection? *Circulation*. 2002;106(12 Suppl 1):I218-228.

131. Jex R, Schaff HV, Piehler JM, Ilstrup D. Early and late results following repair of dissections of the descending thoracic aorta. *J Vasc Surg*. 1986(3):226-236.

132. Verdant A, Cossette R, Page A, et al. Aneurysms of the descending thoracic aorta: three hundred sixty-six consecutive cases resected without paraplegia. *J Vasc Surg*. 1995;21(3):385-390; discussion 390-391.

133. Glower DD, Speier RH, White WD, et al. Management and long-term outcome of aortic dissection. *Ann Surg*. 1991;214(1):31-41.

134. Miller DC, Mitchell RS, Oyer PE, et al. Independent determinants of operative mortality for patients with aortic dissections. *Circulation*. 1984;70(3 Pt 2):I153-I164.

135. Svensson LG, Crawford ES, Hess KR, et al. Dissection of the aorta and dissecting aortic aneurysms. Improving early and long-term surgical results. *Circulation*. 1990;82(5 Suppl):IV24-38.

136. Elefteriades JA, Hartleroad J, Gusberg RJ, et al. Long-term experience with descending aortic dissection: the complication-specific approach. *Ann Thorac Surg*. 1992;53(1):11-20; discussion 20-21.

137. Bortone AS, De Cillis E, D'Agostino D, de Luca Tupputi Schinosa L. Endovascular treatment of thoracic aortic disease: four years of experience. *Circulation*. 2004;110(11 Suppl 1):II262-267.

138. Dake MD, Kato N, Mitchell RS, et al. Endovascular stent-graft placement for the treatment of acute aortic dissection. *N Engl J Med*. 1999;340(20):1546-1552.

139. Nienaber CA, Fattori R, Lund G, et al. Nonsurgical reconstruction of thoracic aortic dissection by stent-graft placement. *N Engl J Med*. 1999;340(20):1539-1545.

140. Onitsuka S, Akashi H, Tayama K, et al. Long-term outcome and prognostic predictors of medically treated acute type B aortic dissections. *Ann Thorac Surg*. 2004;78(4):1268-1273.

141. Erbel R, Oelert H, Meyer J, et al. Effect of medical and surgical therapy on aortic dissection evaluated by transesophageal echocardiography. Implications for prognosis and therapy. The European Cooperative Study Group on Echocardiography. *Circulation*. 1993;87(5):1604-1615.

142. Eggebrecht H, Nienaber CA, Neuhauser M, et al. Endovascular stent-graft placement in aortic dissection: a meta-analysis. *Eur Heart J*. 2006;27(4):489-498.

143. Xu SD, Huang FJ, Yang JF, et al. Endovascular repair of acute type B aortic dissection: early and mid-term results. *J Vasc Surg.* 2006;43(6):1090-1095.

144. White RA, Donayre CE, Walot I, Kopchok GE. Intraprocedural imaging: thoracic aortography techniques, intravascular ultrasound, and special equipment. *J Vasc Surg.* 2006;43(Suppl A):53A-61A.

145. Mossop PJ, McLachlan CS, Amukotuwa SA, Nixon IK. Staged endovascular treatment for complicated type B aortic dissection. *Nat Clin Pract Cardiovasc Med.* 2005;2(6):316-321; quiz 322.

9

Abdominal Aortic Aneurysmal Disease

Tikva S. Jacobs and Michael L. Marin

Abdominal aortic aneurysm (AAA) is the most common type of true arterial aneurysm. Over the last 2 decades the incidence has been increasing; partially due to the aging population and partially due to improvements in diagnostic modalities and the use of screening programs. Since the first description of an AAA by the physician Andreas Vesalius in the sixteenth century, there have been major advances in diagnosis and treatment of this disease. From the first successful ligation of an aorta for an AAA by Rudolph Matas in 1923, to relining the aorta with an endovascular stent graft, the treatment of AAA has made remarkable advances, along with the understanding of the disease process.

Epidemiology

Abdominal aortic aneurysms are generally a disease of older white males. The annual incidence is less than 1 in 1000 people younger than 60 years of age and peaks at approximately 7 in 1000 in people in their mid-60s. The prevalence of AAA is 5 to 6 times more common in men than women and 3.5 times more common in whites than blacks.[1,2] In the Veterans Administration (VA) screening study of more than 73,000 patients aged 50 to 79, the prevalence of an AAA at least 3 cm was 4.6% and an AAA of ≥ 4 cm was 1.4%.[3] Numerous studies, using ultrasonography or autopsy data, have been collected to determine the prevalence of AAAs. These numbers all vary depending on the population studied. However, the prevalence of AAAs in men over the age of 50 in the western world is 3% to 10%.[4]

The prevalence of AAA in a population depends on risk factors that are associated with AAA, including male gender, positive family history, older age, smoking, coronary artery disease, hypertension, peripheral vascular disease, white race, and hypercholesterolemia.[5] Multiple studies have tried to elicit which risk factor has the highest impact on the prevalence of AAAs. In the VA screening study the most strongly associated risk factor for AAAs was smoking. The relative risk of an AAA of 4 cm or larger was 5.6-fold higher in smokers than in nonsmokers, and the risk increased significantly with the number of years of smoking.[3] Several other studies have also shown a strong clinical association between tobacco use and

Vascular Disease: Diagnostic and Therapeutic Approaches. © 2011 Michael R. Jaff and Christopher J. White, editors. Cardiotext Publishing, ISBN: 978-1-935395-16-4.

abdominal aortic aneurysms.[6-10] In a systematic review conducted by Lederle and colleagues,[11] the relative risk for aortic aneurysm in current smokers was generally 3 to 6 compared with 1 to 2 for coronary artery disease and cerebrovascular disease.

Besides smoking, the VA study also found associations between AAA and male gender (4.5-fold risk) white race (2-fold), and family history (2-fold). Patients with diabetes were found to have a decreased risk of having an AAA (0.5-fold less).[3] Madaric et al[12] looked at the prevalence of AAA in patients older than 60 with coronary artery disease and concluded that the prevalence of AAA was higher in those with than those without coronary artery disease.

Familial clustering is also considered one of the main risk factors for AAA. Fifteen percent to 25% of patients undergoing an AAA repair have a first-degree relative with a clinically apparent AAA compared with 2% to 3% of age-matched control patients without AAAs.[13] First-degree relatives of a patient with an AAA have a 12-fold increased risk for aneurysm development themselves,[14] and brothers of a patient with an AAA have an 18-fold increased risk for AAA development, highest in the 50- to 60-year-old range and decreasing thereafter.[15] On average these patients with familial aneurysms tend to be 5 to 7 years younger.[13,15] However, the genetic cause for AAA remains elusive and seems to be a multifactorial combination of genetic and environmental factors.[16]

Pathophysiology

An aneurysm is defined as a widening or dilatation of a vessel. In 1991, the Society for Vascular Surgery and the International Society for Cardiothoracic Surgery Ad Hoc Committee on Standards in reporting on AAAs proposed that the infrarenal diameter should be 1.5 times the expected diameter.[17] The normal diameter of the aorta varies with age, sex, and body weight. Therefore, there is no definite diameter; however, it is conventionally diagnosed when the infrarenal aorta has a transverse diameter of at least 30 mm. The dilatation affects all 3 layers of the aorta and is usually fusiform (affecting the whole circumference) (Figure 9.1).

Although the pathogenesis of an AAA remains poorly understood, the development is clearly associated with alterations of the connective tissue in the aortic wall. The aortic wall contains vascular smooth muscle cells as well as matrix proteins—elastin and collagen. In the normal aorta these are arranged in concentric layers to withstand arterial pressure, and there is a gradual but marked reduction in the number of medial elastin layers from the proximal thoracic aorta to the infrarenal aorta. Besides this structural change of a "thinning" media, there is a decrease in the collagen and elastin content from the proximal to distal aorta.[18] Histologic features of an aneurysm wall shows fragmentation of elastic fibers in the media. This degradation of elastin appears to be the initiating process of aneurysm formation, by causing a dilatation of the medial wall at which point the adventitia, which is primarily made up of collagen, becomes responsible for the strength of the aorta. Collagen degradation is the ultimate cause of rupture.

The alteration in collagen and elastin in the aortic wall is dependent on production of proteases by medial smooth muscle cells, adventitial fibroblasts, and the cells of the lymphomonocytic infiltrate.[19,20] *Matrix metalloproteinases (MMPs)* digest both collagen and elastin, however MMP-2, -7, -9, and -12 are generally considered to be primarily elastases. MMP-9 is found in abundance in medial smooth muscle cells as well as inflammatory cells, and increased levels have been found in the aortic wall and serum in up to 50% of patients with aortic aneurysms. Elevated levels of these MMPs have been shown to occur in aneurysmal aortic wall compared with normal aorta.[21-23] *Tissue inhibitors of matrix metalloproteinases (TIMPs)* are also increased in the wall of the aneurysm. However, the balance between proteases and antiproteases is in favor of proteolysis.[24,25]

The question remains, what initiates the proteases and causes a breakdown of collagen

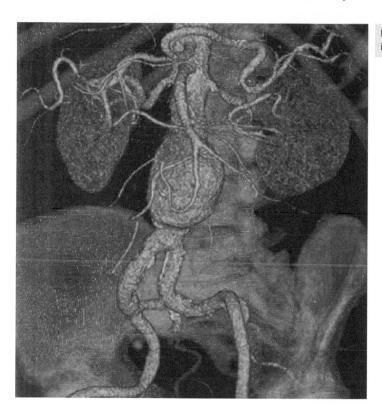

Figure 9.1 3D reconstruction of an infrarenal aortic aneurysm.

and elastin in the media? MMPs are produced in high concentrations by macrophages, and transmural inflammation seems to be central to the development of AAA, but its cause is not clearly understood.

Hemodynamics, structural and autoimmune factors unique to the infrarenal aorta, have also been implicated.[26,27] Reflected waves from the aortic bifurcation increase pulsatility and wall tension in the distal, less compliant atherosclerotic aorta. Absence of vasa vasorum has been suggested to reduce nutrient supply and to potentiate degeneration.[21] Smoking may induce MMP production by macrophages.[11] Overall the exact pathophysiology of AAA formation is likely a combination of structural, cellular, and hemodynamic changes.

Natural History

AAA may be asymptomatic for years; however, approximately 30% will go on to rupture if left untreated. The majority of patients with ruptured aneurysms die before making it to the hospital or the operating room. Those who make it to surgery have a high morbidity and mortality and only 10% to 25% will ultimately survive until discharge.[28]

The risk of rupture is related to the size of the aneurysm. Multiple studies have agreed that the risk of rupture increases to a point that elective repair is warranted when the diameter reaches 5.0 to 5.5 cm. The real controversy is how to manage small aneurysms. In the past, elective repair was advocated for patients with an AAA ≥ 4.0 cm or greater who did not have medical contraindications to surgery.[29] Since then 2 studies have been done to determine the management of these small aneurysms: the UK Small Aneurysm Trial and the US Veterans Affairs Medical Center ADAM trial. Both were randomized, controlled clinical trials that showed no benefit from early repair of patients with aneurysms < 5.5 cm in diameter.[30,31] There was no benefit because the rate of rupture was low (0.6%/year). This rate was consistent with other population-based studies[32,33] and was obtained by using an active surveillance program where patients were urged to return for imaging studies at 6-month intervals.[31]

Diameter of the AAA is not the only isolated factor in risk of rupture; small aneurysms do rupture and larger ones remain stable for long periods of time. Studies have shown that a larger initial diameter, COPD, and hypertension have all been independent predictors of rupture.[34] Female gender (women having a 3-fold higher risk of rupture than men),[28,35,36] familial AAAs, and smoking have also been implicated.[6,8]

Until further studies are done on rupture risks, the current thinking suggests that rupture is dependent on diameter. AAAs < 4 cm have a 0% per year rupture rate. Aneurysms 4 to 5 cm have a 0.5% to 5.0% risk of rupture. Five- to 6-cm aneurysms have a 3% to 15% rupture risk; 6 to 7 cm, 10% to 20% rupture risk per year. Abdominal aortic aneurysms 7 to 8 cm have a 20% to 40% rupture risk per year.[37] In summary, for any given aneurysm size, one must take into consideration gender, hypertension, COPD, and current smoking status. Patients with familial aneurysms or those with rapid expansion are also at higher risk for rupture than their counterparts.

Diagnostic Evaluation

History and Physical Exam

Most AAAs are asymptomatic, therefore, when taking a history the physician must focus on the past medical history of the patient to look for risk factors. Questions should include the history of hypertension, COPD, coronary artery disease, and smoking. Family history of aneurysms, especially AAAs, is also essential. The physician should examine the supraumbilical region with bimanual palpation to try to assess the actual size of the aorta. However, depending on the size of the aneurysm and the body habitus of the patient, it may be missed on physical exam. Sensitivity for being able to palpate the aorta increases with the diameter of the lesion: 61% for 3.0 to 3.9 cm, 69% for 4.0 to 4.9 cm, and 82% for 5 cm or greater.[38] Occasionally an AAA can be seen on plain radiography, if there are calcifications in the aortic wall. Today the majority of AAAs are diagnosed as incidental findings on imaging studies done for other reasons. However, now that the US Preventative Services Task Force has agreed that screening for men ages 65 to 75 who are smokers should be done, some AAAs might be diagnosed earlier.[39]

Noninvasive Imaging

Ultrasonography is the easiest and least expensive diagnostic procedure and can accurately measure the size of the aorta. It is often used as the initial assessment to confirm an AAA and then for follow-up as well as for screening. Ultrasonography is limited in looking at the suprarenal aorta and the iliac arteries and cannot rule out rupture. Computed tomography angiography (CTA) is more accurate for diameter and gives the reader a lot more information about the aorta (Figure 9.2). CT scanning can map out the entire aorta to delineate the extent of the aneurysm. It also gives information about the aorta and iliac vessels to help with operative planning. CTA is extremely good for anatomic features of the aorta, such as thrombus, calcifications, anomalous veins (retro-aortic renal vein), and tortuous iliacs, allowing for precise decisions on what operative technique would work best. CTA can also rule out rupture in a patient with a known AAA and abdominal pain, while looking for other abdominal pathology to explain the symptoms (Figure 9.3). However, CTA is more expensive than ultrasonography and exposes the patient to radiation and intravenous contrast. MRA also be used for operative planning; however, the test is longer and more expensive than CTA, and cannot be used in patients with pacemakers (Figure 9.4). It too, like CTA, gives a lot of information about the anatomic features of the aneurysm, but unlike CTA, has poor sensitivity for the detection of calcium.

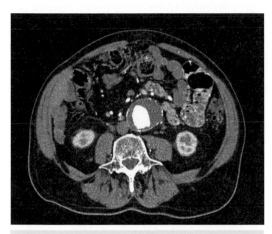

Figure 9.2 CTA, axial image of an abdominal aortic aneurysm, showing the mural thrombus.

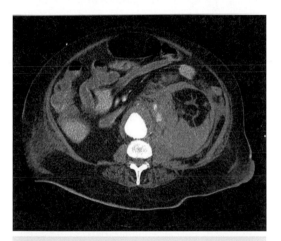

Figure 9.3 CTA of a 76-year-old male who presented with abdominal pain, showing large retroperitoneal hematoma with extravasation of contrast into the hematoma. The patient was taken emergently to the OR and repaired with a bifurcated stent graft.

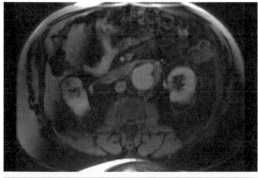

Figure 9.4 MRA of a patient with an abdominal aortic aneurysm.

Invasive Imaging

Conventional angiography is rarely used as a first-line diagnostic tool for AAA, since it too exposes the patient to contrast and radiation and is an invasive procedure. However, it is often used to help with the workup of a patient for endovascular stent-graft repair. Conventional angiography sometimes allows for more precise length measurements of the proximal neck or of the entire aneurysm, especially if the iliac arteries are very tortuous (Figure 9.5). Certain institutions will use angiography prior to the operating room in patients where adjunct procedures are needed, such as renal artery stents or internal iliac artery embolizations (Figure 9.6).

Common variations to know

When evaluating a patient, whether for open or endovascular repair, some important anatomic features to look for on the imaging studies, whether CTA, MRA, or conventional angiography, are accessory renal arteries, retro-aortic renal vein, or a pelvic kidney. The status of the internal iliac arteries and calcification of the external iliac arteries are also important to evaluate prior to repair.

Therapeutic Options

Medical

With the aging population, increased use of imaging for other pathologies, and the US Preventative Services Task Force now recommending screening in men 65 to 75 years old who ever smoked, the number of AAAs diagnosed will continue to rise. The natural history of AAAs is one of progressive structural deterioration, gradual expansion, and eventual rupture. The question becomes how can we disrupt the natural history of AAAs, and slow or prevent them from progressing to the critical diameter needed for surgical repair.

To target these factors physicians must understand the underlying process of aneurysm development. Certain risk factors cannot be ad-

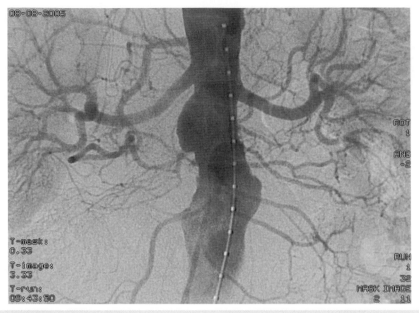

Figure 9.5 Conventional angiogram with a marker catheter to help assess the length of the aorta for preoperative measurements. Each mark is 1 cm apart.

justed, such as male gender and advancing age, so the questions are, what can be done about the modifiable risk factors, and what medical therapy can be aimed at the pathophysiology of the development of AAAs?

Smoking, hypertension, and hypercholesterolemia are some of the modifiable risk factors for the development of AAAs. Smoking is not only a risk factor for the development of an AAA but has also been associated with a higher expansion rate than nonsmokers of 15% to 20%.[9] There is even some evidence of a slow decline of risk after cessation or smoking.[4,9,11] Therefore, smoking cessation should be mandatory in patients with an AAA. Hypercholesterolemia and hypertension have also been implicated, but their association with expansion of AAAs is of uncertain importance.[40]

Multiple medications have been investigated to prevent progression of aortic aneurysms. There was early interest in the use of beta-blockers, specifically propranolol, to try to decrease the rate of dilatation in small AAAs. Two prospective trials were done; both showed a high percentage of patients unable to continue with the drug secondary to side effects (42% and 60%, respectively). In one trial there was no detectable difference between treatment groups with respect to aneurysm growth rate, the need for repair, or mortality.[41] In the other study there was a higher mortality rate in the propranolol group and the study was ended prematurely.[42]

Other trials focused on medical therapy that targeted the pathologic changes observed in AAA: chronic inflammation, destructive remodeling of the extracellular matrix, and depletion of vascular smooth muscle cells. Explant studies, on biopsies of aortic wall taken at the time of aneurysm repair, have highlighted the potential of certain medications to help reduce the production of proteinases and cytokines from human AAA biopsies.[43-45] Indomethacin has been shown to inhibit elastase-induced AAAs in rats, by inhibiting cyclooxygenase (COX-2), which in turn also decreases levels of PGE2, IL-6, and MMP-9.[46] Angiotensin II blockers have been shown to reduce the production of the cytokine osteoprotegerin in aortic aneurysm explants.[47,48] Tetracycline has been shown to reduce MMP production,[49] and statins have reduced levels of MMP-3 and MMP-9 in aortic wall biopsies.[50] Clinical studies to back up these explant studies have been limited.

Nonsteroidal anti-inflammatory drugs have

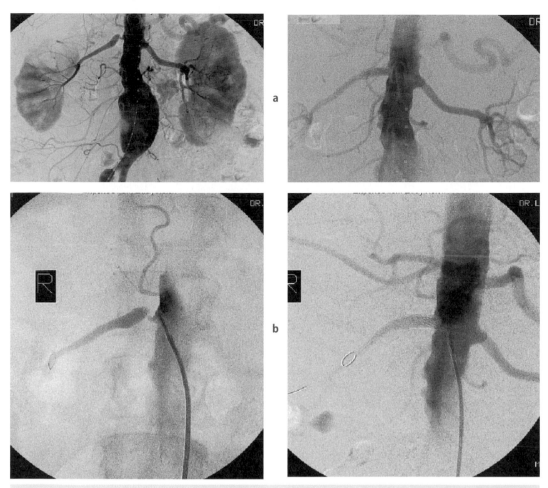

Figure 9.6 Preoperative angiogram. (a, top left and right) Notice the right renal artery with a pinpoint stenosis and then after stent was placed. (b, left and right) Close-up of the stenosis and poststenting angiogram.

been studied in retrospective and cohort studies. Walton and associates[51] found that patients taking NSAIDs had a significantly lower rate of aneurysm expansion compared with the controls (median 1.5 vs. 3.2 mm/year).[51] In the UK Small Aneurysm Trial, a cohort of patients taking nonsteroidal anti-inflammatory medication was noted to have a reduced aortic expansion (1.8 mm/year vs. 3.2mm/year.)[44] Both of these studies were small, and further trials are necessary to determine the true efficacy of NSAIDs in the management of AAAs.

Other investigations have specifically targeted the role of MMPs in aneurysm formation and have focused on suppressing aneurysm development by inhibiting MMPs. Tetracyclines have been successful in explant studies, showing a decrease in the amount of MMPs in the aortic wall as well as in the patient's blood at the time of cross-clamping.[49] Tetracyclines have already shown anti-MMP effects in periodontitis, arthritis, and other conditions.[46] Mosorin et al[52] conducted the first prospective, double-blinded, randomized placebo-controlled study on the effects of doxycycline in patients with small, asymptomatic AAAs. There were 32 patients with AAAs from 3.0 to 5.5 cm. They were randomized to 150 mg of doxycycline daily, for 3 months, and were followed over an 18-month period. Aneurysm expansion rate was significantly lower in the doxycycline group. But it too was a small size and further investigation is needed.[52]

HMG-CoA reductase inhibitors (statins) have also been investigated for their anti-inflammatory properties. They alter the inflammatory status by reducing IL-6 release and may modulate the release of several other substances in the arterial wall, including MMPs.[45,53] Steinmetz and colleagues[54] showed that statins were successful in suppressing the development of experimental AAAs in mice, and there was a relative reduction in wall expression of MMP-9. Human explant studies confirmed a reduction in MMP-9 and MMP-3 in patients treated with statins preoperatively.[45] In a retrospective review of patients in a surveillance program of AAAs, statin users were found to have a decreased growth rate.[53]

Angiotensin-converting enzyme (ACE) inhibitors have been shown to suppress production of elastase in rats.[55] They prevent the expansion and rupture of aortic aneurysms in animal models by preserving medial elastin. Limited human studies are available. In a population-based case-control study looking at patients admitted to the hospital with either a ruptured or an intact abdominal aortic aneurysm, those patients who had been on an ACE inhibitor were significantly less likely to present with a rupture.[56]

The diagnosis and management of small AAAs have come a long way, as has surgical therapies. Further research and trials are needed for potential medical therapies to help stop the natural history of AAAs and to decrease the number of patients who need surgery or those who go on to rupture. Randomized clinical trials are needed to determine if medical treatment can reduce the rate or extent of expansion in patients with small, asymptomatic AAAs.

Indications for Intervention

Randomized clinical trials have determined that aneurysms > 5.5 cm should be repaired. Other indications for surgical intervention include rapid expansion in a short period of time (> 0.7 cm in 6 months) or complications associated with aortic aneurysms: distal embolization, thrombosis, fistulization, and local compression of adjacent organs. Emergent repair is indicated for almost all patients with known or suspected rupture, regardless of the size or the age of the patient. It is also indicated for symptomatic aneurysms in the absence of signs of rupture; such as patients with pain and tenderness over the aneurysms, even if there are no CTA findings suggestive of rupture. The question now becomes how to repair the AAA, and that is dependent on the patient, the physician, and the patient's vascular anatomy.

Surgical Repair

The history of AAA repair dates back to 1923, when Rudolph Matas performed the first successful aortic ligation to treat an aortic aneurysm.[57] It would take over 40 years to come to the endoaneurysmorrhaphy as we know it today. In the 1930s Blakemore and King tried to induce thrombosis of the aneurysm sac by passing a current through wires that were placed into the aneurysm sac.[58] In the 1940s cellophane was used in humans to wrap the aorta to induce periarterial fibrosis, to prevent rupture. It was not until 1951 that Dubost et al[59] performed the first successful aneurysm excision and repair; he used an arterial homograft to replace an aortic aneurysm. Once a successful excision and replacement was done, focus turned to finding a suitable material to use as an aortic graft. Homografts were not always available and deteriorated over time. In 1950 Arthur Voorhes used a material called Vinyon-N in dogs,[60] and in 1953 the first Vinyon-N graft was placed in a human. In 1954, after experimenting with different synthetic materials, Debakey et al[61] performed an AAA repair using Dacron. In the 1950s aneurysms were excised prior to replacing the aorta with a homograft or a synthetic graft. It was not until the 1960s that Oscar Creech[62] popularized the open endoaneurysmorrhaphy that we know today, leaving the back wall of the aneurysm intact and over sewing the lumbar vessels. In the 1990s a whole new population not amenable to open surgical repair was introduced to endovascular stent grafts.

Open Repair

Open repair as we know it today was first described by Creech in the 1960s and was modified and popularized by Debakey.[61,62] The choice of incision can be transperitoneal or retroperitoneal. A midline transperitoneal approach is a rapid approach into the abdomen but may be associated with more pulmonary complications secondary to the postoperative pain and splinting. A retroperitoneal approach is from the lateral rectus margin extending to the tenth or eleventh intercostals space. It affords good exposure of the infrarenal and suprarenal aorta, but limited exposure of the contralateral renal and iliac arteries. It is often the approach used when the patient has had multiple laparotomies in the past and the patient is considered to have a hostile abdomen.

The choice of incision is to some extent personal preference. When making this choice the physician may consider the extent of the aneurysm, the status of the iliac arteries, the degree of obesity and pulmonary disease, previous abdominal surgeries, the speed in which aortic control is needed, and the need to investigate other intraperitoneal organs.

Whichever approach is used, once down on the aorta the rest remains the same. The left renal vein is exposed and retracted superiorly to expose the neck of the aneurysm. Each iliac artery should be exposed as well to define the distal extent of the aneurysm (Figure 9.7). Then enough normal aorta and iliac arteries should be exposed to sufficiently place a clamp on proximally and distally. Heparinization is given prior to cross-clamping. The aneurysm sac is opened longitudinally along the anterior surface away from the IMA (inferior mesenteric artery) in case it requires reimplantation. The proximal aorta is then "t" off horizontally at the level of the proximal anastomosis. Thrombus and debris from the aneurysm sac is then removed from the aneurysm and the patent lumbar vessels are ligated. Once hemostasis within the aneurysm sac is maintained the proximal anastomosis is done. Usually Prolene sutures are used and the graft material is either Dacron or polytetrafluoroethylene (PTFE). Once the proximal anastomosis is completed the graft is clamped and the cross clamp is released to look for any suture line bleeding. The distal anastomosis is then completed; whether it is to the distal aorta or the iliac arteries bilaterally, the same vascular technique is performed. The IMA is inspected for back bleeding, and the sigmoid colon is inspected and if the IMA needs to be reimplanted it is at this point. Once completed the aneurysm sac is closed around the graft. The

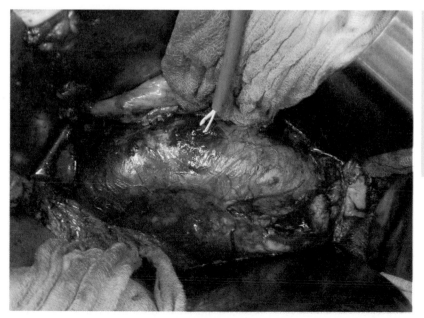

Figure 9.7 Open AAA repair via a transperitoneal approach. The left renal vein is exposed at the left of the picture, marking the proximal neck. The left common iliac artery is at the bottom right and the IMA (inferior mesenteric artery) is controlled with a Rummel.

retroperitoneum is then closed if the transperitoneal approach had been used. The abdominal contents are returned and the wound is closed.

Complications involved with open repair

Despite major improvements in the outcome of elective AAA repair, major complications occur. The mean 30-day mortality rate varies among hospitals and surgeons but has been reported between 1.1% and 7.0%. Myocardial infarction is the single leading single-organ cause of early and late mortality in patients undergoing AAA repair. Renal failure, pulmonary failure, gastrointestinal complications, colonic ischemia, distal embolization, paraplegia secondary to spinal cord ischemia, and impotence are some of the other complications.[63] Late complications are less common after successful aneurysm repair; however, they can occur and include pseudoaneurysms, infection, or thrombosis of an iliac limb.[64]

Besides complications leading to higher rates of morbidity and mortality, functional outcome has been studied as well. Williamson and colleagues[65] reviewed their experience with nonemergent open AAA repair over a 7-year period. Operative mortality rate, technical success, and long-term survival were comparable with other studies. Sixty-four percent of patients reported a full recovery from the operation, with a mean recovery time of 3.9 months, whereas one-third had not fully recovered at an average time of nearly 3 years. Eighteen percent said they would not undergo AAA repair again after knowing the recovery process, despite understanding the implications. Twelve percent of patients were discharged to a skilled nursing facility for an average of 3.7 months. At a mean of 25 months only 64% were fully ambulatory even though they all were ambulatory preoperatively. Although it is difficult to determine the exact role the AAA repair played in this population, the study highlights the high rate of disability after open AAA repair.

The early (30-day) mortality after elective AAA repair in properly selected patients is 5% or less, whereas the early mortality after ruptured AAA is 54%. Five-year survival after successful AAA repair is approximately 70% compared with approximately 80% in the age- and gender-matched general population.[66]

Endovascular Repair

History and design

Endovascular repair (EVAR) for an AAA was first described by Parodi et al[67] in 1991. This technique modeled after work by Dotter et al[68] was initially designed for patients too sick to undergo conventional open aortic repair. The endograft is a vascular prosthetic graft attached to a stent and is delivered to the aorta via a transfemoral route. Under fluoroscopic guidance the device is placed beneath the renal arteries and "deployed"—essentially relining the aorta. Once the endograft is in place the blood travels through the device and excludes the aneurysm sac, preventing rupture. The initial endografts were physician-made, usually consisting of a prosthetic material, for example, Dacron or PTFE, sutured to a balloon-expandable stent. The entire stent graft was then folded, or crimped into a sheath, and then delivered into the aorta through the patient's femoral artery. The first devices were tube grafts with the distal landing zone in the distal aorta.[67] Because of morphologic changes of the aorta this repair had a high rate of failure, which led to the development of the aorto-uniiliac devices, consisting of a distal landing zone in one iliac artery and perfusion of the contralateral leg via a femoral-femoral bypass graft. Soon after these initial devices, the bifurcated, modular device was conceived.[69] Based on the experiences gained with the earlier designs, this device incorporated several critical components necessary for EVAR. The device has stents along its entire length to increase its strength, and the modular component allows for the stent graft to be built within the aortic lumen and additional proximal or distal extension can be added, allowing a broader population to be treated by these newer stent grafts. Additional modifications on bifurcated devices were made. Proximal anchoring devices, such as hooks, as well as uncovered proximal stents both have improved proximal fixation into healthy pararenal aorta.[70]

Indications/contraindications

The initial endografts were used in "high-risk" patients; those patients who were deemed too sick to undergo open repair and for whom EVAR was their only option. Over the years the indications and selection criteria continue to evolve. Any patient who is being considered for an open AAA repair should be evaluated for potential EVAR. Unlike open repair, where the patient's comorbidities have a significant impact on whether or not to do the procedure, EVAR allows patients to undergo an aneurysm repair without general anesthesia, without a large abdominal incision, and without the major blood loss and fluid shifts associated with an open AAA repair. EVAR can be done under regional or even local anesthesia if needed. The contraindications for EVAR are based on anatomical constraints. The physician should review 3 areas when considering a patient for EVAR: the proximal neck, the distal landing zone, and the access vessels. Besides these anatomical constraints there is a strict follow-up regimen of CTA and plain films needed to ensure continued exclusion of the aneurysm sac. The patient should be willing to comply with the surveillance and follow-up protocol.

Proximal neck

The proximal neck is the segment of aorta that is right below the renal arteries and should consist of an undilated segment of aorta of sufficient length to allow for implantation of the proximal portion of the stent graft. Because there are no sutures used with stent grafts, the device relies on the proximal stent (its radial force) and sometimes hooks or barbs to help fix itself into the aortic wall. If there is not a long enough distance between the lowest renal artery and the start of the aneurysm there will not be an adequate fixation zone and the EVAR is set up for failure. The exact length of normal aorta necessary for device implantation varies with device, but it is generally recommended to have at least 1.5 cm of proximal neck to create an adequate seal zone.

Besides the length, the diameter plays a significant role as well. There are 5 commercially available devices to date, 2 of which will treat aneurysms with a neck diameter up to 32mm.

Distal landing zone

The earlier devices were tube grafts and the distal end would end in the aorta above the bifurcation. Over the years the devices have been modified to end in the common or external iliac artery. The vessel where the stent graft is going to end has to be of adequate length and diameter, just like the proximal neck. If the common iliac artery is ectatic or aneurysmal it may not be usable as a distal seal zone, and the graft might have to be extended down into the external iliac artery.

Access vessels

The common and external iliac arteries must be of adequate caliber to allow for passage of the device and its delivery system. Diameter is not the only criteria necessary for a successful access vessel. Tortuosity and calcification of the iliac vessels also contribute to the success of an EVAR. Calcification can make the access vessels stiff and noncompliant, making it difficult to pass the delivery system, and if they are too tortuous the device will not track up into the aorta. At our institution, we have found that delivery of the device is usually successful as long as the access vessels only have one of these challenges. If there are 2 "strikes," for example, calcium and tortuosity, we look for an alternate method of delivering the prosthesis.

Outcomes

Initial outcomes with endovascular stent grafts were promising, showing less operative blood loss, a shorter hospital stay, and fewer postoperative complications.[71,72] However, the reports were retrospective or nonrandomized and often showed similar perioperative mortality rates between open and endovascular groups. A lot of the studies in the literature were single-center experiences or device-specific. It was not long before a randomized controlled clinical trial was conducted.

Clinical Trials

The Endovascular Aneurysm Repair 1 (EVAR-1) trail and the Dutch Randomized Endovascular Aneurysm Management (DREAM) trial were developed to help answer the questions of EVAR versus open surgical repair. The EVAR-1 trial enrolled 1082 patients with an average age of 74 and mean aneurysm size of 6.5 cm. Early results demonstrated short-term survival benefit with EVAR with a 30-day mortality rate of 1.7% versus 4.7%. In-hospital mortality was 2.1% versus 6.2%. The DREAM trial enrolled 345 patients with aneurysms ≥ 5 cm. Although not statistically significant similar end points were seen with a 30-day mortality of 1.2% versus 4.6%. The combined rate for perioperative mortality and severe complications in the endovascular group was roughly half that of the open group: 4.7% versus 9.8%. Early results from both of these studies also confirmed the benefits of the less invasive nature of endovascular repair, including less blood loss, shorter operative times, and shorter hospital stays. The EVAR-1 trial showed at 30 days a higher rate of secondary interventions when compared with open repair, 9.8% versus 5.8%, which is a criticism of endovascular repair. Another concern is the long-term durability. The early data appeared promising; however, the follow-up data are not so clear. At 2 years there was no statistically significant difference in survival rates between the endovascular group and the open repair group in the DREAM trial.[73] Midterm follow-up in the EVAR-1 trial had similar findings; at 4 years the all-cause mortality was similar between the 2 groups, however, there was a difference in aneurysm-related deaths in the endovascular group (4% vs. 7%).[74] Both studies demonstrated a high rate of reintervention following endovascular repair. Seventy-two percent of patients were still alive in the EVAR group at midterm follow-up and will continue to require follow-up, and will likely need some reintervention.

Long-term data from the DREAM and EVAR-1 trials and the ongoing randomized US trial—the Open Versus Endovascular Repair (OVER) trial—will ultimately help physicians decide which patients are likely to benefit from which procedure. However, randomized, controlled clinical trials are becoming harder to complete; with commercially available stent grafts, and educated consumers, patients often come to the doctor already having decided that they want to be treated with a stent graft.[75] The results of the largest prospective randomized trial of open versus endovascular repair of AAA in 1252 patients demonstrated a significantly lower operative mortality with endovascular treatment, but the mortality advantage was lost at the end of follow-up (5 years from the last randomized patient).[76]

Future Devices

Enthusiasm for less invasive therapies for aortic aneurysm repair has been the driving force behind endovascular repair and advancements. Over the 15 years that EVAR has been used, improvements in device delivery systems, device components, and device design has broadened the applicability of these techniques to a much larger patient population. However, anatomic constraints continue to be the limiting factor for EVAR. In the past, aneurysms that involved the visceral vessels would require an open repair, or perhaps a select few could undergo an EVAR coupled with an extra-anatomic bypass. But this also involves open surgery and increases the morbidity of the procedure. Custom-made branched or fenestrated grafts have been developed to allow fixation into healthy aorta while still allowing antegrade blood flow into the visceral vessels. The concept of branched or fenestrated grafts started in the late 1990s in the treatment of type B dissections, and thoracic aneurysms and have been deployed successfully for treatment of thoracoabdominal aneurysms,[77,78] juxtarenal aneurysms,[79,80] and aneurysms that involve the iliac arteries.[81] These procedures are complex and involve precise preoperative imaging and planning, and often require long operative times and more than one access, however, the use of branched stent grafts with renal, superior mesenteric or celiac branches allows a minimally invasive option for high-risk patients with juxtarenal aortic aneurysms.[79,82]

Greenberg et al[80] reported their series of 22 patients who underwent endovascular grafting with a fenestrated Zenith device. Their group achieved successful implantation, including 58 visceral vessels with the acute loss of only a single vessel. They reported a 30-day endoleak rate of 9%, and a decrease in aneurysm sac size was seen in 53% of patients at 6 months and 75% of patients at 12 months. Furthermore, primary and assisted primary patency rates for the 58 vessels were 97% and 98% at 1 month and 94% and 98% at 12 months. Three patients developed renal insufficiency, one of whom went on to require hemodialysis.[80]

Complications

Long-term durability remains a concern for EVAR. The main criticism is the high incidence of endoleaks. An *endoleak* is the persistence of blood flow within the aneurysm sac. The incidence of endoleaks after EVAR has been reported to be 8% to 45%.[77,83-86] Everyone agrees that a type I or III endoleak needs to be fixed immediately (leaks involving an attachment site or a junctional point). Patients with these endoleaks are not protected from aneurysm rupture and are treated as if their aneurysms are not excluded. However, type II endoleaks, which make up the majority of the endoleaks in most series, do not heed such danger. They are related to retrograde flow into the aneurysm sac via patent collateral arteries, usually lumbars or the inferior mesenteric artery. Their treatment remains controversial, primarily because their natural history is not fully elucidated. Studies have shown spontaneous closure without any intervention,[87] and others have reported rupture after documented type II endoleaks.[88] A retrospective review of all EVARs at a single institution over an 8-year period was conducted.

There was a 16% type II endoleak rate, with a mean follow-up time of 22 months. Thirty-six percent of these patients spontaneously sealed their endoleak. Nineteen patients underwent endovascular treatment of their endoleak (12% had evidence of sac enlargement on postoperative imaging studies. Because of the relatively benign natural history of type II endoleaks in this particular study the authors recommend a less aggressive approach to reinterventions for type II endoleaks but recognize the need for diligent follow-up imaging.[87]

Technical Procedural Issues/ Tips and Tricks

Over the last 15 years, endovascular stent grafts for the treatment of AAA has grown and developed to incorporate new techniques and devices. Studies have shown that it is not only feasible but also safe and effective in short- and midterm follow-up. Whether EVAR should be the first-line treatment for all patients with AAA has yet to be determined. Because most patients, and even physicians, do not want to subject themselves to a large open procedure and would rather have a minimally invasive approach to AAA repair, physicians have been pushing the envelope on new and innovative ideas in order to allow more and more patients to undergo EVAR. The only contraindication to EVAR is vascular anatomy, and as more patients are being diagnosed with AAAs, and patients are living longer, more difficult anatomy is being discovered.

Proximal neck

Although it is still recommended to have 15 mm of healthy proximal neck, devices and techniques have been introduced to help extend that limit. Transrenal fixation and fenestrated stent grafts have been employed to increase the number of patients whose anatomy would be amenable to EVAR.

Access vessels

Atherosclerosis is not uncommon in the aging population, and while a physician can be faced with good anatomy for proximal and distal seal zones, the access vessels can be too small, too calcified, or too tortuous to navigate the delivery system and device into the aorta. Conduits have been employed to help bypass the problems of access vessels; an open conduit can be sewn onto a larger common iliac to avoid the small, tortuous external iliac, or an endoluminal conduit can be passed into the iliac to allow for angioplasty of the calcified diseased access vessel.

Summary

Abdominal aortic aneurysms are common in elderly men; the incidence has been rising due to the aging population, improvements in diagnostic modalities, and screening programs. Risk factors include advanced age, smoking, hypercholesterolemia, coronary artery disease, and hypertension. AAA is more common in men than women and family members of patients with AAAs are at increased risk of developing an aneurysm as well. Although a large aneurysm in a thin patient can be felt on physical exam; smaller aneurysms or certain body types make it difficult to rely on physical exam. Knowing which patients are at risk will help physicians care for the patient with a suspected AAA. Ultrasound is the modality of choice for diagnosis and surveillance; however CT scan or MRA is needed for surgical planning.

In general elective surgical repair is recommended in patients with aneurysms larger than 5.5 cm in diameter. Patients with smaller aneurysms should be monitored every 6-12 months depending on the size. Certain risk factor modifications should be employed to help slow the rate of aneurysm growth. Smoking, hypertension, and hypercholesterolemia are some of the modifiable risk factors for the development of AAAs. Although small retrospective studies on statins, antibiotics, ACE inhibitors and Nonsteroidal anti-inflammatory drugs have been positive, randomized clinical trials are needed to determine if medical treatment can reduce the rate of expansion and risk of rupture in patients with small, asymptomatic AAAs.

Open surgical repair has been the gold standard for AAA repair since the 1960s. In 1991 endovascular aneurysm repair (EVAR) was introduced and opened the door to patients who were deemed to sick to undergo conventional open repair. However, EVAR itself has anatomic and device limitations. Earlier devices were constrained by neck diameter, access vessel size, and device fatigue or failure. However it has been almost 2 decades since the first EVAR was implanted to treat an AAA and manufacturers have learned from the shortcomings of the earlier devices. Newer generation devices continue to emerge and push the envelope of who can be treated with an endograft, and perhaps in the not-so-distant future EVAR may become the standard for AAA repair.

References

1. Melton LJ, Bickerstaff LK, Hollier LH, et al. Changing incidence of abdominal aortic aneurysms: a population-based study. *Am J Epidemiol*. 1984;120:379-386.

2. Silverstein MD, Pitts SR, Chaikof EL, Ballard DJ. Abdominal aortic aneurysm (AAA): cost effectiveness of screening, surveillance of intermediate sized AAA, and management of symptomatic AAA. *BUMC Proceedings*. 2005;18:345-367.

3. Lederle FA, Johnson GR, Wilson SE, et al. Prevalence and associations of abdominal aortic aneurysm detected through screening: Aneurysm Detection and Management (ADAM) Veterans Affairs Cooperative Study Group. *Ann Intern Med*. 1997;126:441-449.

4. Wilmink AB, Quick CR. Epidemiology and potential for prevention of abdominal aortic aneurysm. *Br J Surg*. 1998; 85:155-162.

5. Alcorn HG, Wolfson SK Jr, Sutton-Tyrell K, Kuller LH, O'leary D. Risk factors for abdominal aortic aneurysms in older adults enrolled in the cardiovascular health study. *Arterioscler Thromb Vasc Biol*. 1996;16:963-970.

6. MacSweeney ST, Ellis M, Worrell PC, Green-halgh RM, Powell JT. Smoking and growth rate of small abdominal aortic aneurysm. *Lancet.* 1994;344:651-652.

7. Lee AJ, Fowkes FGR, Carson MN, Leng GC, Allan PL. Smoking, atherosclerosis and risk of abdominal aortic aneurysms. *Eur Heart J.* 1997;18:671-676.

8. Brown LC, Powell JT. Risk factors for aneurysm rupture in patients kept under ultrasound surveillance. UK Small Aneurysm Trial Partici-pants. *Ann Surg.* 1999;230:289.

9. Brady AR, Thompson SG, Fowkes GR, Green-halgh RM, Powell JT. Abdominal aortic aneu-rysm expansion. Risk factors and time intervals for surveillance. *Circulation.* 2004;110:16-21.

10. Sakalihasan N, Limet R, Defawe OD. Abdomi-nal aortic aneurysm. *Lancet.* 2005;365:1577-1589.

11. Lederle FA, Nelson DB, Joseph AM. Smokers' relative risk for aortic aneurysm compared with other smoking-related diseases: a systematic review. *J Vasc Surg.* 2003;38:329-334.

12. Madaric J, Vulev I, Bartunek J, et al. Frequency of abdominal aortic aneurysm in patients > 60 years of age with coronary artery disease. *Am J Cardiol.* 2005;96:1214-1216.

13. Darling RC III, Brewster DC, Darling RC, et al. Are familial abdominal aortic aneurysms dif-ferent? *J Vasc Surg.* 1989;10:39-43.

14. Johansen K, Koepsell T. Familial tendency for abdominal aortic aneurysms. *JAMA.* 1986;256:1934.

15. Verloes A, Sakalihasan N, Koulischer L, Limet R. Aneurysm of the abdominal aorta: familial and genetic aspects in three hundred thirteen pedigrees. *J Vasc Surg.* 1995;21:646.

16. Kuivaniemi H, Shibamura H, Arthur C, et al. Familial abdominal aortic aneurysms: col-lection of 233 multiplex families. *J Vasc Surg.* 2003;37:340-345.

17. Johnston KW, Rutherford RB, Tilson MD, Shah DM, Hollier L, Stanley JC. Suggested standards for reporting on arterial aneurysms. Subcom-mittee on Reporting Standards for Arterial Aneurysms, Ad Hoc Committee on Reporting Standards, Society for Vascular Surgery and North American Chapter, International Soci-ety for Cardiovascular Surgery. *J Vasc Surg.* 1991;13:452-458.

18. Halloran BG, Davis VA, McManus BM, Lynch TG, Baxter T. Localization of aortic disease is associated with intrinsic differences in aortic structure. *J Surg Res.* 1995;59:17-22.

19. Holmes DR, Liao S, Parks WC, Thompson RW. Medial neovascularization in abdominal aortic aneurysms: a histopathologic marker of aneu-rysmal degeneration with pathophysiologic implications. *J Vasc Surg.* 1995;21:761-772.

20. Shah PK. Inflammation, metalloproteinases, and increased proteolysis: an emerging patho-physiological paradigm in aortic aneurysm. *Circulation.* 1997;96:2115-2117.

21. Patel MI, Hardman DT, Fisher CM Appleberg M. Current views on the pathogencsis of abdominal aortic aneurysms. *J Am Coll Surg.* 1995;181:371-382.

22. Grange JJ, Davis V, Baxter BT. Pathogenesis of abdominal aortic aneurysms: an update and look toward the future. *Cardiovasc Surg.* 1997;5:256-265.

23. McMillan WD, Tamarina NA, Cipollone M, Johnson DA, Parker MA, Pearce WH. Size matters: the relationship between MMP-9 expression and aortic diameter. *Circulation.* 1997;96:2228-2232.

24. Knox JB, Sukhova GK, Whittemore AD, Libby P. Evidence for altered balance between matrix metalloproteinases and their inhibitors in human aortic disease. *Circulation.* 1997;95:205-212.

25. Defawe OD, Colige A, Lampert CA, et al. TIMP-2 and PAI-1 mRNA levels are lower in aneurysmal as compared to athero-occlusive abdominal aortas. *Cardiovasc Res.* 2003;60:205-213.

26. Halloran BG, Baxter BT. Pathogenesis for aneu-rysms. *Semin Vasc Surg.* 1995;2:85-92.

27. Vorp DA, Raghavan ML, Webster MW. Mechanical wall stress in abdominal aortic aneurysm: influence of diameter and asymme-try. *J Vasc Surg* 1998;27:632-639.

28. Brown MJ, Sutton AJ, Bell PR, Sayers RD. A meta-analysis of 50 years of ruptured abdominal aortic aneurysm repair. *Br J Surg.* 2002;89:714-730.

29. Hollier LH, Taylor LM, Ochsner J. Recommended indications for operative treatment of abdominal aortic aneurysms: report of a subcommittee of the Joint Council of the Society for Vascular Surgery and the North American Chapter of the International Society for Cardiovascular Surgery. *J Vasc Surg.* 1992;15:1046-1056.

30. The UK Small Aneurysm Trial Participants. Mortality results for randomized controlled trial of early elective surgery or ultrasonographic surveillance for small abdominal aortic aneurysms. *Lancet.* 1998;352:1649-1655.

31. Lederle FA, Wilson SE, Johnson GR, et al. For the Aneurysm Detection And Management Veterans Affairs Cooperative Study Group. Immediate repair compared with surveillance of small abdominal aortic aneurysms. *N Engl J Med.* 2002;346:1437-1444.

32. Nevitt MP, Ballard DJ, Hallett JW Jr. Prognosis of abdominal aortic aneurysms: a population-based study. *N Engl J Med.* 1989;321:1009-1014.

33. Glimaker H, Holmberg L, Elvin A, et al. Natural history of patients with abdominal aortic aneurysm. *Eur J Vasc Surg.* 1991;5:125-130.

34. Cronenwett JL, Murphy TF, Zelenock GB, et al. Actuarial analysis of variables associates with rupture of small abdominal aortic aneurysms. *Surgery.* 1985;98:472-483.

35. Semmens JB, Norman PE, Lawrence-Brown MMD, Holman CDJ. Influence of gender on outcome from ruptured abdominal aortic aneurysm. *Br J Surg.* 2000;87:191-194.

36. Lederle FA, Johnson GR, Wilson SE. Abdominal aortic aneurysm in women. *J Vasc Surg.* 2001;34:122-126.

37. Schermerhorn ML, Cronenwett JL. Abdominal aortic and iliac aneurysms. In: Cronenwett JL, et al, eds. *Rutherford Vascular Surgery,* 6th ed. New York: Elsevier; 2005:1419-1420.

38. Fink HA, Lederle FA, Roth CS, Bowles CA, Nelson DB, Haas MA. The accuracy of physical examination to detect abdominal aortic aneurysm. *Arch Intern Med.* 2000;160:833-836.

39. US Preventative Services Task Force. Screening for abdominal aortic aneurysm: recommendation statement. *Ann Intern Med.* 2005;142:198-202.

40. Golledge J, Muller J, Daugherty A, Norman P. Abdominal aortic aneurysm: pathogenesis and implications from management. *Arterioscler Thromb Vasc Biol.* 2006;26:2605-2613.

41. Propanolol Aneurysm Trial Investigators. Propranolol for small abdominal aortic aneurysms: results of a randomized trial. *J Vasc Surg.* 2002;35:72-79.

42. Lindholt JS, Henneberg EW, Juul S, Fasting H. Impaired results of a randomized double blinded clinical trial of propranolol versus placebo on the expansion rate of small abdominal aortic aneurysms. *Int Angiol.* 1999;18:52-57.

43. Franklin IJ, Walton LJ, Greenhalgh RM, Powell JT. The influence of indomethacin on the metabolism and cytokine secretion of human aneurysmal aorta. *Eur J Vasc Endovasc Surg.* 1999;18:35-42.

44. Franklin IJ, Walton LJ, Brown L, Greenhalgh RN, Powell JT. Vascular surgical society of Great Britain and Ireland: nonsteroidal anti-inflammatory drugs to treat abdominal aortic aneurysm. *Br J Surg.* 1999;86:707.

45. Wilson WR, Evans J, Bell PR, Thompson MM. HMG-CoA reductase inhibitors (statins) decrease MMP-3 and MMP-9 concentrations in abdominal aortic aneurysms. *Eur J Vasc Endovasc Surg.* 2005;30:259-262.

46. Steinmetz EF, Buckley C, Thompson RW. Prospects for the medical management of abdominal aortic aneurysms. *Vasc Endovasc Surg.* 2003;37:151-163.

47. Powell JT, Brady AR. Detection, management and prospects for the medical treatment of small abdominal aortic aneurysms. *Arterioscler Thromb Vasc Biol.* 2004;24:241-245.

48. Moran CS, McCann M, Karan M, Norman P, Ketheesan N, Golledge J. Association of osteoprotegerin with human abdominal aortic aneurysm progression. *Circulation.* 2005;111:3119-3125.

49. Franklin IJ, Harley SL, Greenhalgh RM, Powell JY. Uptake of tetracycline by aortic aneurysm wall and its effect on inflammation and proteolysis. *Br J Surg.* 1999;86:771.

50. Kalyanasundaram A, Elmore JR, Manazer JR, et al. Simvastatin suppresses experimen-

tal aortic aneurysm expansion. *J Vasc Surg.* 2006;43:117-124.

51. Walton LJ, Franklin IJ, Bayston T, et al. Inhibition of prostaglandin E2 synthesis in abdominal aortic aneurysms: implications for smooth muscle cell viability, inflammatory processes, and the expansion of abdominal aortic aneurysms. *Circulation.* 1999;100:48-54.

52. Mosorin M, Juvonen J, Biancari F, et al. Use of doxycycline to decrease the growth rate of abdominal aortic aneurysms: a randomized, double-blind, placebo-controlled pilot study. *J Vasc Surg.* 2001;34:606-610.

53. Schouten O, van Lannen JHH, Boersma E, et al. Statins are associated with a reduced infrarenal abdominal aortic aneurysm growth. *Eur J Vasc Endovasc Surg.* 2006;32:21-26.

54. Steinmetz EF, Buckley C, Shames ML, et al. Treatment with simvastatin suppresses the development of experimental abdominal aortic aneurysms in normal and hypercholesterolemic mice. *Ann Surg.* 2005;241:92-101.

55. Liao S, Miralles M, Kelley BJ, Curci JA, Borhani M, Thompson RW. Suppression of experimental abdominal aortic aneurysm in the rat by treatment with angiotensin-converting enzyme inhibitors. *J Vasc Surg.* 2001;33:1057-1064.

56. Hackman DG, Thiruchelvam D, Redelmeier DA. Angiotensin-converting enzyme inhibitors and aortic rupture: a population-based case-control study. *Lancet.* 2006;368:659-665.

57. Matas R. Ligation of the abdominal aorta. *Ann Surg.* 1924;457-464.

58. Blakemoore AH. Progressive constrictive occlusion of the abdominal aorta with wiring and electrothermic coagulation. *Ann Surg.* 1951;133:447-462.

59. Dubost C, Allary M, Oeconomos N. Resection of an aneurysm of the abdominal aorta. Reestablishment of the continuity by a preserved human arterial graft, with results after five months. *Arch Surg.* 1951;64:405-408.

60. Voorhees AB Jr, Jaretzki A, Blakemoore AH. The use of tubes constructed from Vinyon "N" cloth in bridging arterial defects. *Ann Surg.* 1952;135:332-336.

61. DeBakey ME, Cooley DA, Crawford ES, Morris GC Jr. Clinical application of a new flexible knitted Dacron arterial substitute. *Am Surg.* 1958;24:862.

62. Creech O Jr. Endo-aneurysmorrhaphy and treatment of aortic aneurysm. *Ann Surg.* 1966;164:935-946.

63. Ernst CB. Abdominal aortic aneurysm. *N Engl J Med.* 1993;328:1167-1172.

64. Farkas JC, Fichelle JM, Laurian C, et al. Long term follow-up of positive cultures in 500 abdominal aortic aneurysms. *Arch Surg.* 1993;128:284-288.

65. Williamson WK, Nicoloff AD, Taylor LM Jr, Moneta GL, Laudry GJ, Porter JM. Functional outcome after open repair of abdominal aortic aneurysm. *J Vasc Surg.* 2001;33:913-920.

66. Norman PE, Semmens JB, Lawrence-Brown MM. Long-term relative survival following surgery for abdominal aortic aneurysm: a review. *Cardiovasc Surg.* 2001;9:219-224.

67. Parodi JC, Palmaz JC, Barone BD. Transfemoral intraluminal graft implantation for abdominal aortic aneurysms. *Ann Vasc Surg.* 1991;5:491-499.

68. Dotter CT, Judkins MP. Transluminal treatment of arteriosclerotic obstruction. Description of a new technique and a preliminary report of its application. *Radiology.* 1964;30:654-670.

69. Criado FJ, Paroya NA, Lopes JA, Wellons E. Historical evolution of endovascular grafts for the treatment of aortic aneurysm. In: Marin ML, Hollier LH, eds. *Endovascular Grafting: Advanced Treatment for Vascular Disease*, 1-6. Armonk, NY: Future Publishing Company; 2000.

70. Marin ML, Parsons RE, Hollier LH, et al. Impact of transrenal aortic endograft placement on endovascular graft repair of abdominal aortic aneurysms. *J Vasc Surg.* 1998;28:638-646.

71. Zarins CK, White RA, Schwarten D, et al. AneuRx stent graft versus open surgical repair of abdominal aortic aneurysms: multicenter prospective clinical trial. *J Vasc Surg.* 1999; 29:292-308.

72. Lee WA, Carter JW, Upchurch G, Seeger JM, Huber TS. Perioperative outcomes after open and endovascular repair of intact abdominal aortic aneurysms in the United States during 2001. *J Vasc Surg.* 2004;39:491-496.

73. Blankensteijn JD, de Jong SECA, Prinssen M, et al. Two year outcomes after conventional or endovascular repair of abdominal aortic aneurysms. *N Engl J Med.* 2005;352:2398-2405.

74. EVAR trial participants. Endovascular aneurysm repair versus open repair in patients with abdominal aortic aneurysm (EVAR trial 1): randomized controlled trial. *Lancet.* 2005;365:2179-2186.

75. Lederle FA. Endovascular repair of abdominal aortic aneurysm- round two. *N Engl J Med.* 2005;352:2443-2445.

76. The United Kingdom EVAR Trial Investigators. *N Engl J Med* 2010; epub on line April 11, 2010.

77. Chuter TAM, Gordon RL, Reilly LM, Pak LK, Messina LM. Multi-branched stent-graft for type III thoracoabdominal aortic aneurysm. *J Vasc Interv Radio.* 2001;12:391-392.

78. Bleyn J, Schol F, Vanhandenhove I, Vercaeren P. Side-branched modular endograft system for thoracoabdominal aortic aneurysm repair. *J Endovasc Ther.* 2002;9:838-841.

79. Anderson JL, Berce M, Hartley DE. Endoluminal aortic grafting with renal and superior mesenteric artery incorporation by graft fenestration. *J Endovasc Ther.* 2001;8:3-15.

80. Greenberg RK, Haulon S, Lyden SP, et al. Endovascular management of juxtarenal aneurysms with fenestrated endovascular grafting. *J Vasc Surg.* 2004;39:279-287.

81. Abraham CZ, Reilly LM, Schneider DB, et al. A modular multi-branched system for endovascular repair of bilateral common iliac artery aneurysms. *J Endovasc Ther.* 2003;10:203-207.

82. Stanley BM, Semmens JB, Lawrence-Brown M, Goodman MA, Hartley DA. Fenestration in endovascular grafts for aortic aneurysm repair: new horizons for preserving blood flow in branch vessels. *J Endovasc Ther.* 2001;8:16-24.

83. White GH, Yu W, May J, Chaufour X, Stephen MS. Endoleaks as a complication of endoluminal grafting of abdominal aortic aneurysms: classification, incidence, diagnosis and management. *J Endovasc Surg.* 1997;4:152-168.

84. White GH, May J, Waugh RC, Yu W. Type I and type II endoleaks: a more useful classification for reporting results of endoluminal AAA repair. *J Endovasc Surg.* 1998;5:189-191.

85. Van Marrewijk CJ, Fansen G, Laheij RJ, Harris PL, Buth J. EUROSTAR Collaborators. Is a type II endoleak after EVAR a harbinger of risk? Causes and outcome of open conversion and aneurysm rupture during follow-up. *Eur J Endovasc Surg.* 2004;27:128-137.

86. Veith FJ, Baum RA, Ohki T, et al. Nature and significance of endoleaks and endotension: summary of opinions expressed at an international conference. *J Vasc Surg.* 2002;35:1029-1035.

87. Silverberg D, Baril DT, Ellozy SE, et al. An 8-year experience with type II endoleaks: natural history suggests selective intervention is a safe approach. *J Vasc Surg.* 2006;44:453-459.

88. Bernhard VM, Mitchell RS, Matsummura JS, et al. Ruptured abdominal aortic aneurysm after endovascular repair. *J Vasc Surg.* 2002;35:1155-1162.

10

Chronic Mesenteric Ischemia

Jose A. Silva

Chronic mesenteric ischemia (CMI) is an uncommon clinical condition that usually manifests as postprandial abdominal pain and weight loss, which is a result of obstructive atherosclerotic disease of the mesenteric circulation, leading to chronic intestinal ischemia. Although vascular disease-causing intestinal gangrene had been recognized for centuries, and successful surgical treatment of intestinal infarction had been reported in the nineteenth century by Elliot,[1] the condition that we know today as CMI was initially described by Goodman[2] in 1918, who named it "angina abdominis," or abdominal angina, implying a similar pathophysiology to the then recently described symptoms of coronary insufficiency. However, the existence of CMI was not fully accepted until 1936, when a publication by Dunphy provided irrefutable evidence of its existence. In his classic paper, Dunphy[3] described a 47-year-old man who presented with worsening of his chronic postprandial abdominal pain and severe weight loss and suddenly died of acute abdominal pain; the necropsy showed intestinal infarction and severe 3-vessel mesenteric atherosclerotic disease with superimposed thrombotic occlusion of the celiac trunk.

Despite giant steps forward in imaging techniques since the initial descriptions by Goodman and Dunphy, the diagnosis of CMI remains challenging and underrecognized. Historically, the treatment of CMI has been surgical revascularization, however, percutaneous, catheter-based revascularization therapy has recently challenged surgery as the preferred treatment for this condition.

Anatomy of the Mesenteric Arterial Circulation

The mesenteric, or splanchnic, arterial circulation consists of 3 main arteries: the celiac trunk, the superior mesenteric artery (SMA), and the inferior mesenteric artery (IMA). Embryologically, these 3 arteries develop as paired vessels, but they eventually merge, providing the potential for abundant and persistent collateral connections. The celiac trunk arises on the ventral portion of the abdominal aorta at the level of T12 to L1, between the diaphragmatic crura. The SMA arises just distal to the celiac trunk at the level of L1 to L2, also on the ventral portion of the abdominal aorta. The IMA arises on the anterior to left lateral aspect of the abdominal aorta at the level of L3 to L4 about 8 to 10 cm distal to the SMA. The stomach and upper half of the duodenum make up the *foregut* and are supplied by the celiac trunk. The lower half of the duodenum, jejunum, ileum, cecum appendix, ascending colon, and proximal two-thirds of the transverse colon constitute the *midgut* and are supplied by the SMA. The lower third of the transverse colon, sigmoid colon, descending colon, sigmoid colon, rectum, and the upper part of the anal canal constitute the *hindgut* and are supplied by the IMA.

The origin of the celiac trunk is usually encased in the median arcuate ligament of the diaphragm, a fibrous portion of the central and posterior portion of this muscle. The celiac trunk divides soon after its origin into the common hepatic, left gastric, and splenic arteries. The first branch of the SMA is the inferior pancreaticoduodenal artery, which courses superiorly to join the superior pancreaticoduodenal artery (a branch of the gastroepiploic artery), to form one of the most important connections between the celiac trunk and the SMA. The next important branches are the middle colic (supplying flow to the proximal two-thirds of the transverse colon), right colic (for the mid- and distal ascending colon), and the iliocolic arteries (for the distal ilium, cecum, appendix, and proximal and ascending colon). The IMA branches into the left colic artery, which connects with the middle colic artery of the SMA (marginal artery of Drummond), the sigmoid, and superior rectal arteries. The most important branches and anatomical distribution of the 3 mesenteric arteries are described in Figure 10.1.

In about 1% of the population, the SMA arises directly from the celiac trunk, constituting the celiomesenteric trunk. The hepatic artery may also arise from the SMA in about 12% of the cases, and the common hepatic artery may arise directly from the abdominal aorta (usually below the celiac trunk) in about 2% of the cases (Figure 10.2).[4]

There is a rich communication among the 3 mesenteric vessels in normal conditions, which become more important and prominent during chronic ischemia, particularly when one or more mesenteric arteries develops significant stenoses or occlusions.[5] Well-known

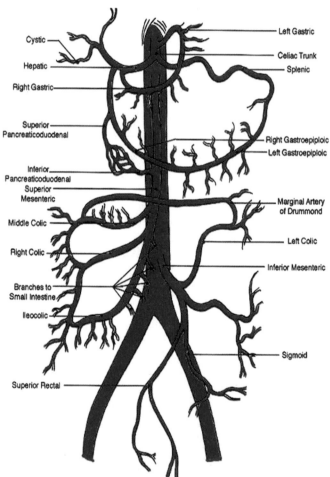

Figure 10.1 Anatomic representation of the mesenteric arterial circulation. (Reproduced with permission from Schwartz LB, Davis RD, Heinle JS, Purut CM, Taylor DC, Brown WC. The vascular system. In: Lyerly HK, Gaynor JW Jr, eds. *The Handbook of Surgical Intensive Care*, 3rd ed. St Louis, MO: Mosby Year Book; 1992:287. Reprinted with permission from Elsevier.)

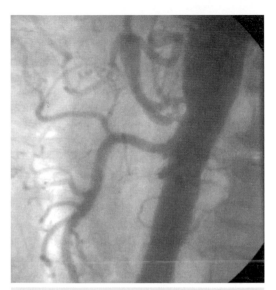

Figure 10.2 Common hepatic artery (middle artery) arising from the abdominal aorta.

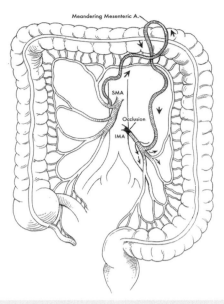

Figure 10.3 The meandering mesenteric artery connecting the superior and the inferior mesenteric arteries.

communications between the celiac trunk and SMA (superior and inferior gastroepiploic arteries), as well as SMA and IMA (marginal artery of Drummond), have been already mentioned. Another important connection between the SMA and IMA is the meandering mesenteric artery, which connects the ascending branch of the left colic artery with a branch of the SMA that arises proximal to the origin of the middle colic artery (Figures 10.1 and 10.3) and often becomes prominent during chronic occlusion of one of these arteries. Other connecting systems among these 3 vessels as well as significant collateral flow to the mesenteric circulation from other aortic branches such as the lumbar intercostal, middle sacral, mammary, and internal iliac arteries are also present.[6]

Prevalence, Etiology, and Natural History

Prevalence

Mesenteric arterial stenoses occur commonly, particularly in the elderly population with estab-

lished atherosclerotic disease. An angiographic study found a prevalence of asymptomatic mesenteric stenosis affecting at least one mesenteric artery in 40%, 29%, and 25% of patients with abdominal aortic aneurysm, aortoiliac obstructive disease, and peripheral athero-oclusive disease of the lower extremities, respectively.[7] A study using duplex ultrasonography in a nonselected group of elderly individuals (> 65 years), found a 17.5% prevalence of significant (> 70%) stenosis, affecting at least one mesenteric artery.[8] Furthermore, patients with renal artery stenosis have a very high (> 50%) prevalence of significant mesenteric artery stenosis.[9] On the other hand, the development of symptoms of chronic mesenteric ischemia is relatively unusual, probably due to the rich communication among the 3 mesenteric vessels as well as the development of collaterals from other arteries. Although it is difficult to estimate the true incidence of this condition, CMI has been reported to occur in 1 in 100,000 individuals.[10]

Etiology

Atherosclerotic disease is responsible for mesenteric arterial stenoses in more than 95% of the cases. These lesions are usually bulky and concentric, located in the ostium or the very proximal portion of the mesenteric artery, and they frequently are caused by progressive atherosclerotic disease of the anterior aortic wall.[11] Other vascular conditions such as fibromuscular dysplasia, Takayasu's arteritis, Buerger's disease, radiation, and autoimmune arteritis are uncommon causes of mesenteric arterial stenoses.[12,13]

The origin of the celiac trunk can be extrinsically compressed by the arcuate ligament of the diaphragm causing significant, sometimes critical, stenosis of this vessel (Figure 10.4).[14] Whether or not isolated, extrinsic compression of the celiac trunk leads to the development of symptomatic chronic mesenteric ischemia, or the so-called celiac axis compression syndrome, has been the subject of great debate.[15] However, careful documentation shows that surgical decompression of this vessel leads to lasting symptom relief.[16]

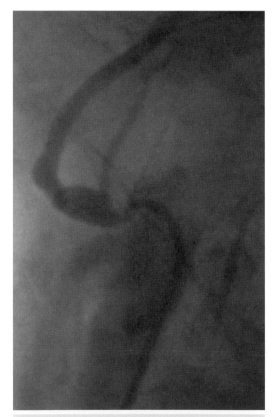

Figure 10.4 Extrinsic compression of the celiac trunk by the median arcuate ligament of the diaphragm.

Natural History

There are scarce data in the literature addressing the progression of mesenteric arterial disease, consequently, the natural history of this condition is still incompletely understood. Some investigators[17] have suggested that progression of atherosclerotic mesenteric arterial stenoses occur at the same pace as that of renal atherosclerotic disease; that is, ~ 20% per year.[18] In asymptomatic patients with established mesenteric atherosclerotic disease, development of symptomatic acute or chronic mesenteric ischemia has recently been shown to occur only in patients with multivessel disease. In a prospective study using invasive abdominal angiography in 980 patients, significant (> 50%) stenosis of at least one mesenteric artery was found in 82 patients.[19] At a mean follow-up of 2.6 years, mesenteric ischemia developed only in the patients with 3-vessel mesenteric arterial stenoses (27% of 15 patients).

The natural history of patients with symptomatic CMI is dire. Some investigators have suggested that 20% to 50% of patients with CMI develop acute mesenteric ischemia, however, the true incidence remains unknown.[20] The other 50% to 80% of the patients continue with symptomatic chronic, postprandial abdominal pain; weight loss; and emaciation; they finally die.[21] It is possible that a portion of these patients may have attenuation or spontaneous relief of symptoms, however, this has not been documented yet.

Physiology, Pathophysiology, and Symptoms

Physiology

Chronic mesenteric ischemia occurs as a result of insufficient oxygen delivery—that is, insufficient arterial blood supply—to the gut tissue, which is necessary to maintain normal intestinal function such as secretion, absorption, and the increased motility that follows food ingestion.

In normal individuals, the intestine receives 10% to 20% of the cardiac output and up to 35% after meals, with 70% of this output supplying the intestinal mucosa.[22] The splanchnic circulation has been shown to be subjected to significant decrease in its arterial flow or to the development of ischemia in conditions of hypovolemia, shock, or extreme physical exercise.[22-24]

Studies using duplex ultrasonography have demonstrated that after a 1000-calorie meal, flow velocities at the SMA increase from 22.2 to 57.0 cm/sec, and interestingly, the Doppler waveform changes from a high-resistance (triphasic) to a low-resistance pattern with high increased end-diastolic velocity.[25] These changes in arterial flow velocities are the result of highly sophisticated and complex mechanisms that control vascular resistance that include intrinsic and neurohormonal mechanisms as well as extrinsic mechanisms. Among the intrinsic mechanisms of splanchnic blood-flow autoregulation, it has been shown that reduction in perfusion pressure leads to the release of adenosine and other metabolites of ischemia, which directly produces a relaxation effect in the arteriolar smooth muscle of the splanchnic arterioles.[22] In addition, during periods of hypoperfusion, the intestinal mucosa is capable of extracting larger amounts of oxygen. A study has shown that the human intestine has a fairly constant oxygen extraction, until blood flow reaches a critical limit of 30 mL/min/100 g.[26] Extrinsic mechanisms of splanchnic flow regulation include neural (the sympathetic nervous system) and hormonal (the renin-angiotensin system, and vasopressin). Sympathetic tone is mainly provided by the preganglionic cholinergic fibers of the greater splanchnic nerves, which synapse in the paired celiac ganglia adjacent to the celiac trunk. On the other hand, parasympathetic fibers of the vagi also innervate the intestine, but probably exert negligible effect on the mesenteric vasculature.[27] The renin-angiotensin system is stimulated under conditions of low extracellular flow volume, which promotes vasoconstriction through the direct action of angiotensin II and indirect action of adrenergic stimulation. Likewise, vasopressin is released from the pituitary gland triggering mesenteric arterial vasoconstriction and venorelaxation in conditions of blood loss and hyperosmolarity.[28]

Pathophysiology

The development of symptoms of CMI usually results when at least 2 mesenteric vessels are affected by hemodynamically significant stenoses. Atherosclerosis, the most common cause of mesenteric arterial stenosis, progresses slowly in the majority of the cases, and thereby enables the recruitment of normally existing connections among the 3 mesenteric arteries, or the development of *de novo* collaterals. Consequently, single-vessel stenosis rarely causes CMI, unless these mesenteric arterial interconnections are congenitally poorly developed, in acute or subacute stenoses where little time is available for the development of collaterals, or in patients in whom they have previously been interrupted as a result of previous abdominal surgery or intestinal resection.

Based of the previous discussion, the existence of CMI with single-vessel mesenteric arterial stenosis, particularly, with isolated celiac trunk stenosis due to extrinsic compression (Figure 10.4) by the median arcuate ligament of the diaphragm has been the subject of intense debate. This condition was initially described in 1963 by Harjola.[29] Later, Bron and Redman[30] showed that almost half of the patients with isolated significant celiac artery stenosis or occlusion had abdominal symptoms. However, in a review of the literature, Szilagyi et al[31] argued that in no single case could the existence of the celiac compression syndrome be conclusively proven, and that postdecompression symptom relief was placebo mediated. In the past 3 decades since that review, other investigators have provided careful documentation of the existence of this condition with lasting symptom relief after surgical decompression.[32]

It is important to understand that although the rich interconnection among the 3 mesenteric arteries has a protective effect against the development of intestinal ischemia, it may also promote a vascular steal phenomenon, a mechanism that appears to play a very important role in the pathophysiology of CMI. In an experimental dog model, using a 50% fixed stenosis of the celiac trunk in the SMA, the intramural pH in the small intestine (using tonometry) significantly decreased after the dogs were fed and the food reached the stomach. The interpretation for the drop in the intestinal pH was that blood was diverted from the intestine (which becomes ischemic) to the stomach to satisfy the stomach metabolic demands stimulated by food.[33] This experiment is important, because it explains the relatively early occurrence of abdominal pain (20–30 minutes after food intake) experienced by most patients with CMI, long before it has reached the intestinal wall. This blood shifting, or *intramesenteric steal,* has also been proposed as the mechanism of abdominal pain or nonspecific abdominal symptoms endured by patients with celiac trunk compression syndrome.[34] Furthermore, intramesenteric steal has been reported to cause colon ischemia.[35]

In addition, certain medications, in particular digoxin, are known to cause mesenteric vasoconstriction and may potentially lead to mesenteric ischemia, especially in patients with known mesenteric arterial stenosis.[36,37]

Symptoms

The typical symptoms of CMI include abdominal pain usually triggered by food ingestion, weight loss, and an abdominal bruit localized in the epigastrium.[2,3] The abdominal pain is usually described as "dull aching" or sometimes as "crampy" in the periumbilical area. It begins within 1 hour (most frequently within 20–30 minutes) after food ingestion and subsides 1 to 2 hours later. Due to the postprandial abdominal pain, patients develop the so-called "fear for food" and gradually decrease the amount of food and caloric intake, which leads to weight loss that in some of cases may be profound. It is not unusual for patients with typical CMI to have a 20- to 40-pound weight loss by the time the diagnosis is made.

More recent reports have shown that ischemic gastropathy and ischemic colitis have been described to be manifestations of chronic mesenteric ischemia. Ischemic gastropathy usually manifests as nausea, vomiting, fullness, right upper quadrant discomfort, abdominal pain, and weight loss.[38-40] Ischemic colitis usually manifests as abdominal pain, gastrointestinal bleeding, and/or hematochezia.[35,41] A mechanism of vascular stealing appears to play an important role in this type of presentation.[35]

Other less-specific symptoms include nausea and change in the bowel habits, with development of diarrhea and/or constipation, which in some instances may be related to intestinal malabsorption.

Diagnosis, Noninvasive Imaging Studies, and Conventional Angiography

The diagnosis of CMI may often be quite challenging, and the typical symptoms and presentation of postprandial abdominal pain, weigh loss, and epigastric bruit, in patients with ≥ 2-vessel mesenteric arterial stenoses, may not always present. Some investigators have reported that only 50% of the patients with CMI develop these typical symptoms.[42] We have reported on a series of 59 patients with CMI and found typical presentation in 78% and ischemic gastropathy or ischemic colitis in 22% of the patients (Figures 10.5 through 10.8).[43]

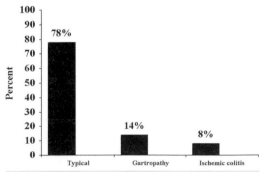

Figure 10.5 Clinical presentation in 59 patients with chronic mesenteric ischemia. (From Silva et al. *J Am Coll Cardiol.* 2006; 47: 944-950. Reprinted with permission from Elsevier.)

Chronic mesenteric ischemia remains a clinical diagnosis based on the presence of clinical symptoms of ischemic origin and hemodynamic stenoses in ≥ 2-vessel mesenteric stenoses. As discussed previously, the presence of CMI in a patient with single-vessel mesenteric artery stenosis, although possible, is unusual and should be made only when other causes of abdominal pain have been excluded. In some patients with atypical or nonspecific symptoms, the diagnosis is often made retrospectively, based on the clinical success of revascularization therapy. Due to these difficulties, some investigators advocate a multidisciplinary team approach for the diagnosis and management of this challenging condition.[44]

Noninvasive and Invasive Imaging Studies

The typical patients referred for noninvasive diagnostic imaging studies usually have significant peripheral, renal, coronary, and neurovascular atherosclerotic disease, as well as presumptive symptoms of chronic intestinal ischemia. It is not uncommon for some of these patients to have endured abdominal symptoms with or without weight loss for years before the clinician considers CMI as a possible diagnosis. Technical improvement in duplex ultrasonography, as well as the introduction of computed tomography angiography (CTA) and magnetic resonance angiography (MRA), is in the majority of the cases accurate enough to establish the diagnosis of mesenteric arterial stenosis. Conventional angiography is at present recommended for patients with a inconclusive noninvasive imaging study, or in whom revascularization therapy is being entertained.

Duplex Ultrasonography

Duplex ultrasonography plays an important role in the diagnosis of mesenteric arterial stenosis; however, the success of a technically adequate examination is highly operator dependent. In addition, patients with abdominal distention, with distended bowel loops, may yield suboptimal images. Overall, in experienced hands with the appropriate patients, an adequate visualization of the celiac trunk and SMA can be obtained in 80% to 95% of the patients.[45] Moneta et al[46] reported that a peak systolic velocity of ≥ 200 cm/sec in the celiac trunk and ≥ 275 cm/sec in the SMA corresponds to ≥ 70% stenosis. In addition, Zwolak and his colleges[47] reported that an end-diastolic velocity of ≥ 55 cm/sec in the celiac trunk and ≥ 45 cm/sec in the SMA corresponds to > 50% arterial stenosis. Although postprandial scanning has been suggested as a means of increasing the sensitivity of the test, it only marginally improves it and at present is not routinely performed in most laboratories.[48]

Computed Tomography Angiography

Computed tomography angiography (CTA) is emerging as one of the most important diagnostic imaging modalities in vascular medicine. Recent developments in image processing with 3-dimensional reconstruction allows for a detailed visualization of specific areas, from different angles. Although not systematically evaluated yet in the mesenteric circulation for CMI, CTA has shown to yield high sensitivities and specificities for detecting stenoses in other vascular territories such as the renal, carotid, and peripheral circulation. In addition, CTA is very sensitive and specific for assessing vascular patency after endovascular stent placement, without the undesired artifact effect seen with other modalities such as MRA (see Figure 10.8).[49-51] The major disadvantages of this image modality are the cost, the need for external beam radiation, and the need for iodinated contrast, which may be contraindicated in patients with renal insufficiency, in particular those with concomitant diabetes mellitus.

Magnetic Resonance Angiography

The introduction of contrast-enhanced magnetic resonance angiography (MRA) into clinical practice has allowed detailed visualization of stenotic areas of the arterial vasculature by obtaining multiple slices in the coronal and vertical planes of the vessel of interest, in a single breath-hold of 20 to 25 seconds. Atherosclerotic disease in the celiac trunk, SMA, and IMA is usually well visualized with this technology, and, as is the case for CTA, 3-dimensional reconstruction, and attainment of images in any desired plane, is possible using maximum-intensity projections or surface-rendering techniques. All this technical sophistication enables clinicians to visualize the ostium and the rest of the target mesenteric artery with a great deal of detail. In a study of 14 patients using simultaneous conventional angiography as a control, stenosis was found in 7 celiac trunks, 6 SMAs, and 4 IMAs. In 2 cases the IMA stenosis was overestimated. The sensitivity and specificity of MRA in this small study was 100% and 95%, respectively.[52] The major disadvantages of this technology are that it may occasionally overestimate the degree of stenosis, development of disease in endovascular stents is not possible, patients with claustrophobia do not tolerate the acquisition of images, and the cost.

Functional Tests

Duplex ultrasonography, CTA, and MRA, as well as conventional angiography provide only anatomical information regarding whether or not stenosis is present in a particular mesenteric artery. They do not provide any physiological information on intestinal ischemia or the patients' symptoms. Tonometry and magnetic resonance imagining (MRI) are capable of providing functional information of intestinal ischemia, although their use has been limited to the research arena. Their development and clinical applicability are going to be of utmost importance since they are going help clinicians to better select patients who require revascularization procedures, particularly those with atypical presentation or with single-vessel disease.

Tonometry measures intestinal mucosa Pco_2 with a *tonometer,* a balloon-tip catheter that is inserted and placed in contact with the stomach or the intestinal mucosa. The balloon is silicone gas-permeable and enables carbon dioxide to equilibrate freely between the gastric or intestinal mucosa and the balloon lumen. The rational for the use of this functional test is that a decrease in intestinal blood flow promotes anaerobic metabolism, leading to increase in Pco_2, which is going to be detected and measured by the tonometer balloon after Pco_2 equilibrates.[53-55] The diagnostic value of postprandial Pco_2 is being debated, whereas postexercise gastric tonometry appears as a promising provocative test for the diagnosis of gastrointestinal ischemia.[56-58]

MRI is also capable of providing functional information of the mesenteric blood flow. Flow velocities and total flow volumes, using 2-dimensional cine-phase contrast velocity mapping can be measured in the mesenteric vessels with MRI. Some studies have shown that compared to healthy volunteers, patients with CMI have decreased postprandial flow volume augmentation.[59-61] MRI has also been used to measure the oxygen saturation of hemoglobin in the superior mesenteric vein using magnetic resonance oximetry. The principle behind this technology is that deoxyhemoglobin in erythrocytes is paramagnetic, whereas oxyhemoglobin is not. Consequently, magnetic resonance oximetry can calculate the percentage of circulating oxyhemoglobin in the superior mesenteric vein. As blood flow decreases, oxygen extraction augments to compensate and keep constant the total amount of oxygen delivery to the intestinal tissue. It has been shown that compared to normal volunteers, in whom the percent oxyhemoglobin increases after ingestion of meals, in patients with CMI, postprandial percent oxyhemoglobin decreases.[62]

Conventional Angiography

Invasive nonselective and selective mesenteric angiography, with or without digital subtraction imaging, has remained the gold standard, against which all other image modalities are compared for the diagnosis of mesenteric arterial stenosis. In the last few years, however, with the improvement of image quality in CTA, MRA, and duplex ultrasonography, this historical tenet is being challenged, and clinicians rely less frequently on conventional angiography for the diagnosis of mesenteric arterial stenoses. At present, the main indications for performing invasive angiography are when patients have equivocal or contradictory noninvasive imaging results, or when revascularization is being considered. It is common practice to take patients to the catheterization suite, with the diagnosis of mesenteric arterial stenosis by a noninvasive image study, for confirmatory angiographic diagnosis with the purpose of proceeding with endovascular therapy during the same session. Alternatively, vascular surgeons may prefer confirmatory invasive angiography prior to surgical revascularization.

Because the mesenteric arteries arise in the ventral portion of the abdominal aorta, it is crucial to obtain images in the lateral view, since the anteroposterior view may easily miss the diagnosis—stenoses in these arteries are more frequently located at the ostium or the very proximal portion of the artery. For the IMA, which often arises from the left anterolateral aspect of the aorta, the right anterior oblique view (± 20°–30° caudal) shows well the ostium and the very proximal portion, which otherwise may be missed in the anteroposterior or lateral views. After a nonselective abdominal aortogram has been obtained, it is our practice to proceed with selective angiography to better outline these vessels, and to minimize overlapping with other abdominal arteries.

Therapy for Chronic Mesenteric Ischemia

Medical Therapy

Patients with CMI, like other patients with atherosclerotic vascular disease, should be treated with aggressive lipid-lowering therapy, smoking cessation, optimization of blood pressure, diabetes control, and the use of antiplatelets such as aspirin. Because of the experimental data of angiotensin II leading to splanchnic vasoconstriction, there may be a theoretical role in the use of ACE inhibitors and/or ARB in these patients.[28] In addition, due to the detrimental actions of digoxin in the splanchnic circulation causing vasoconstriction and ischemia, this drug must be avoided in these individuals.[36,37]

Although it is possible that a small proportion of patients with CMI may have improvement or relief of symptoms with medical therapy, this has not been documented yet, and as a general rule, these patients have progression of disease (see "Natural History") toward development of acute mesenteric ischemia, or inanition and death, unless revascularization is carried out. For this reason the current ACC/AHA Guidelines are that all patients with CMI should be referred for revascularization therapy, either endovascular or surgical.[63]

Surgical Revascularization

After CMI became an established clinical entity in 1936,[3] Mikkelson[64] showed in 1957 that patients with this condition could be successfully be treated with surgery. Since then, the traditional treatment for CMI has been surgical revascularization, with antegrade or retrograde aortomesenteric bypass graft or transthoracic endarterectomy.

Although surgery usually carries lasting symptom relief in the majority of the patients who are successfully discharged from the hospital, the procedural mortality and morbidity are high. In Table 10.1 we have summarized the outcome of 12 surgical studies, showing a mortality rate ranging from 0% to 29% and a morbidity rate ranging from 9% to 62%.[65-76] These results have been confirmed by a surgical study of 336 patients from the Nationwide Inpatients sample as part of the Healthcare Cost and Utilization Project, showing that surgical revascularization for CMI in-hospital mortality was 14.7% and complication rate was 44.6%, with a median hospital stay of 14 days.[77]

	N	Procedural Mortality	Procedural Morbidity	Symptoms Relief	Symptoms Recurrence	Follow-up (years)
Hollier et al[65]	56	8.9%	-	96%	26.5%	3.0
Cunningham et al[66]	85	12%	47%	97%	14%	5.0
Cormier et al[67]	103	4%	-	-	4%	5.5
McAfee et al[68]	58	10%	49%	96%	10%	3.3
Christensen et al[69]	53	0			30%	
Gentile et al[70]	23	0%	—	100%	10%	3.3
Johnston et al[71]	21	0%	19%	—	14%	
Taylor et al[72]	58	0%	9%	—	4%	4.5
Mateo et al[73]	85	8%	33%	81%	24%	4.8
Foley et al[74]	49	12%	35%	—	21%	3.5
Cho et al[75]	25	4%	60%	—	21%	5.3
English et al[76]	58	29%	62%	94%	43%*	3.0

Table 10.1 Results of Surgical Revascularization. (*Death or recurrence of symptoms.)

Patients with CMI are a very sick group of individuals, and the majority have significant coronary, neurovascular, renal, and peripheral atherosclerotic disease. It is not surprising that they frequently develop postoperative vascular events such as myocardial infarction, stroke, renal failure, or noncardiogenic pulmonary edema, causing death or a difficult postoperative course and a very prolonged hospital stay. However, of the patients who were discharged from the hospital, the majority had lasting symptoms relief, with a recurrence rate of 10% to 30% at a follow-up of 3.0 to 5.5 years (Table 10.1).

Endovascular Therapy

Percutaneous, catheter-based revascularization techniques have profoundly changed the management of obstructive atherosclerotic disease in the coronary and in the peripheral circulation and are at present accepted as alternatives to surgery in a significant proportion of patients. Endovascular therapy offers several distinct advantages over surgical revascularization. It may be performed with local anesthesia, enabling the treatment of patients who are at high risk for general anesthesia. The morbidity and mortality from endovascular therapy is very low when compared to surgical revascularization. Problems secondary to angioplasty are generally related to vascular access. Following endovascular therapy, patients are usually ambulatory on the day of treatment and unlike vascular surgery can often return to normal activity within 24 to 48 hours of an uncomplicated procedure. Finally, endovascular therapies may be repeated if necessary, generally without increased difficulty or increased patient risk compared to the first procedure, and prior angioplasty does not preclude surgery if required at a later date.

Patients with CMI are usually malnourished and have significant atherosclerotic disease in other vascular territories, such as the coronary and neurovascular circulation. In addition, stenoses of the mesenteric arteries are usually focal, preferentially located in the ostium or the very proximal portion of these vessels. These clinical and vascular characteristics of patients with CMI make percutaneous transluminal intervention a very attractive treatment modality for this condition.

Percutaneous Transluminal Angioplasty

Since the initial publication of *percutaneous transluminal angioplasty* in a superior mesenteric artery by Furrer and Gruntzing in 1980,[78] the use of percutaneous revascularization in the mesenteric circulation has been reported only in small series with relatively short follow-up. These studies have shown that balloon angioplasty yields a high procedural success, with low morbidity and mortality rates. For this reason, endovascular therapy has become an important alternative treatment to surgical revascularization in selected patients. The reported procedural success rate for balloon angioplasty is between 79% and 100%, with clinical success rates between 63% and 91%. Symptoms reoccurred in 5% to 7%, however, the number of patients treated in these series was smaller and the follow-up shorter than the surgical studies.[79-87]

Endovascular Stent Placement

Aorto-ostial stenoses are difficult to treat with balloon angioplasty alone due to elastic recoil. Stent placement minimizes this recoil, resulting in a larger final lumen diameter and higher procedural success rate than for balloon dilation alone. In renal artery atherosclerotic aorto-ostial stenoses, the use of stents has been shown to be superior to balloon angioplasty alone.[88,89] There are insufficient data in the literature addressing the role of endoluminal stents for the treatment of CMI (Table 10.2). In one of the initial studies of 33 patients (47 arteries) with CMI undergoing percutaneous transluminal angioplasty (12 patients and 15 vessels received stents), the technical success rate was 81% for balloon angioplasty alone and 100% for stenting. Complete or partial resolution of symptoms occurred in 82% and 6% of the patients, respectively.[85]

In another study of 12 patients treated with stent placement,[90] the reported technical success rate was 92%. One patient developed bowel infarction and died in the hospital despite a technically successful procedure. The primary and the primary-assisted patency rates were 74% and 83%, respectively, and the secondary patency rate was 83%.

In a more recent study of 25 patients and 26 arteries treated with primary stenting,[91] technical success was obtained in 96% and symptom relief in 88%. There was no procedural mortality and the only complications were the development of a pseudoaneurysm (n = 2) and renal failure (n = 1). At a mean follow-up of 15 months, the primary clinical benefit (no recurrence symptoms) was 83%, and the restenosis rate was 18%.

Our results with primary stent placement for CMI in 59 patients (79 vessels) are also quite favorable.[43] The angiographic and the procedural success rates were 97% and 96%,

Study	N	Procedural Success	Symptom Relief	In-Hospital Mortality	Procedural Complications	Symptom Recurrence	Primary Patency Rate	Follow-up (months)
Sheeran et al[90]	12	92%	83%	8.0%	0%	18%	83%*	15.7
Sharafuddin et al[91]	25	96%	88%	0%	12.0%	17%	92%*	15.0
AbuRahma et al[92]	22	96%	95%	0%	0%	34%	30%	26.0
Resch et al[93]	17	94%	82%	5.8%	5.8%	17%	69%	14.0
Brown et al[94]	14	100%	100%	0%	0%	50%	43%	13.0
Schaefer et al[95]	19	96%	78%	10.0%	0%	22%	82%	17.0
Silva et al[43]	59	96%	88%	1.7%	2.5%	17%	71%	38.0

Table 10.2 Studies of Patients with CMI Treated with Stent Placement. *Primary assisted

respectively, with symptom relief in 88% of patients. We were unable to cross 2 chronic total occlusions in one patient. One patient died in the hospital due to sepsis and renal failure, despite an angiographically successful procedure. At a mean follow-up of 38 ± 15 months, 17% had recurrence of symptoms but none developed acute mesenteric ischemia and all underwent successful revascularization without any complication. Follow-up was achieved in 90% of the patients and 90% of the vessels with angiographic CT, conventional angiography, or duplex ultrasonography, showing a restenosis rate of 29%. Other investigators have obtained comparable results.[92-95]

Although there are no prospective controlled data comparing outcomes of balloon angioplasty versus stent placement for the treatment of mesenteric arterial stenoses, recent studies suggest that endovascular stent placement confers superior immediate and long-term results than balloon angioplasty alone, for which stent revascularization should be the percutaneous treatment of choice.

Technical aspects

Aspirin is started at least 1 day prior to the procedure. Heparin is given after vascular access had been obtained to achieve an activated clotting time (ACT) of > 250 seconds. We often use retrograde common femoral arterial (CFA) access, however, in cases in which the origin of the mesenteric vessel is significantly caudally oriented, the brachial arterial access is preferred.

We obtain anteroposterior and lateral views for the nonselective aortogram. Selective mesenteric arterial imaging is performed with 4- to 6-Fr (internal mammary, cobra, Simmons, Sos, or Judkins' right configuration) catheters using hand injections of contrast. A soft-tip exchanged-length 0.035-in guide wire (Wholey wire, Mallinckrodt) is then exchanged over the Wholey wire for an 8-Fr hockey stick angioplasty guiding catheter and positioned in contact with the ostium of the vessel. Some of the 6-Fr renal angioplasty guiding catheters can also be used, with a 0.014-in steerable guide to cross the lesion.

When the brachial arterial access is used, a 6- or 7-Fr, 90-cm long vascular sheath (Daig) is advanced over the guide wire and positioned in the abdominal aorta immediately above the target mesenteric artery. A 6-Fr multipurpose diagnostic catheter is then introduced through the long arterial sheath and used to engage the mesenteric artery. A soft-tip exchanged-length 0.035-in steerable guide wire (Wholey wire, Mallinckrodt) is used to cross the mesenteric artery. Alternatively 0.014-in guide wires can be used if the operator plans to use 6-Fr compatible balloon and stent systems. Keeping the 6-Fr multipurpose diagnostic catheter engaging the ostium of the mesenteric artery, and the Wholey wire distally, branch of the mesenteric artery, the arterial sheath is advanced over the multipurpose catheter and positioned in contact with the ostium of the target mesenteric artery. The 6-Fr multipurpose diagnostic catheter is then removed, leaving the guide wire in the mesenteric artery branch, and the arterial sheath in contact with the ostium of the vessel.

After the reference vessel diameter (RVD) is measured with online quantitative angiography, a peripheral angioplasty balloon (4–8 mm in diameter, 2 cm long) is advanced over the Wholey wire (or an 0.014-in guide wire) and positioned at the lesion site. The lesion is then dilated with a balloon sized 1:1 with the RVD, using the lowest pressure that will fully expand the balloon. A balloon-expandable stent, long enough to cover the lesion, is used to scaffold the lesion and maximize the angiographic result. The balloon-expandable stent is advanced over the guide wire, still within the sheath or guiding catheter, to the lesion site. The sheath or the guiding catheter is withdrawn, uncovering the stent, and with contrast injections through the sheath or the guiding catheter, the stent is positioned at the lesion site. The stent is deployed at 6 to 8 atmospheres, and then the balloon is withdrawn into the sheath or the guiding catheter. Angiography is then performed and if inadequate expansion of the stent is observed, the operator repeats dilation of the stent at a higher inflation pressure or with a larger balloon (see Figures 10.6, 10.7, and 10.8).

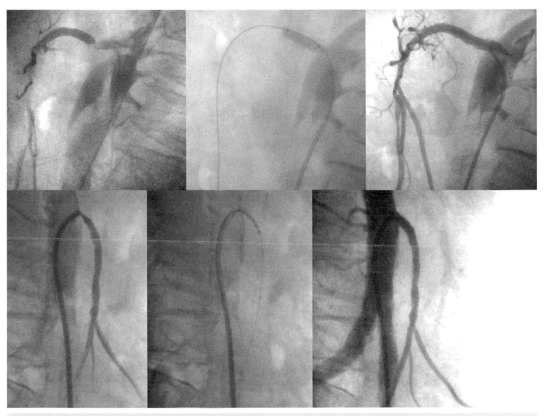

Figure 10.6 A 72-year-old with typical symptoms of chronic mesenteric ischemia and critical stenoses of the superior and inferior mesenteric arteries, successfully treated with a biliary (SMA) and a coronary (IMA) stent. (From Silva JA, White CJ, Collins TJ, et al. Endovascular therapy for chronic mesenteric ischemia. *J Am Coll Cardiol*. 2006;47: 944-950. Reprinted with permission from Elsevier.)

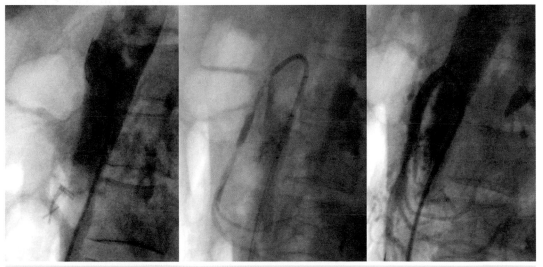

Figure 10.7 A 61-year-old female with symptoms of ischemic gastropathy for over 1 year, consisting of persistent nausea, poor appetite, easy fullness, vomiting, and abdominal pain only occasionally related to food intake. She had lost over 40 pounds before she underwent an abdominal aortogram showing total occlusion of all 3 mesenteric arteries. The superior mesenteric artery was successfully recanalized and stented, with immediate resolution of her chronic symptoms, and she experienced a weight gain. (From Silva JA, White CJ, Collins TJ, et al. Endovascular therapy for chronic mesenteric ischemia. *J Am Coll Cardiol*. 2006;47: 944-950. Reprinted with permission from Elsevier.)

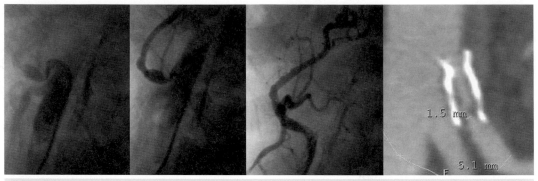

Figure 10.8 A 38-year-old female with a long-standing history of cramping abdominal pain who was awakened from sleep by severe abdominal pain followed by bloody diarrhea. Colonoscopy and biopsy demonstrated ischemic colitis. Angiography revealed extrinsic compression of the celiac trunk with total occlusion during inspiration. The patient refused surgical decompression and underwent successful stent placement with resolution and no recurrence of symptoms. The 6-month CTA (far right) revealed > 50% in-stent restenosis but patency of the stent and no inspiratory collapse. She has had no recurrence of symptoms at more than 3 years of follow-up. (From Silva JA, White CJ, Collins TJ, et al. Endovascular therapy for chronic mesenteric ischemia. *J Am Coll Cardiol.* 2006;47: 944-950. Reprinted with permission from Elsevier.)

Surgical Versus Endovascular Therapy

The growing application of percutaneous, catheter-based techniques for the treatment of peripheral arterio-occlusive disease, as well as the recent publication of studies demonstrating endovascular therapy as an important revascularization therapy for CMI, has given way to an intense debate regarding the best revascularization strategy for this condition. Unfortunately, there are no controlled, prospective randomized studies comparing these 2 treatment modalities and therefore, firm conclusions cannot be drawn with the existing data.

From the previous discussion it is clear that because patients with CMI are a very sick group of individuals—that is, malnourished and frequently with severe coronary and neurovascular disease—and because of the characteristics of their disease, such as proximity and focal nature of the atherosclerotic lesions, this group of patients is ideally suited for endovascular therapy. Results from surgical and endovascular stent series as well as comparative studies show that in the majority of patients, the immediate clinical success and the procedural morbidity and mortality are superior in the endovascular group (see Tables 10.1 and 10.2). Another situation in which percutaneous intervention may be superior over surgery is when graft failure after surgery often presents abruptly, as sudden

occlusion, either in the early postoperative period or at follow-up, leading to bowel infarction and death in the majority of the patients.[65,66,73] This occurrence is rare after percutaneous treatment. In our series of 59 patients treated with endovascular stent revascularization, in no single case did the development of in-stent restenosis lead to mortality. None of our patients had acute mesenteric ischemia, either early after the procedure or at follow-up. There were no acute or subacute postprocedural stent thrombosis events, and the cases of in-stent restenosis led to gradual development of symptoms.[43]

The major controversy stems from whether a particular treatment option confers superior lasting clinical benefits. Four nonrandomized retrospective studies have attempted to compare surgical revascularization and endovascular treatment for CMI.[86,87,94,96] One small study compared the outcomes in 9 patients treated with bypass graft and 8 patients treated with balloon angioplasty alone.[96] Although the immediate and long-term outcomes were comparable in the 2 groups, it is difficult to draw meaningful conclusions from this small study. A second study compared the results of 28 patients treated percutaneously (23 patients received stents) and 85 patients treated with surgery.[86] The patients in the endovascular treatment group were older and had a significantly higher prevalence of coronary artery disease. The procedural-related mortality was 10.7% for the endovascular treatment group and 8.2% for the surgical group (*P* = 0.71), however, serious complications were significantly less common (19% vs. 40%, *P* = 0.03), and hospital stay shorter (5 vs. 13 days, *P* = 0.08) in the percutaneously treated group. The long-term mortality and patency rates were similar in the 2 groups. Recurrence of symptoms was more frequent in the endovascularly treated group than in the surgically treated group (34% vs. 13%, *P* = 0.001), however, the large majority (86%) of the patients with recurrent symptoms in the endovascular treatment group had patent vessels, whereas 90% of the patients with recurrence of symptoms in the surgical group had graft or vessel occlusion.

A more recent study comparing outcomes of 60 patients treated with surgery (n = 41) or endovascular therapy (n =19, 89% received stents) found a much lower morbidity rate and a shorter in-hospital stay in the percutaneously treated group. The 30-day mortality and 3-year cumulative survival were similar in both groups. The 6-month symptom recurrence was significantly higher in the percutaneously treated group despite similar cumulative patency rates (83% vs, 68%, *P* = NS). Comparable results were obtained in a study of 14 patients treated with stent revascularization. At a mean follow-up of 13 months, 50% developed recurrence of symptoms, and 57% developed in-stent restenosis requiring repeat endovascular treatment.[94] When the authors compared their results with historical surgical controls at the same institution, vessel patency was significantly higher in the surgically treated group. These results, however, contrast with our study of 59 patients and 79 arteries, where we found an in-stent restenosis rate of 29% of the arteries (37% of the patients) at a mean follow-up of 38 ± 15 months (Figure 10.9), which is comparable with most surgical series (see Table 10.1).[43]

Other reports also suggest a strategy of endovascular therapy as bridging to surgical revascularization, thereby allowing patients to improve their surgical risk profile (nutritional status, treatment of comorbidities such as coronary artery disease, etc.) and proceed with more definitive surgical treatment at a later stage, if necessary.[94,97]

More studies—ideally prospective randomized—will be needed to draw a definitive conclusion; however, in light of the current evidence, a large and increasing proportion of practitioners, including the author, refer patients with CMI for endovascular stent therapy as the treatment of choice, reserving surgical

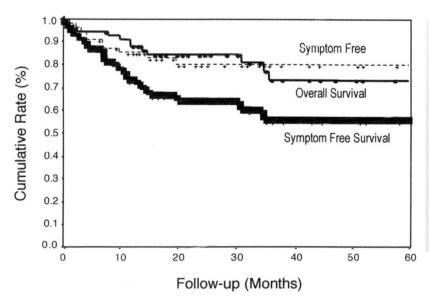

Figure 10.9 Kaplan-Meier survival curves showing the 5-year cumulative probability of overall survival, symptom-free, and symptom-free survival of 59 patients with chronic mesenteric ischemia. (From Silva JA, White CJ, Collins TJ, et al. Endovascular therapy for chronic mesenteric ischemia. *J Am Coll Cardiol.* 2006;47: 944-950. Reprinted with permission from Elsevier.)

revascularization for those patients in whom percutaneous intervention fails (such as patients with chronic total occlusions) or who develop symptom recurrence due to in-stent restenosis, where surgery may be considered instead of repeat percutaneous intervention.

Summary

Atherosclerotic disease affects the mesenteric circulation relatively frequently, however, CMI is an uncommon but complex disease. The natural history of CMI is incompletely understood, but most investigators agree that a proportion of patients develop acute mesenteric ischemia, which carries a very high mortality, and the rest continue toward emaciation and death if it remains undetected.

The diagnosis of this condition is based on the presence of symptoms, usually postprandial abdominal pain with or without weight loss, or other less specific symptoms such as gastroparesis, nausea, vomiting, or colitis in conjunction with the presence of significant mesenteric stenosis (usually ≥ 2 arteries) detected by duplex ultrasonography, CTA, MRA, or conventional angiography. The introduction of functional studies to detect mesenteric ischemia such as tonometry and MRI will very likely help to detect this disease at earlier stages, and refer for revascularization therapy patients with less typical gastrointestinal symptoms.

The traditional treatment for CMI had been surgical revascularization. Surgery provides symptom relief, however, it carries a significant procedural morbidity and mortality. Percutaneous, catheter-based revascularization procedures have been shown to be feasible alternative treatment modalities to surgery for CMI. Recent publications suggest that the use of stents is a safe and effective treatment modality for CMI, yielding low procedural complication and mortality rates and long-term clinical benefits, which are comparable to those of surgical revascularization.

References

1. Elliot J. The operative relief of gangrene of intestine due to occlusion of the mesenteric vessels. *Ann Surg*. 1895;1:9-23.
2. Goodman EH. Angina abdominis. *Am J Med Sci*. 1918;155:524-528.
3. Dunphy JE. Abdominal pain of vascular origin. *Am J Med Sci*. 1936;192:109-112.
4. Kornblith PL, Boley SJ, Whitehoouse BS. Anatomy of the splacnic circulation. *Surg Clin North Am*. 1992;72:1-30.
5. Chiene J. Complete obliteration of the coeliac and mesenteric arteries: viscera and their blood supply through the extra-peritoneal system of vessels. *J Anat Physiol*. 1869;3:65-72.
6. Fisher DF Jr, Fry WJ. Collateral mesenteric circulation. *Surg Gyn Obs*. 1987;164:487-492.
7. Valentine RJ, Martin JD, Myers SI, Rossi MB, Clagett GP. Asymptomatic celiac and superior mesenteric artery stenoses are more prevalent among patients with unsuspected renal artery stenoses. *J Vasc Surg*. 1991;14:195-199.
8. Hansen KJ, Wilson DB, Craven TE, et al. Mesenteric artery disease in the elderly. *J Vasc Surg*. 2004;40:45-52.
9. Valentine RJ, Martin JD, Myers SI, Rossi MB, Clagett GP. Asymptomatic celiac and superior mesenteric artery stenoses are more prevalent among patients with unsuspected renal artery stenoses. *J Vasc Surg*. 1991;14:195-199.
10. Marston A. Diagnosis and management of intestinal ischemia. *Ann R Coll Surg Engl*. 1972;50:29-41.
11. Reiner L, Jimenez FA, Rodriguez FL. Atherosclerosis in the mesenteric circulation: observations and correlations with aortic and coronary atherosclerosis. *Am Heart J*. 1963;66:200-204.
12. Palubinskas AJ, Ripley HR. Fibromuscular hyperplasia in extra-renal arteries. *Radiology*. 1964;82:451-454.
13. Harris MT, Lewis BS. Systemic diseases affecting the mesenteric circulation. *Surg Clin North Am*. 1992;72:245-259.
14. Stanley JC, Fry WJ. Median arcuate ligament syndrome. *Arch Surg*. 1971;103:252-258.
15. Bech FR. Celiac artery compression syndromes. *Surg Clin North Am*. 1997;77:409-424.

16. Reilly LM, Ammar AD, Stoney RJ, et al. Late results following operative repair for celiac artery compression syndrome. *J Vasc Surg.* 1985;2:79-91.

17. van Bockel JH, Geelkerken RH, Wasser MN. Chronic splanchnic ischemia. *Best Pract Res Clin Gastroenterol.* 2001;15:99-119.

18. Zierler RE, Bergelin RO, Isaacson JS, et al. Natural history of atherotic renal artery stenosis: a prospective study with duplex ultrasonography. *J Vasc Surg.* 1994;19:250-257.

19. Thomas JH, Blake K, Pierce GE, Hermreck AS, Seigel E. The clinical course of asymptomatic mesenteric arterial stenosis. *J Vasc Surg.* 1998;27:840-844.

20. Stoney RJ, Cunningham CG. Acute mesenteric ischemia. *Surgery.* 1993;114:372-380.

21. Kwaan JH, Connolly JE. Prevention of intestinal infarction resulting from mesenteric arterial occlusive disease. *Surg Gyn Obst.* 1983;157:321-324.

22. Rosemblum JD, Boyle CM, Schwartz LB. The mesenteric circulation. Anatomy and physiology. *Surg Clin North Am.* 1997;77:289-306.

23. Heer M, Repond F, Hany A, et al. Acute ischemic colitis in long distance runner. *Gut.* 1987;28:896-899.

24. Otte JA, Oostveen E, Geelkerken RH, et al. Heavy exercise of short duration may provoke gastric ischemia in healthy subjects. *Gastroenterology.* 1998;114:A404.

25. Jager K, Bollinger A, Valli C, et al. Measurement of mesenteric blood flow by duplex scanning. *J Vasc Surg.* 1986;3:462-469.

26. Desai TR, Sisley AC, Brown S, et al. Defining the critical limit of oxygen extraction in the human small intestine. *J Vasc Surg.* 1996;23:832-838.

27. Granger DN, Richardson PD, Kvietys PR, et al. Intestinal blood flow. *Gastroenterology.* 1980;78:837-863.

28. Reilly PM, Bulkley GB. Vasoactive mediators and splanchnic perfusion. *Crit Care Med.* 1993;21(2 Suppl):S55-68.

29. Harjola PT. A rare obstruction of the coeliac artery; report of a case. *Annales Gynecologia Fenniae.* 1963;52:547-550.

30. Bron KM, Redman HC. Splanchnic artery stenosis and occlusion. Incidence, arteriographic and clinical manifestations. *Radiology.* 1969;92:323-328.

31. Szilagyi DE, Rian RL, Elliot JP, et al. The coeliac compression syndrome: does it exist? *Surgery.* 1972;72:849-863.

32. Reilly LM, Ammar AD, Stoney RJ. Late results following operative repair for celiac artery compression syndrome. *J Vasc Surg.* 1985;2:79-91.

33. Poole JW, Sammartano RJ, Boley SJ. Hemodynamic basis for the pain of chronic mesenteric ischemia. *Am J Surg.* 1987;153:171-176.

34. Stanley JC, Fry WJ. Median arcuate ligament syndrome. *Arch Surg.* 1971;103:252-258.

35. Geelkerken RH, Schulze Kool LJ, Breslau PJ, et al. Transient colonic ischemia: consequence of a rare anatomical variation of the mesenteric arteries. *Eur J Surg.* 1996;162:827-829.

36. Kim EH, Gewertz BL. Chronic digitalis administration alters mesenteric vascular reactivity. *J Vasc Surg.* 1987;5(2):382-389.

37. Levinsky RA, Lewis RM, Bynum TE, et al. Digoxin induced intestinal vasoconstriction. The effects of proximal arterial stenosis and glucagon administration. *Circulation.* 1975;52(1):130-136.

38. Liberski SM, Koch KL, Atnip RG, Stern RM. Ischemic gastroparesis: resolution after revascularization. *Gastroenterology.* 1990;99:252-257.

39. Babu SC, Shah PM. Celiac territory ischemic syndrome in visceral artery occlusion. *Am J Surg.* 1993;166:227-230.

40. Kathleen MC, Quigley TM, Kozarek RA, Raker EJ. Lethal nature of ischemic gastropathy. *Am J Surg.* 1993;165:646-649.

41. Cappell MS. Intestinal(mesenteric) vasculopathy. II. Ischemic colitis and chronic mesenteric ischemia. *Gastroenterol Clin North Am.* 1998;27:827-858.

42. Geelkerken RH, Van Bockel JH, De Roos WK, et al. Chronic mesenteric vascular syndrome. Results of reconstructive surgery. *Arch Surg.* 1991;126:1101-1106.

43. Silva JA, White CJ, Collins TJ, et al. Endovascular therapy for chronic mesenteric ischemia. *J Am Coll Cardiol.* 2006;47:944-950.

44. Bradbury AW, Brittenden J, McBride K, Ruck-

ley CV. Mesenteric ischaemia: a multidisciplinary approach. *Br J Surg*. 1995;82:1446-1459.

45. Geelkerken RH, Van Bockel JH. Duplex ultrasound examination of splachnic vessels in the assessment of splachnic ischemic symptoms. *Eur J Vasc Endovasc Surg*. 1999;18:371-374.

46. Moneta GL, Lee RW, Yeager RA, Taylor LM, Porter JM. Mesenteric duplex scanning: a blinded prospective study. *J Vasc Surg*. 1993;17:79-86.

47. Zwolak RM, Fillinger MF, Walsh DB, et al. Mesenteric celiac duplex scanning. A validation study. *J Vasc Surg*. 1998; 27:1078-1088.

48. Gentile AT, Moneta GL, Lee RW, et al. Usefulness of fasting and postprandial duplex ultrasound examinations for predicting high-grade superior mesenteric artery stenosis. *Am J Surg*. 1995;169:476-479.

49. Behar JV, Nelson RC, Zidar JP, DeLong DM, Smith TP. Thin-section multidetector CT angiography of renal artery stents. *AJR Am J Roentgenol*. 2002;178:1155-1159.

50. Goldman CK, Morshedi-Meibodi A, White CJ, et al. Surveillance imaging for carotid in-stent restenosis. *Catheter Cardiovasc Interv*. 2006;67:302-308.

51. Maintz D, Tombach B, Juergens KU, et al. Revealing in-stent restenoses of the iliac arteries: comparison of multidetector CT with MR angiography and digital radiographic angiography in a phantom model. *Am J Roentgenol*. 2002;179:1319-1322.

52. Meaney JF, Prince MR, Nostrant TT, et al. Gadolinium-enhanced MR angiography of visceral arteries in patients with suspected chronic mesenteric ischemia. *J Magn Res Imag*. 1997;7:171-176.

53. Dawson AM, Trenchard D, Guz A. Small bowel tonometry: assessment of gut mucosal oxygen tension in dog and man. *Nature*. 1965; 206:943-944.

54. Fiddian-Green RG, Stanley JC, Nostrant T, et al. Chronic gastric ischemia. A cause of abdominal pain or bleeding identified by the presence of gastric mucosal acidosis. *J Cardiovasc Surg*. 1989;30:852-859.

55. Kolkman JJ, Otte JA, Groeneveld AB. Gastrointestinal luminal PCO_2 tonometry: an update on physiology, methodology, and clinical applications. *Br J Anaeth*. 2000;84:74-86.

56. Kolkman JJ, Groeneveld AB, Meuwisen SG. Effect of gastric feeding on intragastric $P(CO_2)$ tonometry in health volunteers. *J Critic Care*. 1999;14:34-38.

57. Geelkerken RH, Schultze Kool LJ, Hermans J, et al. Chronic splachnic ischemia: is tonometry a useful test? *Eu J Surg*. 1997;163:115-121.

58. Kolkman JJ, Groeneveld AB, van der Berg FG, et al. Increased gastric PCO_2 during exercise is indicative of gastric ischemia: a tonometric study. *Gut*. 1999;44:163-167.

59. Li KC, Whitney WS, McDonnell CH, et al. Chronic mesenteric ischemia: evaluation with phase contrast cine MR imaging. *Radiology*. 1994;190:175-179.

60. Burkart DJ, Johnson CD, Reading CC, et al. MR measurements of mesenteric venous flow. Prospective evaluation in healthy volunteers and patients with suspected chronic mesenteric ischemia. *Radiology*. 1995;194:801-806.

61. Dalman RL, Li KC, Moon WK, et al. Diminished postprandial hyperemia in patients with aortic and mesenteric arterial occlusive disease. Quantification by magnetic resonance flow imaging. *Circulation*. 1996;94(9 Suppl):II206-210.

62. Li KC, Dalman RL, Ch'en IY, et al. Chronic mesenteric ischemia: use of in vivo MR imaging measurements of blood oxygen saturation in the superior mesenteric vein for diagnosis. *Radiology*. 1997;204:71-77.

63. Hirsh AT, Haskal ZJ, Hertzer NR, et al. ACC/AHA 2005 guidelines for the management of patients with peripheral arterial disease (lower extremity, renal, mesenteric, and abdominal aortic): executive summary. *J Am Coll Cardiol*. 2006;47:1239-1312.

64. Mikkelsen WP. Intestinal angina: its surgical significance. *Am J Surg*. 1957;94:262-267.

65. Hollier LH, Bernatz PE, Pairolero PC, Payne WS, Osmundon PJ. Surgical management of chronic intestinal ischemia: a reappraisal. *Surgery*. 1981;90:940-946.

66. Cunningham CG, Reilly LM, Rapp JH, Schneider PA, Stoney RJ. Chronic visceral is-

chemia. Three decades of progress. *Ann Surg.* 1991;214:276-288.

67. Cormier JM, Fichelle JM, Vennin J, et al. Atherosclerotic occlusive disease of the superior mesenteric artery: late results of reconstructive surgery. *Ann Vasc Surg.* 1991;5:510-518.

68. McAfee MK, Cherry KJ, Naessens JM, et a;. Influence of complete revascularization on chronic mesenteric ischemia. *Am J Surg.* 1992;164:220-224.

69. Christensen MG, Lorentzen JE, Schroeder TV. Revascularization of atherosclerotic mesenteric arteries: experience in 90 consecutive patients. *Eur J Vasc Surg.* 1994;8:297-302.

70. Gentile AT, Moneta GL, Taylor LM, et al. Isolated bypass to the superior mesenteric artery for intestinal ischemia. *Arch Surg.* 1994;129:926-931.

71. Johnston KW, Lindsay TF, Walker PM, Kalman PG. Mesenteric arterial bypass grafts: early and late results and suggested surgical approach for chronic and acute mesenteric ischemia. *Surgery.* 1995;118:1-7.

72. Taylor LM, Porter JM. Treatment of chronic visceral ischemia. In Rutherford, RB (ed): *Vascular surgery.* Philadelphia, WB Saunders, 1995

73. Mateo RB, O'Hara PJ, Hertzer NR, Mascha EJ, Beven EG, Krajewski LP. Elective surgical treatment of symptomatic chronic mesenteric occlusive disease: early results and late outcomes. *J Vasc Surg.* 1999;29:821-832.

74. Foley MI, Moneta GL, Abou-Zamzam AM, et al. Revascularization of the superior mesenteric artery alone for the treatment of intestinal ischemia. *J Vasc Surg.* 2000;32:37-47.

75. Cho JS, Carr JA, Jacobsen G, Shephard AD, Nypaver TJ, Reddy DJ. Long-term outcome after mesenteric artery reconstruction: a 37-year experience. *J Vasc Surg.* 2002;35:453-460.

76. English WP, Pearce JD, Craven TE, et al. Chronic visceral ischemia: symptom-free survival after open surgical repair. *Vasc Endovasc Surg.* 2004;38:493-503.

77. Derrow AE, Seeger JM, Dame DA, et al. The outcome in the United States after thoracoabdominal aortic aneurysm repair, renal artery bypass, and mesenteric revascularization. *J Vasc Surg.* 2001;34:54-61.

78. Furrer J, Gruntzig J, Kugelmeir J, Goebel N. Treatment of abdominal angina with percutaneous dilatation of an arteria mesenteric superior stenosis. *Cardiovasc Interv Radiol.* 1980;3:43-44.

79. Allen RC, Martin GH, Rees CR, Rivera FJ, et al. Mesenteric angioplasty in the treatment of chronic mesenteric ischemia. *J Vasc Surg.* 1996;24:415-423.

80. Hallisay MJ, Deschaine J, Illescas FF, et al. Angioplasty for the treatment of visceral ischemia. *J Vasc Interv Radiol.* 1995; 6:785-791.

81. Matsumoto AH, Tegtmeyer CJ, Fitzcharles EK, et al. Percutaneous transluminal angioplasty of visceral arterial stenoses: results and long-term clinical follow-up. *J Vasc Interv Radiol.* 1995;6:165-174.

82. Sniderman KW. Transluminal angioplasty in the management of chronic intestinal ischemia In: Strandness DE, van Breda A, eds. *Vascular Diseases: Surgical and Interventional Therapy.* New York: Churchill Livingston; 1994:803-809.

83. Simonetti G, Lupetelli L, Urigo F, et al. Interventional radiology in the treatment of acute and chronic mesenteric ischemia. *Radiol Med.* 1992;84:98-105.

84. Nyman U, Ivancev K, Lindh M, Uher P. Endovascular treatment of chronic mesenteric ischemia: report of five cases. *Cardiovasc Intervent Radiol.* 1998;21:305-313.

85. Matsumoto AH, Angle JF, Spinosa DJ, et al. Percutaneous transluminal angioplasty and stenting in the treatment of chronic mesenteric ischemia: results and long-term clinical follow up. *J Am Coll Surg.* 2002;194:S22-S31.

86. Kasirajan K, O'Hara PJ, Gray BH, et al. Chronic mesenteric ischemia. Open surgery versus percutaneous angioplasty and stenting. *J Vasc Surg.* 2001;33:63-71.

87. Sivamurthy N, Rhodes JM, Lee D, et al. Endovascular versus open mesenteric revascularization: immediate benefits do not equate with short term functional outcomes. *J Am Coll Surg.* 2006; 202:859-867.

88. Van de ven PJ, Kaatee R, Beutler JJ, et al. Arterial stenting and balloon angioplasty in ostial atherosclerotic renovascular disease: a randomized trial, *Lancet.* 1999;353:282-286.

89. Leertouwer TC, Gussenhoven EJ, Bosch JL, et al. Stent placement for renal artery stenosis: where do we stand? A meta-analysis. *Radiology.* 2000;216:78-85.

90. Sheeran SR, Murphy TP, Khwaja A, Sussman SK, Hallisay MJ. Stent placement for the treatment of mesenteric artery stenosis or occlusions. *J Vasc Interv Radiol.* 1999;10:861-867.

91. Sharafuddin MJ, Olson CH, Sun S, Kresowik TF, Corson JD. Endovascular treatment of celiac and mesenteric arteries stenoses: applications and results. *J Vasc Surg.* 2003; 38:692-698.

92. AbuRahma AF, Stone PA, Bates MC, et al. Angioplasty/stenting of the superior mesenteric artery and celiac trunk: early and late outcomes. *J Endovasc Ther.* 2003;10:1046-1053.

93. Resch T, Lindh M, Dias N, et al. Endovascular recanalisation in occlusive mesenteric ischemia—feasibility and early results. *Eur J Endovasc Surg.* 2005;29:199-203.

94. Brown DJ, Schermerhorn ML, Powell RJ, et al. Mesenteric stenting for chronic mesenteric ischemia. *J Vasc Surg.* 2005;42:268-274.

95. Schaefer PJ, Schaefer FK, Hinrichsen H, et al. Stent placement with the monoriel technique for treatment of mesenteric artery stenosis. *J Vasc Interv Radiol.* 2006;17:637-643.

96. Rose SC, Quigley TM, Raker EJ. Revascularization for chronic mesenteric ischemia: comparison of operative bypass grafting and percutaneous transluminal angioplasty. *J Vasc Interv Radiol.* 1995;6:339-349.

97. Biebl M, Oldenburg WA, Paz-Fumagalli R, et al. Endovascular treatment as a bridge to successful surgical revascularization for chronic mesenteric ischemia. *Am Surg.* 2004;70:994-998.

11

Renal Artery Disease

Christopher J. White and Michael R. Jaff

Although generally believed to be a rare cause of hypertension, atherosclerotic *renal artery stenosis (RAS)* is a common finding in selected patient populations. In the general population of hypertensive patients, 1% to 6% of patients have some element of RAS.[1] However, several clinical clues would suggest a greater likelihood of RAS in certain subsets of patients, including the presence of coronary, carotid, abdominal aortic, and lower-extremity arterial occlusive disease. In patients with aortoiliac occlusive disease or abdominal aortic aneurysmal disease, the prevalence of significant bilateral renal artery disease ranges from 33% to 45%.[2,3]

Similar findings have been described in patients with significant extracranial carotid atherosclerosis, where in one study of 60 patients with significant RAS, 46% had 50% to 100% stenosis of an internal carotid artery.[4] Coronary artery atherosclerosis is a similar marker for RAS. In 346 patients with aneurysmal or occlusive vascular disease prompting arteriography, 28% had significant RAS. Of the patients with RAS, 58% had clinically overt coronary artery disease. In those patients without RAS, the incidence of coronary artery disease was only 39%.[5] In a prospective study of 1302 patients under-

going coronary arteriography, abdominal aortography demonstrated significant RAS in 15% of patients. The number of coronary arteries involved with atherosclerosis also predicted the likelihood of RAS in this series. For example, if one coronary artery demonstrated atherosclerosis, the prevalence of significant RAS was 10.7%. If 3 coronary arteries demonstrated atherosclerotic involvement, the prevalence of RAS was 39%.[6]

The prevalence of RAS in black patients has been reported to be low. In a retrospective study of 819 patients referred to the Cleveland Clinic for RAS, only 40 (4.9%) were black. Despite the fact that the location and severity of RAS was equivalent in the 2 groups, more black patients with RAS had severe or refractory hypertension and were more likely to be active tobacco users than their white counterparts. In addition, diffuse atherosclerosis (ie, coronary, cerebrovascular, and peripheral arterial disease) was found in 95% of black patients with RAS and in only 70% of white patients.[7]

Fibromuscular dysplasia (FMD) is the second most likely etiology of RAS, accounting for 40% of cases.[8] FMD is generally felt to represent a congenital arterial abnormality of the

Vascular Disease: Diagnostic and Therapeutic Approaches. © 2011 Michael R. Jaff and Christopher J. White, editors. Cardiotext Publishing, ISBN: 978-1-935395-16-4.

fibrous, muscular, and elastic segments. There are several types: primary intimal fibroplasia, medial fibroplasia (most common, representing 75%–80% of cases), perimedial fibroplasia, fibromuscular hyperplasia, and periadventitial fibroplasia (extremely rare).[9]

When compared to patients with atherosclerotic RAS, patients with FMD of the renal artery are younger, and more likely to be female and had hypertension for shorter periods of time. FMD involves the mid- and distal segments of the main renal artery, as well as the branch renal arteries. These patients rarely have renal dysfunction on the basis of FMD of the renal arteries.[10]

Natural History

End-stage renal disease (ESRD), regardless of the etiology, results in shortened life expectancy. The most frequent cause of death in patients committed to ESRD is related to cardiovascular disease, and the mortality rates of patients with ESRD continues to rise at alarming rates.[11] For example, elderly patients requiring dialytic support because of diabetic glomerulosclerosis have dismal survival rates. In one secondary survival analysis, no elderly patient with ESRD due to diabetes mellitus survived 5 years.[12]

The prevalence of unsuspected, significant RAS in patients with renal insufficiency is surprisingly high, up to 24% in one series.[13] The 5-year survival of patients aged 65 to 74 years of age who have ESRD due to hypertension is 20%, and is only 9% in those patients ≥ 75 years. Among those patients with hypertensive ESRD, 83 of 683 dialysis patients had significant RAS.[14] The 15-year survival of patients with ESRD because of RAS was 0%, compared with 32% in patients on dialysis due to, for example, polycystic kidney disease. In a prospective angiographic trial, RAS was the cause of ESRD in 14% of new patients beginning dialysis.[15]

Once RAS is discovered, the clinical course and natural history may help predict clinical benefit from revascularization. Although there remains controversy about the true natural history of RAS, in one independent arteriographic series, 39% of patients demonstrated progression of RAS.[16] In a pooled review of 5 arteriographic trials, 49% of the renal arteries demonstrated progression of stenosis.[17] Fourteen percent of these vessels progressed to occlusion.

In a retrospective series of 85 patients with RAS followed for a mean of 52 months, 44% demonstrated progression of RAS and 16% demonstrated progression to total occlusion, with progression occurring within the first 2 years in 46% of renal arteries.[18] In the same series, 78 initial renal arteries with < 50% stenosis were followed. Of these renal arteries, 69% demonstrated no significant progression of stenosis. However, of 18 renal arteries with baseline stenosis of > 75% to 99% stenosis, 39% progressed to occlusion on sequential arteriography. Finally, deterioration in renal function as measured by increase in the serum creatinine occurred in 54% of patients with progressive stenosis of the renal artery, whereas only 25% demonstrated an increase in serum creatinine when there was no progression of disease ($P < 0.02$). Renal size decreased in 70% of patients with progressive disease, and in only 27% in patients without increasing stenosis ($P < 0.001$).

In 1 of only 2 prospective natural history studies for RAS, Dean et al[19] followed 41 patients with RAS whose treatment was medical, that is, control of hypertension and correction of any coexisting renal diseases, if possible. Progression of RAS occurred when blood pressure was well controlled; 40% of patients developed an increase in serum creatinine, and 37% of patients demonstrated a decrease in renal mass. The second prospective study involved the use of *renal artery duplex ultrasonography (RADUS).* In this study, 84 patients with at least one abnormal renal artery, whose therapy did not involve revascularization, were included. Of 139 renal arteries over the course of a mean follow-up of almost 13 months, the progression of RAS as documented by RADUS was 42% at 2 years. The occlusion rate at 2 years was 11%. The overall progression rate was 20%.[20]

Until recently, the correlation between progressive RAS and deterioration in renal function had not been demonstrated. This is the critical issue, as many patients presently undergo renal artery revascularization in an effort to preserve renal function. Caps et al[21] demonstrated that untreated RAS leads to renal atrophy. Of 204 kidneys with varying degrees of RAS in 122 patients, followed for a mean of 33 months, the 2-year incidence of renal atrophy (> 1 cm) was 20.8% in patients with severe baseline RAS ($P = 0.009$ compared to normal or mild baseline RAS). Baseline systolic blood pressure > 180 mm Hg and duplex ultrasonography findings suggestive of significant RAS also predicted a higher likelihood of progressive renal atrophy. Of greatest importance, these data revealed that patients who demonstrated bilateral renal atrophy also suffered a greater rise in serum creatinine than in those patients who were found to have no renal atrophy ($P = 0.03$).

This natural history suggests progression of moderate RAS to a more severe degree, and severe baseline RAS to occlusion, with a gradual deterioration in serum creatinine and renal mass. In patients requiring hemodialysis, whose renal parenchyma is being supplied by stenotic renal arteries,[22,23] or in patients with recurrent flash pulmonary edema and/or angina pectoris with RAS,[24-26] early revascularization seems appropriate. However, the "wait-and-see" approach[27] may lead to dialysis dependence with a worse outcome.

Diagnosis

Although a number of noninvasive methods of diagnosis in RAS have been proposed, none have obviated the role of the gold standard, renal arteriography. Each "screening" test has significant limitations that prevent widespread acceptance. Plasma renin activity was considered several years ago but has inadequate sensitivity and specificity to be used as the sole diagnostic test for RAS, even with stimulation with an angiotensin-converting enzyme inhibitor. Captopril-stimulated nuclear renal flow scanning is an accurate screening test for the diagnosis of unilateral RAS in a patient with normal renal function. However, in cases of bilateral RAS, and in patients with impaired renal function, the accuracy of this test decreases and cannot be used in screening. Renal vein renin ratios can be helpful, however, this is an invasive diagnostic test that also requires that most, if not all, antihypertensive agents be withdrawn prior to sampling. Given that many of these patients have poorly controlled hypertension, this would require hospitalization and the use of parenteral antihypertensive agents to adequately perform this test.

Several investigators have demonstrated the validity of duplex ultrasonography to diagnose RAS (Figure 11.1). In one prospective series, 29 patients (58 renal arteries) underwent duplex ultrasonography and contrast arteriography. The sensitivity of renal artery duplex ultrasonography was 84%, with a specificity of 97% and positive predictive value of 94% for a detection of > 60% stenosis.[28] Utilizing criteria of peak systolic velocity within the renal artery > 180 cm/sec, duplex scanning was able to discern between normal and diseased renal arteries with sensitivity of 95% and specificity of 90%.[29] The ratio of peak systolic velocity (PSV) in the area of RAS compared to the PSV within the aorta (renal to aortic ratio, RAR) of > 3.5 predicts the presence of > 60% RAS. Using this criterion, renal artery duplex ultrasonography demonstrated a sensitivity of 92%.

In a large prospective series of 102 consecutive patients who underwent both duplex ultrasonography and contrast arteriography within 1 month of each other, 62 of 63 arteries with < 60% stenosis, 31 of 32 arteries with 60% to 79% stenosis, and 67 of 69 arteries with 80% to 99% stenosis were correctly identified by duplex ultrasonography. Occluded renal arteries were correctly identified by ultrasonography in 22 of 23 cases. The overall sensitivity of duplex ultrasonography was 98%, specificity 99%, positive predictive value 99%, and negative predictive value 97%.[30]

Limitations of direct visualization of the renal arteries include body habitus and overlying

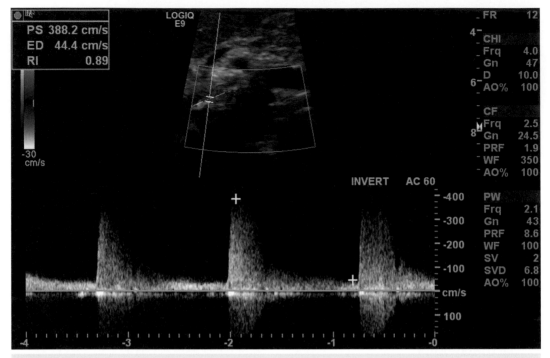

Figure 11.1 Renal artery duplex ultrasound study demonstrating severe right renal artery stenosis.

bowel gas obscuring identification of the renal arteries. Some authors have suggested that renal hilar scanning is easier and as accurate as complete interrogation of the renal arteries.[31] However, direct comparison of both techniques has revealed limitations of hilar scanning, including low sensitivity, inability to discriminate between stenosis and occlusion, and inadequate determination of accessory renal arteries. The sensitivity was 67% for hilar scanning, with a specificity of 89% to 99%.[32] Given that many patients have both main renal artery disease and intraparenchymal disease, the addition of resistive indices within the parenchyma may help predict which patients will benefit from revascularization.[33]

Magnetic resonance angiography (MRA) has the potential to become the ideal diagnostic test for RAS. Minimally invasive, requiring only a peripheral intravenous cannula, and the use of nonnephrotoxic contrast, the results of renal MRA have been very impressive. However, approximately 10% of patients cannot undergo MRA due to implanted metal (eg, permanent pacemakers) or claustrophobia. Finally, in patients who have undergone renal revas-

cularization with metallic endoluminal stents, MRA cannot be used to determine patency of the stent due to signal dropout from the metal. Computerized tomographic arteriography (CTA) has also been utilized to diagnose renal artery stenosis. Although the images are quite impressive, this test requires iodinated contrast and external beam radiation. Therefore, CTA is not an appropriate test for serial assessment of renal artery stenosis (Figure 11.2).[34]

Duplex ultrasonography is the ideal method of determining the adequacy of revascularization.[35] Given the proliferation of endovascular therapy (percutaneous angioplasty with stent deployment),[36] duplex ultrasonography is helpful in detecting important areas of restenosis.

Therapeutic Alternatives

Controversy exists among experts regarding the utilization of renal artery revascularization for renal artery stenosis. Optimal outcomes following percutaneous renal intervention (PRI) are

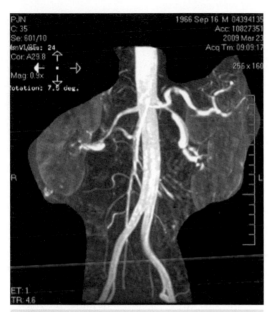

Figure 11.2 Computerized tomographic arteriography of the renal arteries, suggesting segmental arterial mediolysis with stenosis and pseudoaneurysm formation of the renal arteries.

obtained by maximizing the safety and efficacy of the procedure (Table 11.1). Current technology has advanced such that the success rate for endovascular renal artery stent placement is achievable in a very high percentage of patients (Table 11.2).[37-43] Further improvement in the efficacy and safety of renal intervention will require improvement in patient selection, and new technical and pharmacologic approaches to minimize complications related to vascular access and protecting the kidney from atheroembolic injury.

Medical Therapy

A review of medical therapy for renovascular diseases is beyond the scope of this text, however, best medical therapy contrasted with renal revascularization strategies will be discussed in the "Endovascular Therapy" section. Advances in medical therapy have greatly increased the numbers of hypertensive patients who can be controlled with medical therapy alone. The impact of modern antiatherosclerotic approaches with statin therapy and antiplatelet therapy remain to be determined.[44] While aggressive medical therapy may be associated with intolerable side effects in some patients and a serious cost burden in others, the current standard of care is to attempt treatment with medical therapy before considering a revascularization strategy.

Benefit	Risk
Control of hypertension	Progressive loss of renal function
Salvage of renal function	Procedural complications
Control of heart failure/angina	Restenosis

Table 11.1 Risk-to-Benefit Assessment of Renal Revascularization

Reference	Patients (n)	Procedure Success (%)	Death (%)	Dialysis (%)	Major Complication* (%)
Tuttle et al[36]	148	98	0	0	4.10
Rocha-Singh et al[37]	150	97.3	0.6	0	2.60
Blum et al[38]	68	100	0	0	0
White et al[39]	100	99	0	0	1.00
Dorros et al[93]	163	99	0.6	0	1.80
Ivanovic et al[41]	179	98	0.5	0.6	4.10
Zeller et al[42]	215	100	0	0	2.80
Total/Avg	1023	98.8 ± 1	0.24 ± 0.2	0.09 ± 0.2	2.3 4± 1.5

Table 11.2 Technical Success Rate and Complications of Renal Intervention
*Death, myocardial infarction, emergency surgery, need for dialysis, or blood transfusion

The conservative approach requires failure of at least 3 maximally tolerated doses of antihypertensive medications, one of which should be a diuretic, before considering a patient for renal artery revascularization (surgery or stent). Other experts suggest that failure of 2-drug therapy may be considered an indication for renal artery stenting in an anatomically suitable patient.

There is quantifiable patient risk for recommending "conservative" or medical management of significant RAS (Figure 11.3).[45] With medical therapy, progressive loss of renal function (atrophy) occurs in approximately 20% of patients with significant RAS (Figure 11.4).[46] Furthermore, progression to complete renal artery occlusion in 10% or more of patients treated with medical therapy has been documented in several trials.[47,48]

The ongoing Cardiovascular Outcomes in Renal Atherosclerotic Lesions (CORAL) trial will randomize RAS patients to medical therapy or stenting to determine the event-free survival from cardiovascular and renal adverse events, defined as a composite of cardiovascular or renal death, stroke, myocardial infarction (MI), hospitalization for congestive heart failure (CHF), progressive renal insufficiency, or need for permanent renal replacement therapy. The CORAL trial employs a medical treatment regimen designed to control blood pressure, to treat dyslipidemia and diabetes, to promote smoking cessation, to add an antiplatelet agent, and to pay attention to the complications of renal insufficiency. Some opponents of intervention suggest that with aggressive use of modern medical management it is quite possible that revascularization, no matter how well performed, will provide little additional benefit to most patients.[49]

Surgical Therapy

Catheter-based therapy for hemodynamically significant RAS has largely replaced surgical revascularization in patients with suitable anatomy. A recent survey of Medicare patients suggests that renal surgery decreased by almost half in the year 2000, while catheter-based therapy increased by 2.4-fold.[50] Surgical revascularization of atherosclerotic RAS is an effective treatment for renovascular hypertension.[51] However, renovascular surgery is associated with the morbidity and hospital stay of a major operation as well as with complications, including bypass graft thrombosis and nephrectomy in up to 4% and operative mortality rates of up to 3% of patients.[52,53]

In a study of 17 patients with volume-dependent renovascular hypertension and bilateral RAS treated with surgical revascularization, pulmonary edema occurred in 65% prior to surgery despite a normal left ventricular ejection fraction. Bilateral disease was present in 94% of the patients and an occluded renal artery was present in 54%. A variety of surgical approaches were selected including bypass, endarterectomy, and angioplasty in one patient. Contralateral nephrectomy was performed in 41% and concomitant aortic reconstruction was performed

- 204 kidneys, 122 pts, f/u 33 mos.
- RAS followed q6 mos with ultrasound.
- Atrophy = reduction in kidney length (1 cm).

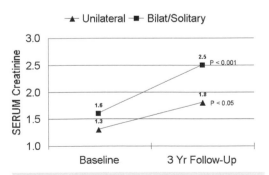

Figure 11.3 Progression of renal failure with medical therapy.[44]

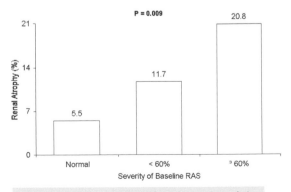

Figure 11.4 Progressive loss of renal tissue (atrophy) with medical therapy and RAS.[45]

in 24%.[54,55] The clinical outcomes after surgery were excellent. Two of the 3 patients requiring dialysis before surgery did not require dialysis after the procedure. After 2 years of follow-up, 1 (6%) patient had hypertension cured, and 16 (94%) patients had hypertension improvement. Only one patient had recurrence of pulmonary edema during follow-up. The authors stressed that in occluded renal arteries ≥ 7 cm in length, every attempt should be made to revascularize the kidney before nephrectomy is considered. Finally, the investigators stressed that patients presenting with pulmonary edema and renovascular hypertension frequently have bilateral RAS, left ventricular hypertrophy, renal insufficiency, and uncontrolled hypertension.

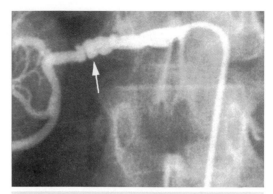

Figure 11.5 Angiogram of fibromuscular dysplasia with the typical appearance of "stacked coins."

Endovascular Therapy

Procedural efficacy is defined by technical and clinical end points. Technical success occurs when stent deployment results in anatomic and physiologic relief of the obstruction to renal blood flow. Progressive equipment and device evolution (including downsizing from older peripheral vascular 0.035-in systems to the coronary 0.014-in systems and new renal guiding catheter shapes), and advanced balloon-expandable stent designs (many are off-label devices approved for other anatomic regions), have led to excellent technical success rates for renal stenting in skilled operators' hands (Table 11.2).

Clinical success following PRI is manifested by a lower blood pressure, improved or stabilized renal function, and/or control of CHF depending on the indication for the procedure. A key principle is that clinical benefit from PRI directly results from correcting renal hypoperfusion. Published meta-analyses suggest that a very high PRI technical success rate (> 95%) is accompanied by modest and inconsistent clinical improvement.[56,57] The discordance between the high technical success and the inconsistent clinical response to revascularization suggests that some successfully revascularized RAS lesions were not causing symptomatic renal hypoperfusion, or that the symptoms being treated with renal revascularization were not

the result of renal hypoperfusion. Improved selection of truly ischemia-producing RAS lesions for revascularization will increase the clinical response rate of PRI.

Indications for Renal Intervention

Provisional renal stent placement (the placement of a stent for a failed or unsatisfactory balloon angioplasty result) is the treatment of choice for fibromuscular dysplasia (Figure 11.5).[58] For atherosclerotic RAS, primary stenting is the procedure of choice (Figure 11.6).[59,60] The current ACC/AHA Guidelines for PRI in hypertensive patients (systolic blood pressure > 140 mm Hg; 130 mm Hg in diabetics) or a diastolic pressure greater than 90 mm Hg (80 mm Hg in diabetics) with hemodynamically significant RAS and a viable kidney (linear length > 7 cm) include (1) accelerated hypertension, (2) refractory hypertension (failure of 3 appropriate drugs, one of which should be a diuretic),[61] (3) hypertension with a small kidney, or (4) hypertension with intolerance to medications (Class IIa, Level of Evidence B).[62] A hemodynamically significant stenosis requires demonstration of a > 70% RAS by visual estimation or by intravascular ultrasonography measurement, or a 50% to 70% RAS with a resting translesional systolic gradient of ≥ 20 mm Hg or a mean translesional gradient of ≥ 10 mm Hg (Figure 11.7).[63]

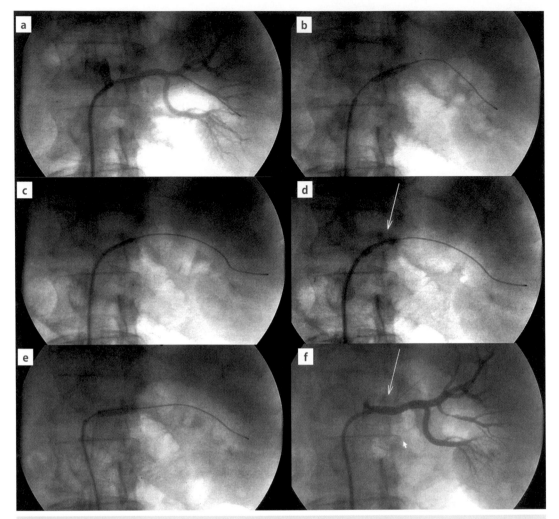

Figure 11.6 (a) Baseline angiogram of severe ostial RAS. (b) Predilation with 5.5x15.0-mm balloon to confirm an expandable lesion. (c) Positioning a 6x15-mm balloon expandable stent across the lesion. (d) Initial inflation to create dumbbell appearance to prevent stent migration during inflation. (e) Complete deployment of stent, with horizontal positioning of stent. (f) Final angiogram (note spasm in branch artery due to wire placement).

The current ACC/AHA Guidelines for catheter-based therapy to preserve renal function concludes that renal intervention is reasonable for patients with RAS and progressive chronic kidney disease with bilateral RAS or a RAS to a solitary functioning kidney (Class IIa, Level of Evidence: B). PRI may also be considered on an individual basis for patients with RAS and chronic renal insufficiency with unilateral RAS (Class IIb, Level of Evidence: C).[62]

Percutaneous revascularization is a Class I (Level of Evidence: B) indication for patients with hemodynamically significant RAS and recurrent, unexplained CHF or sudden, unexplained pulmonary edema. For patients with hemodynamically significant RAS and unstable angina, the ACC/AHA Guidelines recommend percutaneous revascularization (Class IIa, Level of Evidence: B).[62]

Contraindications to Renal Intervention

Contraindications to renal angioplasty and stenting are relative and not absolute. The risk versus benefit of the procedure for each in-

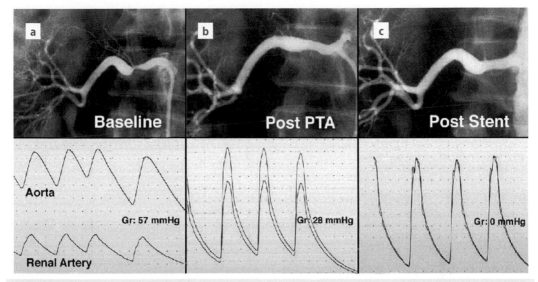

Figure 11.7 (a) Baseline RAS with resting translesional gradient of 57 mm Hg. (b) Following balloon angioplasty, the stenosis is improved, but the gradient remains significant (28 mm Hg). (c) Following stent placement, the stenosis is only slightly improved, but the gradient is now resolved.

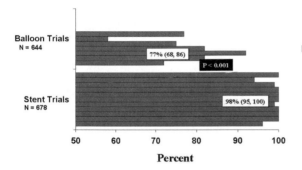

Figure 11.8 Meta-analysis of stent vs. balloon success for percutaneous renal intervention.[56]

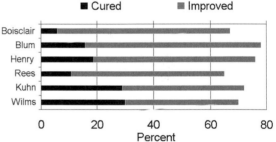

Figure 11.9 Meta-analysis of blood pressure response after renal artery intervention.[38,56,62-66]

dividual must be weighed. Patients with atheroembolic disease, or a "shaggy" aorta, are at increased risk of cholesterol emboli with catheter manipulation in the aorta. Severe contrast reactions and renal impairment are serious procedural risks that should be carefully weighed. Patients with renal artery aneurysms are at risk of rupture, and surgical correction should be considered. Patients with "undilatable" lesions are not suitable candidates for stent therapy unless balloon expansion can be facilitated with a cutting balloon or rotational atherectomy.

Outcomes for Renovascular Hypertension

The response rate for blood pressure improvement or cure after successful renal stenting is about 70%.[39,57,63-68] The discordance between the high procedure success (> 95%) (Figure 11.8) and the modest clinical response (Figure 11.9) for renal stents suggests that either the RAS was not causally related to the hypertension or the revascularization procedure did not correct the renal hypoperfusion.[57]

The "Achilles heel" of renal intervention is

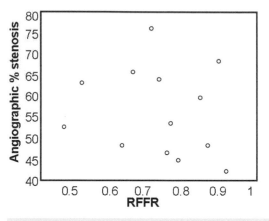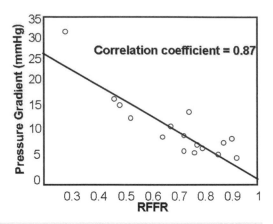

Figure 11.10 Left: No correlation between quantitative angiography and renal fractional flow reserve (RFFR), Right: Excellent correlation of pressure gradient and RFFR.[68]

the use of invasive angiography to measure the severity of RAS. Even quantitative assessment angiography is inadequate to discriminate between nonobstructive RAS and clinically significant RAS that causes renal hypoperfusion (Figure 11.10).[69] Most would agree that operators are able to identify "critical" narrowings, with stringlike lumens, but for less severe RAS, physiological confirmation of the severity of the narrowing is necessary.

Atherosclerotic RAS usually involves the ostial and proximal portions of the main renal artery, and these complex lesions can be

difficult to visualize with 2-dimensional angiography. The errors made with angiographic assessment are increased when operators use visual estimation to determine lesion severity.[70] Under the best of circumstances, visual estimation of angiographic stenoses lacks reproducibility and precision. With larger renal arteries compared to smaller coronary arteries, these errors are magnified.

There has been interest in quantitative angiographic measurements of renal blood flow with renal frame counts (RFC) for arterial flow and renal blush grades (RBG) for microvascu-

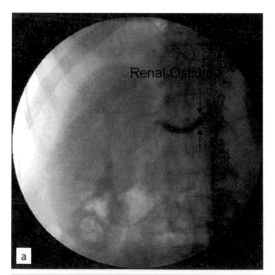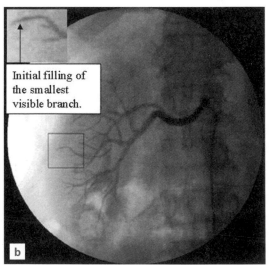

Figure 11.11 (a) First frame as contrast fills ostium of the renal artery. (b) Last frame as contrast fills the smallest visible branch (films at 30 frames/sec).[70]

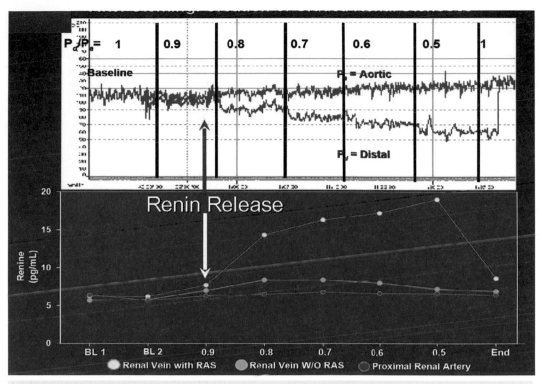

Figure 11.12 Correlation of unilateral renal vein renin release with a translesional pressure ratio (P_a/P_d) of > 0.9.[73]

lar flow. Normal patients can be differentiated from patients with fibromuscular dysplasia of the renal arteries with RFC (Figure 11.11).[71] Building on that work, Mahmud et al[72] confirmed that hypertensive patients with RAS have decreased renal perfusion as measured by RFC and RBG. In a series of patients they were able to demonstrate separation between hypertensive patients without RAS (RFC = 20.1 ± 5.4) and hypertensive patients with RAS (RFC = 26.6 ± 9.1) who returned toward the control group values following stent placement (RFC = 21.4 ± 6.7). Clinical responders (systolic blood pressure fell by ≥ 15 mm Hg after intervention) tended to have higher baseline RFCs than nonresponders and had significantly greater improvement in their RFC values following renal stenting. Three-quarters of the blood pressure responders had a baseline RFC ≥ 25, and of those patients with an improvement in the RFC > 4, 79% were responders to intervention.

Biomarkers

The original biomarker for renovascular hypertension was renin. Renin may be measured invasively, from the renal veins, or noninvasively in peripheral blood usually following a stimulatory test with captopril. While renin release is certainly a direct result of hypoperfusion of the kidney, it has been very difficult to use in clinical practice. Measurements of plasma renin activity have been plagued by a lack of sensitivity and specificity for renovascular disease.[73] Invasive renal vein renin measurements can detect unilateral elevations of renin, but to improve accuracy, all medications that affect renal renin secretion must be stopped for 2 weeks including all antihypertensive agents, diuretics, and nonsteroidal anti-inflammatory drugs. Renin measurement is further complicated by the patient's volume status, the degree of renal insufficiency, and whether they have unilateral or bilateral disease.

An excellent example of the use of selective

renal vein renin measurements is the study by De Bruyne and colleagues,[74] who demonstrated a threshold for unilateral renal vein renin release determined by a ratio of pressure distal to graduated RAS (P_d) created with incremental balloon inflation and the pressure measured in the aorta (P_a) (Figure 11.12). However, to ensure accuracy of the renin measurement, there remain too many confounders in clinical medicine to support its use in everyday practice.

Another biomarker for renovascular disease is brain natriuretic peptide (BNP), a neurohormone released from the myocardium under conditions of myocardial volume or pressure overload.[75-77] BNP promotes diuresis, natriuresis, and arterial vasodilation and antagonizes renin.[75] BNP may be increased in patients with renovascular hypertension, a condition known to promote activation of the renal angiotensin system and the release of angiotensin II.

BNP was increased in patients with severe (> 70%) RAS and an elevated baseline BNP level of > 80 pg/mL (pg = picogram) correlated with a blood pressure response to renal stenting.[78] BNP was measured in 27 patients without other causes of BNP elevation who had refractory hypertension and significant (≥ 70%) RAS before and after successful stenting. BNP was elevated (187 [89, 306] [median, 25%, 75%] pg/mL) before stent placement and fell within 24 hours of the successful stent procedure (96 [61, 182] pg/mL, $P = 0.002$). Clinical improvement in hypertension correlated with a baseline BNP > 80 pg/mL (n = 22) in 17 patients (77%) compared to none (0%) of the patients with a baseline BNP ≤ 80 pg/mL (n = 5) ($P = 0.001$) (Figure 11.13).[78]

Data are supported by results from the Prospective Randomized Evaluation of Celecoxib Integrated Safely Versus Ibuprofen or Naproxen (PRECISION) study in which 55 patients with severe RAS were treated with a new

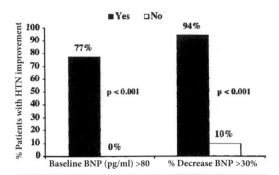

Figure 11.13 Baseline BNP level predicts blood pressure improvement after renal intervention.[77]

stent.[79] While it is not clear from the manuscript that patients were screened for other causes of elevated BNP, that is, clinical heart failure or acute coronary syndromes, the baseline BNP was elevated at 251 ± 282 pg/mL (range 5–1300) and significantly decreased after successful intervention to 188 ± 219 pg/mL (range 10–758, $P = 0.046$). There was a trend for higher levels of BNP in blood pressure responders (BNP = 202 ± 240) compared with patients who did not respond (BNP = 85 ± 89, $P = 0.2$).

Hemodynamic assessment

The important work of De Bruyne and colleagues[74] established a firm *in vivo* relationship between a threshold hemodynamic gradient ($P_d/P_a < 0.9$) and ipsilateral renal vein renin release (see Figure 11.12) and provides fundamental understanding of the threshold hemodynamic value for RAS. Neither resting baseline gradients nor hyperemic pressure gradients separated blood pressure responders from nonresponders after successful PRI in our series (Table 11.3).[80] However, we were able to demonstrate that an abnormal renal fractional flow reserve (RFFR, < 0.8) independently predicted a beneficial blood pressure response to PRI (Figure 11.14).

	Peak (mm Hg)	Mean (mm Hg)	Hyperemic (mm Hg)
Responders (n = 9)	28.6 ± 26	10.6 ± 13.8	15.5 ± 17.9
Nonresponders (n = 7)	30.7 ± 26.9	9.5 ± 8.1	18.9 ± 10.9
P value	0.88	0.85	0.64

Table 11.3 Borderline Pressure Gradients Do Not Correlate with Blood Pressure Response After Renal Stenting[79]

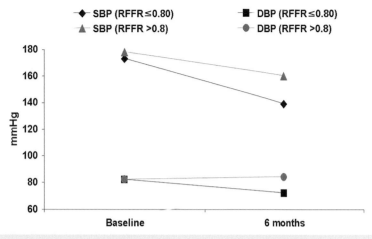

Figure 11.14 Improvement in blood pressure with RFFR ≤ 0.80 compared with RFFR > 0.80.[79]

In a larger series of patients the best correlation with blood pressure improvement after successful PRI is the baseline hyperemic translesional pressure gradient.[81] In 62 patients with RAS who also had angiographic and intravascular ultrasonography (IVUS) measurements performed, a hyperemic systolic gradient of > 21 mm Hg measured with an 0.014-in pressure wire following intrarenal injection of 30 mg of papaverine was the best predictor of improved blood pressure response after PRI. Hypertension improvement at 1 year occurred in 84% of those with HSG (hyperemic systolic gradient) ≥ 21 mm Hg compared with 36% with HSG < 21 mm Hg ($P < 0.01$). Once again, this information needs to be tested in a larger series of patients.

Outcomes for Renal Function Preservation

Patient selection
Ischemic nephropathy—its incidence and its reversibility—is a source of debate among experts.[68,82] The number of patients with atherosclerotic renovascular disease requiring dialysis therapy is increasing.[83] Opponents of aggressive revascularization of RAS patients with renal insufficiency contend that the kidney is supplied with an excess of nutrient blood flow and therefore few kidneys will benefit from revascularization. There is no "stress test" for a kidney that can tell the clinician how much renal

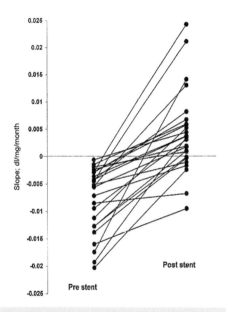

Figure 11.15 Improvement in renal function. Slopes of plots of reciprocal of serum creatinine measured before and after renal artery stent deployment in 25 patients with global renovascular disease and chronic renal failure. Negative and positive slopes depict deteriorating and improving renal function, respectively.[85]

function remains to be salvaged, leading some to contend that there is little to be gained and a definite procedural risk for revascularizing chronically damaged kidneys.

The literature is replete with patient series in which stenting improves renal function (Figure 11.15),[84-88] as well as counterbalancing reports of worsening of renal failure (Figure 11.16).[56,89,90] There are no well-designed, large, randomized studies demonstrating the benefit

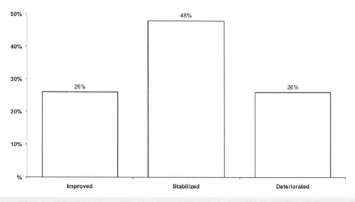

Figure 11.16 Renal function following renal intervention shows that 25% improve, 25% worsen, and about half stay the same.[55] Pooled 10 renal stent studies with abnormal baseline serum creatinine (>133 μmol/l)

of revascularization over medical therapy alone. Poorly designed trials, such as the recently completed STAR trial (STent placement and blood pressure and lipid-lowering for the prevention of progression of renal dysfunction caused by Atherosclerotic ostial stenosis of the Renal artery), do very little to advance science in this area.[91] STAR compared renal stenting plus best medical therapy (BMT) to BMT alone in patients with RAS and impaired renal function. Unfortunately, methodological problems, such as enrolling study patients with mild (< 50%) RAS and allowing significant treatment crossover (30% of the stent group did not get a stent) invalidated this "intention to treat" trial. The RAS lesions (in both groups) were milder than expected. Renal stent placement would not be expected to benefit nonischemic kidneys with mild stenoses. Moreover, the BMT-only group would not be expected to suffer any decline due to the mild nature of the RAS. Once again, as was the case for the Dutch Renal Artery Stenosis Intervention Cooperative (DRASTIC) trial,[48] the methodological errors inflated the benefits of "conservative" therapy and biased this trial against revascularization therapy.[92]

Another poorly designed and conducted trial, the Angioplasty and Stenting for Renal Artery Lesions (ASTRAL) trial, was published demonstrating little or no benefit for patients with mild RAS, undergoing renal intervention by inexperienced operators, to improve their almost normal renal function. The investigators enrolled patients with "uncertain" indications for revascularization. They did not enroll

patients who might actually benefit from renal stent placement. The major adverse event rate of 9% in ASTRAL is way out of line with the 2% major complications reported in contemporary renal stent studies (see Table 11.2).[93]

To design a trial and make it difficult or impossible for renal stents to perform better than medical therapy, researchers would need to (1) enroll patients with milder RAS that is not causing significant renal ischemia, and for whom the RAS is unlikely to worsen without a stent; (2) make sure that a large number of the patients randomized to the stent group do not receive stents; and (3) make sure there are no core laboratories looking over your shoulder to discover the errors made by the onsite investigators, the same group whose complication rate was almost 4 times higher than published renal stent studies (see Table 11.2).[37-40,42,43,94] This is exactly what was done in the ASTRAL trial.

A large, nonrandomized matched cohort study compared patients with RAS and chronic kidney disease from 2 European centers.[95,96] One center offered patients (n = 182) BMT only and the other center offered renal stent plus BMT (n = 348). Patients were matched for the degree of renal dysfunction and outcomes were compared over 5 years. Patients who underwent intervention had a marked reduction in mortality (relative risk [RR] 0.55; 95% CI, 0.34–0.88; P = 0.013) by multivariate Cox regression analysis. When analyzed according to the degree of renal impairment, there were striking improvements in renal function after endovascular therapy for the patients with moderate to severe

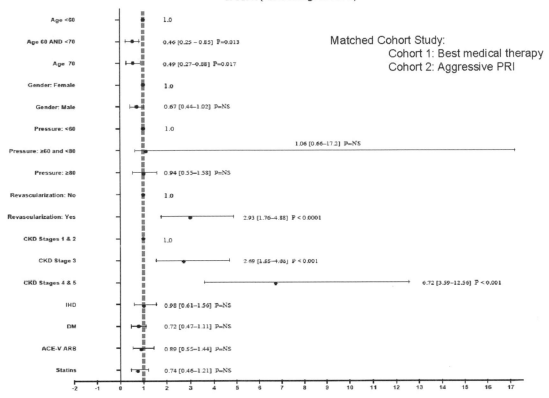

Figure 11.17 Graphical assessment of likelihood of renal function improvement after intervention.[96]

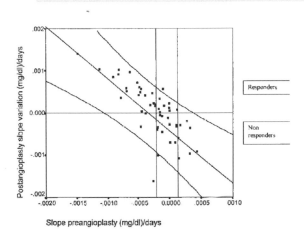

Figure 11.18 Graphic demonstrating that rate of decline in renal function correlates with likelihood of response to PTRA.[86]

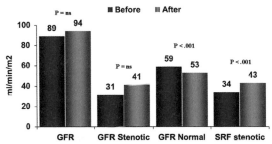

Figure 11.19 Improvement in renal function after unilateral renal artery PTRA. The eGFR of the normal kidney returns to normal and the split renal function shows a positive response in the stenotic kidney.[101]

renal impairment (Figure 11.17).[95] The authors concluded that patients with RAS and impaired renal function can improve renal function in advanced chronic kidney disease (stages 4–5), and that this can provide a survival advantage.

To improve renal function with revascularization, there must be an obstructive RAS lesion causing hypoperfusion to the kidney. Patients with rapidly declining renal function, as opposed to those with stable renal failure, have the most to gain from revascularization (Figure 11.18).[87,97] The more renal tissue at risk, the more likely there will be a response. Patients with bilateral RAS and solitary kidney RAS are traditionally thought to be most likely to improve. Patients with small kidneys (< 7 cm) and those with significant proteinuria are less likely to benefit from revascularization.[98]

There is now a significant body of literature describing renal function improvement with revascularization of unilateral RAS (Figure 11.19).[99-101] For chronic renal insufficiency to manifest in a patient with unilateral RAS, there must be impaired function of the nonstenotic kidney resulting in decreased overall renal function. Multiple clinical trials have demonstrated improvement in overall renal function in patients with predominantly unilateral RAS.[43,79,87] Renal intervention with unilateral RAS improved the split-renal function of the stenotic kidney.[99,101,102] Concomitant hyperfiltration, often seen in the nonstenotic kidney, was also corrected after successful intervention resulting in decreased proteinuria due to hyperfiltration on the nonobstructive side.[99,101]

The rate of decline in renal function, determined as the slope of the regression line of serum creatinine over time, is a strong predictor of benefit with revascularization.[87] In their multivariate analysis, the only significant predictor of benefit following revascularization was the rate of decline of renal function that preceded the procedure (Figure 11.19). Baseline creatinine, the presence of proteinuria, renal size, and diabetes were not significant predictors of improvement in this study.

Cardiac Disturbance Syndromes

Cardiac disturbance syndromes attributable to RAS include exacerbations of coronary ischemia and CHF due to peripheral arterial vasoconstriction and/or volume overload. The importance of renal artery stent placement in the treatment of cardiac disturbance has been described in a series of patients presenting with either CHF or an acute coronary syndrome.[103] Successful renal stent placement resulted in a significant decrease in blood pressure and control of symptoms in 88% (42 of 48) of all patients. Some patients underwent both coronary and renal intervention, while others had only renal artery stent placement due to coronary lesions unsuitable for revascularization. Assessment of the treatment effects acutely and at 8 months using the Canadian Cardiovascular Society (CCS) angina classification and the New York Heart Association (NYHA) functional classification were not different between the combined coronary and renal revascularization group compared to those who had only renal stent placement, suggesting that renal revascularization was the most significant intervention (Figure 11.20).[103]

In another study, 39 patients underwent renal artery stent implantation for control of CHF,[104] which represented 19% of the renal artery stent population. Eighteen (46%) patients had bilateral RAS and 21 (54%) patients had stenosis to a solitary functioning kidney. Renal artery stent implantation was technically

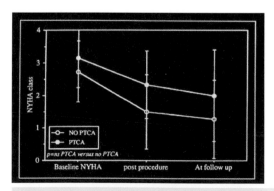 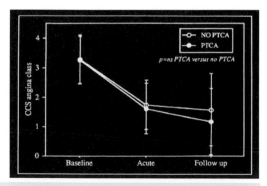

Figure 11.20 Cardiac disturbance: Benefit in both groups was independent of the coronary procedure and driven by renal revascularization.[103]

successful in all 39 patients. Blood pressure improved in 72% of patients. Renal function improved in 51% and was stable in 26% of patients. As has been reported in other series, following intervention, renal function deteriorated in 23% of patients. The mean number of hospitalizations for CHF prior to stenting was 2.37 + 1.42 (range 1–6) and after renal stenting was 0.30 + .065 (range–3, $P < 0.001$). Seventy-seven percent of patients had no further hospitalizations after renal artery stenting over a mean follow-up period of 21.3 months. The mechanism by which RAS causes CHF and pulmonary edema is not well defined. The improvement following revascularization may in part be related to the ability to use ACEI (angiotensin converting enzyme inhibitor) or ARB (angiotensin receptor blocker), especially for those with impaired left ventricle function and the ability to better control volume.

Technical and Procedure Issues

Catheter-based therapy for hemodynamically significant RAS has largely replaced surgical revascularization in patients with suitable anatomy. A recent survey of Medicare patients suggests that renal surgery decreased by almost half in the year 2000, while catheter-based therapy increased by 2.4-fold.[50] The overall procedural success rates for catheter-based therapy are very high (98%, 95% CI, 95–100), the overall complication rates are acceptable (11%, 95% CI, 6%–16%), and the serious complication rates are low (see Table 11.2).[57]

Balloon angioplasty versus renal stent

Balloon angioplasty has been the traditional treatment of choice for renal artery fibromuscular dysplasia (see Figure 11.5).[58] Atherosclerotic RAS predominantly affects the most proximal or ostial portion of the renal artery. This atherosclerotic plaque is often in continuity with aortic wall plaque. The lesions are typically bulky and calcified. Balloon angioplasty often fails in these lesions predominantly due to recoil of the bulky aortorenal plaque. Balloon angioplasty is associated with a restenosis rate that approaches 50% due to the significant recoil.[105,106]

Dorros and colleagues[59] demonstrated a superior hemodynamic result for stents compared to balloons in atherosclerotic RAS. A randomized trial comparing balloon angioplasty versus stent placement in 85 patients with atherosclerotic RAS and hypertension demonstrated a higher success rate and superior long-term patency rate with stent placement compared to balloon angioplasty.[60] At six months the angiographic restenosis rate for the balloon angioplasty group was 48% compared with only 14% ($P < 0.01$) for the stent group. The authors calculated that a provisional stent strategy (bailout) would avoid a stent 40% of the time. However, 45% of the patients would ultimately require a second procedure due to restenosis, making the strategy of primary stent placement more efficient. For the balloon group to achieve a 90% patency rate at 6 months, 62% of all patients would ultimately require a stent and 57% of all patients would need a second or third procedure. To obtain a 90% 6-month patency rate in the primary stent group, only 12% would need a second procedure. This randomized controlled trial clearly demonstrated the superiority of renal stents over balloons in hypertensive patients with atherosclerotic RAS for procedure success, late patency, and cost-effectiveness.[60]

A meta-analysis of 10 renal stent studies performed between 1991 and 1997 demonstrated procedural success rates ≥ 96% with a procedure-related mortality of < 1%.[56] The average restenosis rate was 16%. A second meta-analysis, comparing renal stent placement to balloon angioplasty, for atherosclerotic RAS was performed by Leertouwer and colleagues.[57] They confirmed a significantly higher procedural success rate for stents (98%) than for balloon angioplasty (77%, $P < 0.001$) and a lower restenosis rate for stents (17%) than for balloon angioplasty (26%, $P < 0.001$) (see Figure 11.8).

Avoiding Complications

Restenosis

Two meta-analyses of renal artery intervention have demonstrated average restenosis rates after stent placement of 16%[56] and 17%.[57] More recent reports suggest that with optimal deployment techniques, restenosis rates of less than 15% can be achieved.[38,39,107,108]

Renal artery restenosis after stent placement related to both acute gain and late loss, similar to restenosis after coronary artery intervention. We performed quantitative angiography on a series of 100 consecutive patients and found that patients with patent renal arteries at 8-month follow-up had significantly larger renal stent minimal lumen diameters (MLD) (4.3 ± 0.7 mm vs. 4.9 ± 0.9 mm, $P = 0.025$) and had significantly less late loss (1.3 ± 0.9 mm vs. 3.0 ± 1.4 mm, $P < 0.001$).[40]

In the largest single series of renal stent implantation, Lederman et al[109] found that a larger reference vessel diameter (RVD) and larger acute gain (ie, poststent MLD) after stent deployment were strongly associated with a lower incidence of restenosis. For example, restenosis in a vessel with a RVD of < 4.5 mm was 36% compared with only 6.5% for an artery with a RVD of > 6.0 mm (Figure 11.21).

The type of stent, or composition of the stent, has been shown to have an impact on restenosis. One report described a 1-year restenosis rate for gold-coated stents (NIRoyal, BSC) of 31% in 59 patients compared with 16% ($P = 0.012$) for stainless steel stents in 38 patients.[110] Of interest, the rate of restenosis increased over time, with the 2-year patency rate for gold-coated stents at 61% compared with 22% in stainless steel stents. Using a multivari-

ate analysis, the use of gold-coated stents was the strongest predictor of restenosis ($P = 018$; HR 3.3; 95% CI, 1.2–8.7).

Renal stents have been shown to have excellent long-term patency rates. Blum and colleagues[39] reported a cumulative primary patency rate of 84.5% and a secondary patency rate of 92.4% at 5 years. These results were confirmed by Henry and associates,[107] who reported a cumulative primary patency rate of 78.8% and a secondary patency rate of 97.8% at 6 years (72–78 months) follow-up.[107]

Atheroembolism and embolic protection

The issue of atheroembolism has been difficult to define. There is no available surrogate biomarker, such as troponin for the heart, to detect renal embolic injury. The evidence for atheroemboli associated with carotid intervention and manipulation of the plaque has been well documented with noninvasive studies.[111] It is likely that the same is true for renal arteries.[112]

Renal atheroembolism in individuals with no aortorenal intervention or surgery performed has been described in autopsy studies in up to 20% of patients with severe atherosclerosis.[113] Clinically evident acute atheroembolic renal disease has a dramatically negative impact on prognosis.[114,115] However, the majority of atheroembolic renal disease is subclinical and chronically progressive, rather than acutely catastrophic.[112] A major milepost on the journey to safely revascularize kidneys will be our ability to avoid causing atheroembolism to the renovascular bed. With the reported frequency of visible atherosclerotic debris recovered after renal stenting with embolic protection devices (EPDs) well above 50%, it is not surprising that 25% of successfully revascularized kidneys have a decline in renal function.[116-124]

In a meta-analysis, Isles and colleagues[56] determined that in patients with abnormal renal function who undergo renal artery stent placement, roughly one-quarter improve their renal function, one-quarter worsen their renal function, and one-half remain unchanged. The 2 most likely reasons for deterioration of renal function after intervention are contrast-

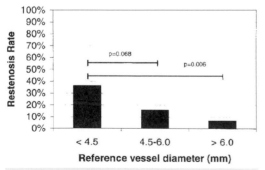

Figure 11.21 Restenosis after intervention and reference vessel diameter.[109]

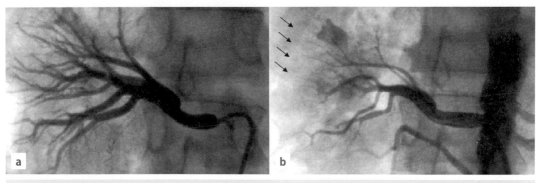

Figure 11.22 Renal angiogram with massive embolization. (a) Baseline angiogram. (b) Poststent angiogram showing loss of small vessels (arrows).

induced nephropathy and atheroembolization. The bulky aorto-ostial plaque is a likely source of emboli, but the incidence has been difficult to determine (Figure 11.22).

Henry and colleagues[117] placed renal stents in 65 renal arteries in 56 patients using emboli protection devices. They noted debris retrieval following renal stent deployment in 100% of the patients with distal balloon occlusion (PercuSurge [n = 38], Medtronic) and in 80% of the filter cases (FilterWire [n = 26], BSC; Angioguard [n = 1], Cordis). Particulate analysis demonstrated atheromatous debris measuring 201 ± 76 μm in diameter. Interestingly, there was no difference in the size or number of particles whether or not balloon predilation was performed. There were 2 episodes of renal artery spasm, relieved with vasodilators. There were no dissections or major complications related to the use of the protection device. Holden and colleagues[118] also reported a retrospective series involving 46 renal stents and 37 patients who had abnormal renal function. This group used the Angioguard filter device and found visible debris present in 65% of the cases.

A small, nicely done, randomized comparative trial compared 2b3a antiplatelet antagonists, EPDs, both, and neither during renal stent placement.[125] There was no benefit for the EPD or 2b3a antiplatelet agent alone, however, there was benefit for the 2b3a antiplatelet antagonists and the EPD together (Figure 11.23). The reasons for this interaction are speculative, and be-

cause the number of patients studied was small it will require confirmation in larger numbers of patients.

It is interesting to note that in coronary disease patients, 2b3a antiplatelet antagonists are beneficial for native coronary interventions,[126] but they are not in saphenous vein graft interventions;[127] the reverse is true for EPDs.[128,129] Is it possible that renal angioplasty shares elements of both procedures? The aorto-ostial plaque is similar to the bulky plaque found in saphenous vein grafts, and the kidney's microvascular bed may need to be protected, similar to the native coronary artery's runoff with antiplatelet therapy. Further work in this area is needed, however, it is tempting to offer for patients with underlying renal dysfunction (eGFR ≤ 60 mL/min) the empiric protection of an off-label EPD if their renal artery anatomy is suitable.

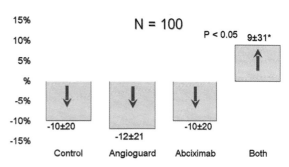

Figure 11.23 Data from the RESIST trial showing percent in eGFR and the interaction between the emboli protection device and the antiplatelet therapy.[125]

One approach to reducing renal athero-embolization is to reduce the risk of catheter trauma to the aorta, or scraping the aorta during endovascular procedures.[130] This is particularly relevant for RAS with bulky aorto-ostial disease, when trying to engage a guiding catheter. The likelihood of trauma to the aorto-ostial plaque during direct guiding catheter engagement is high. Two approaches may be used to reduce guiding catheter trauma. The first is the telescoping guide or exchange technique, with a 4-Fr diagnostic internal mammary catheter placed within a 6-Fr guiding catheter, with its tip protruding. The 4-Fr catheter and guide catheter are advanced over a 0.035-in wire to the level of the target renal artery. The soft, atraumatic diagnostic 4-Fr catheter is used to engage the renal ostium. A guide wire is advanced across the lesion and safely into the distal renal artery. The guide catheter is then advanced over the 4-Fr catheter and atraumatically engages the renal artery ostium.

The second technique is the "no touch" technique.[130] A 0.035-in J-wire is advanced into the descending thoracic aorta above the renal arteries. The renal guide catheter is advanced over the J-wire until it is near the renal ostium. By gently advancing and/or withdrawing the 0.035-in wire, the tip of the guide catheter can be manipulated closer to the renal artery ostium. When the guide is near the ostium, a 0.014-in steerable guide wire is advanced into the renal artery and across the stenosis into the distal portion of the renal artery. As the 0.035-in guide wire is withdrawn, the guide catheter will atraumatically engage the renal ostium over the 0.014-in wire.

During carotid stenting it has been documented that embolic signals are produced with every manipulation of the stenosis.[111] The *in vitro* work of Hiromoto et al[131] leaves little doubt that atheroemboli are also a common accompaniment of renal intervention. Multiple trials describing the performance of the various EPDs confirm the high frequency of embolic material.[116-124]

Why do we need a comparative trial to prove that removal of atheroembolic debris is better than allowing that debris to flow downstream to the kidney? If the devices are safe, and the multiple registry reports attest to their safety, why not use EPDs to prevent renal atheroembolization? The argument for randomized trials reminds one of the sarcastic argument made by Smith and Pell[132] regarding the effectiveness of "parachutes" among those who skydive. Do we need a randomized trial to prove that parachutes improve the survival of skydivers? This level of proof (debris removal and safety in registry studies) met the requirements to get carotid EPDs approved by the Food and Drug Administration and mandated for coverage by Medicare.[133]

Vascular access

The predominant access site for renal intervention is the common femoral artery with retrograde access via the infrarenal aorta. Published trials for renal intervention report femoral vascular access complications ranging from 4.4% to 28%.[39,48,60,125,134] In a recent report of 179 renal stent interventions, serious vascular access site complications were reported in 7.4% of patients.[42] The most common vascular complication was pseudoaneurysm (4.6%) formation. The adoption of smaller 6-Fr guiding catheters with 0.014-in wire systems to replace the traditional 8-Fr guiding catheters with the larger 0.035-in wire systems is expected to further lower the rate of vascular access complications.

The "secret" to avoiding vascular access complications is to use the radial artery for access. The coronary interventional literature has demonstrated a marked reduction in vascular access complications with radial artery access compared to femoral artery access.[135] Using 6-Fr guiding catheters allows the radial artery approach to be an option.[136] The radial artery approach has several advantages, including avoiding vascular access complications, increased patient acceptance, and improved catheter engagement due to the frequent downward or caudal orientation of most renal arteries. The radial approach does require some investment in time by the operator, as there is a learning curve. The undeniable benefit, however, is a major reduction in the vascular access–related complications.[137]

In-stent restenosis

The optimal treatment of renal artery in-stent restenosis is uncertain. An initial report described the feasibility and late follow-up in 15 patients with 20 stents with recurrent stenosis who were treated with either balloon angioplasty (n = 18) or restenting (n = 2).[138] Follow-up angiography was available in 16 (80%) of the arteries at slightly less than 1 year and showed a restenosis rate of 25%. Other methodologies such as cutting balloons and brachytherapy have also been reported, but no systemic studies of their comparative efficacy are available.[139-141] Wöhrle and colleagues[142] reported a 21.7% recurrence rate at 6 months following balloon angioplasty of in-stent restenosis in 46 patients. They also noted that balloon angioplasty of in-stent restenosis was associated with a much lower rate of recurrence in matched pairs who underwent repeat balloon angioplasty after renal angioplasty restenosis (41.3%, $P < 0.042$).

Summary

Atherosclerotic renal artery stenosis is a common disorder, most evident among those patients with evidence of coronary and/or peripheral artery disease. Methods of diagnosis have advanced to the point that renal artery stenosis is now quite easy to identify. The challenge is determining the appropriate patients for the treatment of renal artery stenosis with endovascular strategies. No data currently available provides adequate guidance for the treatment of patients with renal artery stenosis. It is our hope that the CORAL trial will provide insights into this, however, until this data is available, consider use of translesional pressure gradients and BNP levels to predict clinical response to intervention.

References

1. Simon N, Franklin SS, Bleifer KH, Maxwell MH. Clinical characteristics of renovascular hypertension. *JAMA*.1972;220:1209-1218.

2. Olin JW, Melia M, Young JR, et al. Prevalence of atherosclerotic renal artery stenosis in patients with atherosclerosis elsewhere. *Am J Med*. 1990;88:46N-51N.

3. Missouris CG, Buckenham T, Cappucio FP, MacGregor GA. Renal artery stenosis: a common and important problem in patients with peripheral vascular disease. *Am J Med*. 1994;96:10-14.

4. Louie J, Isaacson JA, Zierler RE, et al. Prevalence of carotid and lower extremity arterial disease in patients with renal artery stenosis. *Am J Hypertens*. 1994;7:436-439.

5. Valentine RJ, Clagett GP, Miller GL, et al. The coronary risk of unsuspected renal artery stenosis. *J Vasc Surg*. 1993;18:433-440.

6. Harding MB, Smith LR, Himmelstein SI, et al. Renal artery stenosis: prevalence and associated risk factors in patients undergoing routine cardiac catheterization. *J Am Soc Nephrol*. 1992;2:1608-1616.

7. Novick AC, Zaki S, Goldfarb D, Hodge EE. Epidemiologic and clinical comparison of renal artery stenosis in black patients and white patients. *J Vasc Surg*. 1994;20:1-5.

8. Olin JW, Novick AC. Renovascular disease. In: Young JR, Olin JW, Bartholomew JR, eds. *Peripheral Vascular Diseases*, 2nd ed. Philadelphia: Mosby, 1996:321-342.

9. Harrison HG, McCormack LJ. Pathologic classification of renal artery disease in renovascular hypertension. *Mayo Clin Proc*. 1971;46:161-173.

10. Luscher TF, Lie JT, Stanson AW, et al. Arterial fibromuscular dysplasia. *Mayo Clin Proc*. 1987;62:931-952.

11. Huting J. Cardiovascular survival of patients undergoing long-term dialysis. *Prim Cardiol*. 1994;20:21-28.

12. Byrne C, Vernon P, Cohen JJ. Effect of age and diagnosis on survival of older patients beginning chronic dialysis. *JAMA*. 1994;271:34-36.

13. O'Neil EA, Hansen KJ, Canzanello VJ, et al.

Prevalence of ischemic nephropathy in patients with renal insufficiency. *Am Surg.* 1992;58:485-490.

14. Mailloux LU, Napolitano B, Bellucci AG, et al. Renal vascular disease causing end-stage renal disease, incidence, clinical correlates, and outcomes: a 20-year clinical experience. *Am J Kid Dis.* 1994;24:622-629.

15. Scoble JE, Maher ER, Hamilton G, et al. Atherosclerotic renovascular disease causing renal impairment—a case for treatment. *Clin Nephrol.* 1989;31:119-122.

16. Meaney TF, Dustan HP, McCormack LJ. Natural history of renal arterial disease. *Radiology.* 1968;9:877-887.

17. Greco BA, Breyer JA. The natural history of renal artery stenosis: who should be evaluated for suspected ischemic nephropathy? *Semin Neph.* 1996;16:2-11.

18. Schreiber MJ, Pohl MA, Novick AC. The natural history of atherosclerotic and fibrous renal artery disease. *Urol Clin N Am.* 1984;11:383-392.

19. Dean RH, Kieffer RW, Smith BM, et al. Renovascular hypertension: anatomic and renal function changes during therapy. *Arch Surg.* 1981;116:1408-1415.

20. Zierler RE, Bergelin RO, Isaacson JA, et al. Natural history of atherosclerotic renal artery stenosis: a prospective study with duplex ultrasonography. *J Vasc Surg.* 1994;19:250-258.

21. Caps MT, Zierler RE, Polissar NL, et al. Risk of atrophy in kidneys with atherosclerotic renal artery stenosis. *Kidney Int.* 1998;53:735-742.

22. Novick AC, Pohl MA, Schreiber M, et al. Revascularization for preservation of renal function in patients with atherosclerotic renovascular disease. *J Urol.* 1983;129:907-912.

23. Kaylor WM, Novick AC, Ziegelbaum M, Vidt DG. Reversal of end stage renal failure with surgical revascularization in patients with atherosclerotic renal artery occlusion. *J Urol.* 1989;141:486-488.

24. Pickering TG, Devereux RB, James GD, et al. Recurrent pulmonary edema in hypertension due to bilateral renal artery stenosis: treatment by angioplasty or surgical revascularisation. *Lancet.* 1988;Sept:551-552.

25. Messina LM, Zelenock GB, Yao KA, Stanley JC. Renal revascularization for recurrent pulmonary edema in patients with poorly controlled hypertension and renal insufficiency: a distinct subgroup of patients with arteriosclerotic renal artery occlusive disease. *J Vasc Surg.* 1992;15:73-82.

26. Tami LF, McElderry MW, Al-Adli A, et al. Renal artery stenosis presenting as crescendo angina pectoris. *Cath Cardiovasc Diag.* 1995;35:252-256.

27. Scoble JE. Is the "wait-and-see" approach justified in atherosclerotic renal artery stenosis? *Nephrol Dial Trans.* 1995;4:588-589.

28. Taylor DC, Kettler MD, Moneta GL, et al. Duplex ultrasound scanning in the diagnosis of renal artery stenosis: a prospective evaluation. *J Vasc Surg.* 1988;7:363-369.

29. Strandness DE. Duplex imaging for the detection of renal artery stenosis. *Am J Kid Dis.* 1994;24:674-678.

30. Olin JW, Piedmonte MR, Young JR, et al. The utility of duplex ultrasound scanning of the renal arteries for diagnosing significant renal artery stenosis. *Ann Intern Med.* 1995;122:833-838.

31. Munier MNS, Hoballah JJ, Miller EV, et al. Renal hilar Doppler analysis is of value in the management of patients with renovascular disease. *Am J Surg.* 1997;174:164-168.

32. Isaacson JA, Zierler RE, Spittell PC, Strandness DE. Noninvasive screening for renal artery stenosis: comparison of renal artery and renal hilar duplex scanning. *J Vasc Tech.* 1995;19:105-110.

33. Cohn EJ, Benjamin ME, Sandager GP, et al. Can intrarenal duplex waveform analysis predict successful renal artery revascularization? *J Vasc Surg.* 1998;28:471-481.

34. Liu PS, Platt JF. CT angiography of the renal circulation. *Radiol Clin N Am* 2010;48:347-365.

35. Eidt JF, Fry RE, Clagett GP, et al. Postoperative follow-up of renal artery reconstruction with duplex ultrasound. *J Vasc Surg.* 1988;8:667-673.

36. Dorros G, Jaff M, Mathiak L, et al. Four-year follow-up of Palmaz-Schatz stent revascularization as treatment for atherosclerotic renal artery stenosis. *Circulation.* 1998;98:642-647.

37. Tuttle KR, Chouinard RF, Webber JT, et al. Treatment of atherosclerotic ostial renal artery stenosis with the intravascular stent. *Am J Kidney Dis.* 1998;32:611-622.

38. Rocha-Singh KJ, Mishkel GJ, Katholi RE, et al. Clinical predictors of improved long-term blood pressure control after successful stenting of hypertensive patients with obstructive renal artery atherosclerosis. *Catheter Cardiovasc Interv.* 1999;47:167-172.

39. Blum U, Krumme B, Flugel P, Gabelmann A, et al. Treatment of ostial renal-artery stenoses with vascular endoprostheses after unsuccessful balloon angioplasty [see comments]. *N Engl J Med.* 1997;336:459-465.

40. White CJ, Ramee SR, Collins TJ, Jenkins JS, Escobar A, Shaw D. Renal artery stent placement: utility in lesions difficult to treat with balloon angioplasty. *J Am Coll Cardiol.* 1997;30:1445-1450.

41. Dorros G, Jaff MR, Mathiak L, et al. Stent revascularization for atherosclerotic renal artery stenosis. 1-year clinical follow-up. *Tex Heart Inst J.* 1998;25:40-43.

42. Ivanovic V, McKusick MA, Johnson CM III, et al. Renal artery stent placement: complications at a single tertiary care center. *J Vasc Interv Radiol.* 2003;14:217-225.

43. Zeller T, Frank U, Muller C, et al. Predictors of improved renal function after percutaneous stent-supported angioplasty of severe atherosclerotic ostial renal artery stenosis. *Circulation.* 2003;108:2244-2249.

44. Silva VS, Martin LC, Franco RJ, et al. Pleiotropic effects of statins may improve outcomes in atherosclerotic renovascular disease. *Am J Hypertens.* 2008;21:1163-1168.

45. Chabova V, Schirger A, Stanson AW, McKusick MA, Textor SC. Outcomes of atherosclerotic renal artery stenosis managed without revascularization. *Mayo Clin Proc.* 2000;75:437-444.

46. Caps MT, Zierler RE, Polissar NL, et al. Risk of atrophy in kidneys with atherosclerotic renal artery stenosis. *Kidney Int.* 1998;53:735-742.

47. Caps M, Perissinotto C, Zierler R, et al. Prospective study of atherosclerotic disease progression in the renal artery. *Circulation.* 1998;98:2866-2872.

48. van Jaarsveld B, Krijnen P, Pieterman H, et al. The effect of balloon angioplasty on hypertension in atherosclerotic renal artery stenosis. *N Eng J Med.* 2000;342:1007-1014.

49. Dworkin LD, Cooper CJ. Clinical practice. Renal-artery stenosis. *N Engl J Med.* 2009;361:1972-1978.

50. Murphy TP, Soares G, Kim M. Increase in utilization of percutaneous renal artery interventions by medicare beneficiaries, 1996-2000. *AJR Am J Roentgenol.* 2004;183:561-568.

51. Weibull H, Bergqvist D, Bergentz SE, Jonsson K, Hulthen L, Manhem P. Percutaneous transluminal renal angioplasty versus surgical reconstruction of atherosclerotic renal artery stenosis: a prospective randomized study. *J Vasc Surg.* 1993;18:841-850; discussion 850-842.

52. Hansen KJ, Starr SM, Sands RE, Burkart JM, Plonk GW Jr, Dean RH. Contemporary surgical management of renovascular disease. *J Vasc Surg.* 1992;16:319-330; discussion 330-311.

53. Novick AC, Ziegelbaum M, Vidt DG, Gifford RW Jr, Pohl MA, Goormastic M. Trends in surgical revascularization for renal artery disease. Ten years' experience. *JAMA.* 1987;257:498-501.

54. Messina L, Zelenock G, Yao K, Stanley J. Renal revascularization for recurrent pulmonary edema in patients with poorly controlled hypertension and renal insufficiency: a distinct subgroup of patients with arteriosclerotic renal artery occlusive disease. *J Vasc Surg.* 1992;15:73-82.

55. Libertino J, Beckman C. Surgery and percutaneous angioplasty in the management of renovascular hypertension. *Urol Clin N Am.* 1994;21:235-243.

56. Isles CG, Robertson S, Hill D. Management of renovascular disease: a review of renal artery stenting in ten studies. *Quart J Med.* 1999;92:159-167.

57. Leertouwer TC, Gussenhoven EJ, Bosch JL, et al. Stent placement for renal arterial stenosis: where do we stand? A meta-analysis. *Radiology.* 2000;216:78-85.

58. Slovut DP, Olin JW. Fibromuscular dysplasia. *N Engl J Med.* 2004;350:1862-1871.

59. Dorros G, Prince C, Mathiak L. Stenting of a renal artery stenosis achieves better relief of the obstructive lesion than balloon angioplasty. *Cathet Cardiovasc Diagn*. 1993;29:191-198.

60. van de Ven PJ, Kaatee R, Beutler JJ, et al. Arterial stenting and balloon angioplasty in ostial atherosclerotic renovascular disease: a randomised trial. *Lancet*. 1999;353:282-286.

61. Chobanian AV, Bakris GL, Black HR, et al. Seventh report of the Joint National Committee on Prevention, Detection, Evaluation, and Treatment of High Blood Pressure. *Hypertension*. 2003;42:1206-1252.

62. Hirsch AT, Haskal ZJ, Hertzer NR, et al. ACC/AHA 2005 guidelines for the management of patients with peripheral arterial disease (lower extremity, renal, mesenteric, and abdominal aortic): executive summary a collaborative report from the American Association for Vascular Surgery/Society for Vascular Surgery, Society for Cardiovascular Angiography and Interventions, Society for Vascular Medicine and Biology, Society of Interventional Radiology, and the ACC/AHA Task Force on Practice Guidelines (Writing Committee to Develop Guidelines for the Management of Patients With Peripheral Arterial Disease) endorsed by the American Association of Cardiovascular and Pulmonary Rehabilitation; National Heart, Lung, and Blood Institute; Society for Vascular Nursing; TransAtlantic Inter-Society Consensus; and Vascular Disease Foundation. *J Am Coll Cardiol*. 2006;47:1239-1312.

63. Boisclair C, Therasse E, Oliva VL, et al. Treatment of renal angioplasty failure by percutaneous renal artery stenting with Palmaz stents: midterm technical and clinical results. *AJR Am J Roentgenol*. 1997;168:245-251.

64. Henry M, Amor M, Henry I, et al. Stent placement in the renal artery: three-year experience with the Palmaz stent. *J Vasc Interv Radiol*. 1996;7:343-350.

65. Rees CR, Palmaz JC, Becker GJ, et al. Palmaz stent in atherosclerotic stenoses involving the ostia of the renal arteries: preliminary report of a multicenter study. *Radiology*. 1991;181:507-514.

66. Kuhn FP, Kutkuhn B, Torsello G, Modder U. Renal artery stenosis: preliminary results of treatment with the Strecker stent. *Radiology*. 1991;180:367-372.

67. Wilms GE, Peene PT, Baert AL, et al. Renal artery stent placement with use of the Wallstent endoprosthesis. *Radiology*. 1991;179:457-462.

68. Safian RD, Textor SC. Renal-artery stenosis. *N Engl J Med*. 2001;344:431-442.

69. Subramanian R, White CJ, Rosenfield K, et al. Renal fractional flow reserve: a hemodynamic evaluation of moderate renal artery stenoses. *Catheter Cardiovasc Interv*. 2005;64:480-486.

70. Topol EJ, Nissen SE. Our preoccupation with coronary luminology: the dissociation between clinical and angiographic findings in ischemic heart disease. *Circulation*. 1995;92:2333-2342.

71. Mulumudi MS, White CJ. Renal frame count: a quantitative angiographic assessment of renal perfusion. *Catheter Cardiovasc Interv*. 2005;65:183-186.

72. Mahmud E, Smith TW, Palakodeti V, et al. Renal frame count and renal blush grade: quantitative measures that predict the success of renal stenting in hypertensive patients with renal artery stenosis. *JACC Cardiovasc Interv*. 2008;1:286-292.

73. Maxwell MH, Rudnick MR, Waks AU. New approaches to the diagnosis of renovascular hypertension. *Adv Nephrol Necker Hosp*. 1985;14:285-304.

74. De Bruyne B, Manoharan G, Pijls NH, et al. Assessment of renal artery stenosis severity by pressure gradient measurements. *J Am Coll Cardiol*. 2006;48:1851-1855.

75. Mukoyama M, Nakao K, Hosoda K, et al. Brain natriuretic peptide as a novel cardiac hormone in humans. Evidence for an exquisite dual natriuretic peptide system, atrial natriuretic peptide and brain natriuretic peptide. *J Clin Invest*. 1991;87:1402-1412.

76. Morrison LK, Harrison A, Krishnaswamy P, Kazanegra R, Clopton P, Maisel A. Utility of a rapid B-natriuretic peptide assay in differentiating congestive heart failure from lung disease in patients presenting with dyspnea. *J Am Coll Cardiol*. 2002;39:202-209.

77. ten Wolde M, Tulevski II, Mulder JW, et al. Brain natriuretic peptide as a predictor of

adverse outcome in patients with pulmonary embolism. *Circulation*. 2003;107:2082-2084.

78. Silva JA, Chan AW, White CJ, et al. Elevated brain natriuretic peptide predicts blood pressure response after stent revascularization in patients with renal artery stenosis. *Circulation*. 2005;111:328-333.

79. Rastan A, Krankenberg H, Muller-Hulsbeck S, et al. Improved renal function and blood pressure control following renal artery angioplasty: the renal artery angioplasty in patients with renal insufficiency and hypertension using a dedicated renal stent device study (PRECISION). *EuroIntervention*. 2008;4:208-213.

80. Mitchell J, Subramanian R, White C, et al. Predicting blood pressure improvement in hypertensive patients after renal artery stent placement. *Catheter Cardiovasc Interv*. 2007;69:685-689.

81. Leesar MA, Varma J, Shapira A, et al. Prediction of hypertension improvement after stenting of renal artery stenosis: comparative accuracy of translesional pressure gradients, intravascular ultrasound, and angiography. *J Am Coll Cardiol*. 2009;53:2363-2371.

82. Textor SC, Lerman L, McKusick M. The uncertain value of renal artery interventions: where are we now? *JACC Cardiovasc Interv*. 2009;2:175-182.

83. Foley RN, Collins AJ. End-stage renal disease in the United States: an update from the United States Renal Data System. *J Am Soc Nephrol*. 2007;18:2644-2648.

84. Harden P, MacLeod M, Rodger R, et al. Effect of renal artery stenting on progression of renovascular renal failure. *Lancet*. 1997;349:1133-1136.

85. Rimmer JM, Gennari FJ. Atherosclerotic renovascular disease and progressive renal failure. *Ann Intern Med*. 1993;118:712-719.

86. Watson P, Hadjipetrou P, Cox S, Piemonte T, Eisenhauer A. Effect of renal artery stenting on renal function and size in patients with atherosclerotic renovascular disease. *Circulation*. 2000;102:1671-1677.

87. Muray S, Martin M, Amoedo M, et al. Rapid decline in renal function reflects reversibility and predicts the outcome after angioplasty

in renal artery stenosis. *Am J Kidney Dis*. 2002;39:60-66.

88. Beutler JJ, Van Ampting JM, Van De Ven PJ, et al. Long-term effects of arterial stenting on kidney function for patients with ostial atherosclerotic renal artery stenosis and renal insufficiency. *J Am Soc Nephrol*. 2001;12:1475-1481.

89. Dejani H, Eisen TD, Finkelstein FO. Revascularization of renal artery stenosis in patients with renal insufficiency. *Am J Kidney Dis*. 2000;36:752-758.

90. Textor SC. Ischemic nephropathy: where are we now? *J Am Soc Nephrol*. 2004;15:1974-1982.

91. Bax L, Algra A, Mali WP, Edlinger M, Beutler JJ, van der Graaf Y. Renal function as a risk indicator for cardiovascular events in 3216 patients with manifest arterial disease. *Atherosclerosis*. 2008;200:184-190.

92. White C. Fight the stupids! *Catheter Cardiovasc Interv*. 2009;74:530-532.

93. Rocha-Singh K, Jaff MR, Rosenfield K, and the ASPIRE 2 Investigators. Evaluation of the safety and effectiveness of renal artery stenting after unsuccessful balloon angioplasty: the ASPIRE-2 study. *J Am Coll Cardiol*. 2005;46:776-783.

94. Dorros G, Jaff M, Mathiak L, et al. Four-year follow-up of Palmaz-Schatz stent revascularization as treatment for atherosclerotic renal artery stenosis. *Circulation*. 1998;98:642-647.

95. Kalra PA, Chrysochou C, Green D, et al. The benefit of renal artery stenting in patients with atheromatous renovascular disease and advanced chronic kidney disease. *Cathet Cardiovasc Intervent*. 2009;75:1-10.

96. Kalra P, Green D, Cheung CM, et al. Medical therapy versus primary renal artery stenting—a twin centre study of outcome in atherosclerotic renovascular disease. *Nephrol Dial Transplant*. 2007;22:vi8(A).

97. Rivolta R, Bazzi C, Stradiotti P, Paparella M. Stenting of renal artery stenosis: is it beneficial in chronic renal failure? *J Nephrol*. 2005;18:749-754.

98. Chrysochou C, Cheung CM, Durow M, et al. Proteinuria as a predictor of renal functional outcome after revascularization in athero-

sclerotic renovascular disease (ARVD). *QJM*. 2009;102:283-288.

99. Coen G, Moscaritolo E, Catalano C, et al. Atherosclerotic renal artery stenosis: one year outcome of total and separate kidney function following stenting. *BMC Nephrology*. 2004;5:15.

100. Marone LK, Clouse WD, Dorer DJ, et al. Preservation of renal function with surgical revascularization in patients with atherosclerotic renovascular disease. *J Vasc Surg*. 2004;39:322-329.

101. La Batide-Alanore A, Azizi M, Froissart M, Raynaud A, Plouin PF. Split renal function outcome after renal angioplasty in patients with unilateral renal artery stenosis. *J Am Soc Nephrol*. 2001;12:1235-1241.

102. Leertouwer TC, Derkx FH, Pattynama PM, Deinum J, van Dijk LC, Schalekamp MA. Functional effects of renal artery stent placement on treated and contralateral kidneys. *Kidney Int*. 2002;62:574-579.

103. Khosla S, White CJ, Collins TJ, Jenkins JS, Shaw D, Ramee SR. Effects of renal artery stent implantation in patients with renovascular hypertension presenting with unstable angina or congestive heart failure. *Am J Cardiol*. 1997;80:363-366.

104. Gray B, Olin J, Childs M, Sullivan T, Bacharach J. Clinical benefit of renal artery angioplasty with stenting for the control of recurrent and refractory congestive heart failure. *Vasc Med*. 2002;7:275-279.

105. Sos TA, Pickering TG, Sniderman K, et al. Percutaneous transluminal renal angioplasty in renovascular hypertension due to atheroma or fibromuscular dysplasia. *N Engl J Med*. 1983;309:274-279.

106. Plouin P, Darne B, Chattelier G, et al. Restenosis after a first transluminal percutaneous renal angioplasty. *Hypertension*. 1993;21:89-96.

107. Henry M, Amor M, Henry I, et al. Stents in the treatment of renal artery stenosis: long-term follow-up. *J Endovasc Surg*. 1999;6:42-51.

108. Tuttle KR, Puhlman ME, Cooney SK, Short R. Urinary albumin and insulin as predictors of coronary artery disease: an angiographic study. *Am J Kidney Dis*. 1999;34:918-925.

109. Lederman R, Mendelsohn F, Santos R, Phillips H, Stack R, Crowley J. Primary renal artery stenting: characteristics and outcomes after 363 procedure. *Am Heart J*. 2001;142:314-323.

110. Nolan BW, Schermerhorn ML, Powell RJ, et al. Restenosis in gold-coated renal artery stents. *J Vasc Surg*. 2005;42:40-46.

111. Al-Mubarak N, Roubin GS, Vitek JJ, Iyer SS, New G, Leon MB. Effect of the distal-balloon protection system on microembolization during carotid stenting. *Circulation*. 2001;104:1999-2002.

112. Scoble JE. Do protection devices have a role in renal angioplasty and stent placement? *Nephrol Dial Transplant*. 2003;18:1700-1703.

113. Thurlbeck WM, Castleman B. Atheromatous emboli to the kidneys after aortic surgery. *N Engl J Med*. 1957;257:442-447.

114. Modi KS, Rao VK. Atheroembolic renal disease. *J Am Soc Nephrol*. 2001;12:1781-1787.

115. Scolari F, Ravani P, Pola A, et al. Predictors of renal and patient outcomes in atheroembolic renal disease: a prospective study. *J Am Soc Nephrol*. 2003;14:1584-1590.

116. Henry M, Klonaris C, Henry I, et al. Protected renal stenting with the PercuSurge Guard-Wire device: a pilot study. *J Endovasc Ther*. 2001;8:227-237.

117. Henry M, Henry I, Klonaris C, et al. Renal angioplasty and stenting under protection: the way for the future? *Catheter Cardiovasc Interv*. 2003;60:299-312.

118. Holden A, Hill A. Renal angioplasty and stenting with distal protection of the main renal artery in ischemic nephropathy: early experience. *J Vasc Surg*. 2003;38:962-968.

119. Henry M, Henry I, Polydorou A, Rajagopal S, Lakshmi G, Hugel M. Renal angioplasty and stenting: long-term results and the potential role of protection devices. *Expert Rev Cardiovasc Ther*. 2005;3:321-334.

120. Hagspiel KD, Stone JR, Leung DA. Renal angioplasty and stent placement with distal protection: preliminary experience with the FilterWire EX. *J Vasc Interv Radiol*. 2005;16:125-131.

121. Edwards MS, Craven BL, Stafford J, et al. Distal embolic protection during renal artery angioplasty and stenting. *J Vasc Surg*. 2006;44:128-135.

122. Holden A, Hill A, Jaff MR, Pilmore H. Renal

artery stent revascularization with embolic protection in patients with ischemic nephropathy. *Kidney Int.* 2006;70:948-955.

123. Edwards MS, Corriere MA, Craven TE, et al. Atheroembolism during percutaneous renal artery revascularization. *J Vasc Surg.* 2007;46:55-61.

124. Henry M, Henry I, Polydorou A, Hugel M. Embolic protection for renal artery stenting. *J Cardiovasc Surg* (Torino). 2008;49:571-589.

125. Cooper C, Haller S, Colyer W, et al. Embolic protection and platelet inhibition during renal artery stenting. *Circulation.* 2008;117:2752-2760.

126. Topol EJ, Lincoff AM, Kereiakes DJ, et al. Multi-year follow-up of abciximab therapy in three randomized, placebo-controlled trials of percutaneous coronary revascularization. *Am J Med.* 2002;113:1-6.

127. Roffi M, Mukherjee D, Chew DP, et al. Lack of benefit from intravenous platelet glycoprotein IIb/IIIa receptor inhibition as adjunctive treatment for percutaneous interventions of aortocoronary bypass grafts: a pooled analysis of five randomized clinical trials. *Circulation.* 2002;106:3063-3067.

128. Baim DS, Wahr D, George B, et al. Randomized trial of a distal embolic protection device during percutaneous intervention of saphenous vein aorto-coronary bypass grafts. *Circulation.* 2002;105:1285-1290.

129. Stone GW, Rogers C, Hermiller J, et al. Randomized comparison of distal protection with a filter-based catheter and a balloon occlusion and aspiration system during percutaneous intervention of diseased saphenous vein aorto-coronary bypass grafts. *Circulation.* 2003;108:548-553.

130. Feldman RL, Wargovich TJ, Bittl JA. No-touch technique for reducing aortic wall trauma during renal artery stenting. *Catheter Cardiovasc Interv.* 1999;46:245-248.

131. Hiramoto J, Hansen KJ, Pan XM, Edwards MS, Sawhney R, Rapp JH. Atheroemboli during renal artery angioplasty: an ex vivo study. *J Vasc Surg.* 2005;41:1026-1030.

132. Smith GCS, Pell JP. Parachute use to prevent death and major trauma related to gravi-tational challenge: systematic review of randomised controlled trials. *BMJ.* 2003;327:1459-1461.

133. Clarification on Billing Requirements for Percutaneous Transluminal Angioplasty (PTA) Concurrent With the Placement of an Investigational or FDA-Approved Carotid Stent. Available at: http://www.cms.hhs.gov/transmittals/downloads/R53ncd.pdf

134. Plouin PF, Chatellier G, Darne B, Raynaud A. Blood pressure outcome of angioplasty in atherosclerotic renal artery stenosis: a randomized trial. Essai Multicentrique Medicaments vs Angioplastie (EMMA) Study Group. *Hypertension.* 1998;31:823-829.

135. Kiemeneij F, Laarman GJ, Odekerken D, Slagboom T, van der Wieken R. A randomized comparison of percutaneous transluminal coronary angioplasty by the radial, brachial and femoral approaches: the access study. *J Am Coll Cardiol.* 1997;29:1269-1275.

136. Kessel DO, Robertson I, Taylor EJ, Patel JV. Renal stenting from the radial artery: a novel approach. *Cardiovasc Intervent Radiol.* 2003;26:146-149.

137. Trani C, Tommasino A, Burzotta M. Transradial renal stenting: why and how. *Cathet Cardiovasc Intervent.* 2009;76:951-956.

138. Bax L, Mali WP, Van De Ven PJ, Beek FJ, Vos JA, Beutler JJ. Repeated intervention for in-stent restenosis of the renal arteries. *J Vasc Interv Radiol.* 2002;13:1219-1224.

139. Munneke GJ, Engelke C, Morgan RA, Belli AM. Cutting balloon angioplasty for resistant renal artery in-stent restenosis. *J Vasc Interv Radiol.* 2002;13:327-331.

140. Spratt JC, Leslie SJ, Verin V. A case of renal artery brachytherapy for in-stent restenosis: four-year follow-up. *J Invasive Cardiol.* 2004;16:287-288.

141. Ellis K, Murtagh B, Loghin C, et al. The use of brachytherapy to treat renal artery in-stent restenosis. *J Interv Cardiol.* 2005;18:49-54.

142. Wöhrle J, Kochs M, Vollmer C, Kestler HA, Hombach V, Hoher M. Re-angioplasty of in-stent restenosis versus balloon restenoses—a matched pair comparison. *Int J Cardiol.* 2004;93:257-262.

Part 5

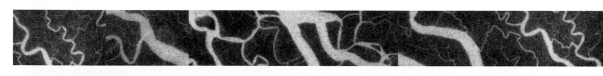

Lower-Extremity Artery Disease

12

Acute Limb Ischemia

Kenneth Ouriel and Vikram S. Kashyap

Acute limb ischemia occurs when blood flow to an extremity is abruptly arrested. This can occur from thrombosis or embolism; the former is much more common, especially occurring as a result of a failed arterial bypass graft or of a percutaneous intervention. The severity of symptoms depends on the severity of hypoperfusion. The process can develop abruptly, and when the patient presents soon after its onset the entity is said to represent *acute limb ischemia*. Acute limb ischemia is differentiated from those patients with an insidious onset of symptoms; these patients tend to present late and the term *chronic limb ischemia* is used to identify such a scenario. In chronic limb ischemia, atherosclerotic disease within a native artery is the most common mechanism and symptoms are often less severe than those associated with acute occlusions.

Epidemiology and Pathophysiology

Acute limb ischemia commonly occurs in elderly individuals with atherosclerotic occlusive disease. Patients are more often male than female, and the entity is particularly common in smokers and in diabetics.

The severity of symptoms is extremely variable in patients with acute limb ischemia. In mild cases the patient may experience symptoms only with increased activity, such as occurs with walking—an entity known as *intermittent claudication*. Patients with symptoms of claudication alone are at low risk for amputation, even without treatment. Alternatively, inadequate oxygen delivery occurs even without activity in patients with severe hypoperfusion. Such patients experience pain at rest and particularly at night, marking the onset of so-called limb-threatening symptoms, a situation associated with significant risks of limb loss and even death if the hypoperfusion progresses unchecked (Table 12.1, p. 246).

There exist a variety of causes for the development of acute limb ischemia. By and large, however, the process can be subdivided into those cases occurring as the result of embolization and those occurring as the result of a primary thrombotic process (Table 12.2). Emboli originate from the heart in over 90% of cases[6] and normally lodge at the site where the arterial

Vascular Disease: Diagnostic and Therapeutic Approaches. © 2011 Michael R. Jaff and Christopher J. White, editors. Cardiotext Publishing, ISBN: 978-1-935395-16-4.

Study	Year Published	Severity of Ischemia	Amputation Rate	Mortality Rate
Blaisdell et al[1]	1978	Not specified	25%	30%
Jivegård et al[2]	1988	Not specified	Not specified	20%
Rochester (Ouriel et al[3])	1994	Class IIb	14%	18%
STILE (STILE investigators[4])	1994	Class I, IIa, IIb	5%	6%
TOPAS (Ouriel et al[5])	1996	Class IIa, IIb	2%	5%

Table 12.1 Outcome of Patients Presenting with Acute Limb Ischemia (Note: Morbidity and mortality are dependent on the severity of ischemia, with a suggestion of improved results in the more recent studies.)

channel normally narrows—most commonly at an arterial bifurcation. Thus, the most common sites of emboli include the common femoral arterial bifurcation and the popliteal trifurcation.

The decreasing prevalence of rheumatic heart disease underlies a diminishing proportion of embolic versus thrombotic causes for acute limb ischemia. When embolization occurs, it usually does so in the setting of atrial fibrillation or acute myocardial infarction, when portions of atrial or ventricular mural thrombus detach and embolize to the arterial tree. Paradoxical embolism through a patent foramen ovale is a less frequent etiology. Thrombosis as an etiology for acute limb ischemia is a much more diverse etiologic category compared to embolization. With the increased use of peripheral arterial bypass grafts for chronic limb ischemia and the finite patency rate of any bypass graft conduit, it is not surprising that acute graft occlusion is now the most frequent cause of acute lower-extremity ischemia in most centers.[7]

Irrespective of the etiology of ischemia, the end result is the buildup of toxic by-products within the ischemic tissue bed. These toxins include the free radical, oxygen-derived, chemically reactive molecules that are responsible for the injury that occurs after ischemia and reperfusion. Ischemia induces leakage of protein and fluid from the capillary bed, resulting in tissue edema.[8] Hydrodynamic pressure in the extravascular space rises to a level that competes with venous outflow, perpetuating a viscous cycle that can eventually impede arterial inflow. At first, this process occurs at a microscopic level

Classification of Acute Limb Ischemia
Bypass graft occlusion
Prosthetic conduit
Intimal hyperplasia at the anastomoses (usually distal)
Occlusion without a demonstrable lesion
Autogenous conduit (eg, saphenous vein graft)
Retained valve cusp of an *in situ* graft
Stenosis at the site of a prior venous injury (eg, superficial phlebitis)
Native arterial occlusion
Thrombosis at the site of an atherosclerotic stenotic lesion
Embolism to an arterial bifurcation
Thrombosis within a near-normal artery, usually as the result of a hypercoagulable state
Arterial inflammatory diseases such as giant cell arteritis (Takayasu's arteritis)
Thrombosis of an aneurysm (popliteal common)
Rare etiologies (popliteal entrapment syndrome, adventitial cystic disease of the popliteal artery)

Table 12.2 Classification of Acute Limb Ischemia

but may progress to the development of high tissue pressures at a regional level and the clinical entity known as the *compartment syndrome*. The development of a compartment syndrome is hastened by the abrupt reperfusion of a previously ischemic tissue bed, a phenomenon that explains the relatively frequent need for fasciotomy after lower-extremity surgical revascularization for severe limb ischemia.[9]

Diagnostic Algorithm

Acute limb ischemia is a clinical diagnosis; there are few diagnostic tests. The patients complain of numbness and pain in the extremity, progressing in severe cases to motor loss and muscle rigidity. Examination will reveal the absence of palpable pulses, and the location of the pulse deficit allows the physician to predict the site of arterial occlusion. The "5 Ps" have been used as a mnemonic to remember the presentation of a patient with acute limb ischemia; *paresthesia, pain, pallor, pulselessness,* and *paralysis.* In some cases, a sixth "P" is added; *poikilothermia,* meaning equilibration of the temperature of the limb to that of the ambient environment (coolness). The process is sometimes confused with deep venous thrombosis by an inexperienced observer. While a deep venous thrombosis may manifest as limb ischemia when severe (phlegmasia cerulea dolens), profound lower-extremity edema is uncommon in pure arterial ischemia. Occasionally, a patient with arterial ischemia and pain at rest will keep the extremity in a dependent position and edema may develop; such a scenario will be apparent if an adequate history is obtained.

In an effort to classify the extent of acute ischemia to standardize reporting of outcome, the Society of Vascular Surgery/International Society of Cardiovascular Surgery (SVS/ISCVS; now SVS) ad hoc committee was established and published what has now come to be known as the *Rutherford criteria*, after Dr. Robert Rutherford, the lead author of the article.[10] Three classes were defined: Class I, where the limb is viable and will remain so even without therapeutic intervention; Class II for limbs that are threatened and will require revascularization for salvage; and Class III for those limbs that are irreversibly ischemic, and infarction has developed such that salvage is not possible. The initial work of the reporting standards commit-

tee was revised several years later, dividing the middle category into 2 subclassifications: 2A for limbs that are not immediately threatened, and 2B for those limbs that are severely threatened to the point where urgent revascularization is necessary for salvage.[11]

As examples, a patient with a palpable femoral pulse but absent popliteal pulse is likely to have a superficial femoral artery occlusion. An absence of a femoral pulse signifies disease above the inguinal ligament, within the iliac arterial segment or the aorta itself. Patients with common femoral artery emboli will maintain an easily palpable femoral pulse, sometimes even augmented with a "water hammer" characteristic, until such time as the absence of outflow in the external iliac artery causes this vessel to thrombose and the femoral pulse to disappear. Patients with popliteal emboli, by contrast, will usually have a palpable popliteal pulse but no palpable pulses below (dorsalis pedis or posterior tibial). Lastly, a patient with leg ischemia secondary to a popliteal aneurysm will usually demonstrate a very large and easily palpable popliteal pulse, concurrent with severe calf and foot ischemia. The popliteal pulse is maintained in these patients as a result of the events leading to occlusion—the aneurysm is associated with serial embolic events to the 3 crural vessels, occluding them one by one until, at the time of the last occlusion, the leg becomes ischemic. The aneurysm itself, however, remains palpable due to the somewhat static column of blood and absent outflow.

Even the most astute clinicians will sometimes have difficulty in discerning their own digital pulse from the patient's pedal pulse. For this reason, the use of a Doppler instrument is advantageous to document flow within the smaller arteries and, most importantly, to provide an objective and quantitative assessment of the extent of arterial insufficiency through the calculation of a Doppler-derived ankle-brachial index (ABI) (Table 12.3). Normally, the ABI is greater than 1.0.[12] The index is decreased to 0.5 to 0.8 in patients with claudication and to lower levels in patients with pain at rest or tissue loss. The ABI may be normal in some patients with mild arterial narrowing; treadmill exercise has been used in these cases to increase the sensitivity of the test.[13] Patients with diabetes mellitus or renal failure may have calcific lower-leg arteries, rendering them incompressible and causing a falsely elevated ABI; in these cases a toe-brachial pressure index can be measured and is more predictive of significant arterial disease.[14] Transcutaneous oxygen tension has also been used to assess the severity of peripheral arterial occlusion,[15] as well as to predict the most appropriate level of amputation.

The anatomic level of the arterial stenoses can be predicted from palpation of pulses in the femoral, popliteal, and ankle regions. For example, patients with disease confined to the superficial femoral artery will have a normal femoral pulse but no palpable popliteal or ankle pulses below, whereas patients with aortoiliac disease will have absent femoral pulses as well. Doppler segmental pressures are also useful in defining the level of involvement; a drop in pressure of 30 mm Hg or more between 2 segments predicts arterial occlusion between the 2 levels.[16] For example, a superficial femoral arterial occlusion would be suggested in a patient with a systolic pressure of 120 mm Hg at the proximal thigh pressure cuff and 90 mm Hg at the above-knee cuff.

Contrast arteriography remains the gold standard with which all other tests must be compared. Even today, standard arteriography is the most accurate test for all but the occasional patient with such slow flow in the tibial or foot vessels that digital subtraction imaging fails to demonstrate a patent artery. Arteriography is, however, a semi-invasive modality and as such its use should be confined to those patients for whom a surgical or percutaneous intervention is contemplated. Patients with borderline renal function may experience contrast-induced nephrotoxicity, and in this subgroup the use of alternate contrast agents such as gadolinium or carbon dioxide have been employed.[17,18]

Duplex ultrasonography has been used in some centers to define the anatomic extent of peripheral artery disease (PAD).[19] While duplex ultrasonography has been useful in documenting the patency of a single arterial segment, such as a stented superficial femoral artery or a bypass graft, evaluation of the entire lower-extremity arterial tree remains imprecise, and its adequacy as the sole diagnostic modality for planning a percutaneous or open surgical intervention remains controversial. Magnetic resonance angiography (MRA) is being used with greater frequency in patients with PAD.[20] Using gadolinium as an MRA contrast agent, the specificity and sensitivity of the test exceeds that of duplex ultrasonography and approaches the accuracy of standard arteriography. MRA has been effective in demonstrating patent tibial arteries undetected with less-sensitive conventional arteriography, identifying potential target vessels for an otherwise unfeasible lower-extremity reconstructive bypass procedure. Today, MRA is widely employed in patients with chronic renal insufficiency to limit the dye load. Another noninvasive imaging modality, computed tomography angiography (CTA), is gaining appeal as a means of delineating anatomy to provide a means of localizing the extent and severity of occlusive disease.[21] With future improvements in hardware and software technology, it is likely that MRA and CTA will effectively replace conventional diagnostic ar-

Clinical Category	Ankle-Brachial Index (ABI)
Normal	> 0.97 (usually 1.10)
Claudication	0.40–0.80
Rest pain	0.20–0.40
Ulceration, gangrene	0.10–0.40
Acute ischemia	Usually inaudible Doppler signals

Table 12.3 Characteristic ABI in Patients Presenting with Lower-Limb Ischemia

teriography, and arterial cannulation will be reserved solely for percutaneous interventional therapies.

Therapeutic Alternatives

Unlike the situation in patients with chronic limb ischemia, where observation alone is a common and quite appropriate treatment option, patients presenting with acute limb ischemia often require revascularization to salvage the leg. In fact, this is why they present acutely and are often able to identify the precise time of the occlusive event, similar to the manner that a patient with a perforated peptic ulcer will know exactly when it occurred. In many cases, the paucity of preexisting collateral channels renders the limb very ischemic after thrombotic or embolic occlusion of the main arterial segment, and symptoms occur with severity and rapidity, forcing the patient to seek treatment almost immediately.

Once the diagnosis is made, adequate systemic anticoagulation is instituted. A bolus of unfractionated heparin is standard, followed by a continuous infusion to maintain the activated partial thromboplastin time (aPTT) in a therapeutic range. The goal of anticoagulation is 2-fold: to decrease the risk of thrombus propagation, and in the case of presumed embolic occlusion, to prevent recurrent embolization. Occasionally, if early angiographic evaluation is feasible, heparinization can be withheld, pending the establishment of arterial access. Otherwise, a micropuncture technique (small localizing needle, guide wire, and a 4-Fr sheath) is utilized to gain access or the anticoagulation is withheld to allow the aPTT to fall to within 1.5x control.

There exist several basic therapeutic options to pursue in patients with acute limb ischemia (Figure 12.1). The first option is anticoagulation alone. If the ischemia is nonthreatening (eg, Rutherford Class I or IIa), such a nonaggressive course may be appropriate. Angiographic evaluation and elective revascularization may then be

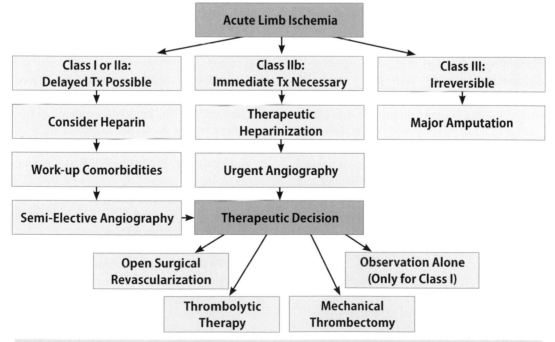

Figure 12.1 A treatment algorithm for patients with acute limb ischemia. The rapidity of therapy is chosen on the basis of the severity of ischemia at presentation; the procedure is dependent, among other factors, on the anatomic appearance of the process.

undertaken after the patient has been fully pre-pared and other comorbidities such as concurrent coronary artery disease have been addressed.

Patients who present with more severe ischemia (Rutherford Class IIb) will require some form of intervention to prevent progression to irreversible ischemia and limb loss. These patients should undergo early angiographic evaluation with adequate imaging of the affected and the unaffected extremity. Arterial access is accomplished at a site distant from the ischemic extremity using a contralateral femoral artery or brachial approach to avoid the creation of needle entry sites in an artery that might subsequently be infused with a thrombolytic agent.

Early angiographic imaging should be undertaken in all patients, with the sole exception of those patients with common femoral emboli. These individuals can be taken directly to the operating room for embolectomy, but completion angiography is necessary to rule out retained thromboembolic material.[22]

Once adequate diagnostic information has been obtained from the angiogram, the clinician is in a position to make a decision about whether or not to pursue a percutaneous or open surgical option.

Thrombolytic therapy

Thrombolytic therapy with the plasminogen activators (urokinase, alteplase, reteplase, or tenecteplase) has been demonstrated to lower the morbidity and mortality when compared with a traditional approach of immediate operative revascularization.[3,4] These benefits appear to be especially prominent in patients with "hyperacute" ischemia, where revascularization is necessary within just a few hours. The complication rate is high when such patients are taken urgently to open surgical revascularization; a finding that is explained by the frequency and magnitude of comorbid conditions in this frail group of patients.

Percutaneous mechanical thrombectomy

Removal of intra-arterial thrombus with a mechanical device has gained popularity over the last several years.[23,24] Some devices rely on hydrodynamic, rheolytic forces to extract the thrombus, while others utilize a rotating basket to fragment the clot. Percutaneous mechanical thrombectomy (PMT) devices can be used in conjunction with pharmacologic thrombolysis. While the devices do result in clearing of much of the occluding thrombus, an infusion of thrombolytic agent is still necessary in many cases, to remove smaller amounts of retained mural thrombus. In a single-center retrospective study of 57 patients with acute limb ischemia treated with PMT, complete thrombus removal was only noted in 61% of cases.[25] However, with 31% of patients receiving adjuvant catheter-directed thrombolytic therapy, the in-hospital limb salvage rates was over 96%.

Immediate open surgical revascularization

Early operation has been remarkably effective in restoring adequate blood flow to an ischemic extremity. The relatively simple procedure of balloon catheter thromboembolectomy, however, has fallen into disfavor for all but true embolic occlusions. The underlying lesion responsible for the thrombotic event must be identified and corrected to avoid early reocclusion. For this reason, long, atherosclerotic occlusions are best treated with the placement of a bypass graft.[26] As well, patients with occlusion of a bypass graft as the cause of ischemia are best served with the placement of a new bypass graft, if at all possible.[27]

Unfortunately, immediate open surgical interventions have been associated with an unexpectedly high risk of major morbidity and mortality. Blaisdell et al[1] first reported this finding, noting a 30% perioperative mortality rate in a review of over 3000 patients in the published works from the 1960s and 1970s. While the results have improved since the publication of Blaisdell's landmark review, mortality rates continue to remain undesirably high.[28] This observation appears to relate to the relatively common occurrence of cardiopulmonary complications developing in these medically compromised patients—patients who are ill-prepared to undergo early operative intervention.[3] The severity of ischemia precludes adequate preoperative preparation of the patient, and complications such as perioperative myocardial infarction, cardiac arrhythmia, or pneumonia appear to underlie the unacceptable mortality rate in these patients.

The mortality rate from open surgical treatment of acute limb ischemia has been reconfirmed in numerous studies published after Blaisdell's landmark series. Dale[29] reviewed cases of nontraumatic extremity ischemia and observed an 11% mortality rate in those with embolism, versus 3% in those with acute thromboses. Several years later, Jivegård et al[2] documented a mortality rate of 20% in patients presenting with acute arterial embolism or thrombosis, a finding that was explained by preexisting cardiac disease in these patients. A study by Edwards and colleagues[27] reported a 1-year mortality rate of 38% in patients undergoing the placement of new autogenous vein grafts for treatment of failed prior grafts in the same leg, with an amputation rate of 6% over the same time frame.

Noting the high morbidity from primary open surgical revascularization in patients suffering from true limb-threatening lower-limb ischemia, 3 randomized, prospective clinical trials were organized to compare thrombolytic therapy and immediate open surgical revascularization. The first study, the Rochester series, compared urokinase to primary operation in a single-center experience of 114 patients presenting with what has subsequently been called *hyperacute ischemia*.[3] Patients enrolled in this trial all had severely threatened limbs (Rutherford Class IIb) with mean symptom duration of

approximately 2 days. After 1 year of follow-up, 84% of patients randomized to urokinase were alive, compared with only 58% of patients randomized to primary operation (Figure 12.2). By contrast, the rate of limb salvage was identical at 80%. A closer inspection of the raw data revealed that the defining variable for mortality differences was the development of cardiopulmonary complications during the periprocedural period. The rate of long-term mortality was high when such periprocedural complications occurred but was relatively low when they did not occur. It was only the fact that such complications occurred more commonly in patients taken directly to the operating theater that explained the greater long-term mortality rate in the operative group.

The second prospective, randomized analysis of thrombolysis versus surgery was the Surgery or Thrombolysis for the Ischemic Lower Extremity (STILE) trial.[4] Genentech, the manufacturer of the Activase brand of rt-PA, funded the study. At its termination, 393 patients were randomized to 1 of 3 treatment groups, rt-PA, urokinase, or primary operation. Subsequently, the 2 thrombolytic groups were combined for purposes of data analysis when the outcome was found to be similar. While the rate of the composite end point of untoward events was higher in the thrombolytic patients, the rates of the more relevant and objective end points of amputation and death were equivalent (Figure 12.3). There appeared articles consisting of subgroup analyses of the STILE data, one relating to native artery occlusions[30] and

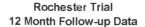

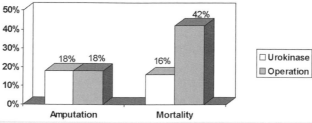

Figure 12.2 The rate of amputation was identical in the 2 treatment groups in the Rochester trial, but the mortality rate was significantly lower in patients assigned to the thrombolytic arm.[3]

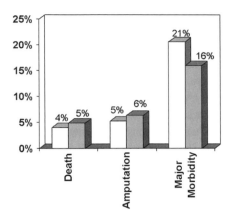

Figure 12.3 Outcome measures from the STILE data after 30 days of follow-up. Importantly, the rates of death and amputation are similar.[4]

one to bypass graft occlusions.[31] Thrombolysis appeared more effective in patients with graft occlusions. The rate of major amputation was higher in native arterial occlusions treated with thrombolysis (10% thrombolysis vs. 0% surgery at 1 year). By contrast, amputation was lower in patients with acute graft occlusions treated with thrombolysis. These data suggest that thrombolysis may be of greatest benefit in patients with acute bypass graft occlusions of less than 14 days.

The third and final randomized comparison of thrombolysis and surgery was the Thrombolysis or Peripheral Arterial Surgery (TOPAS) trial, funded by Abbott Laboratories. Following completion of a preliminary dose-ranging trial in 213 patients,[5] 544 patients were randomized to a recombinant form of urokinase or primary operative intervention.[7] After a mean follow-up period of 1 year, the rate of amputation-free survival was identical in the 2 treatment groups: 65.0% and 69.9% in the urokinase and surgical patients, respectively (Table 12.4). While this trial failed to document improvement in survival or limb salvage with thrombolysis, fully 32% of the thrombolytic patients were alive without amputation with nothing more than a percutaneous procedure after 6 months of follow-up. After 1 year, this number had decreased only slightly, with 26% alive, without amputation and with only percutaneous interventions. Thus, the original goal of the TOPAS trial, to generate data on which regulatory approval of recombinant urokinase would be based, was not

Intervention or Outcome	Urokinase Group (N=272)		Surgery Group (N=272)	
	6 mo	1 year	6 mo	1 year
Operative intervention	no. of interventions			
Amputation	48	58	41	51
Above the knee	22	25	19	26
Below the knee	26	33	22	25
Open surgical procedures	315	351	551	590
Major	102	116	177	193
Moderate	89	98	136	145
Minor	124	137	238	252
Percutaneous procedures	128	135	55	70
Worst outcome*	% of patients			
Death	16.0	20.0	12.3	17.0
Amputation	12.2	15.0	12.9	13.1
Above the knee	5.6	6.5	6.1	7.5
Below the knee	6.6	8.5	6.8	5.6
Open surgical procedures	40.3	39.3	69.0	65.4
Major	23.6	24.3	39.3	39.3
Moderate	10.3	8.7	16.3	13.4
Minor	6.4	6.3	13.4	12.7
Endovascular procedures	16.9	15.4	2.1	1.7
Medical treatment alone	14.6	10.3	3.7	2.8

Table 12.4 Results in the TOPAS Trial of Recombinant Urokinase Versus Surgery for Acute Peripheral Arterial Occlusion (From Ouriel K, Veith FJ, Sasahara AA. A comparison of recombinant urokinase with vascular surgery as initial treatment for acute arterial occlusion of the legs. *N Engl J Med*. 1998;338:1105-1111.) *Worst outcome is the most severe event that occurred. over the specified time period. Copyright 1998. Massachusetts Medical Society. All rights reserved.)

achieved. Nevertheless, the findings confirmed that acute limb ischemia could be managed with catheter-directed thrombolysis, achieving similar amputation and mortality rates but avoiding the need for open surgical procedures in a significant percentage of patients.

Summary

Acute limb ischemia develops with the sudden occlusion of a native artery or bypass graft, resulting in hypoperfusion of the distal extremity. Symptoms include pain and sensory loss, progressing to paralysis. Signs include pallor and coolness of the extremity, with absence of palpable pulses distal to the occlusion.

When severe, ischemia progresses to infarction and limb loss, the rapidity of which is dependent on the adequacy of preexisting collateral arterial channels. Treatment is accomplished through the restoration of adequate distal blood flow with open surgical revascularization procedures, pharmacologic thrombolytic therapy, percutaneous mechanical thrombectomy, or combinations of the 3.

Morbidity and mortality rates are high, especially in those patients with medical comorbidities that render them ill-prepared to undergo urgent surgical interventions. The keys to improving outcome lie in rapid diagnosis, effective reperfusion, correction of the culprit lesion that caused the occlusion, and liberal use of antithrombotic therapy.

References

1. Blaisdell F W, Steele M, and Allen RE. Management of acute lower extremity arterial ischemia due to embolism and thrombosis. *Surgery*. 1978;84:822-834.

2. Jivegård L, Holm J, Scherstén T. Acute limb ischemia due to arterial embolism or thrombosis: influence of limb ischemia versus pre-existing cardiac disease on postoperative mortality rate. *J Cardiovasc Surg*. 1988;29:32-36.

3. Ouriel K, Shortell CK, DeWeese JA, et al. A comparison of thrombolytic therapy with operative revascularization in the initial treatment of acute peripheral arterial ischemia. *J Vasc Surg*. 1994;19:1021-1030.

4. STILE investigators. Results of a prospective randomized trial evaluating surgery versus thrombolysis for ischemia of the lower extremity. The STILE trial. *Ann Surg*. 1994;220:251-266.

5. Ouriel K, Veith FJ, Sasahara AA. Thrombolysis or peripheral arterial surgery: phase I results. TOPAS Investigators. *J Vasc Surg*. 1996;23:64-73.

6. Abbott WM, Maloney RD, McCabe CC. Arterial embolism: a 44 year perspective. *Am J Surg*. 1982;143:460-464.

7. Ouriel K, Veith FJ, Sasahara AA. A comparison of recombinant urokinase with vascular surgery as initial treatment for acute arterial occlusion of the legs. *N Engl J Med*. 1998;338:1105-1111.

8. Bulkley GB. Pathophysiology of free radical-mediated reperfusion injury. [Review] [47 refs]. *J Vasc Surg*. 1987;5:512-517.

9. Rush DS, Frame SB, Bell RM, Berg EE, Kerstein MD, Haynes JL. Does open fasciotomy contribute to morbidity and mortality after acute lower extremity ischemia and revascularization? *J Vasc Surg*. 1989;10:343-350.

10. Suggested standards for reports dealing with lower extremity ischemia. Prepared by the Ad Hoc Committee on Reporting Standards, Society for Vascular Surgery/North American Chapter, International Society for Cardiovascular Surgery. *J Vasc Surg*. 1986;4:80-94.

11. Rutherford RB, Baker JD, Ernst C, et al. Recommended standards for reports dealing with lower extremity ischemia: revised version. *J Vasc Surg*. 1997;26:517-538.

12. Ouriel K, Zarins CK. Doppler ankle pressure: an evaluation of three methods of expression. *Arch Surg*. 1982;117:1297-1300.

13. Ouriel K, McDonnell AE, Metz CE, Zarins CK. Critical evaluation of stress testing in the diagnosis of peripheral vascular disease. *Surgery*. 1982;91:686-693.

14. Gunderson J. Segmental measurement of

systolic blood pressure in the extremities including the thumb and the great toe. *Acta Chir Scand.* 1972;(Suppl) 426:1-90.

15. Cina C, Katsamouris A, Megerman J, et al. Utility of transcutaneous oxygen tension measurements in peripheral arterial occlusive disease. *J Vasc Surg.* 1984;1:362-371.

16. Moneta GL, Yeager RA, Lee RW, Porter JM. Noninvasive localization of arterial occlusive disease: a comparison of segmental Doppler pressures and arterial duplex mapping. *J Vasc Surg.* 1993;17:578-582.

17. Kerns SR, Hawkins IFJ, Sabatelli FW. Current status of carbon dioxide angiography. *Radiol Clin North Am.* 1995;33:15-29.

18. Parodi JC, Ferreira LM. Gadolinium-based contrast: an alternative contrast agent for endovascular interventions. *Ann Vasc Surg.* 2000;14:480-483.

19. Proia RR, Walsh DB, Nelson PR, et al. Early results of infragenicular revascularization based solely on duplex arteriography. *J Vasc Surg.* 2001;33:1165-1170.

20. Schoenberg SO, Londy FJ, Licato P, Williams DM, Wakefield T, Chenevert TL. Multiphase-multistep gadolinium-enhanced MR angiography of the abdominal aorta and runoff vessels. *Invest Radiol.* 2001;36:283-291.

21. Rubin GD, Dake MD, Semba CP. Current status of three-dimensional spiral CT scanning for imaging the vasculature. *Radiol Clin North Am.* 1995;33:51-70.

22. Crolla RM, van de Pavoordt ED, Moll FL. Intraoperative digital subtraction angiography after thromboembolectomy: preliminary experience. *J Endovasc Surg.* 1995;2:168-171.

23. Kasirajan K, Gray B, Beavers FP, et al. Rheolytic thrombectomy in the management of acute and subacute limb-threatening ischemia. *J Vas Interv Radiol.* 2001;12:413-421.

24. Kasirajan K, Haskal ZJ, Ouriel K. The use of mechanical thrombectomy devices in the management of acute peripheral arterial occlusive disease. *J Vasc Interv Radiol.* 2001;12:405-411.

25. Ansel GM, Botti CF, Silver MJ. Treatment of acute limb ischemia with a percutaneous mechanical thrombectomy-based endovascular approach: 5-year limb salvage and survival results from a single center series. *Catheter Cardiovasc Interv.* 2008;72:325-330.

26. Dormandy JA, Rutherford RB. Management of peripheral arterial disease (PAD). TASC Working Group. TransAtlantic Inter-Society Consensus (TASC). *J Vasc Surg.* 2000;31:S1-S296.

27. Edwards JE, Taylor LM Jr, Porter JM. Treatment of failed lower extremity bypass grafts with new autogenous vein bypass grafting. *J Vasc Surg.* 1990;11:136-145.

28. Dormandy J, Heeck L, Vig S. Acute limb ischemia. *Semin Vasc Surg.* 1999;12:148-153.

29. Dale WA. Differential management of acute peripheral arterial ischemia. *J Vasc Surg.* 1984;1:269-278.

30. Weaver FA, Comerota AJ, Youngblood M, Froehlich J, Hosking JD, Papanicolaou G. Surgical revascularization versus thrombolysis for nonembolic lower extremity native artery occlusions: results of a prospective randomized trial. The STILE Investigators. Surgery versus Thrombolysis for Ischemia of the Lower Extremity. *J Vasc Surg.* 1996;24:513-521.

31. Comerota AJ, Weaver FA, Hosking JD, et al. Results of a prospective, randomized trial of surgery versus thrombolysis for occluded lower extremity bypass grafts. *Am J Surg.* 1996;172:105-112.

13

Occlusive Diseases of the Abdominal Aorta and Iliac Arteries

Joseph J. Ricotta II and Timothy M. Sullivan

The **TASC II** document (Inter-Societal Consensus for the Management of PAD) provides a framework for the identification, diagnosis, and treatment of patients with peripheral artery disease.[1] Most patients with PAD do have some impairment in their ability to walk, and as such, have decreased level of function and quality of life. Patients who are asymptomatic, however, having had aortic disease diagnosed at the time of investigation of another medical issue, should be managed with risk factor modification; intervention (surgical or endovascular) is not indicated. Those patients with symptomatic disease, however, will typically present with intermittent claudication (which means, literally, "to limp") of varying degrees. Patients may also present with critical limb ischemia (rest pain or tissue loss) when aortic disease is present in combination with iliac and infrainguinal occlusive disease, or in the presence of distal embolization. The most common location of pain, which occurs with ambulation and is relieved by rest, is the calf; patients may, however, experience pain in the thigh and buttocks. The classic triad of intermittent claudication, absent femoral pulses, and impotence was first described by the French surgeon René Leriche.

Physical Examination and Diagnosis

Physical examination should concentrate on the vascular system as a whole and include a complete pulse examination; palpation of the aorta to identify aneurysmal disease; auscultation of the neck, abdomen, and groins to identify bruits; and inspection of the feet and toes for identification of ulceration and discrimination of atheroemboli. Pallor with limb elevation and rubor with dependency suggest a critical degree of chronic limb ischemia. The presence of normal pulses does not, however, rule out the presence of significant disease; a patient may have normal hemodynamics and pulses at rest, only to have decreased pulses and ankle-brachial index (ABI) with exercise. All patients should have noninvasive lower-extremity arterial studies (segmental pressures, with exercise if indicated) performed to establish a baseline and to follow any subsequent interventional procedure. A resting ABI less than 0.9 is considered abnormal. With exercise, a decrease in the ABI of 15% to 20%, associated with a reproduction of symptoms, is considered diagnostic.

Importantly, an abnormal noninvasive study confirms the diagnosis of PAD, can provide for risk stratification, and can prompt the clinician to evaluate patients for associated coronary and cerebrovascular diseases.

The definitive diagnosis can be made by CTA, MRA, or more invasive means, such as catheter angiography. When evaluating the aortoiliac segment, it is important to visualize the visceral vessels (celiac, superior mesenteric, inferior mesenteric, and renal arteries) and to evaluate the distal aorta and iliac vessels with oblique and lateral views, as needed. In patients suspected of having atheromatous embolization from an abdominal aortic source, it may be prudent to perform the angiographic procedure from an upper-extremity approach to avoid further embolic events secondary to catheter manipulation.

The TASC II document categorizes aortoiliac (inflow) disease into 4 types (A through D), based on severity and extent of disease. In the context of *isolated* aortic disease, a short (< 3 cm) stenosis of the infrarenal aorta is considered a TASC A lesion, while infrarenal aortic occlusion is classified as TASC D. TASC A lesions of the aortoiliac segment are generally treated with endovascular means, while TASC D lesions are typically best treated with an open surgical approach. In general, when endovascular and open surgical procedures have equivalent short- and long-term results, the endovascular solution should be instituted first. Of note, patients with thrombosis/complete occlusion of the infrarenal aorta may not have a benign course; several investigators have suggested that these patients may be at increased risk of renal artery thrombosis, due to propagation of thrombus into the renal ostia, when managed expectantly.[2]

Patients presenting with acute aortic occlusion have an especially grave course. Babu et al[3] reported on 48 patients treated for acute aortic occlusion treated over a 19-year period. Presentation was quite variable, with acute limb ischemia (n = 34) being the most common clinical scenario. Other presenting symptoms included acute abdomen, spinal-cord ischemia, and sudden onset of hypertension. Acute thrombosis was secondary to underlying atherosclerotic disease in 36 patients, cardiac embolus in 4, thrombosis of an aortic aneurysm in 2, and hypercoagulable state (with an underlying normal aorta) in 6. The overall mortality rate was 52%; those with poor left ventricular function, thrombosis of the visceral arteries or arteries below the inguinal ligament, and a hypercoagulable state were associated with an ominous prognosis.

Patients having small aortas have been found to be at risk of late graft failure regardless of gender. Valentine et al[4] reviewed 37 young men and 36 young women (age < 49 years) having elective aortic reconstruction for symptomatic aortoiliac occlusive disease over a 15-year period, all of whom had had smaller aortas than a comparable group of controls. Fifty-four percent of women and 47% of men had graft limb occlusions within a mean of 31 months, regardless of angiographic runoff. The authors concluded that young patients with premature atherosclerosis and small aortas have a substantially increased risk of graft failure, and that aortic size is a critical determinant of graft patency. Others have suggested that aortic size, both at the upper and lower distributions of aortic diameter, are both risk factors for developing peripheral arterial disease.[5]

Endovascular Therapy for Isolated Aortic Disease

Isolated, focal stenoses of the infrarenal abdominal aorta secondary to atherosclerotic occlusive arterial disease is a relatively uncommon clinical entity; patients with more diffuse disease of the entire aortoiliac segment are encountered more commonly in clinical practice.[6] In addition to the typical presentation of lower-extremity claudication, patients may also present with *blue toe syndrome*—painful, blue toes secondary to atheromatous embolization. The angiographic appearance of these lesions may underestimate the soft, friable nature of plaque, which may be subject to further embolization during the course of endovascular intervention (Figures 13.1 and 13.2). Nevertheless, many of these lesions are amenable to angioplasty and/or stenting. Elkouri and colleagues[7] described their experience, during an era before the routine use of stents, in treating atherosclerotic lesions of the infrarenal aorta in 46 patients with angioplasty alone. Initial technical success was 83%; of those patients without initial hemodynamic improvement, 4 required surgical revascularization, 2 of which were urgent. Fifty-six percent of patients remained clinically improved at 5-year follow-up. Primary patency was 70% at 4 years and 63% at 5 years. Factors predictive of failure included poor runoff and the presence of concomitant iliac occlusive disease. The addition of stents to angioplasty seems to improve the short- and long-term results of isolated aortic intervention. The largest experience to date has been reported by de Vries and colleagues.[8] They performed angioplasty of the infrarenal aorta on a total of 69 patients with symptomatic disease with only one technical failure in a patient with a near occlusion. They achieved a primary 5-year patency rate of 75% and a secondary patency rate of 97%. Seventeen patients underwent repeat procedures, the majority of which were endovascular in nature. Importantly, they identified a nearly 4:1 female to male ratio; 75% of patients were cigarette smokers.

While endovascular therapy is typically safe and effective in the treatment of most patients with isolated infrarenal atherosclerosis, distal embolization may complicate these procedures, especially in those patients with friable plaque or those with superimposed thrombosis. Karnabatidis et al[9] described an extensive experience in treating 48 patients with angioplasty and stenting of isolated aortic lesions, using distal embolic protection with a nitinol filter device. All patients had particles recovered within the filters; 58% had particles greater than 1 mm in diameter recovered, while 12% had particles greater than 3 mm. The collected particles consisted of platelets, fibrin, erythrocytes, and inflammatory cells. Longer lesions, increased

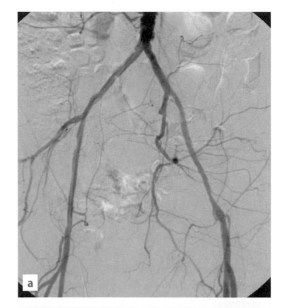

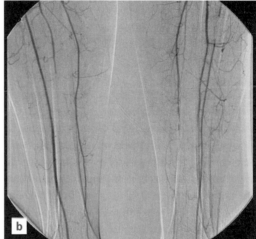

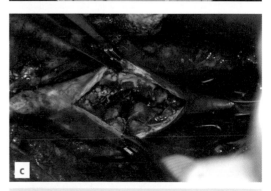

Figure 13.1 (a) Distal aortic irregularity in a young female with atheromatous embolization to both feet. (b) Angiographic evidence of embolic tibial artery occlusion. (c) Operative photograph of soft, friable, cholesterol-laden plaque in the infrarenal aorta.

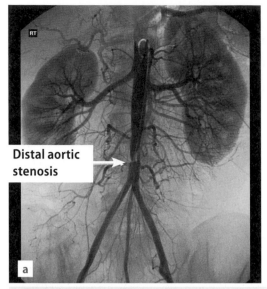
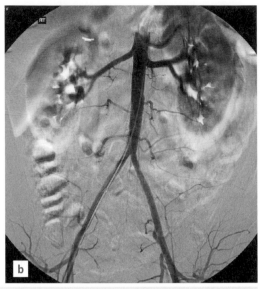

Distal aortic
stenosis

a

b

Figure 13.2 (a) Fifty-year-old female with midaortic lesion presenting with atheromatous embolization to both feet (blue toe syndrome). (b) Successful endovascular therapy with angioplasty and stent placement.

reference vessel diameter, acute thrombosis, and complete occlusions were associated with an increased embolic burden. Chaufour et al[10] have evaluated the risks of using large balloons in the infrarenal aorta. Their study, conducted in cadaveric aortas, suggests that overdilation of the aorta up to 6 mm may be safe in noncalcified vessels; overdilation by 2 mm, at pressures less than 2 atmospheres (atm), may be safe in calcified vessels.

Distal Embolization from an Aortic Source

The heart remains the most frequent source of peripheral embolization, followed by aneurysms of the aorta and peripheral arteries.[10] Previously termed *cryptogenic emboli*, as their origins could not be ascertained, the aorta is increasingly identified as an important source of distal embolization, especially with the increased use of noninvasive imaging modalities, including transesophageal echocardiography (TEE), CTA, and MRA. Kvilekval and colleagues[11] reviewed outcomes in 41 patients having atheroembolic

disease to the abdominal viscera and lower extremities. All patients (30 men, 11 women; mean age 65 years) had a radiographically identified proximal embolic source. The overall mortality rate was 17% in their series, and the rate of recurrent embolization was 15%. Mortality (60% vs. 11%) and recurrent embolic episodes (60% vs. 8%) were significantly more frequent in patients with disease extending above the diaphragm than those whose disease was localized to the infradiaphragmatic aorta. In addition, patients with diffuse disease had higher rates of death and recurrent embolic events than those with a single identified source.

In a prospective study encompassing a 3-year period, Reber et al[12] evaluated 89 patients having acute embolic events with TEE, CTA, or MRA to detect an embolic source. Those patients whose emboli originated from the heart (n = 51), aortoiliac disease (n = 16), or abdominal aortic aneurysms (n = 12) were excluded from analysis. Eight patients (5 women, 3 men; median age 63 years) with bilateral or repetitive embolic events from mural aortic thrombi (MAT) were identified, representing 9% of all patients with arterial thromboembolism in their series. Percutaneous aspiration thrombectomy was performed in 6 patients and surgical thrombectomy in another 2. Two of 8 patients ultimately suffered limb loss (25%). Seven patients underwent definitive surgical therapy, including graft replacement and open thrombectomy or thromboendarterectomy. No recurrent embolic events occurred during a follow-up period of 13 months. The authors recommend an aggressive diagnostic workup in all patients when other, more common sources of embolization have been ruled out.

Localized obstruction of the suprarenal aorta, the aptly-named "coral reef" aorta, was first described by Qvarfordt et al[13] in 1984. Nine patients were identified over a 13-year period with this unique clinical entity that required surgical reconstruction to treat lower-extremity ischemia, hypertension, visceral ischemia, and heart failure. All were found to have eccentric, heavily calcified polypoid lesions originating from the posterior surface of the aorta, typically extending from the diaphragm to the level of the renal arteries. All patients underwent endarterectomy through a thoracoretroperitoneal approach; 2 of 8 died postoperatively, 1 of whom had an emergency operation for aortic thrombosis. The plaque, which grossly resembles a white coral reef, was calcified and exhibited metaplastic bone formation on pathologic analysis.

Embolization to the lower extremities from an isolated mobile thrombus in the aorta has also been repaired via endovascular means, using a covered stent to isolate the thrombus (Figure 13.3).

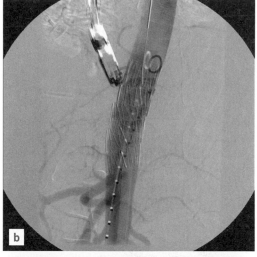

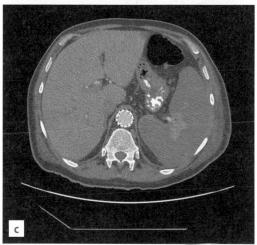

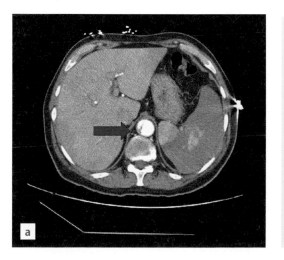

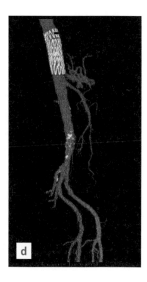

Figure 13.3 (a) Sixty-three-year-old male with emboli to spleen, liver, and kidneys. Supraceliac aortic thrombus (arrow) identified on CT scan. (b) Endovascular repair with placement of 2 covered stents in suprarenal aorta. (c) Follow-up CT scan shows covered stents patent and without evidence of recurrent thrombus. (d) Three-dimensional reconstruction.

Surgical Reconstruction for Aortic Occlusive Disease

History of Aortic Surgery

The history of aortic surgery dates back more than 80 years. In 1923, René Leriche described a syndrome of thigh/buttock claudication, impotence, and absence of femoral pulses (published in 1940), and suggested that resection of the terminal aorta with graft replacement would be an ideal treatment. The operation that Leriche suggested was later performed by Roland Oudot in 1950. In the late 1940s, L. Bazy[14] described aortic endarterectomy, a procedure brought to the United States by E. Jack Wylie.[15] Ultimately, with the advent of prosthetic grafts, endarterectomy was supplanted by bypass. Oudot performed the first extra-anatomic bypass (external iliac to external iliac) in 1950.[15] Early aortic reconstruction was characterized by substantial mortality and morbidity, especially acute renal failure. By the 1960s, however, the risk of renal failure had decreased to < 1%, and the mortality rate had diminished to < 5% for elective cases.

Direct Reconstruction

The gold standard for the treatment of complex (TASC D) aortoiliac occlusive disease is *aortobifemoral bypass grafting*. Some authors have correctly suggested that the widespread adoption of endovascular techniques for the treatment of aortoiliac disease has limited the utility of direct aortic reconstruction to those patients with endovascular failures or those with such severe disease that endovascular intervention is not feasible.

In a report by Hertzer et al,[16] a total of 355 direct aortic reconstructions (aortobifemoral bypass, aortoiliac bypass, and aortoiliac endarterectomy) for occlusive disease were performed from 1976 to 2002. During the same time period, 181 extra-anatomic bypasses (axillofemoral/bifemoral and femoral-femoral bypass) were performed. Simultaneous infrainguinal revascularization procedures were necessary in 36

patients (6.7%). The majority of patients (50%) were treated for claudication, while 48% were treated for advanced lower-extremity ischemia. Those with limb-threatening ischemia were more likely to have superficial femoral artery (SFA) occlusions, a history of prior inflow operations, elevated serum creatinine, and chronic obstructive pulmonary disease (COPD). Of the 355 direct aortic reconstructions, 248 (70%) were performed during the first 8 years of the reporting period; only 107 (30%) were performed during the last 12 years of the study, likely due to the rise of endovascular therapy. Not surprisingly, patients having extra-anatomic bypass were older, and they were more likely to have advanced ischemia, superficial femoral artery occlusion, a history of prior inflow operation, elevated serum creatinine, and COPD. Extra-anatomic bypass was associated with a higher incidence of postoperative death and of graft thrombosis compared to direct reconstruction. In the early postoperative period, women were more likely than men to sustain graft thrombosis or require amputation. For the entire cohort, late survival was 64% at 5 years, 39% at 10 years, and 20% at 15 years; survival was significantly lower in patients requiring extra-anatomic bypass. Primary patency was 95% at 1 year, 85% at 5 years, and 77% at 10 years. The authors conclude that direct reconstruction, including aortofemoral, aortoiliac, or iliofemoral bypass are more durable procedures than extra-anatomic methods and should be chosen for average- or low-risk patients. Patients with severe medical comorbidities that preclude direct reconstruction should be considered for extra-anatomic bypass; in the current era, these patients are typically those high-risk patients in whom an endovascular solution is not feasible.

Cardiac evaluation is an important determinant of risk stratification in patients considered for aortic reconstruction. Although recent studies have questioned the efficacy of aggressive preoperative cardiac testing, the authors continue to consider it an important part of patient evaluation in patients requiring aortic operation. In the Cleveland Clinic series,[16] substantial numbers of patients (n = 263, 49%)

underwent coronary angiography in an attempt to reduce perioperative cardiac events and improve short- and long-term survival. Patients having direct aortic reconstruction were more likely to have had coronary angiography than those having extra-anatomic bypass. Preliminary coronary artery bypass grafting (CABG) or percutaneous transluminal coronary angioplasty (PTCA) were performed in a small minority of patients having direct reconstruction (6.5%) or extra-anatomic bypass (2.2%) prior to their incident procedure.

A study by deVries et al[17] evaluated the results of aortic reconstruction for occlusive disease in more than 6000 patients in a meta-analysis encompassing 23 studies, all of which reported patency rates based on life table analysis. Patency rates (limb-based) were 91% at 5 years and 87% at 10 years for claudicants, compared with 88% and 82% in those operated on for critical limb ischemia. Morbidity and mortality were stratified with respect to date of study publication; aggregate operative mortality was 4.6% in studies started prior to 1975, compared with 3.3% in later studies ($P = 0.01$). Perioperative morbidity was 13.1% in the older studies and 8.3% in the more recent published series ($P < 0.001$). Patency rates were similar over time.

Several studies have evaluated method of aortic exposure as a determinant of important perioperative variables including respiratory morbidity, time to restoration of gastrointestinal function, and hospital length of stay. Cambria et al[18] randomized 113 patients to either transperitoneal or retroperitoneal exposure for aortic reconstruction over an 18-month period. Factors including respiratory morbidity, recovery of gastrointestinal function, requirement for narcotics, metabolic parameters of operative stress, incidence of major and minor complications, and hospital length of stay were similar for the 2 groups. When compared to a retrospectively reviewed cohort having aortic reconstruction at their institution, randomized patients had a highly significant ($P < 0.001$) reduction in postoperative ventilation, transfusion requirements, and length of stay, independent of transperitoneal or retroperitoneal approach, suggesting

that changes in patient care over time, and not operative approach to aortic exposure, were responsible for changes in these variables. Sicard and colleagues,[19] in a similar study, randomized 145 patients over a 3-year period. The incidence of intraoperative complications was the same for both groups. During the postoperative period, however, the incidence of prolonged ileus and small-bowel obstruction was higher in the transabdominal group, whereas the retroperitoneal group had fewer complications, shorter intensive care unit stays, and a trend toward shorter hospitalization and lower hospital cost. There was no difference in pulmonary complications. The retroperitoneal group reported more incisional pain at long-term follow-up. These authors conclude that retroperitoneal aortic exposure for aortic surgery is associated with improved outcomes. Finally, Piquet and colleagues[20] reviewed their experience with a minimally invasive retroperitoneal approach in the treatment of patients with infrarenal aortic disease. Over a 3-year period, 150 patients were treated for aneurysmal or occlusive disease utilizing a small (12-cm) left flank incision for aortic exposure. Perioperative mortality was 0.7%, while nonfatal complications occurred in 8.0%. Conversion to a "standard" exposure was required in only 3 patients. Median return to a regular diet was 2 days, while median hospital length of stay was 8 days. These authors conclude that this approach is safe and effective in the treatment of patients with infrarenal aortic pathology requiring operative intervention.

One of the most novel approaches to aortic reconstruction involves the use of laparoscopic surgery. Coggia and colleagues[21] described their experience in 93 total laparoscopic aortic operations performed for TASC C or D aortoiliac lesions. Aortic exposure, via a left retroperitoneal approach, and the aortic anastomosis were performed with the use of a laparoscope and laparoscopic instruments via 5 or 6 ports. Median operative time was 240 minutes (range 150–450 min); median duration of the aortic anastomosis was 30 minutes (range 12–90 min), with the longer operative and anastomotic times reflecting the early portion of the learning curve.

Operative mortality was 4%; 2 of the 4 deaths occurred secondary to myocardial infarction. Median hospital stay was 7 days. At 19 months mean follow-up, all grafts were patent. The authors conclude that this technique is feasible, with outcomes similar to conventional bypass, and that operative trauma may be reduced following an initial learning curve.

Aortoiliac endarterectomy (AIE) was the preferred treatment of patients with aortoiliac occlusive disease in the 1950s and 1960s, prior to the widespread availability of synthetic grafts. Naylor and colleagues[22] reviewed their experience with this procedure in 57 patients over an 11-year period. Cumulative patency at 2 and 5 years was 94% and 90%, respectively. Advantages of this approach are principally the absence of prosthetic graft material and the ability to treat the internal iliac arteries in males with erectile dysfunction. It may be preferable to aortobifemoral bypass in patients whose disease does not involve the external iliac arteries, in males with erectile dysfunction, in those who may be at increased risk of infection or with small arteries, and in patients with localized disease of the aorta, as well as following removal of an infected aortic graft where an end-to-side anastomosis has been performed. Contraindications to this technique include patients with extensive disease that extends into the external iliac and femoral arteries, and those with aneurysmal dilatation. As suggested by Connolly et al,[23] this operation is infrequently performed, and may be "a lost art" (Figure 13.4).

Extra-Anatomic Bypass

Extra-anatomic bypass has traditionally been used to treat patients with severe aortoiliac disease who are not amenable, due to significant medical comorbidities, to direct aortic reconstruction, and as a precursor to removal of prosthetic aortic grafts due to infection. The axillofemoral and axillobifemoral bypass were first described in the 1960s as an alternative to direct reconstruction.[24,25] Initial enthusiasm for this technique was tempered by lower patency rates and a higher risk of graft infection compared to

direct reconstructive techniques. These grafts frequently required thrombectomy, over time, to maintain patency, with primary patency rates reported in the 40% to 60% range at 3 years. Subsequent reports, using externally supported grafts, have shown improved results. El-Massry and colleagues[26] reviewed their experience with 79 consecutive operations using externally supported Dacron grafts. Operative mortality was 5%, with primary patency rates of 78% at 5 years and 73% at 10 years (mean follow-up, 42 months). Patency was not adversely affected by graft configuration (unifemoral vs. bifemoral), patency of the superficial femoral artery, or indication for operation (claudication vs. limb salvage). Not surprisingly, survival in this group of medically compromised patients was inferior to a concurrent group having aortofemoral bypass (23% vs. 72% at 10 years). Passman and colleagues[27] compared their results with axillofemoral and aortofemoral bypass in 247 patients (108 axillofemoral, 139 aortofemoral); the decision to perform either operation was based on assessment of surgical risk and surgeon's preference. Patients having axillofemoral reconstruction were older, had an increased incidence of heart disease, and were more likely to present with critical limb ischemia. No differences in operative mortality were found, but those having aortic operations were more likely to have major postoperative complications. Five-year primary patency, limb salvage, and survival rates were 74%, 89%, and 45% for axillofemoral bypass, and 80%, 79%, and 72% for aortofemoral bypass. While survival for those patients having extra-anatomic bypass were statistically lower than those having direct reconstruction, primary patency and limb salvage rates were not different. The authors conclude that extra-anatomic bypass, when reserved for patients with limited life expectancy from medical comorbidities, had excellent and comparable patency when compared to direct reconstruction.

Thoracofemoral bypass is another viable option for patients with aortic occlusive disease who have failed axillobifemoral grafts and/or have a hostile abdomen. The Northwestern University group[28] reported on its experience

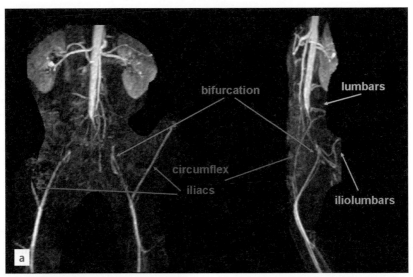

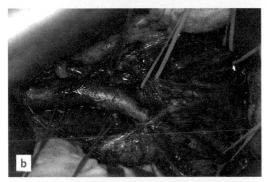

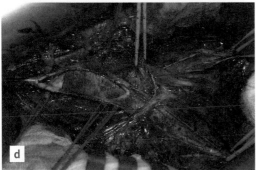

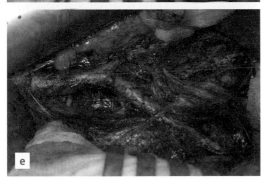

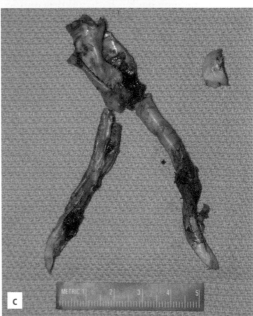

Figure 13.4 (a) Occlusion of the infrarenal aorta and common iliac arteries in a 45-year-old female; MRA. (b) Surgical exposure of the aorta and iliac arteries. (c) Surgical specimen following thromboendarterectomy. (d) Aorta following endarterectomy. (e) Following primary closure of arteriotomy with polypropylene sutures.

with this procedure in 21 patients operated over a 10-year period. In 12 patients, these operations were performed to replace an axillofemoral or axillopopliteal bypass; the remainder were performed following multiple failed attempts at intra-abdominal aortic repair or to avoid abdominal aortic exposure in patients with a hostile abdomen. Surgical technique involved a seventh interspace thoracotomy, a bypass from the descending thoracic aorta to the left femoral artery, and a femoral-femoral crossover graft. There was no operative mortality. Mean hospital length of stay was 15.1 days, including 4.3 days in the intensive care unit. Patency at 4 years was 100%. The authors conclude that this technique is safe and durable, and it is especially useful in patients having had axillofemoral reconstruction for aortic graft infection.

Summary

Diseases of the abdominal aorta are frequently encountered in modern vascular practice. The presence of aortic disease should alert the astute clinician to the presence of atherosclerotic disease of the coronary and cerebrovascular beds. A thorough evaluation, focusing on the multisystem nature of vascular disease, is imperative in the successful long-term management of these patients. The pros and cons, risks/benefits, and long-term results of endovascular and open surgical repair of aortic lesions should be discussed with the patient so that an informed decision can be made regarding type of treatment. A multidisciplinary team of physicians with special interest in peripheral artery disease lends itself to optimal care of these complex patients.

References

1. TASC II. Inter-Society Consensus for the Management of PAD. *J Vasc Surg.* 2007;45:Suppl S.
2. Deriu GP, Ballotta E. Natural history of ascending aortic thrombus of the abdominal aorta. *Am J Surg.* 1983;145:652-657.
3. Babu SC, Shah PM, Nitahara J. Acute aortic occlusion—factors that influence outcome. *J Vasc Surg.* 1995;21:567-575.
4. Valentine RJ, Hansen ME, Myers SI, et al. The influence of sex and aortic size on late patency after aortofemoral revascularization in young adults. *J Vasc Surg.* 1995;21:296-306.
5. van den Bosch MAAJ, van der Graaf Y, Eikelboom BC, et al. Distal aortic diameter and peripheral arterial occlusive disease. *J Vasc Surg.* 2001;34:1085-1089.
6. McPherson SJ, Laing AD, Thomson KR, et al. Treatment of infrarenal aortic stenosis by stent placement: a 6-year experience. *Australas Radiol.* 1999;43:185-191.
7. Elkouri S, Hudon G, Demers P, et al. Early and long-term results of percutaneous transluminal angioplasty of the lower abdominal aorta. *J Vasc Surg.* 1999;30:679-692.
8. de Vries JPPM, van Den Huevel DAF, Vos JA, et al. Freedom from secondary interventions to treat stenotic disease after percutaneous transluminal angioplasty of infrarenal aorta: long-term results. *J Vasc Surg.* 2004;39:427-431.
9. Karnabatidis D, Katsanos K, Kagadis GC, et al. Distal embolism during percutaneous revascularization of infra-aortic arterial occlusive disease: an underestimated phenomenon. *J Endovasc Ther.* 2006;13:269-280.
10. Chaufour X, White GH, Hambly BD, et al. Evaluation of the risks of using an oversized balloon catheter in the human infrarenal abdominal aorta. *Eur J Vasc and Endovasc Surg.* 1998;16:142-147.
11. Kvilekval KHV, Yunis JP, Mason RA, Giron F. After the blue toe: prognosis of noncardiac embolization in the lower extremities. *J Vasc Surg.* 1993;17:328-335.
12. Reber PU, Patel AG, Stauffer E, et al. Mural aortic thrombi: an important cause of peripheral embolization. *J Vasc Surg.* 1999;30:1084-1089.
13. Qvarfordt PG, Reilly LM, Sedwitz MM, et al. Coral reef atherosclerosis of the suprarenal aorta: a unique clinical entity. *J Vasc Surg.* 1984;1:903-909.

14. Bazy L, Reboul H. Technique del'endartériectomie desoblitérante. *J Int Chir.* 1950; 65:196-198.

15. Thompson JE. Early history of aortic surgery. *J Vasc Surg.* 1998;28:746-752.

16. Hertzer NR, Bena JF, Karafa TK. A personal experience with direct reconstruction and extra-anatomic bypass for aortoiliofemoral occlusive disease. *J Vasc Surg.* 2007;45:527-535.

17. de Vries SO, Hunink MGM. Results of aortic bifurcation grafts for aortoiliac occlusive disease; a meta-analysis. *J Vasc Surg.* 1997;26:558-569.

18. Cambria RP, Brewster DC, Abbott WM, et al. Transperitoneal versus retroperitoneal approach for aortic reconstruction: a randomized prospective study. *J Vasc Surg.* 1990;11:314-325.

19. Sicard GA, Reilly JM, Rubin BG, et al. Transabdominal versus retroperitoneal incision for abdominal aortic surgery: report of a prospective randomized trial. *J Vasc Surg.* 1995;21:174-183.

20. Piquet P, Amabile P, Rollet G. Minimally invasive retroperitoneal approach for the treatment of infrarenal aortic disease. *J Vasc Surg.* 2004;40:455-462.

21. Coggia M, Javerliat I, Di Centa I, et al. Total laparoscopic bypass for aortoiliac occlusive lesions: 93-case experience. *J Vasc Surg.* 2004:40;899-906.

22. Naylor AR, Ah-See AK, Engeset J. Aortoiliac endarterectomy: an 11-year review. *Br J Surg.* 1990;77:190-193.

23. Connolly JE, Price T. Aortoiliac endarterectomy: a lost art? *Ann Vasc Surg.* 2006;20:56-62.

24. Louw JH. Splenic-to-femoral and axillary-to-femoral bypass grafts in diffuse atherosclerotic occlusive disease. *Lancet.* 1963;1:1401-1402.

25. Blaisdell FW, Hall AD. Axillary-femoral artery bypass for lower extremity ischemia. *Surgery.* 1963;54:563-568.

26. El-Massry S, Saad E, Sauvage LR, et al. Axillofemoral bypass with externally supported, knitted Dacron grafts: a follow-up through twelve years. *J Vasc Surg.* 1993;17:107-115.

27. Passman MA, Taylor LM, Moneta GL, et al. Comparison of axillofemoral and aortofemoral bypass for aortoiliac occlusive disease. *J Vasc Surg.* 1996;23:263-271.

28. McCarthy WJ, Mesh CL, McMillan WD, et al. Descending thoracic aorta to femoral artery bypass: ten years' experience with a durable procedure. *J Vasc Surg.* 1993;17:336-348.

14

Femoropopliteal Artery Disease

Mitchell J. Silver and Gary M. Ansel

Peripheral artery disease (PAD) of the lower extremities affects a large segment of the adult population, with an age-adjusted prevalence of 12% to 20%.[1,2] PAD, which is strongly age dependent, is increasing in prevalence as the population ages. Data from participants in the Framingham Study, which actually considered incidence as it related to age, found that symptomatic disease onset, as manifest by *intermittent claudication,* increased 10-fold in men from ages 30 to 44 and ages 65 to 74 (with an incidence of 6/10,000 in the former and 61/10,000 in the latter age group). Interestingly, in females, onset increased almost 20-fold from the younger to older age groups (3/10,000, increasing to 54/10,000). It should be noted that the incidence data from the Framingham Study[3] clearly underestimates clinically relevant PAD, as it was limited to symptomatic patients. In fact, data from the Rotterdam Study suggest that the presence of symptoms of intermittent claudication does not have a good predictive value for PAD as defined by noninvasive measurements.[4] The Rotterdam investigators found that only 6.3% of those with an ankle-brachial index (ABI) < 0.9 had classic intermittent claudication. In addition, only 69% of patients with claudication had an ABI of < 0.9.[4] These data illustrate that symptomatic intermittent claudication has only a moderate positive predictive value for the presence of PAD. Asymptomatic PAD is certainly more prevalent than symptomatic disease. Data from the systolic hypertension in the elderly study showed that the ABI was ≤ 0.9 in 25.5% of the 1537 participants.[5] In an ancillary study to the multicenter study of osteoporotic fractures, the ABI was ≤ 0.9 in 5.5% of 1492 women followed in this study.[6]

Pathophysiology

The pathophysiology of the developing atherosclerotic plaque is beyond the scope of this review of *femoropopliteal artery disease.* Instead, a focus on the way in which clinically relevant femoropopliteal artery disease evolves will be detailed.

Atherosclerotic plaque tends to occur on the posterior wall of the lower-extremity arteries. As the plaque matures, circumferential deposition and growth of plaque are common.[7] A very common distribution of atherosclerotic

---

plaque involves the origins of arteries or arterial bifurcations. Common locations for clinically significant atherosclerosis of the lower extremities include the common femoral, distal superficial femoral at the adductor canal, and the tibial-peroneal trunk. Diffuse atherosclerosis is often found along the entire length of the superficial femoral artery, which makes the profundus femoral artery the "lifeline" source of collateral circulation to the lower extremity. As in any artery involved with atherosclerosis, the obstructing plaque becomes flow restrictive, and thrombus may be deposited on the obstructing lesion as well as the adjacent arterial wall. The obstructive plaques become unstable once plaque rupture develops with subsequent intraplaque hemorrhage and thrombosis, ultimately leading to complete closure.[8] In the more common scenario, as atherosclerosis progresses, focal and segmental occlusion of the arterial supply occurs over a chronic period, and perfusion to the lower-extremity skeletal muscle becomes impaired, particularly with walking. Skeletal muscle beds distal to the arterial stenosis or obstruction experience tissue ischemia, the degree of which depends on the location and extent of the arterial occlusion, and most importantly, the status of any collateral vessels. Intermittent claudication most often manifests as calf discomfort with walking, which is most often related to occlusion of the superficial femoral artery. The profundus femoral artery maintains blood flow to the distal tissue beds particularly in chronic progressive superficial femoral artery disease. Most commonly this process is so gradual that the profundus femoral artery collaterals develop to adequately perfuse and maintain the viability of more distal tissue. If there is an acute occlusion, such as thrombosis *in situ* or thrombo-embolism, the onset of symptoms is commonly more severe and dramatic. The geniculate collaterals around the knee also provide an important source of collateral circulation when atherosclerosis more extensively involves both the superficial femoral and popliteal arteries. Because the occlusive process can be so gradual, and the development of collaterals so substantial, patients

may be symptomatic only when walking briskly or over long distances. Critical lower-extremity ischemia such as ischemic rest pain, gangrene, or ischemic ulceration usually occurs when collateral pathways are not developed enough to provide perfusion to maintain tissue viability. This is commonly found when atherosclerosis involves multiple arterial levels, or there is compromise of the collateral circulation, that is, disease of the origin of the profundus femoral artery.

Natural History

Limb-Related Complications

Although a patient with intermittent claudication will fear progression to severe disease and amputation, this is a relatively rare outcome of claudication, with only 1% to 3% of claudicants ever requiring major amputation over a 5-year period. In a study by Cox et al[9] that included 377 patients (520 limbs) with superficial femoral artery disease, the risk for patients requiring surgery or endovascular treatment was 11% at 5 years and 14% at 10 years. In a study from Edinburgh, among those with intermittent claudication at baseline, 8.2% underwent vascular surgery or amputation, and 1.4% developed leg ulceration after 5 years.[10] In regard to the diabetic patient with intermittent claudication, Jonason and Ringquist[11] have studied 224 nondiabetic patients and 47 diabetic patients over a 6-year period. Gangrene occurred in 31% of diabetics as opposed to only 5% of patients without diabetes, and rest pain and/or gangrene occurred in 40% of patients with diabetes mellitus and only in 18% of those without. Interestingly, once a patient manifests the symptom of intermittent claudication, deterioration is most frequent during the first year after diagnosis (6%–9%) compared with 2% to 3% per annum thereafter.

Smoking is the most important risk factor for progression of local disease in the lower extremities, with an amputation rate 11 times greater in smokers than nonsmokers.[12] Diabetes, male gender, and hypertension are also important risk factors for progression.

Long-Term Survival

Intermittent claudication is a marker for a patient's total atherosclerotic burden. In turn, decreases in ABI correlate with long-term cardiovascular mortality (Figure 14.1).[5] Whether PAD is symptomatic or asymptomatic, studies have shown a 20% to 40% increased risk for nonfatal myocardial infarction,[10] a 60% increased risk of progression to congestive heart failure,[13] and a 90% to 500% increased risk of fatal myocardial infarction and coronary artery disease death.[14] Population-based studies and follow-up studies of surgically treated patients indicate that for those individuals with lower-extremity atherosclerosis, the mortality rate at 5 years is approximately 30%, at 10 years 50%, and at 15 years 70% to 75%.[15] It is, therefore, quite evident that intermittent claudication should be regarded as a marker for increased risk from fatal and nonfatal cardiovascular events, and 2% to 4% of claudicants have a nonfatal cardiovascular event every year.

The risk is higher in the first year after developing intermittent claudication than in a long-standing stable claudicant, and the average claudicant is more likely to have a nonfatal myocardial infarction or stroke in the next year than of ever requiring a major amputation for leg ischemia. Certainly these collective data illustrate that there are really 2 important aspects of treating patients with intermittent claudication. The first involves management of leg symptoms and the second involves long-term survival.

Diagnostic Evaluation

History and Physical Examination

It is critical that the initial evaluation of patients with femoropopliteal artery disease include a comprehensive history, including the patient's functional limitations and the presence of ischemic rest pain, nonhealing ulcers, or gangrene. Because intermittent claudication is a marker for systemic atherosclerosis, a thorough review of other atherosclerotic risk factors and screening for aneurysmal disease should be completed.

When both legs and feet are examined and compared with each other, a temperature difference may often be evident. The limb with critical leg ischemia may feel cool, and often an obvious area of demarcation in temperature is present.

A systematic approach should be used to examine all vascular beds in regard to relative strength and quality of arterial pulsation. The presence or absence of arterial bruits should be documented. Leg raising may manifest significant pallor in the patient with significant PAD, and change to rubor in the dependent position. A comparison of blood pressures of the upper extremities should be routinely performed. A sensory examination is very useful, particularly in the diabetic population, where impairment in sensing vibration, pain, and light touch is prevalent.

After the history and physical examination, noninvasive studies should be obtained to provide a more objective and quantitative assessment of the degree of ischemia. The decision about which noninvasive test to perform is dictated in part by the acuity and severity of

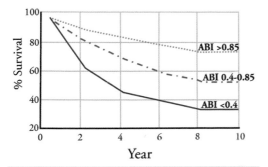

Figure 14.1 Survival according to ankle-brachial index (ABI). (From McKenna M, Wolfson S, Kuller L. The ratio of ankle and arm arterial pressure as an independent predictor of mortality. *Atherosclerosis.* 1991;87:119-128. Reprinted with permission from Elsevier.)

the ischemia. The minimal assessment should include interrogation of the distal artery with a continuous-wave handheld Doppler and measurement of the ABI. An abnormal ABI will also predict a future risk of cardiovascular morbidity and mortality.[16]

Noninvasive Studies

Continuous-Wave Doppler

The audible signal of continuous-wave, nondirectional handheld Doppler can provide useful information. Normal arterial signals are biphasic or triphasic.[17] The first sound corresponds to high-velocity forward flow during systole. The second sound results from reverse flow in early diastole. The third sound represents forward flow in late diastole. In the presence of extremity ischemia, peripheral resistance falls and the

second sound disappears. As ischemia worsens, the signal will become monophasic or absent (Figure 14.2).

Ankle-Brachial Index and Segmental Pressures

The simplest vascular laboratory test for lower-extremity circulation is the ankle-brachial index (ABI). The equipment is inexpensive and consists of an ordinary blood pressure cuff and a Doppler ultrasonic velocity detector. The ABI is obtained by measuring the highest pressure at the ankle using a continuous-wave Doppler and dividing it by the highest arm pressure. The normal ABI averages 1.1 because the pressure in the ankle is 12 to 24 mm greater than the arm in the supine position.[17] The ABI determines whether hemodynamically significant arterial disease is present. A normal ABI makes significant disease unlikely. If the ABI is normal and the clinical index of suspicion remains high, the

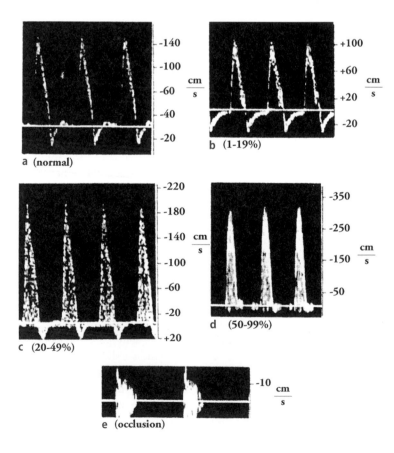

Figure 14.2
Lower-extremity duplex scan velocity patterns seen with varying degrees of involvement with atherosclerosis. (From Silver MJ, Ansel GM. Femoropopliteal occlusive disease: diagnosis, indications for treatment, and results of interventional therapy. *Cather Cardiovasc Interv.* 2002;56:555-561. Reprinted with permission.)

ABI should be repeated after exercise. The increased flow generated by exercise accentuates the pressure drop across a fixed stenosis (Figure 14.3). Medial calcification, as seen in diabetics, results in noncompressible vessels and is one cause of spurious elevated ankle pressures.

Segmental pressures can be measured by placing blood pressure cuffs at the high thigh, calf, and ankle levels to determine the level of occlusive disease. A pressure drop greater than 15 mm Hg from one site to the next suggests that a hemodynamically significant stenosis is present in the artery with the lower pressure.[17]

Pulse Volume Recording

The pulse volume recording (PVR) relies on air plethysmography to produce waveforms that correlate with pulsatile arterial flow. The PVR is particularly useful in 2 settings. The transmetatarsal PVR is helpful in determining the need

Before exercise   **After exercise**

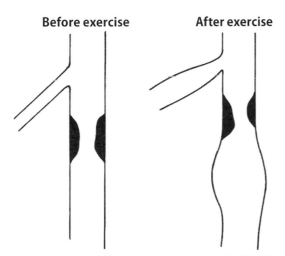

Figure 14.3 At rest (left) there is an area of obstruction that is not severe enough to cause an abnormality in pressure distal to the obstruction. Therefore, the pulses and blood pressure at rest are normal. Exercise increases the metabolic demand to the muscles. However, the obstruction only allows oxygen to be delivered at a fixed rate. In an attempt to compensate, more blood is shunted in the collateral vessels proximal to the obstruction. The vessels distal to the obstruction dilate so less blood is delivered to dilated segments of the distal vessels and the pressure decreases. (From Krajewski LP, Oin JW. Atherosclerosis of the aorta and lower extremity arteries. *Peripheral Vascular Diseases*, 2nd ed. Philadelphia: CV Mosby; 1996:208-233. With permission from Elsevier.)

for revascularization in the diabetic patient with a foot ulcer or gangrene who has a spuriously elevated ABI. The absence of pulsatile arterial flow on PVR in such a patient would indicate severe arterial obstruction. The PVR is also a valuable tool following revascularization, which when performed immediately before and after intervention, can detect an improvement or deterioration in pulsatile arterial flow.

Duplex Ultrasonography

Duplex ultrasonography can assess both arterial anatomy and physiology by combining a real-time, high-resolution image of the vessel wall and lumen with Doppler signal analysis. The ultrasound image is able to localize plaque and characterize its morphology. In addition, other abnormalities such as intraluminal thrombus, intraplaque hemorrhage, aneurysmal disease, or dissection can be characterized using ultrasound imaging. The Doppler analysis includes 3 components: spectral analysis, velocity waveforms, and color-flow imaging. Spectral analysis detects stenosis by identifying abnormalities in blood-flow patterns. Due to the interruption of laminar flow, more random movements of red blood cells occur, and these movements create spectra with wider ranges of frequencies and amplitudes. *Spectral broadening* is a term used to describe the resultant wider frequency ban. Specific criteria have been established for calculating the percent diameter reduction for both the carotid circulation and lower-extremity lesions based on spectral analysis of pulse Doppler signals. Color-flow imaging provides flow information of the entire image in real time. The specific information produced by the color includes the direction of flow and the estimate of the mean frequency. Importantly, color-flow imaging does not allow a precise calculation of the degree of stenosis, as does spectral analysis. In regard to velocity waveforms, a normal lower-extremity artery has a triphasic waveform that corresponds to the audible Doppler signal previously described. With a severe degree of stenosis, the waveform distal to the stenosis becomes monophasic, with a low, rounded peak.

The waveform within the stenosis, on the other hand, would demonstrate a markedly increased peak systolic velocity. For the hemodynamically significant lesions (> 50%), the increase in peak velocity will be > 100% in the stenosis, with loss of reverse flow and the presence of marked spectral broadening.

Magnetic Resonance Imaging

Magnetic resonance imaging (MRI) has been receiving increased attention for studying the peripheral circulation. MRI forms an image of blood flow based on physical differences between moving and stationary protons. The signal intensity is a reflection of the velocity and flow pattern of moving protons within the bloodstream. MRI continues to be plagued by overestimating the degree of stenosis that is present in some vascular beds.

Postprocedure Testing

Lower-extremity duplex scanning is very valuable in the follow-up of patients after endovascular revascularization. As the indications for femoropopliteal artery disease angioplasty and stenting continue to broaden, the noninvasive follow-up of patients following revascularization is extremely important for the early detection of recurrent lesions or restenosis. Importantly, neither clinical symptoms nor the standard ABI are as sensitive as duplex scanning for the detection of recurrent disease or restenosis.[18] A peak systolic velocity > 200 cm/sec, or flow velocities < 45 cm/sec, is quite indicative of a stenosis of ≥ 50%. As the use of self-expanding nitinol stents is becoming more widespread for long occlusive femoropopliteal artery disease, postprocedure testing should include an ABI evaluation prior to discharge, then duplex scanning at 3-, 6-, and 12-month periods. A strict duplex surveillance program should lead to secondary patency rates in excess of 90%.

In a series of 333 patients who underwent femoropopliteal intervention, followed by rigorous duplex ultrasound-based surveillance, to detect restenosis ≥ 80%, the peak systolic velocity was most predictive when ≥ 275 cm/sec with a systolic velocity ratio ≥ 3.5.[19]

Invasive Evaluation

Diagnostic angiography should be considered in a patient who has symptomatic disease, including those with severe lifestyle-limiting claudication, ischemic rest pain, or tissue loss.[20] Currently, with the evolution of endovascular techniques, the safety of diagnostic angiography and femoropopliteal revascularization, even in high-risk patients, has significantly improved, with a major complication rate with an endovascular approach of < 1%. Because of this, the superior safety of an endovascular approach has overridden the continued controversy regarding the long-term efficacy of endovascular versus surgical revascularization. Therefore, the shift in the risk versus benefit ratio provided by endovascular revascularization of the femoropopliteal segment has resulted in a broader population of patients, with less-severe symptoms, to be considered for treatment.

Normal Anatomy

The superficial femoral artery originates in the femoral triangle as a direct continuation of the common femoral artery. The profunda femoral artery typically arises from the posterolateral side of the common femoral artery fairly high in the femoral triangle. The profundus femoral artery is the chief supply to the muscles of the thigh, although the common femoral artery itself gives off occasional small, muscular branches. The superficial femoral artery lies anterior, and medial, to the profundus femoral artery (Figure 14.4). In its proximal extent, the superficial femoral artery courses through the femoral triangle as it reaches the adductor canal. The adductor longus muscle separates the profundus branches from the superficial femoral artery branches. The superficial femoral artery traverses the adductor canal through the tendinous opening in the adductor magnus muscle to reach the popliteal fossa, located in the distal portion of the posterior surface of the femur. Once it emerges from the adductor canal, into the popliteal fossa, the superficial femoral artery becomes the popliteal artery. Atherothrombosis of the superficial femoral artery very frequently starts at the level of the tendinous hiatus and apparently originates as a result of trauma to the vessel wall by the tendon of the adductor magnus.

Important Collateral Circulation

The integrity of the profundus femoral artery should always be evaluated during diagnostic angiography as it is an important collateral vessel to the lower extremity. This is extremely important especially when considering endovascular treatment of the ostium of the superficial femoral artery.

The 2 largest branches of the profundus femoral artery are the lateral and medial femoral circumflex vessels. The *lateral femoral circumflex artery* typically arises from the lateral side of the upper end of the profunda, but in up to 15% of individuals, it arises from the common femoral artery above the profundus femoral artery. The *medial femoral circumflex artery* typically arises from the medial or posteromedial side of the profundus femoral artery, and turns posteriorly between the iliopsoas and pectineus muscles. Perforating muscular branches often originate from the profundus femoral artery in its distal aspect providing perfusion to the muscles of the thigh. Proximally, the medial and lateral circumflex branches have anastomotic connections to the internal iliac artery. Distally, usually the lateral circumflex artery has connections to the collateral circulation at the knee joint, which have connections to the popliteal and tibial arteries. The superficial femoral artery gives off the descending genicular branch, proximal to the adductor canal, which provides an important collateral channel to the infrapopliteal vessels.

Common Variations

Up to 15% of the time, the medial and lateral circumflex femoral branches will arise directly from the common femoral artery. Some individuals may have nonpalpable dorsalis pedis pulses with otherwise normal lower-extremity arterial perfusion. This is most often the result of an anomaly of the infrapopliteal anatomy.[21]

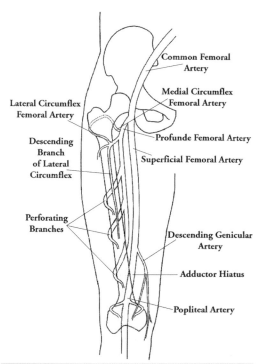

Figure 14.4 Anatomic depiction of superficial femoral artery and major tributaries (right leg).

Labels in figure:
- Common Femoral Artery
- Medial Circumflex Femoral Artery
- Lateral Circumflex Femoral Artery
- Descending Branch of Lateral Circumflex
- Profunde Femoral Artery
- Superficial Femoral Artery
- Perforating Branches
- Descending Genicular Artery
- Adductor Hiatus
- Popliteal Artery

Therapeutic Options

Medical Therapy

Medical therapy for PAD should encompass both symptomatic relief and risk factor modification. In regard to lower-extremity symptoms, 5% to 10% of asymptomatic patients with PAD will become symptomatic over 5 years.[22] Although PAD typically presents with a slow and low rate of local symptoms and complications, it definitely is balanced by ongoing atherogenesis in other vascular territories with a very high rate of mortality (25%–30% within 5 years in symptomatic patients) due mainly to myocardial infarction and stroke.[23]

Improving Leg Symptoms

In patients with stable intermittent claudication, a supervised walking program significantly improves maximal walking time and distance.[24] Walking through the discomfort of claudication is not harmful, and will usually gradually increase walking distance.

A significant role for pharmacotherapy in treating the lower-extremity symptoms of claudication has emerged for the agent cilostazol. Cilostazol has been studied in over 12,000 patients worldwide, and data demonstrate a marked improvement in walking distance over both placebo and pentoxifylline (Table 14.1).[25,26]

Atherosclerotic Risk Factor Modification

Smoking cessation reduces cardiovascular death and improves overall survival at 10 years in the claudicant population.[12] Multiple clinical trials, including the Heart Outcomes Prevention Evaluation (HOPE) and the Appropriate Blood Pressure Control in Diabetes (ABCD) trials have shown that more intensive blood pressure treatment is more effective in patients with PAD than less-intensive blood pressure lowering.[27] The importance of statin therapy in individuals at high vascular risk, irrespective of the initial lipid profile, is reinforced by a large meta-analysis.[28] Antiplatelet therapy should be used in all patients with PAD who do not have a contraindication. Numerous clinical data are available that demonstrate antiplatelet therapy in patients at high risk of atherosclerotic vascular disease reduces the risk of myocardial infarction, stroke, or cardiovascular death by about 25% (Table 14.1).[29]

Surgical Revascularization

Historically, patients with diffuse femoropopliteal artery disease and limb-threatening ischemia have been treated surgically. Prior to the placement of an infrainguinal bypass, the inflow and outflow vessels must be assessed and

Indication	Intervention	Method/Comment
Improving leg symptoms	Smoking cessation	Physician advice Nicotine replacement therapy Bupropion
	Exercise	Consider structured exercise program
	Statin drugs	Benefit appears to be related to noncholesterol-lowering properties of statins
	Blood pressure-lowering drugs	Angiotensin-converting enzyme inhibitors
	Cilostazol	Contraindicated in patients with heart failure
Preventing systemic complications	Smoking cessation	
	Weight loss	Consider in overweight patients with peripheral arterial disease
	Lowering blood pressure	Effect determined by magnitude of blood pressure-lowering effects
	Angiotensin-converting enzyme inhibitors	Possible benefits beyond blood pressure-lowering effects
	Lowering blood cholesterol level	
	Antiplatelet therapy	Aspirin, with clopidogrel as suitable alternative

Table 14.1 Medical Treatment of PAD (From Hankey GJ, Norman PE, Eikelboom JW. Medical treatment of peripheral arterial disease. *JAMA.* 2006;295[5]:547-553. Copyright © 2006 American Medical Association. All rights reserved.)

optimized. Inflow procedures for aortoiliac disease, if needed, must be addressed before going on to either prosthetic or venous infrainguinal bypass. Even minor disease proximal to an infrainguinal bypass graft has been correlated with a decrease in long-term graft patency due to disease progression.[30] Infrainguinal grafts appear to demonstrate improved patency if the proximal anastomosis is made to the native vessel rather than to a proximal graft segment.[31] Patency of infrainguinal bypasses also appears to be improved by extending the graft to the least diseased distal arterial segment even if this extends below the knee in the case of venous conduits.[32,33]

In situ vein or reversed saphenous vein bypass have been shown to outperform prosthetic grafts in the infrainguinal locations. Above-knee expanded polytetrafluoroethylene (ePTFE) grafting in properly selected patient populations is an acceptable alternative.[34] However, extending below the knee joint with the currently available prosthetic grafts is associated with inferior results (4-year primary patency rates of ~ 40%).[35] All variations of vein conduit, including contralateral saphenous vein, arm vein, superficial femoral vein, and spliced combinations, have shown better results than prosthetic materials. However, there is some evidence that heparin-bounded grafts are showing improved results with patency rates approaching that of veins in midterm follow-up.[36-38] Comparison of graft patencies to endoluminal techniques is problematic since the definition of graft patency in the surgical literature has been so heterogeneous.

Maintenance of graft patency without occlusion is very important for long-term patency of venous conduits. Classic teaching is that all venous bypasses should undergo a regular regime of duplex scanning with intervention prior to failure.[39,40] However, randomized data has not confirmed this teaching.[41] Surveillance of prosthetic grafts has also not been as conclusively proven.[42,43] Lesions will usually occur in the body of the venous graft, while prosthetic grafts usually develop lesions at the anastomoses. Surveillance programs should be started immediately postoperatively and continued at regular intervals.

Postbypass antiplatelet therapy in the form of ASA (acetylsalicylic acid) has been shown to be beneficial though somewhat more important in the prosthetic graft.[44] Early data on the use of more aggressive therapy with ticlopidine appears to also show benefit.[45]

Currently, the indications for infrainguinal surgical bypass include vocation-limiting claudication and limb-threatening ischemia. Broadening of the indications would be difficult due the associated surgical morbidities such as infection (15%–25%) and mortality (1%–2%).[46]

Endovascular Revascularization

The surgical morbidity and mortality associated with femoropopliteal artery disease have led to a surge in the use of percutaneous endovascular techniques, which by their nature are inherently lower-risk procedures. Typically endovascular procedures employ one or multiple techniques, including balloon angioplasty, stents, stent grafts, laser, and atherectomy. Controversy over the actual indications exists due to the paucity of reliable controlled and comparable outcome data. However, the BASIL trial has shown the clinical utility of a percutaneous approach for patients with critical limb ischemia (CLI).[47] The use of any technology in the femoropopliteal arterial segment will be challenging since this area is unique in that it experiences a multitude of external forces, including compression, elongation, and twisting.

The application of the various endovascular techniques in the appropriate patient population certainly may affect procedure durability. Variables that may affect outcome durability include lesion length, vessel diameter, diabetes, renal insufficiency, smoking, and quality of distal runoff.[48,49]

Percutaneous Transluminal Angioplasty and Cryoplasty

Closely examining previous controlled endovascular trials can assist in defining the durability for balloon angioplasty. The IntraCoil stent versus balloon angioplasty femoropopliteal trial allowed for lesion lengths up to 16 cm.[50] However, investigators usually enrolled patients with focal disease leading to a short average lesion length of 3.3 cm. The 9-month angiographic restenosis (≥ 50%) rate for the balloon control arm was 33.7%. The Peripheral Arteries Radiation Investigational Study (PARIS) trial compared stand-alone percutaneous transluminal angioplasty (PTA) to PTA with adjunctive brachytherapy.[51] With an average lesion length of 5.8 cm the 9-month angiographic restenosis rate for stand-alone PTA was 28%. Cejna et al[52] randomized patients to PTA or Palmaz stenting for lesions < 5 cm. The 1-year angiographic restenosis rate for the balloon arm was 47%. For more diffuse femoropopliteal artery disease the results of balloon angioplasty have been best characterized by the Vienna-3 (brachytherapy) and Peripheral Excimer Laser Angioplasty (PELA) trials. The Vienna-3 trial, with a mean lesion length of 10.3 cm, showed the 12-month angiographic restenosis rate for stand-alone PTA to be 64%.[53] The PELA trial with the longest and most complex lesion lengths (20-cm occlusions) demonstrated a 9-month restenosis rate for PTA of 85%.[54]

Registry data evaluating the use of near-freezing balloon technology (cryoplasty) has been published. This system has been shown in laboratory data to bring about apoptosis (planned cell death), which may limit intimal hyperplasia. This registry allowed for up to 10-cm lesions (mean enrolled lesion length 4.7 cm) and showed the 9-month, duplex-controlled restenosis rate to be similar to plain balloon angioplasty of short lesions, that is, 30%.[55]

In order to improve procedural and long-term patency, some have espoused the technique of subintimal angioplasty. This technique establishes a channel between the intima and media with wire re-entry into the native vessel lumen beyond the distal edge of the occlusion. A meta-analysis of 23 studies, including over 1500 patients, resulted in technical success of 80% to 90% and primary patency at 1 year of only 50%, with procedural complication rates between 8% and 17%.[56]

Excimer Laser and Directional Atherectomy

Atherectomy and excimer laser have been shown to be excellent tools for debulking; unfortunately neither have shown any improved patency over balloon angioplasty.[57-59]

The role of these devices is yet to be fully defined, but certainly they may play a role in areas where current technology options are limited, such as the common femoral, ostial superficial femoral, and popliteal vessels. Broader application of atherectomy may be affected by the risk of embolization and perforation inherent in the procedure.

Bare Metal Stents

Bare metal stents have been utilized in an effort to decrease clinically significant restenosis by increasing the postprocedural vessel luminal diameter (Figure 14.5). Early stainless steel stents did not show much clinical utility for a multitude of reasons, including poor study design.[60,61] The first FDA-approved stent for the femoropopliteal arterial bed was a nitinol coil stent. This stent in a randomized study against balloon angioplasty did not show a restenosis benefit but did show that a primary stent approach was associated with a lower complication rate (1.8% vs. 8.7%).[35] More promising results have been reported for tubular nitinol stents.[62] However, not all of the available tubular nitinol stents appear to act the same after placement. Some nitinol stents experience a clinically relevant higher rate and complexity of stent fracture. European data certainly suggest that some nitinol stents may develop less-clinically significant simple strut fractures, while others appear to be prone to complex fractures that result in decreased patency.[63,64] In general, nitinol stents have demonstrated good clinical utility and acceptable restenosis rates at short- and midterm follow-up.

In a randomized trial of a nitinol stent

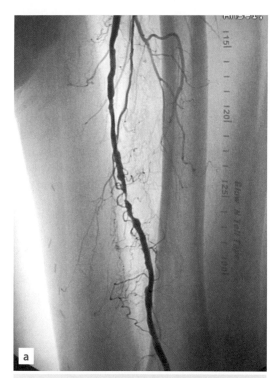

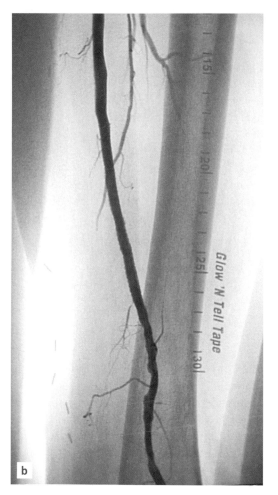

Figure 14.5 (a) Present angiography demonstrating diffuse femoropopliteal disease. (b) Angiogram post-stent demonstrating significant luminal gain.

compared to percutaneous transluminal angioplasty in relatively short lesions (mean lesion length 4.5 cm), there was no improvement in patency at 1 year or target lesion revascularization in the stent-treated patients.[65] However, in a randomized trial of a different nitinol stent compared to balloon angioplasty, patency and exercise tolerance were superior at 1 year in those patients treated with stents.[66] Interestingly, at 2 years, the patency advantage of nitinol stents was preserved, but the exercise improvement was lost.[67]

The longest follow-up of nitinol stent fractures suggested that in 239 patients, stent fracture resulted in significant reduction in primary patency at 2 years of follow-up. However, at 4 years, there was no further deterioration in patency. The multicenter Bilateral Lower Arterial Stenting Employing Reopro (BLASTER) study of complex superficial femoral disease showed a 9-month duplex restenosis rate of 24%.[68] Functional outcome was improved as well with

significantly improved treadmill study in 88% of patients.[69] Prospective longer-term data on these nitinol tubular stents has been lacking. One retrospective study of long lesions (> 10 cm) with duplex follow-up appears to show an approximately 40% restenosis rate at 2 years.[70] The addition of the restenosis-inhibiting agent sirolimus to a self-expanding nitinol stent has demonstrated early but not sustained significant benefit possibly due to problematic drug elution rates and better-than-expected results with bare nitinol stents.[71,72] Randomized studies of more flexible and possibly fracture-resistant stents and stents with other types of drug elution such as paclitaxel are currently underway. Longer-term follow-up > 2 years is needed to more fully assess the role of stents in this vascular bed.

Covered Stents

Covered stents were originally utilized for exclusion of arterial aneurysm. However, interest in covered stents for atherosclerotic disease has emerged in an effort to improve longer-term restenosis rates (Figure 14.6). The potential uses for a covered stent include the treatment of aneurysms, *de novo* atherosclerotic lesions, in-stent restenosis, treatment of a failing surgical bypass, and percutaneous extravascular arterial bypass. Early covered stents included devices such as the Cragg system (Min Tec)

and Wallgraft (Boston Scientific) for the treatment of atherosclerotic disease. Clinical efficacy in the femoropopliteal artery was suboptimal, with low patency and significant thrombosis rates.[73,74] The early covering materials such as Dacron seem to elicit a significant inflammatory response with associated poor patency rate and high thrombosis rate.[75]

Subsequently, most industry attention has been directed to the use of stents covered with polytetrafluoroethylene (PTFE). The efficacy of PTFE in surgical bypass is well documented, and

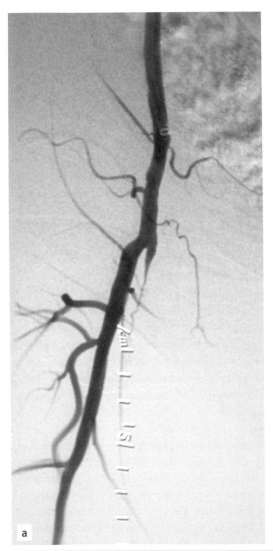
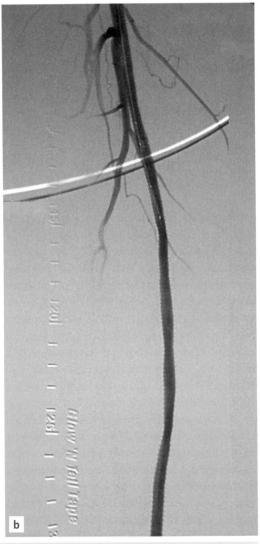

Figure 14.6 (a) Preprocedure angiogram demonstrating long, diffuse total occlusion of the superficial femoral artery. **(b)** Poststent graft angiography demonstrating reestablishment of flow.

this material has shown favorable tissue interaction. Complete neointima formation has been documented, though for long-segment disease this process may take many months.[76] Up until recently there were 3 PTFE-covered stents commercially available in the United States: the biliary-approved Fluency (C.R. Bard), the FDA-approved VIABAHN (W.L. Gore and Associates), and the recently discontinued spiral configured aSpire (Vascular Architects).

An international feasibility trial of the earlier version of the current VIABAHN named the Hemobahn (W.L. Gore and Associates) was associated with very high technical success and a 79% primary patency at 1 year.[77] Though no large multicenter randomized trial results have been published evaluating the current VIABAHN stent graft, several published registries have reported 1- and 2-year patencies of approximately 82% and 77%, respectively.[78-80] Though the majority of patients in these studies were claudicants, the lesions were complex, with average lesion lengths > 10 cm. In contrast are 4 studies that have shown poor results with short-term patencies of < 70%, however, these studies have many procedural shortcomings, including not covering the entire angioplasty zone, ballooning outside the area of stent deployment, heavily calcified lesions, poor runoff (< 1–2 vessels), suboptimal antiplatelet therapy, and limited balloon dilation poststent deployment.[81-83] More recent prospective data have shown comparable results in short lesions (mean < 5 cm) in both the iliac and femoropopliteal segments.[84] Surgical series typically enter patients with a preponderance of CLI, so the findings in many of these series that appear to compare very favorably with prosthetic femoropopliteal bypass must be kept in perspective. There are 3 small published series that have evaluated the VIABAHN PTFE-covered stent in patient populations with primarily CLI. Railo et al,[85] in a small series of 15 patients (73% with CLI) with relatively short lesions (4–10 cm) reported a primary patency at 1 and 2 years of 93% and 84%, respectively. Bauermeister[86] evaluated the use of the VIABAHN in 35 patients with more diffuse disease, with a mean lesion length of 22 cm (74% with CLI). In this series 40% also underwent common femoral surgical patching, and 20% ring-stripper disobliteration showed a 1-year primary patency of 73% by duplex scanning. The only randomized comparison of claudicants versus CLI treated with the Hemobahn reported similar 1-year primary patencies of 81.3% and 88.9%, respectively. The average lesion lengths were similar at 9.8 cm and 11.7 cm, respectively. The tibial outflow status and treatment were significantly different between these 2 groups. Poor runoff defined as 0 to 1 patent tibial vessel was present in only 18.7% of the claudicants, whereas 88.9% of the CLI group had poor runoff. Outflow treatment was completed in only 6.3% of the claudicants versus 66.7% of the CLI cohort.[87]

The etiology of endovascular procedure failure is related to the amount of time that has lapsed since the procedure. Early procedural failure may be related to lack of periprocedural anticoagulation, hypercoagulable state, hypoperfusion, or hypotension. Technical failure may include suboptimal lesion dilation, stent-graft oversizing leading to material redundancy, and unrecognized proximal or distal dissection. These failures can be minimized by appropriate sizing of balloons, stents, and stent grafts and covering all dilated areas with stents or stent grafts. Pressure gradient measurement may be utilized to assess adequacy of lesion treatment.

An intermediate time for procedural failure (6–24 months) is most commonly due to excessive intimal hyperplasia within bare metal stents and at the ends of stent grafts. Late stent-graft failure is commonly secondary to progression of proximal or distal vascular occlusive disease.

Technical Considerations

Though possibly more important for stent grafts, as with surgical grafts adequate inflow is important for any endovascular femoropopliteal procedure. Iliac disease should be treated before undertaking the femoropopliteal segment.

Status of distal runoff vessels has been shown to affect the durability of endovascular procedures. Intervention with 2- to 3-vessel distal runoff is associated with significant improvement in patency compared to patients with 0- to 1-vessel runoff.[88,89] Tibial patency that is usually present in claudicants may explain why both surgical and endovascular procedures appear to be more durable in this population.

Data on crossing the knee with bare metal stents are insufficient presently for evaluation. However, anatomic position is an important consideration with stent grafts. Though not currently studied in the occlusive disease population, studies evaluating covered stent grafting of popliteal aneurysms have seen stent-graft occlusion to occur in 20% to 22% (1 year).[90,91] One must weigh the risk/benefit of crossing a diseased but potential collateral source in order to end the stent graft in a less-diseased, more distal vessel.

Special attention to antiplatelet therapy may be beneficial, though comparative data are lacking. A placebo-controlled randomized trial comparing nitinol stenting with abciximab showed no benefit to this aggressive approach beyond aspirin and clopidogrel.[69]

Emerging Therapies

Recently there has been increasing enthusiasm for the use of percutaneous transluminal angioplasty with balloons coated with antirestenosis agents. Obvious advantages include the lack of need for placement of metallic stents in segments of the femoropopliteal arteries and impregnating a drug at the angioplasty site that will theoretically prolong the durability of procedures. Two publications using balloon catheters coated with paclitaxel demonstrated encouraging results when compared to bare balloons. In the Local Taxan with Short Time Exposure for Reduction of Restenosis in Distal Arteries (THUNDER) trial, 154 patients were randomly assigned to 1 of 3 strategies: bare balloon, bare balloon with paclitaxel dissolved in contrast media, and a paclitaxel-coated balloon. The late lumen loss was significantly lower in the segments treated with the coated balloon for mean lesion lengths of 7.5 cm.[92] In a second study, 87 patients were randomized to bare balloon versus paclitaxel-coated balloon, and in mean lesion lengths ranging from 5.7 to 6.1 cm, late lumen loss and target lesion revascularization were significantly lower in the coated balloon-treated segments.[93]

Many trials using different drug and coating technologies are currently being planned, and these investigations may result in a significant alteration in treatment strategies for patients with femoropopliteal artery disease.

Summary

Endovascular revascularization techniques continue to evolve. Angioplasty has been the cornerstone of therapy but randomized trials have demonstrated superiority of both stents and stent grafts. However, patency of stents and stent grafts is still suboptimal and techniques of successfully treating restenosis have yet to be defined. Other, more niche techniques have been successfully utilized but currently there is no randomized data to allow us to compare to even angioplasty or stents. Drug-eluting balloons and possible stents are currently being studies with positive early trials.

References

1. Hiatt WR, Marshall JA, Baxter J, et al. Diagnostic methods for peripheral arterial disease in the San Luis Valley Diabetes Study. *J Clin Epidemiol.* 1990;43:597-606.

2. Crigni MH, Frank A, Barret-Connor E, Klauber MR, Gabriel S, Goodman D. The prevalence of peripheral arterial disease in a defined population. *Circulation.* 1985;71:510-515.

3. Kannel W, Skinner JJ, Schwartz M, et al. Intermittent claudications: incidence in the Framingham Study. *Circulation.* 1970;41:875-883.

4. Meijer WT, Hoes AW, Rutgers D, et al. Peripheral arterial disease in the elderly: the Rotterdam Study. *Arterioscler Thromb Vasc Biol.* 1998;18:185-192.

5.   Newman AB, Sutton-Tyrrell K, Vogt MT, Kuller LH. Morbidity and mortality in hypertensive adults with a low ankle/arm blood pressure index. *JAMA*. 1993;270:487-489.

6.   Vogt MT, Cauley JA, Newman AB, Kuller LH, Hulley SB. Decreased ankle/arm blood pressure index and mortality in elderly women. *JAMA*. 1993;270:465-469.

7.   Stary HC. Natural History and Histologic Classification of Atherosclerotic Lesions: an Update. *Arterioscler Thromb Vasc Biol*. 2000 May; 20(5): 1177-1178.

8.   Mecley M, Rosenfield K, Kaufman J, Langevin RE Jr, Razvi S, Isner JM. Atherosclerotic plaque hemorrhage and rupture associated with crescendo claudication. *Ann Intern Med*. 1992;117:663-666.

9.   Cox GS, Hertzer NR, Young JR, et al. Non-operative treatment of superficial femoral artery disease: long term follow-up. *J Vasc Surg*. 1993;17:172-182.

10. Leng GC, Lee AJ, Fowkes FG, et al. Incidence, natural history and cardiovascular events in symptomatic and asymptomatic peripheral arterial disease in the general population. *Int J Epidemiol*.1996;25:1172-1181.

11. Jonason T, Ringquist I. Diabetes mellitus and intermittent claudication. Relation between peripheral vascular complications and location of occlusive atherosclerosis in the legs. *Acta Med Scand*. 1985;218:217-221.

12. Jonason T, Bergstrom R. Cessation of smoking in patients with intermittent claudication: effects on the risk of peripheral vascular complications, myocardial infarction, and mortality. *Acta Med Scand*. 1987;221:253-260.

13. Newman A, Shemanski L, Manolio T, et al. Ankle-arm index as a predictor of cardiovascular disease and mortality in the cardiovascular health study. *Arterioscler Thromb Vasc Biol*. 1999;19:538-545.

14. Kornitzer M, Dramaix M, Sobolski, J, et al. Ankle-arm pressure index in asymptomatic middle-aged males: an independent predictor of ten-year coronary heart disease mortality. *Angiology*. 1995;46:211-219.

15. Coffman JD. Intermittent claudication: not so benign. *Am Heart J*. 1986;112:1127.

16. Vogt MT, McKenna M, Wolfson SK, Kuller LH. The relationship between ankle brachial index, other atherosclerotic disease, diabetes, smoking and mortality in older men and women. *Atherosclerosis*. 1993:101:191-202.

17. Summer D. Objective diagnostic techniques: the role of the vascular laboratory. In: Rutherford R, ed. *Vascular Surgery*. Philadelphia: W.B. Saunders; 1989:110-111.

18. Idu MM, Blankenstein JD, de Gies P. Impact of a color flow duplex surveillance program on infrainguinal vein graft patency: a five year experience. *J Vasc Surg*. 1993;17:42-53.

19. Baril DT, Rhee RY, Kim J, et al. Duplex criteria for determination of in-stent stenosis after angioplasty and stenting of the superficial femoral artery. *J Vasc Surg*. 2009;49:133-139.

20. Dormandy JA, Rutherford RB. Management of peripheral arterial disease. TASC working group. TransAtlantic Inter-Society Consensus (TASC). *J Vasc Surg*. 2000;31:51-S296.

21. Kim D, Orron DE, Skillman JJ. Surgical significance of popliteal arterial variants and a unified angiographic classification. *Ann Surg*. 1989;210:776.

22. Hooi JD, Stoffers HE, Knottnerus JA, van Ree JW. The prognosis of non-critical leg ischemia: a systematic review of population-based epidemiological evidence. *Br J Gen Pract*. 1999:490:49-55.

23. Crigui M, Langer R, Fronck A, et al. Mortality over a period of 10 years in patients with peripheral arterial disease. *N Engl J Med*. 1992;326:381-386.

24. Leng GC, Fowler B, Ernst E. Exercise for intermittent claudication. *Cochrane Database Syst Rev*. 2000; (2):CD000990 doi:10.1002/14651858.

25. Dawson DL, Cutler BS, Meissner MH, et al. Cilostazol has beneficial effects in treatment of intermittent claudication. *Circulation*. 1998;98:678-686.

26. Money JR, Herd JA, Isaacsohn JL, et al. Effect of Cilostazol on walking distances in patients with intermittent claudication caused by peripheral vascular disease. *J Vasc Surg*. 1998;28:267-275.

27. Mehler PS, Coll JR, Estacia R, Esler A, Schrier

RW, Hiatt WR. Intensive blood pressure control reduces the risk of cardiovascular events in patients with peripheral arterial disease and type 2 diabetes. *Circulation*. 2003; 107:753-756.

28. Cholesterol Treatment Trialists (CTT) Collaborators. Efficacy and safety of cholesterol lowering treatment: prospective meta analysis of data from 90,056 participants in 14 randomized trials of statins. *Lancet*. 2005;366:1267-1278.

29. Antithrombotic Trialists Collaboration. Collaborative meta analysis of randomized trials of antiplatelet therapy for prevention of antiplatelet therapy for infarction and stroke in high risk patients. *BMJ*. 2002;324:71-81.

30. Rosenbloom MS, Walsh JJ, Schuler JJ, et al. Long-term results of infragenicular bypasses with autologous vein originating from the distal superficial femoral and popliteal arteries. *J Vasc Surg*. 1988;7:691-696.

31. Lam E, Landry G. Risk factors for autogenous infrainguinal bypass occlusion in patients with prosthetic inflow grafts. *J Vasc Surg*. 2004;39:336-342.

32. Conti MS, Belkin M, Donaldson MC, et al. Femorotibial bypass claudication: do results justify an aggressive approach? *J Vasc Surg*. 1995;21:873-880.

33. Veith FJ, Gupta SK, Ascer E, et al. Six-year prospective multicenter randomized comparison of autologous saphenous vein and expanded polytetrafluoroethylene grafts in infrainguinal arterial reconstruction. *J Vasc Surg*. 1986;3:104-114.

34. Hunink MGM, Wong JB, Donaldson MC, et al. Patency results of percutaneous and surgical revascularization from femoropopliteal arterial disease. *Med Decis Making*. 1994;14:71-81.

35. Schweiger H, Klein P, Lang W. Tibial bypass grafting for limb salvage with ringed polytetrafluoroethylene prostheses: results of primary and secondary procedures. *J Vasc Surg*. 1993;18:867-874.

36. Bosiers M, Deloose K, Verbist J, et al. Heparin-bonded expanded polytetrafluoroethylene vascular graft for femoropopliteal and femorocrural bypass grafting: 1-year results. *J Vasc Surg*. 2006;43:313-318.

37. Devine C, McCollum C, North West Femoro-Popliteal Trial Participants. Heparin-bonded Dacron or polytetrafluoroethylene for femoropopliteal bypass: five-year results of a prospective randomized multicenter trial. *J Vasc Surg*. 2004;40:924-931.

38. Battaglia G, Tringale R, Monaca V. Retrospective comparison of a heparin bonded ePTFE graft and saphenous vein for infragenicular bypass: implications for standard treatment protocol. *J Cardiovasc Surg*. 2006;47:41-47.

39. Cohen JR, Mannick JA, Couch NP, Whittemore AD. Recognition and management of impending graft failure: importance for long-term patency. *Arch Surg*. 1986;121:758-759.

40. Visser K, Idu MM, Buth J, et al. Duplex scan surveillance during the first year after infrainguinal autologous vein bypass grafting surgery: costs and clinical outcomes compared with other surveillance programs. *J Vasc Surg*. 2001;33:123030.

41. Davies AH, Hawdon AJ, Sydes MR, et al. Is duplex surveillance of value after leg vein bypass grafting? Principal results of the vein graft surveillance randomized trial (VGST). *Circulation*. 2005;112:1985-1991.

42. Lalak NJ, Hanel KC, Hunt J, Morgan A. Duplex-scan surveillance of infrainguinal prosthetic grafts. *J Vasc Surg*. 1994;20:637-641.

43. Dunlop P, Sayers RD, Naylor AR, et al. The effect of a surveillance programme on the patency of prosthetic infrainguinal bypass grafts. *Eur J Vasc Endovas Surg*. 1996;11:441-445.

44. Green RM, Roedersheimer LR, DeWeese JA. Effects of aspirin and dipyridamole on expanded polytetrafluoroethylene graft patency. *Surgery*. 1982;92:1016-1026.

45. Becquemin JP. Effect of ticlopidine on the long term patency of saphenous vein bypass grafts in the legs. *N Engl J Med*. 1997;337:1726-1731.

46. Conte MM, Belkin M, Upchurch GR, et al. Impact of increasing comorbidity on infrainguinal reconstruction: a 20-year perspective. *Ann Surg*. 2001;233:445-452.

47. Adam DJ, Beard JD, Cleveland T, et al. Bypass versus angioplasty in severe ischemia of the leg (BASIL): multicenter, randomized controlled trial. *Lancet*. 2005;366:1925-1934.

48. Johnson KW. Femoral and popliteal arteries: reanalysis of results of balloon angioplasty. *Radiology.* 1992;183:767-771.

49. Muradin G, Bosch J, Stijnen T, Hunink MG. Balloon dilation and stent implantation for treatment of femoropopliteal arterial disease: meta-analysis. *Radiology.* 2001;221:137-145.

50. FDA Intracoil data. Food and Drug Administration: Cardiovascular and Radiologic Health Advisory Board. April 23, 2001.

51. Waksman R. Paris: Brachytherapy IR 192 offers no benefit 2004. http://www.tctmd. com/csportal/appmanager/tetmd/main?_ nfpb=true&_pageLabel=TCTMDContent&hd Con=920795.

52. Cejna M, Thurnher S, Illiasch H, et al. PTA versus Palmaz stent placement in femoropopliteal artery obstructions: a multicenter prospective randomized study. *J Vasc Interv Radiol.* 2001;12:23-31.

53. Pokrajac B, Potter R, Roswitha M, et al. Endovascular brachytherapy prevents restenosis after femoropopliteal angioplasty: results of the Vienna-3 randomized multicenter trial. *Radiother Oncol.* 2005;74:3-9.

54. Laird J. Laser applications in the periphery 2005. http://www.tctmd.com/csportal/appmanager/tctmd/main?_nfpb=tru3&_pageLabel=TC TMDContent&hdCon=86311.

55. Laird J, Jaff MR, Biamino G, et al. Cryoplasty for the treatment of femoropopliteal arterial disease: results of a prospective, multicenter registry. *J Vasc Interv Radiol.* 2005;16:1067-1073.

56. Met R, Van Lieden KP, Koelemay MJW, et al. Subintimal angioplasty for peripheral arterial occlusive disease: a systematic review. *Cardiovasc Intervent Radiol.* 2008;31:687-697.

57. Scheinert D, Laird J, Schroeder M, et al. Excimer laser-assisted recanalization of long, chronic superficial femoral artery occlusions. *J Endovasc Ther.* 2001;8:156-166.

58. Tielbeek AV, Vroegindeweij D, Bluth J, Landman GH. Comparison of balloon angioplasty and Simpson atherectomy for lesions in the femoropopliteal artery: angiographic and clinical results of a prospective randomized trial. *J Vasc Interv Radiol.* 1996;7:837-844.

59. Zeller T, Rastan A, Schwarzwalder U, et al. Percutaneous peripheral atherectomy of femoropopliteal stenoses using a new-generation device: six-month results from a single-center experience. *J Endovasc Ther.* 2004;11:676-685.

60. Martin EC, Katzen BT, Benenati JF, et al. Multicenter trial of the wallstent in the iliac and femoral arteries. *J Vasc Interv Radiol.* 1995;6:843-849.

61. Gray BH, Sullivan TM, Childs MB, et al. High incidence of restenosis/reocclusion of stents in the percutaneous treatment of long-segment superficial femoral artery disease after suboptimal angioplasty. *J Vasc Surg.* 1997;25:74-83.

62. Sabeti S, Schillinger M, Amighi J, et al. Primary patency of femoropopliteal arteries treated with nitinol versus stainless steel self-expanding stents: propensity score-adjusted analysis. *Radiology.* 2004;232:516-521.

63. Scheinert D, Scheinert S, Sax J, et al. Prevalence and clinical impact of stent fractures after femoropopliteal stenting. *Am Coll Cardiol.* 2005;45:312-315.

64. Scheinert D. Nitinol stent fractures in different nitinol self-expanding stents: a prospective evaluation. http://www.tctmd.com/csportal/ appmanager/tctmd/main?_nfpb=true&_page Label=TCTMDContent&hdCon=808868.

65. Krankenburg H, Schluter M, Steinkamp HJ, et al. Nitinol stent implantation versus percutaneous transluminal angioplasty in superficial femoral artery lesions up to 10 cm in length. *Circulation.* 2007;116:285-292.

66. Schillinger M, Sabeti S, Loewe C, et al. Balloon angioplasty versus implantation of nitinol stents in the superficial femoral artery. *N Engl J Med.* 2006;354:1879-1888.

67. Schillinger M, Sabeti S, Dick P, et al. Sustained benefit at 2 years of primary femoropopliteal stenting compared with balloon angioplasty with optional stenting. *Circulation.* 2007;115.

68. Iida O, Nanto S, Uematsu M, et al. Influence of stent fracture on the long-term patency in the femoro-popliteal artery. *J Am Coll Cardiol Interv.* 2009;2:665-671.

69. Ansel GM, Silver MJ, Botti CF Jr, et al. Functional and clinical outcomes of nitinol stenting with and without abciximab for complex super-

ficial femoral artery disease: a randomized trial. *Catheter Cardiovasc Interv.* 2006;67:288-297.

70. Mewissen MW. Self-expanding nitinol stents in the femoropopliteal segment: technique and mid-term results. *Tech Vasc Interv Radiol.* 2004;7:2-5.

71. Duda SH, Pusich B, Richter G, et al. Sirolimus-eluting stents for the treatment of obstructive superficial femoral artery disease: six-month results. *Circulation.* 2002;106:1505-1509.

72. Duda SH, Bosiers M, Lammer J, et al. Sirolimus-eluting versus bare nitinol stent for obstructive superficial femoral artery disease: the SIROCCO II trial. *J Vasc Interv Radiol.* 2005;16:331-338.

73. Cragg AH, Dake MD. Treatment of peripheral vascular disease with stent-grafts. *Radiology.* 1997;205:307-314.

74. Henry M, Amor M, Cragg A, et al. Occlusive and aneurysmal peripheral arterial disease: assessment of a stent-graft system. *Radiology.* 1996; 201:717-724.

75. Ahmadi R, Schillinger M, Maca T, et al. Femoropopliteal arteries: immediate and long-term results with a Dacron-covered stent-graft. *Radiology.* 2002;223:345-350.

76. Marin J, Veith F, Cynamon J, et al. Human transluminal placed endovascular stented grafts: preliminary histopathologic analysis of healing grafts in aortoiliac and femoral artery occlusive disease. *J Vasc Surg.* 1995;21:595-604.

77. Lammer J, Dake MD, Bleyn J, et al. Peripheral arterial obstruction: prospective study of treatment with a transluminally placed self-expanding stent-graft. International Trial Study Group. *Radiology.* 2000;217(1):95-104.

78. Tielbeek AV, Vroegindeweij D, Bluth J, Landman GH. Comparison of balloon angioplasty and Simpson atherectomy for lesions in the femoropopliteal artery: angiographic and clinical results of a prospective randomized trial. *J Vasc Interv Radiol.* 1996;7:837-844.

79. Zeller T, Rastan A, Schwarzwalder U, et al. Percutaneous peripheral atherectomy of femoropopliteal stenoses using a new-generation device: six-month results from a single-center experience. *J Endovasc Ther.* 2004;11:676-685.

80. Martin EC, Katzen BT, Benenati JF, et al.

Multicenter trial of the Wallstent in the iliac and femoral arteries. *J Vasc Interv Radiol.* 1995;6:843-849.

81. Deutschmann HA, Schedlbauer P, Berczi V, et al. Placement of Hemobahn stent-grafts in femoropopliteal arteries: early experience and midterm results in 18 patients. *J Vasc Interv Radiol.* 2001;12(8):943-950.

82. Bray PJ, Robson WJ, Bray AE. Percutaneous treatment of long superficial femoral artery occlusive disease: efficacy of the Hemobahn stent-graft. *J Endovasc Ther.* 2003;10(3):619-628.

83. Daenens K, Maleux G, Fourneau I, et al. Hemobahn stent-grafts in the treatment of femoropopliteal occlusive disease. *J Cardiovasc Surg.* 2005;46:25-29.

84. Wiesinger B, Beregi JP, Oliva VL, et al. PTFE-covered self-expanding nitinol stents for the treatment of severe iliac and femoral artery stenoses and occlusions: final results of a prospective study. *J Endovasc Ther.* 2005;12:240-246.

85. Railo M, Roth WD, Edgren J, et al. Preliminary results with endoluminal femoropopliteal thrupass. *Ann Chir Gynaecol.* 2001;90(1):15-18.

86. Bauermeister G. Endovascular stent-grafting in the treatment of superficial femoral artery occlusive disease. *J Endovasc Ther.* 2001;8(3):315-320.

87. Hartung O, Otero M, Dubuc M, et al. Efficacy of Hemobahn in the treatment of superficial femoral artery lesions in patients with acute or critical ischemia: a comparative study with claudicants. *Eur J Vasc Endovasc Surg.* 2005;30:300-306.

88. Gallino A, Mahler F, Probst P, et al. Percutaneous transluminal angioplasty of the arteries of the lower limbs: a 5 year follow-up. *Circulation.* 1984;70:619-623.

89. Jeans WD, Armstrong S, Cole SEA, et al. Fate of patients undergoing transluminal angioplasty for lower-limb ischemia. *Radiology.* 1990;177:559-564.

90. Tielliu IF, Verhoeven EL, Prins TR, et al. Treatment of popliteal artery aneurysms with the Hemobahn stent-graft. *J Endovasc Ther.* 2003;10:111-116.

91. Tielliu IF, Verhoeven EL, Zeebregts CJ, et al. Endovascular treatment of popliteal artery

aneurysms: results of a prospective cohort study. *J Vasc Surg.* 2005;41:561-567.

92. Tepe G, Zeller T, Albrecht T, et al. Local delivery of paclitaxel to inhibit restenosis during angioplasty of the leg. *N Engl J Med.* 2008;358:689-699.

93. Werk M, Langner S, Reinkensmeier B, et al. Inhibition of restenosis in femoropopliteal arteries: paclitaxel-coated versus uncoated balloons: femoral paclitaxel randomized pilot trial. *Circulation.* 2008;118:1358-1365.

15

Critical Limb Ischemia: Limb Salvage, Angiogenesis

Ashequl M. Islam and Kenneth Rosenfield

Chronic critical limb ischemia (CLI) occurs as a result of reduced arterial blood flow, resulting in ischemic limb pain at rest, nonhealing ischemic ulceration, or gangrene. The criteria for diagnosis (Figure 15.1) includes either (1) more than 2 weeks of recurrent foot pain at rest that requires regular use of analgesics and is associated with an ankle systolic pressure of 50 mm Hg or less, (2) a toe systolic pressure of 30 mm Hg or less, or (3) a nonhealing wound or gangrene of the foot or toes, with similar hemodynamic measurements.[1] These criteria meet requirements of stage III and IV of the Fontaine classification and Rutherford 4, 5, and 6 categories in the new SVS and SVS-ISCVS Recommendation of Reporting Standards (Table 15.1).[2]

Pathophysiology

The majority of patients with CLI suffer from advanced atherosclerotic disease. Other clinical conditions such as atheroembolism, *in situ* thrombosis, and arteritides such as thromboangiitis obliterans can also cause CLI. The patho-physiology of CLI in humans is not well established. The basic macrocirculatory abnormality involves atherosclerotic obstructive lesions in the arterial tree. Patients with both proximal (such as aortoiliac) and distal (such as femoral or subcrural) lesions are more likely to develop CLI than are those with an isolated lesion, even when seemingly adequate collateral circulation is present. The final precipitating event may involve a thromboembolic phenomenon. Gradual decrease in perfusion pressure may result from increasing atherosclerosis, and a more rapid deterioration in perfusion may result from local thrombosis. Rupture of a thin fibrous cap of a lipid-rich plaque results in platelet and coagulation cascade activation in acute coronary syndrome. The same mechanism may be responsible for causing CLI in some patients.[3] In some cases the hemodynamic consequences of arterial obstruction is compounded by significant chronic venous insufficiency or low cardiac output.

Microcirculatory pathophysiology is more complex in CLI. The etiology of rest pain and trophic changes in CLI is critically reduced microcirculation to the skin as opposed to intermittent claudication caused by the reduction

Vascular Disease: Diagnostic and Therapeutic Approaches. © 2011 Michael R. Jaff and Christopher J. White, editors. Cardiotext Publishing, ISBN: 978-1-935395-16-4.

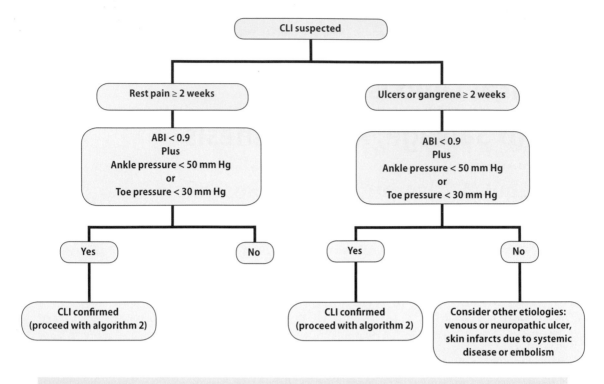

Figure 15.1 Algorithm 1: Clinical diagnosis in patients with critical limb ischemia.

Fontaine		Rutherford			
Stage	Clinical	Grade	Category	Clinical	Objective Criteria
I	Asymptomatic	0	0	Asymptomatic	Normal treadmill or reactive hyperemia test
IIa	Mild claudication	I	1	Mild claudication	
IIb	Moderate–severe claudication	I	2	Moderate claudication	AP after exercise > 50 mm Hg but ≥ 20 mm Hg lower than resting value
		I	3	Severe claudication	
III	Ischemic rest pain	II	4	Ischemic rest pain	Resting AP < 60 mm Hg, ankle or metatarsal PVR flat or barely pulsatile; TP < 40 mm Hg
IV	Ulceration or gangrene	III	5	Minor tissue loss	Resting AP < 60 mm Hg, ankle or metatarsal PVR flat or barely pulsatile; TP < 40 mm Hg
		IV	6	Ulceration or gangrene	

Table 15.1. Classification Schemes for PAD

Abbreviations: AP = ankle pressure; PVR = pulse volume recording; TP = toe pressure
(Norgren L, Hiatt WR, Dormandy JA, Nehler MR, Harris KA, Fowkes FR, on the behalf of the TASC II Working Group. Inter-society consensus for the management of peripheral arterial disease [TASC II]. J Vasc Surg. 2007;45: S29A. Reprinted with permission from Elsevier.)

in muscle blood flow during exercise. In CLI, a more advanced cutaneous microcirculatory deterioration has been described, with a more severely impaired post-ischemic hyperemia, a reduced cPO2 and a severely impared skin flow-motion in the diseases limb.[4] The normal function of the skin's microcirculation is dependent on a complex microvascular-flow regulatory system and a series of defense mechanisms. The microvascular-flow-regulating system is a result of the interplay among extrinsic neurogenic mechanisms, intrinsic local mediators, and the modulation by circulating humoral and blood-borne factors. The endothelium also plays an integral part in the regulation of flow by the release of vasodilatory mediators such as prostacyclin, the endothelium-derived relaxing factor nitric oxide, and several endothelium-derived contractile factors (eg, endothelin). The mechanism that may result in impaired microcirculatory blood flow in CLI includes abnormal vasomotor, endothelial swelling; microthromboses; interstitial edema; platelet aggregation; and red and white blood cell adhesions. In addition to the microvascular-flow-regulating system there are several microvascular defense mechanisms. An imbalance between the defense mechanisms and an inappropriate activation of hemostasis and inflammation play a central role in the pathophysiology of CLI.

Endothelial dysfunction in CLI may be associated with an increased level of endothelin, a potent vasoconstrictor, and a decreased level of nitric oxide, an endothelial vasodilator. Dysfunctional endothelium also contributes to a procoagulant environment characterized by the decreased secretion of tissue plasminogen activator, increased secretion of plasminogen activator inhibitor-1 (PAI-1), increased reactivity and activation of platelets, local production of tissue factor, and exposure to collagen.[5] Also, increasing evidence exists that leukocytes play an important role in ischemic disease. Activated leukocytes are abnormally rigid and therefore candidates for microvascular occlusion. CLI is often associated with local infections, which may in turn amplify leukocyte activation and result in cellular and immunological responses due to toxins.[6] There are abnormally high levels of fibroblast growth and von Willebrand factor associated with CLI. It is postulated that high levels of von Willebrand factor is indicative of endothelial damage.[7]

Natural History

The antecedent natural history of CLI is not clearly understood. The Fontaine classification system for CLI has 4 categories: stage I (asymptomatic), stage II (claudication), stage III (rest pain), and stage IV (tissue necrosis). However, many studies on natural history of Fontaine stage II disease showed only a small percentage of patients ever progress to CLI and only 4% of the patients are at risk of limb loss.[8] An exception to this rule occurs in patients with claudication and subsequent failure of angioplasty or bypass graft with increased risk for development of CLI.[9] Therefore, in most patients CLI progresses directly from Fontaine stage I to stages III and IV. It is no longer possible to clearly delineate the natural history of CLI because most patients now undergo some form of revascularization. In a multicenter prospective prostacyclin trial of more than 700 patients with below-knee amputations, Dormandy et al[10] demonstrated that 50% of the enrolled patients were asymptomatic 6 months before major amputation because of CLI. Based on a national survey by the Vascular Surgery Society of Great Britain and Ireland the annual incidence of CLI is approximately 400 per million per year.[11]

Patients with CLI have significant increased long-term mortality (10%–30%) than patients with intermittent claudication.[12-14] The 5-, 10-, and 15-year mortality rates for patients with intermittent claudication are approximately 30%, 50%, and 70%.[15] The 5-year survival rate in CLI patients in surgical literature is only 50% to 60%.[16-20] Mortality of patients presenting with rest pain reaches 70% at 5 years and 85% at 10 years.[21] Prognosis is poorer in selected series of patients.[22,23] In a large cohort of patients with CLI, age $\geq$ 70 years, history of prior stroke and major amputation were significantly associated with increased mortality.[22] Diabetic patients with peripheral artery occlusive disease are about 10 times more likely to have amputation than nondiabetic patients with this disease. The prevalence of gangrene is 20 to 30 times higher in diabetic compared to nondiabetic patients. Following bypass surgery limb salvage, graft patency and survival were lower for diabetic than for nondiabetic patients, though the difference was solely caused by diabetic women in the study.[24] Another study based on a large Finnish registry showed diabetes was not an independent risk factor for early postoperative mortality in CLI, though it led to more morbidities such as below-knee amputations.[25] CLI patients with chronic renal insufficiency or end stage renal disease were found to have very poor survival in several studies.[18,26] Approximately 80% of patients with peripheral artery disease (PAD) die from cardiovascular or cerebrovascular events: more than 60% from coronary artery disease and 10% from strokes.[27]

Clinical Presentation

Chronic CLI usually occurs due to severely reduced arterial blood flow to the tissue, often as a result of combination of inflow (refers to suprainguinal) and outflow (refers to infrainguinal) disease. Clinical manifestations of severe tissue ischemia are rest pain or nonhealing ulcers and in more extreme cases gangrene.

Ischemic rest pain is characteristically described as a burning pain in the ball of the foot and toes or in the vicinity of an ischemic ulcer or gangrenous toe. The pain is often partially relieved by dependent position and worsened by elevation or cold temperature. Often, patients sleep with their ischemic leg dangling over the side of the bed, or sitting in an armchair; as a result patients may develop ankle or foot edema. In more severe cases, patients are unable to sleep through the night since rest pain sets in only after short periods in a supine position in bed. As a result, there is progressive deterioration of the patient's general and psychological condition. Sometimes, peripheral ischemic

neuropathy causes severe, sharp, shooting pain usually more pronounced in the distal part of the extremity. This may often occur at night and can last minutes to hours with constant diffuse pain lasting in between.

Nonhealing ulcers or gangrene usually develop in digits or the heels in bedridden patients due to pressure points. It is usually initiated with minor trauma such as use of new and ill-fitting shoes in patients with neuropathy. In diabetic patients silent progression of ischemic ulcers can occur without having any rest pain. Thus an undiagnosed and asymptomatic patient can rapidly progress to CLI. Superimposed infection can cause rapid deterioration of a threatened limb. Gangrenous tissue, if not infected, can lead to eschar formation and shrink and eventually mummify, and spontaneous amputation can then follow if the underlying circulation is adequate. Identification of subclinical patients and instituting preventive measures can prevent CLI or at least prompt early referral if patients develop CLI. Physical findings in CLI usually include absent or diminished pulses, collapsed veins, loss of hair, and other integuments leading to shiny skin and cool, pale, or cyanotic distal parts of extremities. Patients with CLI often have brittle and damaged toenails and muscle wasting of the calves. Decreased capillary filling of the toes, edema of ankles or feet, elevation pallor, and dependent rubor are commonly present in patients with CLI.

Noninvasive Evaluation

Segmental Pressures and Pulse Volume Recordings

An objective measure of blood flow can easily be obtained using a handheld Doppler probe and blood pressure cuff. As mentioned earlier, an ankle systolic pressure of ≤ 50 mm Hg and a toe systolic pressure of ≤30 mm Hg would suggest the presence of CLI. The ankle-brachial index (ABI) is often used to classify patients with CLI. ABI is calculated as the ratio of the higher of the dorsalis pedis or posterior tibialis systolic pressure and left or right brachial arterial systolic pressure. In general, an ABI of 0.5 to 0.8 indicates moderate and 0.4 severe or critical limb ischemia. ABI is, however, unreliable in patients with noncompressible arteries due to medial calcification leading to falsely elevated lower-extremity pressures. In diabetics approximately one-third will have a falsely elevated ABI. In these instances, a toe-brachial index instead should be obtained. A normal toe brachial pressure index is 0.8 to 0.9.

In vascular laboratories continuous-wave Doppler probes are also used to measure segmental pressures to aid in localizing stenoses and occlusions. A series of limb pressure cuffs are placed on the thigh, calf, ankle, and transmetatarsal region of the foot and digit. ABI is measured first. The Doppler probe is placed on the pedal vessel and the cuff pressure is gradually reduced to detect the peak systolic pressure of each segment. In general a segmental systolic pressure difference of > 20 mm Hg would be an indication of occlusive arterial disease above the pressure cuff. In addition a difference of 20 to 30 mm Hg between 2 limbs at the same cuff level would also indicate significant arterial stenosis or occlusion proximal to the cuff.[28]

In vascular laboratories standard treadmill exercise at 2 mph on a 12% grade is usually used to evaluate an exercise-induced response in ABI. Walking on the treadmill is continued for 5 minutes or until the patient is forced to stop. Ankle and arm cuffs are kept on during exercise and ABI is measured before and immediately after exercise. A normal response to exercise is a slight increase or no change in the ankle systolic pressure after exercise. If ankle pressure is decreased immediately after exercise, the test is considered positive and repeat measurements are done at 1- to 2-minute intervals for up to 10 minutes. The magnitude of the immediate decrease in ankle pressure and the time to recovery to baseline are 2 important components during the study. Ankle pressure is usually < 60 mm Hg when a patient is forced to stop walking due to arterial occlusive disease. Patients with CLI and rest pain may have unrecordable ankle pressure for 15 minutes or more.

Reactive hyperemia testing is occasionally used as an alternative to standard treadmill exercise when patients cannot exercise. A pneumatic cuff is inflated at thigh level above the systolic pressure for 3 to 5 minutes. Following release of the cuff, normally there is a transient drop in systolic pressure by 17% to 34%, possibly due to vasodilatation response to ischemia.[29] In patients with arterial occlusive disease there is in general a good correlation between the maximum pressure drop with reactive hyperemia and the maximum pressure drop after treadmill exercise. The usefulness in patients with CLI, however, is not clear.

A pulse volume recording (PVR) is a plethysmographic tracing that detects changes in the volume of tissue in the extremities due to volume of blood flowing through the limb. Using the pressure cuffs in the segments of the lower extremities as previously described, cuffs are inflated to between 10 and 65 mm Hg and plethysmographic tracing is recorded at various levels.[30] A PVR indicates changes of volume of lower-extremity tissue during the cardiac cycle. Normally there is a systolic upstroke due to overall increase in tissue volume, which is in turn due to higher arterial inflow compared to venous outflow. A diastolic downslope occurs due to lower arterial inflow compared to the diastole outflow, and a brief period of retrograde flow in peripheral arteries causes the dicrotic notch in the downslope. With proximal arterial occlusive disease, obliteration of the dicrotic notch is one of the earliest changes. When the disease is more severe, the upstroke is slower, the peak is more rounded, and the downslope is bowed away from the baseline. Segmental PVR measurements are especially useful in patients with incompressible arteries with artificially elevated systolic pressures due to medial calcification.

In CLI with ulcers, healing is unlikely if ankle pressure is < 55 mm Hg in nondiabetics and < 80 mm Hg in diabetics.[31] However, toe pressure may be a better predictor of ulcer or amputation healing in CLI patients. In one study, only 5% of limbs had healing of foot ulcers, and toe or transmetatarsal amputations when the toe pressure was < 30 mm Hg. On the other hand, 90% of limbs healed if the toe pressure was ≥ 30 mm Hg.[32]

Duplex Ultrasonography

Qualitative and quantitative Doppler flow analysis is commonly used in modern vascular practices (see Chapter 4). A normal Doppler velocity pattern of extremity arteries shows characteristic triphasic form. When a Doppler probe is placed distal to the area of arterial stenosis, the waveform becomes flat and rounded with the peak systolic velocity lower than normal and loses its triphasic form. When the Doppler probe is placed directly on the area of stenosis, the signal has an abnormally elevated peak systolic velocity. The character of Doppler waveform obtained proximal to the stenosis depends on the extent of collateral circulation. If there are well-developed collaterals between the probe and point of obstruction, the waveform may be normal as compared to a harsh-quality signal described as a "thumping" sound when there is no collateral flow.[33] Duplex ultrasonography has the advantage of not involving radiation. Although it has proved to be useful in selected arterial segments, assessing the entire lower-extremity arterial tree would be an arduous task. Patients with CLI frequently need to be evaluated for abdominal aortic and entire lower-extremity arterial disease. In addition, duplex ultrasonography does not provide a "road map" for endovascular or surgical revascularization and has lower sensitivity and specificity.

Tissue Oxygen Pressure and Saturation

A transcutaneous oxygen pressure (TcPO2) measurement might be a good indicator of CLI and of the subsequent need for vascular intervention. In a study of 147 patients with CLI, 44 with palpable pulses underwent successful surgery, such as major and minor amputations, incision, and drainage.[34] One hundred three patients had decreased or absent pulses, of whom 14 patients had TcPO2 values $\geq$ 30 mm Hg and had major or minor amputation with 91% complete healing. Of the 90 patients with TcPO2 values < 30 mm Hg, 22 did not have any revascularization and only 50% of them showed primary healing after minor amputation or debridement. Sixty-seven patients underwent revascularization, 95% showed improvement of TcPO2 > 30 mm Hg and of these 91% had healing of minor amputation or debridement sites ($P < 0.05$).

Tissue (muscle) oxygen saturation (StO2) of gastrocnemius muscle, measured by the InSpectra tissue spectrometer (Hutchinson Technology), is a new technique to evaluate patients with PAD. In a study of 35 normal and 14 PAD patients, StO2 was similar and 65% in both groups at rest.[35] After standard treadmill exercise the peak exercise StO2 was significantly lower, and absolute change in StO2 and the percent change in StO2 were significantly greater in PAD patients ($P < 0.045$). The amounts of time to 50% of StO2 recovery to baseline (T_{50}) and complete recovery to baseline (T_{100}) were longer in the PAD patients compared with normal subjects ($P = 0.001$ and 0.002, respectively). A $T_{50} > 70$ seconds yielded a sensitivity of 89% and a specificity of 85% for PAD. This technique would appear to have usefulness in CLI and patients with intermittent claudication and compartment syndrome.

Magnetic Resonance Angiography

Magnetic resonance angiography (MRA) is one of the most commonly used noninvasive imaging evaluations of PAD (see Chapter 2). The main advantages are the relative noninvasive nature of the imaging and the fact that there is no need for ionizing radiation and nephrotoxic contrast agents. There are 2 main categories of MRA in clinical use: the more traditional *2-dimensional (2D) time-of-flight MRA (TOF-MRA)* and the *contrast-enhanced MRA (CE-MRA)*. TOF-MRA has the advantage of visualizing the entire arterial area of the lower extremities from abdominal aorta to the feet. In general the sensitivity and specificity of detecting > 50% stenosis in extremity arteries are 85% to 92% and 81% to 88%, respectively.[36,37] However, excessive scan time of more than 2 hours is a major limitation. Additionally, artifacts caused by pulsatile arterial flow and venous contamination in below-the-knee arteries are major drawbacks encountered with TOF-MRA.

CE-MRA combines use of a heavily T1-weighted gradient echo sequence and the intravenous injection of a gadolinium-based agent to achieve high-quality arterial imaging. Several published protocols involve use of short-repetition-time 3D spoiled gradient echo acquisitions from the abdomen to the feet that performed sequentially to perform angiography during the first pass of intravenous contrast material. This technique offers high-quality MRA images, which correlate well with x-ray angiogram to detect hemodynamically significant stenoses.[38,39] Several limitations still exist in CE-MRA, including prolonged acquisitions, venous enhancement–related contamination, motion artifacts, and decreased contrast to noise ratio (CNR). The limitations affect below-the-knee arterial imaging the most. In one study as many as 43% of calf station images were nondiagnostic.[40] Standard CE-MRA involves relatively fast scanning with some compromise in image resolution to reduce acquisition time. Although this results in sufficient image resolution for vessels in pelvic and thigh stations, the smaller vessels below the knee require submillimeter resolution. Therefore, different approaches, as described next, have been developed to increase the temporal and spatial resolution in calf stations.

Wang and associates[40] examined a hybrid MRA using contrast-enhanced, dynamic 2D acquisition at the feet and calf and bolus-chase 3D acquisition from the abdominal aorta to the calf in 89 consecutive patients with PAD. The bolus-chase 3D acquisition was of diagnostic quality in 100% of the acquisitions in the abdomen, 96% in the thigh, and only 43% in the calf. By using the dynamic 2D acquisition, diagnostic-quality images were obtained in 100% of the acquisitions in the calf and 98% in the feet. Another group of investigators described a hybrid MRA technique that included submillimeter dual-phase 3D gadolinium-enhanced MRA in the lower calf and foot, and 4-station bolus-chase MRA in the pelvis, thigh, and upper calf in patients with CLI.[41] There was excellent or

adequate image quality in 18 (95%) of 19 limbs and no substantial venous overlay was present. Three readers were involved in interpreting all the MRA and digital subtraction angiography (DSA) images. Agreement of all 3 readers was superior with use of MRA for determination of inflow segments (72%) and outflow segments (68%), compared with agreement with use of DSA (68% of inflow segments and 53% of outflow segments). Agreement in therapy decision was higher with DSA (79%) than with MRA (61%). One possible explanation for the higher agreement among readers with DSA imaging could be a result of more familiarity with DSA than MRA.

Another study compared multi-injection time-resolved imaging of contrast kinetics (TRICKS) and single-injection bolus-chase MRA in 10 volunteers and 10 grade IIA and IIB PAD on the basis of the Fontaine classification.[42] Image quality and venous phase contamination of major vessels of the abdomen, thigh, and calf were evaluated. Overall, 69.2% of the images were classified as diagnostic on TRICKS images compared with 48.9% on bolus-chase MRA images ($P < 0.05$). A significantly reduced frequency of venous contamination was noted using TRICKS compared with bolus-chase MRA ($P < 0.007$).

Another technique to increase the temporal and spatial resolution in calf stations is to combine dynamic 2D and 3D bolus-chase MRA in patients with PAD.[43,44] In one study, 3 radiologists retrospectively reviewed x-ray angiography and MRAs in 30 consecutive patients, 15 of whom were evaluated for limb salvage.[43] They used a 2D MRA of the area from the adductor canal to the middle portion of the foot combined with 3-station 3D bolus-chase MRA in a single examination. Comparing x-ray and MRA, the mean percentage of agreement for 3 readers were 91%, 91%, and 95%, respectively, for inflow segments and 91%, 91%, and 97%, respectively, for outflow segments.

Technical improvements such as use of dedicated peripheral phased array coil systems have improved acquisition time and spatial resolution in lower leg vessels.[45] Hagspiel and associates[46] examined the impact of integrated parallel acquisition technique (iPAT) on signal to noise ratio (SNR) and contrast to noise ratio (CNR), venous contamination and overall image interpretability using a dedicated phased array coil system in all 3 stations (pelvis, thigh, calf) in 38 consecutive patients. They found that compared with conventional MR angiography, iPAT MRA significantly reduced SNR ($P < .007$) and CNR ($P < .01$) in the pelvis and thigh stations and venous contamination ($P < .003$) in the calf station. There was a significantly better confidence of interpretability with iPAT MRA in the calf station due to an improvement in the temporal gain ($P < .008$).

It is often challenging to obtain diagnostic pretreatment MRA imaging in CLI patients due to overall debility, frequent rest pain, and early arteriovenous shunt time resulting from delayed arterial outflow. However, with technical improvements, CE-MRA may even be better than intraarterial DSA in patients with CLI or diabetes. DSA carries additional risks because of the invasive nature of the procedure and the use of ionizing radiation and potentially nephrotoxic contrast agents. Several studies have suggested the superiority of CE-MRA over DSA for identifying patent runoff arteries in the lower calf and foot.[41,47-52]

Computed Tomography Angiography

Lower-extremity computed tomography angiography (CTA) using multiple-detector row computed tomography scanners is the latest technique for peripheral arterial imaging. With multiple-row scanners, it is possible to image the entire lower-extremity arterial tree with a single acquisition and single intravenous contrast medium injection. CTA has the advantages of widespread and increasing availability, high spatial resolution, and relative freedom from operator dependence. The major disadvantages include the need for a relatively large amount of potentially nephrotoxic iodinated contrast agent and exposure to ionizing radiation. Multiple published articles compared

CTA and DSA in patients with peripheral arterial occlusive disease.[53-59] All of these studies report overall good sensitivities and specificities for the detection of hemodynamically significant steno-occlusive disease. Most of these used 4-channel CTA in comparison to DSA. In general, sensitivity and specificity are greater for arterial occlusive disease than for stenosis. Willmann et al[59] compared 16-detector-row CTA with DSA and found that the overall sensitivities, specificities, and accuracies for aortoiliac, femoral, and popliteocrural steno-occlusive disease were all greater than 96%. There was loss of diagnostic performance in popliteocrural branches. When compared to MRA, multi-detector-row CTA has significantly lower average diagnostic costs.[60] In patients with CLI, delineation of inflow and outflow arterial diseases suitable for possible percutaneous intervention or target vessels for possible bypass graft surgery is essential. With the newest-generation 64-channel CTA machines, it is expected that further improvement in spatial resolution will allow better visualization of small crural and pedal vessels.

Invasive Evaluation

Digital Subtraction Angiography

Intra-arterial digital subtraction angiography (DSA) is still the benchmark for evaluation of PAD. It has replaced traditional static film-changer angiography. However, cross-sectional imaging studies (MRA, CTA, and ultrasonography) are used in increasing frequency. The main disadvantages of DSA include use of potentially nephrotoxic contrast agents, exposure to ionizing radiation, cost, and higher vascular complication rates. Use of angiography for diagnostic purposes is reserved only for clarification of inadequate and conflicting results from physiologic testing and cross-sectional vascular imaging. Despite a paradigm shift away from conventional angiography as a purely diagnostic technique, its use in intervention has increased dramatically.[61] For the foreseeable future, DSA will likely remain the cornerstone technology in PAD intervention. Patients with CLI present special challenges often due to the presence of multiple steno-occlusive lesions in the "inflow" and "runoff" segments in the lower-extremity arterial tree. Several studies have shown that DSA may fail to show the runoff vessels in patients with severe PAD associated with diabetes.[47,48] This results from dilution of contrast medium below the long segmented or multiple lesions in patients with CLI, leading to insufficient enhancement of distal vessels. Several studies with hybrid MRA[40-45,49] and multi-detector-row CTA[53-59] have reported the usefulness of the cross-sectional imaging in diagnosis and treatment planning in patients with significant PAD. In patients with diabetes and CLI, hybrid MRA visualizes lower-extremity vessels that are not seen by DSA.[49]

The diagnostic performance of DSA can be increased by more selective arterial injections without an increased amount of potentially nephrotoxic contrast medium and exposure to radiation. DSA provides high resolution of imaging compared to current cross-sectional imaging modalities. It also provides access to individual arterial segments and direct physiologic assessment of lesions before and after any intervention and a platform for intervention. Recent developments such as bolus chasing, rapid image acquisition, vessel measurements, image stacking, regional pixel shifting, 3D reconstruction, rotational angiogram, and angioscopic representation have improved the usefulness of DSA in patients with PAD.[62-64] Nonnephrotoxic CO_2 and less nephrotoxic gadolinium chelates can be used with DSA in patients with higher risk of contrast-medium-induced renal failure.[65,66] Use of vasodilating agents during DSA has been reported in an attempt to improve image quality, without any convincing evidence.[67,68] Patients with CLI are likely to have already maximally dilated calf and foot vessels due to severe ischemia, and the usefulness of vasodilating agents is questionable.

Management of Critical Limb Ischemia

Overall Strategy

Next to ensuring adequate blood flow, treatment goals for patients with CLI are pain control, wound care to expedite ulcer healing, limb salvage, improved function and quality of life, and prolonged survival. For all patients, aggressive cardiovascular risk factor modification is essential. In case of infection superimposing an ischemic ulcer or gangrene, appropriate wound care and antibiotic therapy may be needed. Patients should be promptly referred to vascular specialists experienced in caring for patients with advanced vascular disease. A need for appropriate revascularization procedures should be considered in a timely manner (Figure 15.2). Many of these patients will need aggressive care for other comorbidities. Some patients will not be eligible for any revascularization due to severe systemic disease or poor anatomy. For them primary amputation may be quite appropriate.

Pain Control

Pain control is an essential part of management of patients with CLI. The source of pain is usually ischemic skin and sometimes may be bony structures. Often patients have partial pain relief with dependency to increase tissue perfusion. Therefore, tilting the leg end of the bed may be important in bedridden patients. Ideally, pain relief is accomplished by increased tissue perfusion by revascularization. While revascularization is being planned, patients may require appropriate analgesics, such as acetaminophen, nonsteroidal anti-inflammatory agents, or narcotic analgesics. Those without any revascularization option or failed revascularization will likely require narcotic analgesics, often for prolonged periods. It is important to evaluate pain control on a daily basis and make changes as appropriate. Patients with chronic pain are often depressed, and better pain control is achieved by treating depression simultaneously.

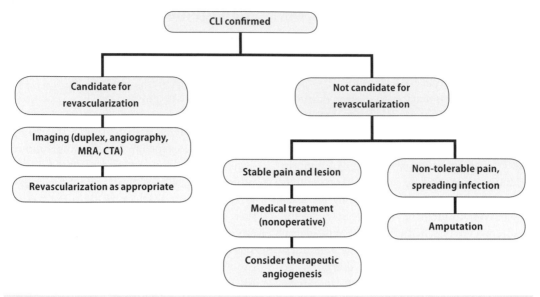

Figure 15.2 Algorithm 2: Management of patients with CLI. (Modified from Norgren L, Hiatt WR, Dormandy JA, Nehler MR, Harris KA, Fowkes FR, on the behalf of the TASC II Working Group. Inter-society consensus for the management of peripheral arterial disease [TASC II]. *J Vasc Surg.* 2007;45:S35. With permission from Elsevier.)

Wound Management

Patients with CLI and ischemic ulcers or tissue loss often need a multidisciplinary approach including revascularization and local wound care. Basic principles of ischemic foot care involve off-loading before and after revascularization to enhance wound healing. Off-loading of the affected limb can be achieved by shoe modification, orthotics, and casting techniques. Special care should be given to prevent repetitive trauma from ill-fitting shoes. General care of ischemic ulcers includes keeping the wound moist, removing necrotic or fibrotic tissues, and treating infection when present. Often revascularization is delayed until acute infection is adequately controlled. Systemic signs of toxicity such as fever and elevated C-reactive protein are uncommon in patients with CLI. Rapid diagnosis of infection and treatment are of prime importance since infection could spread aggressively. In diabetics infection is usually polymicrobial involving gram-positive cocci, gram-negative rods, and anaerobic organisms. Empiric broad-spectrum antibiotics should be started while waiting for culture and sensitivity. A prior history of infection with specific organisms sometimes can help to select initial antibiotics of choice.

Limb Salvage Procedures

Limb salvage after revascularization is defined as preservation of some or all of the foot. It is generally recommended to wait at least 3 days after revascularization to allow sufficient time for restoration of perfusion and tissue demarcation before planning for any salvage procedures. Natural history of minor foot amputation should be kept in mind while planning for salvage procedures. Great toe and/or first-ray amputation has a high likelihood of a second amputation either of the same foot or the contralateral foot compared to amputation of lateral toes or rays (fourth and fifth digits). Sometimes debridement procedures and bone excision such as exostectomy, arthroplasty, metatarsal head excision, and calcanectomy are needed to salvage a revascularized limb.

Amputation

Contemporary care of CLI frequently involves aggressive limb salvage attempts by surgical or endovascular means. In highly specialized centers as many as 90% of patients presenting with CLI undergo some type of revascularization in an effort to salvage limbs. *Primary amputation* is defined as amputation without any antecedent revascularization attempt and is usually undertaken in patients with unconstructable arterial disease. The primary major amputation (above-the-ankle) rate varies in the range of 10% in specialized centers to as high as 40% in more community-based facilities. It is believed that aggressive limb salvage strategy over the last 3 decades has led to lower amputation rates in patients with CLI. However, there is ongoing controversy over whether this approach can lead to improved patient survival. In a fixed population in Sweden, studied over 8 years, a significant decrease was found in primary amputation, from 42% to 27%, due to increased revascularization. This led to an overall decrease in amputation from 61% to 47%.[69] In the United States and United Kingdom major amputation estimates are approximately 280 and 300 million per annum, respectively. As per the joint vascular research group in Britain study, patients with CLI with gangrene or ulceration are twice as likely to require a major amputation as those with rest pain alone.[70] However, a study reported more than 50% of patients with lower-extremity ischemia who needed below-the-knee major amputation were asymptomatic for limb ischemia in the previous 6 months.[10]

Several studies reported high mortality rates in patients with recent diagnosis of CLI.[22,70] Wolfe[70] reported a 1-year mortality of approximately 20% in unselected patients with CLI. Patients who have no options or failed revascularization will have a very poor prognosis. The fate of these patients can be postulated from several multicenter, randomized placebo-controlled studies of pharmacologic therapy. The results for this subgroup reveal the grave prognosis that approximately 40% will lose a leg within 6 months, whereas up to 20% will die.[71-73] In most of these studies, less than half of the patients were alive without a major amputation after 6 months.

Several studies have shown that the ankle-brachial index (ABI) is a strong predictor of survival without amputation in patients with CLI.[74,75] It is not surprising since the ABI has already been strongly associated with survival in patients with intermittent claudication. ABI is an overall measure of atherosclerotic disease burden in these patients. A majority of patients with CLI suffer from cardiovascular deaths. Cardiovascular risk factor modification is therefore strongly recommended in patients with CLI. In a report from Britain ABI was a good predictor of survival in CLI patients with rest pain and added little additional value in patients with more advanced disease with ulceration or gangrene.[70] Many believe an aggressive limb salvage strategy offers better quality of life if not survival than primary amputation in patients with CLI. Major amputation has significant perioperative mortality in the range of 3% to 10% with below-the-knee amputations and 15% to 20% with above-the-knee amputations. These rates are believed to be due to older and high-risk patients with more extensive arterial disease undergoing above-the-knee amputations in an attempt to achieve primary healing. Higher perioperative mortality was not significantly associated with diabetes or cardiovascular, cerebrovascular, or respiratory diseases.[75] The difference continues for up to 2 years, with mortality rates of 25% to 35% for patients with below-the-knee amputations and 45% for above-the-knee amputations.[76-78] Five years after a below-the-knee amputation, 30% of the patients have a major contralateral amputation, 50% will be dead, and only 20% will be alive with one intact leg.

A patient with major amputation will require a prosthesis. Meticulous technique is essential to ensure a well-perfused and well-formed stump with soft tissue covering and an appropriate prosthesis. Patients require physical and occupational rehabilitation to promote successful return to independent ambulation and their former quality of life. Overall success of independent ambulation is higher with below-the-knee compared with above-the-knee amputation (< 50%).

Pharmacotherapy

Pharmacotherapy is considered to increase distal microcirculatory perfusion pressure, especially in patients who have failed or no options of revascularization. Several agents have been investigated in patients with CLI. Pharmacotherapy may be particularly important in asymptomatic patients before they develop any foot lesions or in those with shallow lesions due to borderline perfusion pressures.

Prostanoids prevent platelets and leukocyte activation and protect vascular endothelium. They are administered parentally over several weeks. Their role in CLI was studied in several randomized studies with PGE_1 or PGI_2.[72,79-84] Although there was a decrease in ulcer size, no evidence of improvement in clinical outcomes was seen using PGE_1. Studies using PGI_2 showed mixed data. A recent placebo-controlled trial using lipo-ecraprost showed no significant benefit in reducing death or amputation during 6-month follow-up data.[85]

Other pharmacologic agents such as direct vasodilators have no proven role in patients with CLI. These agents typically improve blood flow in nonischemic areas. Antiplatelet agents such as aspirin, ticlopidine, or clopidogrel were not specifically studied in CLI patients. Dual antiplatelet agents using aspirin and ticlopidine or clopidogrel have been found to reduce cardiovascular events in several trials. In modern practice, all CLI patients should be on dual antiplatelet therapy unless risk of bleeding is prohibitive. There is no clear role of antithrombin or defibrinating agents in care of patients with CLI. Unfractionated heparin is frequently used as prophylaxis and during revascularization procedures. In patients with severe steno-occlusive disease with superimposed thromboembolic phenomenon, anticoagulation is usually indicated at least for the short term.

Vasoactive drugs such as intravenous naftidrofuryl was studied in several trials. It is a 5-hydroxytryptamine type 2 antagonist and may improve muscle metabolism and reduce red blood cell and platelet aggregation. A Cochrane review of these trials did not show any significant benefit in reducing symptoms in CLI patients.[86] Pentoxifylline lowers fibrinogen levels, improves red cell and white cell deformability, and thus lowers blood viscosity. In 2 placebo-controlled trials with patients with CLI, pentoxifylline offered no benefit.[87,88]

Other Treatments

Spinal Cord Stimulation

In patients with CLI, spinal cord stimulation has been shown to improve blood flow, reduce pain, heal ulcers, and increase activity.[89-91] The main disadvantages include the invasive nature of the procedure and high expense. *Transcutaneous electrical nerve stimulation (TENS)* has also been reported to improve lower-extremity blood flow.[92,93] TENS is noninvasive, simple, and cheap, however, it causes paresthesia. Therefore, double-blind studies are difficult to perform using this technique. *Transcutaneous spinal electroanalgesia (TSE)* is a method to deliver transcutaneous spinal cord stimulation using pulses of short wavelength, high frequency, and relatively high voltage without causing peripheral nerve stimulation. In a randomized double-blind crossover study using this technique daily for 1 week, there was no improvement in microcirculation, pain, or activity in patients with CLI.[94]

Intermittent Pneumatic Compression

In patients with CLI, it is believed that the arterioles are "maximally dilated," a phenomenon known as *vasomotor paralysis*. The result is an increase in tissue blood flow in critically ischemic limbs. *Intermittent pneumatic compression* temporarily increases the arterial blood possibly by increasing the lower-extremity arteriovenous gradient and reversing vasomotor paralysis. In a prospective pilot study of 33 limbs with CLI, and a mean follow-up of 3 months, 58% of the legs were salvaged, rest pain was improved in 40% of patients, 26% of foot ulcers healed, and toe pressures improved significantly.[95]

Hyperbaric Oxygen

A Cochrane review concluded that hyperbaric therapy significantly reduces the risk of major amputations in diabetic patients with ischemic ulcers.[96] However, due to methodological shortcomings, absence of proven benefit, and high cost, this therapy is not always recommended. It may be useful in patients who have not responded to, or are not candidates for, any revascularization.

Surgical Revascularization

The 5-year survival rate in CLI patients undergoing surgical bypass is only 50% to 60%.[16-20] As mentioned earlier, primary amputation carries a high perioperative mortality. Only about two-thirds of those who survive the operations have successful rehabilitation.[97,98] Many, if not most, patients with CLI have multilevel disease. Brewster et al[99] reported that 49% of patients undergoing aortobifemoral bypass grafts would have occlusion of the superficial femoral artery. It is generally accepted that any hemodynamically significant aortoiliac disease should be treated before performing any outflow procedure. Sometimes only inflow revascularization would be enough to relieve rest pain, and healing of ulcers leading to limb salvage. The need for subsequent bypass has been estimated to be as high as 21% to 25%. We consider a peak systolic pressure gradient of $\geq$ 10 mm Hg at rest and $\geq$ 15-20 mm Hg after vasodilator challenge across an aortoiliac obstruction to be hemodynamically significant. In patients with CLI, aortofemoral bypass surgery has a robust long-term primary patency of 87.5% at 5 years and 81.8% at 10 years and an operative mortality of 3.3%.[100]

In a study over 12 years (1987–1998) with 256 consecutive patients with CLI who underwent pedal bypass grafting using autologous veins, in-hospital mortality rate was 1.6%.[17] Seventy-five percent of the patients were diabetic and 20% had renal insufficiency. The rates of primary and secondary patency, limb salvage, and survival at 5 years were 58%, 71%, 78%, and 60%, respectively. In a mean follow-up of 2.7 years (range 0.1–10.1 years) 57% of limbs required additional interventions. Survival after amputation was only 79%, 53%, and 26% at 1, 3, and 5 years, respectively. End stage renal disease and composite vein grafts predicted limb loss significantly in this study.

A more modern and retrospective analysis of 1032 dorsalis pedis bypass procedures using autologous veins for CLI, 30-day mortality was 0.9%.[18] Ninety-two percent of the patients were diabetic. The rates of primary and secondary patency, limb salvage, and survival were 56.8%, 62.7%, 78.2%, and 48.6%, respectively, at 5 years and 37.7%, 41.7%, 57.7%, and 23.8% at 10 years. Saphenous vein grafts performed significantly better than all other conduits with a secondary patency of 67.6% versus 46.3% at 5 years. This study provided evidence in favor of routine use of pedal bypasses in patients with diabetes and CLI. It was also proven that dorsalis pedis bypass using venous conduits is durable, with high likelihood of limb salvage over many years.

Chung et al[101] retrospectively studied 334 consecutive patients with CLI who had undergone infrainguinal bypass using reversed saphenous vein conduits. At 1 year and 3 years the primary patency was 63% and 50%, assisted primary patency was 80% and 70%, limb salvage was 85% and 79%, and survival was 89% and 74%, respectively. The mean follow-up was 30 ± 23 months. Despite these expected results, 25% of patients did not achieve wound healing at 1 year of follow-up, 19% lost ambulatory function, and 5% lost independent living status.

Endovascular Therapy

Endovascular therapy for CLI (Figures 15.3 and 15.4) has become increasingly common and has several advantages over surgical revascularization. These include less invasiveness of the procedure, lower risk of wound infection, shorter hospital stay, potential cost advantage, repeatability, and lower risks of mortality. Even if the treatment site reoccludes following ulcer healing, often no symptoms or intervention are needed. The "tide over" concept is that less blood flow is needed to maintain healed tissue than required for initial healing. Schwarten[102] reported infrapopliteal angioplasty in 96 patients (112 limbs). There were 31 total occlusions and 95 multiple stenoses. The primary success rate was 97%, and the 2-year limb salvage rate was 83%. The results of angioplasty were comparable to 320 femorodistal bypasses done at the same period. Soder et al[103] prospectively analyzed efficacy of infrapopliteal percutaneous transluminal angioplasty (PTA) in 72 limbs of 60 patients with CLI. The major complication rate was 2.8%. The patients were followed for 12 to 24 months. The primary success rates were 84% and 61% and restenosis rates 32% and 52%, respectively. A cumulative limb salvage rate was comparable with surgical techniques—80% at 18 months.

Dorros et al[104] examined tibioperoneal angioplasty as primary treatment in 235 patients with CLI. The procedure was successful in 95% of the limbs, of which 59% also required dilatation of ipsilateral inflow obstructions. At 5 years clinical follow-up, bypass surgery was needed in 8% and amputation in 9%; the limb salvage

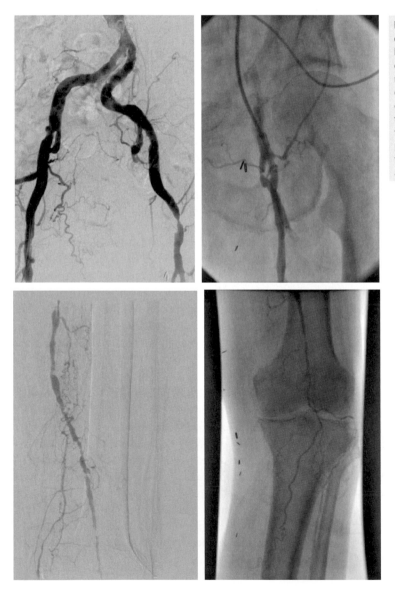

Figure15.3 DSA of a 76-year-old diabetic patient with left lower-extremity CLI and severe common and superficial femoral, popliteal, and below-knee disease. The patient had undergone profunda and superficial femoral artery angioplasty and failed recanalization of left popliteal and tibioperoneal trunk and needed below-knee amputation.

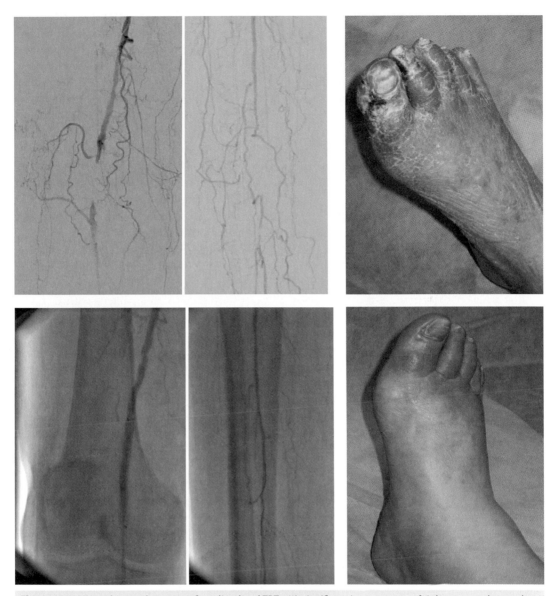

Figure 15.4 PTA and stent placement of popliteal and TPT with significant improvement of right great and second toe ulceration in a diabetic patient. (Courtesy of Douglas Drachman, MD.)

rate was 91% and overall survival was 56%. This study established a definitive role for percutaneous endovascular treatment as the initial and effective revascularization therapy in patients with CLI.

The early trials of infrapopliteal angioplasty were limited mainly due to the absence of prospective design, rigorous tallying, adjudication of clinical outcomes, and comparison to surgical bypass. The Bypass Versus Angioplasty in Severe Ischemia of the Leg (BASIL) trial, a multicenter, randomized controlled trial, randomly assigned 452 patients with CLI to receive surgery or angioplasty as the first therapy.[105] During the first year of follow-up, 86% of patients assigned to bypass surgery and 96% of patients assigned to balloon angioplasty underwent an attempt at intended therapy. Follow-up finished when a patient reached an end point of amputation of trial leg above the ankle, or death. At the end of 5.5 years of follow-up, 55% of patients were alive without and 8% alive with amputation of the trial leg, and 29% were dead without amputation. The surgery-first group had significantly longer duration of hospitalization, intensive care, or high-dependency unit stay compared to the angioplasty-first group. There was no difference in health-related quality of life between the 2 groups. However, in the first year, there was significantly higher hospital cost in the surgery-first strategy than the angioplasty-first strategy. In conclusion, this randomized controlled trial comparing surgery-first and angioplasty-first strategies in CLI patients showed broadly similar outcomes in terms of amputation-free survival at a higher short-term cost due to longer hospitalizations.

In addition to balloon angioplasty, excimer laser angioplasty, stents, atherectomy, and thrombolytic therapy are often used in infrainguinal endovascular interventions in patients with CLI. None of these technologies have proven to make any definitive impact on long-term outcome and primary durability. However, each has extended physicians' ability to treat difficult infrainguinal lesions. Laird[106] and Boisers et al[107] examined the usefulness of excimer laser-assisted angioplasty in high-risk patients with CLI who were poor candidates for surgical revascularization. In 48 patients 51 chronically ischemic limbs were treated with excimer laser-assisted angioplasty, with or without adjunctive balloon angioplasty or stenting. There were 6 deaths, 4 major amputations, and 4 repeat interventions in 6 months. Among survivors, limb salvage rate was 90.5% with freedom from critical ischemia in 86.0% at 6 months follow-up.

Yancey and colleagues[108] reported their experience of using FoxHollow SilverHawk atherectomy in 16 consecutive patients with 17 limbs with critical ischemia. All of the patients had more than one level of arterial obstructions. Initial resolution of symptoms was achieved in 12 limbs, partial healing was achieved in 2 others, and early amputation was needed in the remaining 3 patients. Two additional patients

required amputations in 6 months of follow-up. Stenosis-free patency of the femoropopliteal segment was only 22% at 12 months. It is not clear that these adjunctive techniques add anything other than cost to the procedure of angioplasty with or without stenting.

The aim of endovascular treatment is to reestablish a straight-line, pulsatile flow to the foot. Feiring et al[109] reported stent-supported angioplasty in 82 patients and 92 limbs with CLI (68%) and severe lifestyle-limiting claudication (32%). Technical success was achieved in 94% of the *de novo* lesions without any 1-month death, myocardial infarction, major unplanned amputation, need for surgical revascularization, or major bleeding. At 30 days, relief of rest pain and healing of ulcerations and amputations were seen in 96% patients with CLI who underwent successful intervention. At 1-year follow-up, there were 2 planned major amputations and no deaths or myocardial infarctions in patients who presented with CLI. This study demonstrated early and midterm safety and efficacy of primary below-the-knee stent-supported angioplasty for both CLI and severe lifestyle-limiting claudication.

Therapeutic Angiogenesis

A large percentage of patients with CLI still suffer from major amputations and death within 1 year because of insufficient response to pharmacotherapy and percutaneous or surgical revascularization. New pharmacological and angiogenic therapies need to be explored given the severe morbidity and mortality of this condition. The first phase of angiogenesis therapies in patients with coronary or peripheral ischemia were aimed at delivering angiogenic factors, such as vascular endothelial growth factors (VEGF) and fibroblast growth factor-2 to ischemic tissues by using recombinant proteins or vectors encoding these factors. In early nonrandomized clinical trials, encouraging results were obtained. However, results of controlled clinical trials have not been consistent.[110]

The second phase of therapeutic angiogenesis included identification of circulating bone-marrow-derived endothelial progenitor cells (EPCs), such as hematopoietic progenitor cells (CD34, c-kit) and endothelial cells (VEGFR2), which participate in ischemia-induced angiogenesis. The EPCs are believed to be recruited to the sites of ischemia and differentiate into the endothelial cells and smooth muscle cells leading to new blood vessel formation. Many of the *angiogenic growth factors* identified in the first phase were shown to function as vasculogenic cytokines in the second phase. Administration of cytokines such as granulocyte-macrophage colony-stimulating factor (GM-CSF), which promote the mobilization of the bone-marrow-derived EPCs was studied in the START trial. This study involved patients with limb ischemia and showed no efficacy of GM-CSF in therapeutic angiogenesis.[111]

In the third phase, the bone-marrow-derived cells were identified in the ischemic sites, more specifically in the perivascular location. Their participation in tissue vascularization was limited to an instructive role by producing *paracrine factors*. More recently, Tateno et al[112] reported the possible usefulness of peripheral blood mononuclear cells (PB-MNC) when transplanted in critically ischemic limbs in 29 "no option" patients. Approximately 10 billion PB-MNCs were collected from each patient by peripheral blood apheresis and injected at approximately 100 sites. The procedure was repeated about 1 month later. The patients were assessed at 2, 9, and 12 months after treatment according to increase in maximum walking distance, healing of ischemic ulcers, ABI, and decrease in rest pain and amputations. In 21 of 29 patients, improvement in at least one of these categories was noted. This is in contrast to the findings in another study, in which injection of PB-MNCs was performed as a negative control in the contralateral limb of patients treated with injections with bone marrow MNCs.[113] Tateno et al[112] found that the responders had increased plasma levels of angiogenic factors, in particular interleukin-1B. The authors suggested that transplanted PB-MNCs promoted tissue vascularization by stimulating skeletal muscles in ischemic limbs to increase production of inter-leukin-1B and other angiogenic cytokines. The efficacy of PB-MNCs in neovascularization in patients with CLI should be studied in a double-blind placebo controlled randomized study.

Summary

CLI results from multiple occlusive lesions in limb arteries coupled with structural and functional changes in microcirculation leading to inadequate tissue perfusion and ulcers or necrosis. The principal aim of therapy should be directed toward the correction of arterial obstructions by endovascular or surgical revascularization and local wound care. Pharmacotherapy may enhance the result of revascularization by normalizing or improving the microcirculation, and may be the only option in patients who are not candidates for or have failed revascularization. Future treatment strategies involving gene and cell therapies have shown promising results.

References

1. Dormandy J, Verstraete M, Andreani D, et al. Second European consensus document on chronic critical leg ischemia. *Circulation*. 1991;84(Suppl 4):1-26.

2. Ad Hoc Committee on Reporting Standards. Suggested standards for reports dealing with lower extremity ischemia. *J Vasc Surg*. 1986;4:80-94.

3. Makin A, Silverman SH, Lip GY. Peripheral vascular disease and Virchow's triad for thrombogenesis. *QJM*. 2002;95:199.

4. Rossi M, Carpi A. Skin microcirculation in peripheral arterial obliterative disease. *Biomed. Pharmacother*. 58 (2004); 427-431.

5. Behrendt D, Ganz P. Endothelial function. From vascular biology to clinical applications. *Am J Cardiol*. 2002;90:40L-48L.

6. Mantovani A, Dejana E. Cytokines as communication signals between leukocytes and endo-

thelial cells. *Immunol Today.* 1989;10:370-375.

7.   Boneu B, Abbal M, Plante J, et al. Letter: Factor-VIII complex and endothelial damage. *Lancet.* 1975;1:1430.

8.   Dormandy J, Heeck L, Vig S. The natural history of claudication: risk to life and limb. *Semin Vasc Surg.* 1999;12:123-137.

9.   Nehler MR, Mueller RJ, McLafferty RB, et al. Outcome of catheter directed thrombolysis for lower extremity arterial bypass occlusion. *J Vasc Surg.* 1999;12:123-137.

10. Dormandy J, Belcher G, Broos P, et al. Prospective study of 713 below-knee amputations for ischemia and the effect of a prostacyclin analogue on healing. Hawaii Study Group. *Br J Surg.* 1994;81:33-37.

11. The Vascular Society of Great Britain and Ireland. Critical limb ischemia: management and outcome. Report of a national survey. *Eur J Vasc Endovasc Surg.*1995;10:108-113.

12. Dormandy JA, Rutherford RB. Management of peripheral arterial disease (PAD). TASC Working group. TransAtlantic Inter-Society Consensus (TASC*). J Vasc Surg.* 2000;31(1 Pt 2):S1-S296.

13. Taylor LM Jr, Porter JM. Clinical and anatomic considerations for surgery in femoropopliteal disease and the results of surgery. *Circulation.* 1991;83 (2 Suppl):I63-I69.

14. Crawford ES, Bomberger RA, Glaeser DH, Saleh SA, Russell WL. Aortoiliac occlusive disease: factors influencing survival and function following reconstructive operation over a twenty-five-year period. *Surgery.* 1981;90:1055-1067.

15. Muluk SC, Muluk VS, Kelley ME, et al. Outcome events in patients with claudication: a 15-year study in 2777 patients. *J Vasc Surg.* 2001;33:251-257.

16. Feinglass J, Perace WH, Martin GJ, et al. Postoperative and amputation-free survival outcomes after femorodistal bypass grafting surgery: findings from the Department of Veterans Affairs National Surgical Quality Improvement Program. *J Vasc Surg.* 2001;34:283-290.

17. Karla M, Gloviczki P, Bower TC, et al. Limb salvage after successful pedal bypass grafting is associated with improved long-term survival. *J Vasc Surg.* 2001;33:6-16.

18. Pomposelli FB Jr, Kansal N, Hamdan AD, et al. A decade of experience with dorsalis pedis artery bypass: analysis of outcome in more than 100 cases. *J Vasc Surg.* 2003;37:307-315.

19. Taylor LM Jr, Hamre D, Dalman RL, Porter JM. Limb salvage vs amputation for critical ischemia: the role of vascular surgery. *Arch Surg.* 1991;126:1251-1257.

20. Abou-Zamzam AM Jr, Lee RW, Moneta GL, Taylor LM Jr, Porter JM. Functional outcome after infrainguinal bypass for limb salvage. *J Vasc Surg.* 1997;25:287-295.

21. Walker SR, Yusuf SW, Hopkinson BR. A 10-year follow-up of patients presenting with ischemic rest pain of the lower limbs. *Eur J Vasc Endovasc Surg.* 1998;15:478-482.

22. Long-term mortality and its predictors in patients with critical leg ischemia. The I.C.A.I. Group (Gruppo di Studio dell'Ischemia Cronica Critica delgi Arti Inferiori). The Study Group of Critical Chronic Ischemia of the Lower Extremities. *Eur J Vasc Endovasc Surg.* 1997;14:91-95.

23. Nehler MR, Moneta GL, Edwards JM, Yeager RA, Taylor LM Jr, Porter JM. Surgery for chronic lower extremity ischemia in patients eighty or more years of age: operative results and assessment of post-operative independence. *J Vasc Surg.* 1993;18:618-624.

24. Luther M, Lepäntalo M. Femorotibial reconstructions for chronic critical leg ischemia: influence on outcome by diabetes, gender and age. *Eur J Vasc Endovasc Surg.* 1997;13:569-577.

25. Virkkunen J, Heikkinen M, Lepäntalo M, Metsänoja R, Salenius J. Diabetes as an independent risk factor for early postoperative complications in critical limb ischemia. *J Vasc Surg.* 2004;40:761-767.

26. Albers M, Romiti M, Braganca Pereira CA, Fonseca RL, da Silva JM. A meta-analysis of infrainguinal arterial reconstruction in patients with end-stage renal disease. *Eur J Vasc Endovasc Surg.* 2001;22:294-300.

27. Regensteiner JG, Hiatt WR. Current medical therapies for patients with peripheral arterial disease: a critical review. *Am J Med.* 2002;112:49-57.

28. Strandnes DE Jr. Noninvasive vascular laboratory and vascular imaging. In: Young JR, Olin

JW, Bartholomew JR, eds. *Peripheral Vascular Disease.* St. Louis, MO: Mosby; 1996:369-374.

29. Hummel BW, Hummel BA, Mowbry A, et al. Reactive hyperemia vs treadmill exercise testing in arterial disease. *Arch Surg.* 1978;113:95-98.

30. MacDonald NR. Pulse volume plethysmography. *J Vasc Tech.* 1994;18:241-248.

31. Raines JK, Darling RC, Both K, et al. Vascular laboratory criteria for the management of peripheral vascular disease of the lower extremities. *Surgery.* 1976;79:21-29.

32. Ramsey DE, Manke DA, Sumner DS. Toe blood pressure – a valuable adjunct to blood pressure measurement fro assessing peripheral arterial disease. *J Cardiovasc Surg.* 1983;24:43-48.

33. Strandness DE, Schultz RD, Sumner DS, et al. Ultrasonic flow detection: a useful technique in the evaluation of peripheral vascular disease. *Am J Surg.* 1967;113:295-297.

34. Bunt TJ, Holloway GA. TcPO2 as an accurate predictor of therapy in limb salvage. *Ann Vasc Surg.* 1996;10:224-227.

35. Comerota AJ, Throm RC, Kelly P, Jaff M. Tissue (muscle) oxygen saturation (StO2): a new measure of symptomatic lower-extremity arterial disease. *J Vasc Surg.* 2003;38:724-729.

36. Baum RA, Rutter CM, Sunshine JH, et al. Multicenter trial to evaluate vascular magnetic resonance angiography of the lower extremity. American College of Radiology Rapid Technology Assessment Group. *JAMA.* 1995;274:875.

37. Yucel EK, Kaufman JA, Geller SC, et al. Atherosclerotic occlusive disease of the lower extremity: prospective evaluation with two dimensional time-of-flight MR angiography. *Radiology.* 1993;187:637.

38. Ho KY, Leiner T, deHann MW, Kessels AG, Kitslaar PJ, van Engleshoven JM. Peripheral vascular tree stenosis: evaluation with moving-bed infusion tracking MR angiography. *Radiology.* 1998;206:683-692.

39. Meaney JF, Ridway JP, Chakraverty S, et al. Stepping-table gadolinium-enhanced digital subtraction MR angiography of the aorta and lower extremities: preliminary experience. *Radiology.* 1999;211:59-67.

40. Wang Y, Priscilla A, Winchester PA, et al. Contrast-enhanced peripheral MR angiography

from the abdominal aorta to the pedal arteries: combined dynamic two-dimensional and bolus-chase three-dimensional acquisitions. *Invest Radiol.* 2001;36:170-177.

41. Meissner OA, Rieger J, Weber C, Siebert U, et al. Critical limb ischemia: hybrid MR angiography compared with DSA. *Radiology.* 2005;235:308-318.

42. Hany TF, Carroll TJ, Omary RA, et al. Aorta and runoff vessels: single-injection MR angiography with automated table movement compared with multiinjection time-resolved MR angiography – initial results. *Radiology.* 2001;221:266-272.

43. Khilnani NM, Winchester PA, Prince MR, et al. Peripheral vascular disease: combined 3D bolus chase and dynamic 2D MR angiography compared with X-ray angiography for treatment planning. *Radiology.* 2002;224:63-74.

44. Zhang HL, Khilnani NM, Prince MR, et al. Diagnostic accuracy of time-resolved 2D projection MR angiography for symptomatic infrapopliteal arterial occlusive disease. *AJR Am J Roentgenol.* 2005;184:938-947.

45. Huber A, Scheidler J, Wintersperger B, et al. Moving-table MR angiography of the peripheral runoff vessels: comparison of body coil and dedicated phased array coil systems. *AJR Am J Roentgenol.* 2003;180:1365-1373.

46. Hagspiel KD, Yao L, Shih MP, Burkholder B, Bissonette E, Harthun NL. Comparison of multistation MR angiography with integrated parallel acquisition technique versus conventional technique with a dedicated phased-array coil system in peripheral vascular disease. *J Vasc Interv Radiol.* 2006;17:263-269.

47. Kreitner KF, Kalden P, Neufang A, et al. Diabetes and peripheral arterial occlusive disease: prospective comparison of contrast-enhanced three-dimensional MR angiography with conventional digital subtraction angiography. *AJR Am J Roentgenol.* 2000;174:171-179.

48. Dorweiler B, Neufang A, Kreitner KF, Schmiedt W, Oelert H. Magnetic resonance angiography unmasks reliable target vessels for pedal bypass grafting in patients with diabetes mellitus. *J Vasc Surg.* 2002;35:766-772.

49. Lapeyre M, Kobeiter H, Desgranges P, Rahmouni A, Becquemin J, Luciani A. Assessment

of critical limb ischemia in patients with diabetes: comparison of MR angiography and digital subtraction angiography. *AJR Am J Roentgenol.* 2005;185:1641-1650.

50. Loewe C, Schoder M, Rand T, et al. Peripheral vascular occlusive disease: evaluation with contrast-enhanced moving-bed MR angiography versus digital subtraction angiography in 106 patients. *AJR Am J Roentgenol.* 2002;179:1013-1021.

51. Morasch MD, Collins J, Pereles FS, et al. Lower extremity stepping-table magnetic resonance angiography with multilevel contrast timing and segmented contrast infusion. *J Vasc Surg.* 2003;37:62-71.

52. Owens RS, Carpenter JP, Baum RA, Perloff LJ, Cope C. Magnetic resonance imaging of angiographically occult runoff vessels in peripheral arterial occlusive disease. *N Engl J Med.* 1992;326:1577-1581.

53. Ofer A, Nitecki SS, Linn S, et al. Multidetector CT angiography of peripheral vascular disease: a prospective comparison with intraarterial digital subtraction angiography. *AJR Am J Roentgenol.* 2003;180:719-724.

54. Martin ML, Tay KH, Flak, et al. Multidetector CT angiography of the aortoiliac system and lower extremities: a prospective comparison with digital subtraction angiography. *AJR Am J Roentgenol.* 2003;180:1085-1091.

55. Catalano C, Fraioli F, Laghi A, et al. Infrarenal aortic and lower-extremity arterial disease: diagnostic performance of multiple-detector row CT angiography. *Radiology.* 2004;231:555-563.

56. Ota H, Takase K, Igarashi K, et al. MDCT compared with digital subtraction angiography for assessment of lower extremity arterial occlusive disease: importance of reviewing cross-sectional images. *AJR Am J Roentgenol.* 2004;182:201-209.

57. Edwards AJ, Wells IP, Roobottom CA. Multidetector row, CT angiography of the lower limb arteries: a prospective comparison of volume-rendered techniques and intra-arterial digital subtraction angiography. *Clin Radiol.* 2005;60:85-95.

58. Portugaller HR, Schoellnast H, Hausegger KA, et al. Multislice spiral CT angiography in peripheral arterial occlusive disease: a valuable tool in detecting significant arterial lumen narrowing? *Eur Radiol.* 2004;14:1681-1687.

59. Willmann JK, Baumert B, Schertler T, et al. Aortoiliac and lower extremity arteries assessed with 16-detector row CT angiography: prospective comparison with digital subtraction angiography. *Radiology.* 2005;236:1083-1093.

60. Ouwendijk R, de Vries M, Pattynama PM, et al. Imaging peripheral arterial disease: a randomized controlled trial comparing contrast-enhanced MR angiography and multi-detector row CT angiography. *Radiology.* 2005;236:1094-1103.

61. Oiln JW, Kaufman JA, Bluemke DA, et al. Atherosclerotic Vascular Disease Conference: Writing Group IV: Imaging. *Circulation.* 2004;109:2626-2633.

62. Unno N, Mitsuka H, Takei Y, et al. Virtual angioscopy using 3-dimensional rotational digital subtraction angiography for endovascular assessment. *J Endovasc Ther.* 2002;9:529-534.

63. Bosanac Z, Miller RJ, Jain M. Rotational digital subtraction carotid angiography: technique and comparison with static digital subtraction angiography. *Clin Radiol.* 1998;53:682-687.

64. Seymour HR, Matson MB, Belli AM, et al. Rotational digital subtraction angiography of the renal arteries: technique and evaluation in the study of native and transplant renal arteries. *Br J Radiol.* 2001;74:134-141.

65. Spinosa DJ, Kaufman JA, Hartnell GD. Gadolinium chelates in angiography and interventional radiology: a useful alternative to iodinated contrast media for angiography. *Radiology.* 2002;223:319-325.

66. Oliva VL, Denbow N, Therasse E, et al. Digital subtraction angiography of the abdominal aorta and lower extremities: carbon dioxide versus iodinated contrast material. *J Vasc Interv Radiol.* 1999;10:723-731.

67. London NJ, Varty K, Sayers RD, Thompson MM, Bell PR, Bolia A. Percutaneous transluminal angioplasty for lower-limb critical ischaemia. *Br J Surg.* 1995;82:1232-1235.

68. Alson MD, Lang EV, Kaufman JA. Pedal arterial imaging. *J Vasc Interv Radiol.* 1997;8:9-18.

69. Karlström L, Bergqvist D. Effects of vascular surgery on amputation rates and mortality. *Eur J Vasc Endovasc Surg*. 1997;14:273-283.

70. Wolfe JN. Defining the outcome of critical ischaemia: a one year prospective study. *Br J Surg*. 1986;73:321.

71. Lowe GD, Dunlop DJ, Lawson DH, et al. Double-blind controlled clinical trial of ancrod for ischemic rest pain of the leg. *Angiology*. 1982;33:46-50.

72. Norgen L, Alwmark A, Angqvist KA, et al. A stable prostacyclin analogue (Iloprost) in the treatment of ischemic ulcers of the lower limb: a Scandinavian-Polish placebo-controlled randomized multicenter study. *Eur J Vasc Surg*. 1990;4:463-467.

73. Bliss B, Wilkins D, Campbell WB, et al. Treatment of limb threatening ischemia with intravenous Iloprost: a randomized double-blind placebo-controlled study. *Eur J Vasc Surg*. 1991;5:511-516.

74. Belcher G. Effects of iloprost and factors affecting outcome in patients with severe inoperable lower limb ischaemia. In: Schrör K, ed. *Prostaglandins in the Cardiovascular Symptom*. Basel: Karger; 1992:354-359.

75. Kihn RB, Warren R, Beebe GW. The "geriatric" amputee. *Ann Surg*. 1972;176:305-314.

76. Whitehouse FW, Jurgensen C, Block MA. The later life of the diabetic amputee: another look at the fate of the second leg. *Diabetes*. 1968;17:520-521.

77. Norgren L. Definition, incidence and epidemiology. In: Dormandy JA, Stock G, eds. *Critical Leg Ischaemia. Its Pathophysiology and Management*. Berlin: Springer-Verlag, 1990:7-13.

78. Gregg RO. Bypass or amputation? Concomitant view of bypass arterial grafting and major amputations. *Am J Surg*. 1985;149:397-402.

79. Brock FE, Abri O, Baitsch G, et al. Iloprost in the treatment of ischemic tissue lesions in diabetics. Results of a placebo-controlled multicenter study with a stable prostacyclin derivative. *Schweiz Med Wochenschr*. 1990;120:1477-1482.

80. Diehm C, Abri O, Baitsch G, et al. Iloprost, a stable prostacycline derivative, in stage 4 arterial occlusive disease. A placebo-controlled multicenter study. *Dtsch Med Wochenschr*. 1989;114:783-788.

81. Sakaguchi S. Prostaglandin E_1 intra-arterial infusion therapy in patients with ischemic ulcers of the extremities. *Int Angiol*. 1984;3:39-42.

82. Guilmot J, Diot E. For the French Iloprost Study Group. Treatment of lower limb ischemia due to atherosclerosis in diabetic and nondiabetic patients with iloprost, a stable analogue of prostacycline: results of French Multicenter trial. *Drug Invest*. 1991;3:351-359.

83. Ciprostene Study Group. The effect of ciprostene in patients with peripheral vascular disease (PVD) characterized by ischemic ulcers. *J Clin Pharmacol*. 1991;31:81-87.

84. UK Severe Limb Ischemia Study Group. Treatment of limb threatening ischemia with intravenous Iloprost: a randomized double-blind placebo controlled study. *Eur J Vasc Surg*.1991;5:511-516.

85. Brass EP, Anthony R, Dormandy J, et al. Parenteral therapy with lipo-ecraprost, a lipid-based formulation of a PGE1 analog, does not alter six-month outcomes in patients with critical leg ischemia. *J Vasc Surg*. 2006;43:752-759.

86. Smith FB, Bradbury AW, Fowkes FG. Intravenous naftidrofuryl for critical limb ischemia. *Cochrane Database Syst Rev* 2000;CD002070.

87. European Study group. Intravenous pentoxifylline. *Eur J Vasc Endovasc Surg*. 1995;9:426-436.

88. Norwegian Pentoxifylline Multicenter Trial Group. Efficacy and clinical tolerance of parenteral pentoxifylline. *Ant Angiol*. 1996;15:75-80.

89. Cook AW, Oyger A, Baggenstos P. Vascular disease of extremities: electrical stimulation of spinal cord and posterior roots. *NYS J Med*. 1976;69:1309-1311.

90. Augustinsson LE, Carlsson CA, Holm J, Jivegard L. Epidural electrical stimulation of severe limb ischemia. *Ann Surgery*. 1985;202:104-111.

91. Broseta J, Barbera J, de Vera JA, et al. Spinal cord stimulation in peripheral arterial disease. *J Neurosurg*. 1986;64:71-80.

92. Frost T, Pfutzner A, Bauersachs R, et al. Comparison of the microvascular response to TENS and post-occlusive ischaemia in the diabetic foot. *J Diabetes Complications*. 1997;11:291-297.

93. Cosma P, Svenson H, Bornmyr S, Wikstrom S. Effects of TENS on the microcirculation in chronic leg ulcers. *Scand J Plastic Reconstr Hand Surg.* 200;34:61-64.

94. Simpson KH, Ward J. A randomized, double-blind, crossover study of the use of transcutaneous spinal electroanalgesia in patients with pain from chronic critical limb ischemia. *J Pain Symptom Manage.* 2004;28:511-516.

95. Louridas G, Saadia R, Spelay J, et al. The ArtAssist device in chronic lower limb ischemia. A pilot study. *Int Angiol.* 2002;21:28-35.

96. Krake Pea. *Cochrane Database Syst Rev.* 2004;CD004123.

97. Dormandy JA, Ray S. The natural history of peripheral arterial disease. In: Tooke JE, Lowe GD, eds. *A Textbook of Vascular Medicine.* London: Arnold; 1996:162-175.

98. Hobson RW, Lynch TG, Jamil Z, et al. Results of revascularization and amputation in severe lower extremity ischemia: a five-year clinical experience. *J Vasc Surg.* 1985;2:174-185.

99. Brewster DC, Perler BA, Robinson JG, Darling RC. Aortofemoral graft for multilevel occlusive disease. Predictors of success and need for distal bypass. *Arch Surg.* 1982;117:1593-1600.

100. de Vries SO, Hunink MG. Results of aortic bifurcation grafts for aortoiliac occlusive disease: a meta analysis. *J Vasc Surg.* 1997;26:558-569.

101. Chung J, Bartelson BB, Hiatt WR, et al. Wound healing and functional outcomes after infrainguinal bypass with reversed saphenous vein for critical limb ischemia. *J Vasc Surg.* 2006;43:1183-1190.

102. Schwarten DE. Clinical and anatomical considerations for non-operative therapy in tibial disease and the results of angioplasty. *Circulation.* 1991;83[Suppl I]:I86-I90.

103. Soder HK, Manninen HI, Jaakkola P, et al. Prospective trial of infrapopliteal artery balloon angioplasty for critical limb ischemia: angiographic and clinical results. *JVIR.* 2000;11:1021-1031.

104. Dorros G, Jaff MJ, Dorros AM, Mathiak LM, He T. Tibioperoneal (outflow lesion) angio-plasty can be used as primary treatment in 235 patients with critical limb ischemia: five-year follow-up. *Circulation.* 2001;104:2057-2062.

105. Bypass versus angioplasty in severe ischaemia of the leg (BASIL): multicenter, randomized controlled trial. BASIL trial investigators. *Lancet.* 2005;366:1925-1934.

106. Laird JL. Laser angioplasty for critical limb ischemia phase 2: final results. International Society of Endovascular Therapy 2003 Conference, Miami, FL. January 2003.

107. Boisers M, Peeters P, Elst FV, et al. Excimer laser assisted angioplasty for critical limb ischemia: results of the LACI Belgium study. *Eur J Vasc Endovasc Surg.* 2005;29:613-619.

108. Yancey AE, Minion DJ, Rodriguez C, Patterson DE, Endean ED. Peripheral atherectomy in Trans-Atlantic Inter-Society Consensus type C femoropopliteal lesions for limb salvage. *J Vasc Surg.* 2006;44:503-509.

109. Feiring AJ, Wesolowski AA, Lade S. Primary stent-supported angioplasty for treatment of below-knee critical limb ischemia and severe claudication: early and one-year outcomes. *J Am Coll Cardiol.* 2004;44:2307-2314.

110. Yla-Hertualla S, Alitalo K. Gene transfer as a tool to induce therapeutic vascular growth. *Nat Med.* 2003;9:694-701.

111. van Royen N, Schirmer SH, Atasever B, et al. START Trial: a pilot study on STimulation of ARTeriogenesis using subcutaneous application of granulocyte-macrophage colony-stimulating factor as a new treatment for peripheral vascular disease. *Circulation.* 2005;112:1040-1046.

112. Tateno K, Minamino T, Toko H, et al. Critical roles of muscle-secreted angiogenic factors in therapeutic neovascularization. *Circ Res.* 2006;98:1194-1202.

113. Tateishi-Yuyama E, Matsubara H, Murohara T, et al. Therapeutic Angiogenesis Using Cell Transplantation (TACT) Study Investigators. Therapeutic angiogenesis for patients with limb ischemia by autologous transplantation of bone-marrow cells: a pilot study and a randomized controlled trial. *Lancet.* 2002;360:427-435.

16

Vascular Access Complications and Treatment

Stephen R. Ramee and John P. Reilly

The access site for endovascular procedures performed for the diagnosis and treatment of peripheral artery disease (PAD) remains a common source for complications. Increasingly complex procedures balanced by advances in technology and techniques have resulted in little change in the incidence of vascular access site complications.[1-4] The reported rate of access site complications from endovascular procedures ranges from 0.7% to 9%.[4-7] As many as 75,000 surgical procedures a year are performed related to access site complications.[8]

Arterial Puncture Technique

Appropriate attention must be directed toward avoiding complications before they occur. The patient's history should be reviewed with particular attention to factors that may predispose to vascular access complications: thrombocytopenia, renal insufficiency, use of anticoagulants, known PAD, previous access site complications, or history of vascular surgery involving the proposed access site. Prior to the procedure, a complete examination of the access site is mandatory. This examination should include an evaluation of the quality of the pulse as well as all downstream pulses of the extremity, a determination of the presence of thrills or bruits over the proposed access site, a look at the appearance of the entire extremity, and an assessment of the soft tissue over the site, for example, scar tissue. The proposed procedure should be kept in mind when interpreting the findings of the preprocedural examination. If the access site appears inappropriate for the proposed procedure—for example, if the vessel appears to be too small or diseased to accept the sheath that will be required—another strategy for vascular access should be adopted, or a noninvasive imaging test considered to demonstrate that the initial strategy is appropriate. A complete examination prior to the procedure aids in the interpretation of postprocedural findings should a complication arise. At the completion of all successful procedures, the access site should be examined, as well as distal pulses of the extremity checked in the event of complications presenting later.

Meticulous attention to technique when gaining access reduces the probability of complications. Single-, front-wall puncture of the

Vascular Disease: Diagnostic and Therapeutic Approaches. © 2011 Michael R. Jaff and Christopher J. White, editors. Cardiotext Publishing, ISBN: 978-1-9353951-6-4.

vessel on the first attempt ensures the greatest likelihood of a complication-free procedure. Particular attention must be paid to anatomic landmarks, keeping in mind that the inguinal crease bears no consistent relationship to the inguinal ligament or the pelvis. Performing fluoroscopic imaging prior to obtaining femoral artery access avoids arterial punctures that are too high or too low, thereby reducing complications.[9,10]

Similarly, care must be paid when performing popliteal puncture. Arterial puncture should be performed mediolaterally 6 cm above the fluoroscopically identified knee joint to reduce the risk of creating an arteriovenous fistula.[11] Some authors have recommended ultrasonography of the popliteal fossa to determine the level where the artery and vein are no longer overlapped.[12] We prefer obtaining contralateral access, positioning a 4-Fr diagnostic catheter in the ipsilateral external iliac or common femoral artery. The patient is then placed in a prone position, and the back of the ipsilateral leg is prepped and sterilized. An angiogram is performed through the diagnostic catheter to locate the popliteal artery prior to puncture. Once the course of the artery has been angiographically demonstrated, a front-wall puncture is performed.

Retrograde femoral artery access is the most common vascular access for diagnostic angiography and catheter-based intervention. The larger caliber of the femoral artery accepts larger sheaths and catheters relative to radial or brachial artery access. This may be of greater significance for peripheral intervention, which may require larger-caliber sheaths relative to coronary angiography. Femoral artery access allows more efficacious manual compression against the femoral head after sheath removal. Vascular access complications are more likely to be related to bleeding with femoral artery access, while brachial and radial artery access complications are more likely to be ischemic.

Radial artery access is used in only a minority of endovascular procedures in the United States, although it is used more widely outside the United States.[13] As with femoral artery access, preprocedural examination of the pulse should be performed to characterize the quality and caliber of the radial artery. An Allen's test may be performed in order to assess the integrity of the palmar arch. An abnormal Allen's test, however, need not preclude radial artery access. Arterial lines are frequently placed in radial arteries in intensive care unit settings without performing an Allen test. There is no predictive power of an abnormal Allen test and ischemic injuries.[14,15] Radial arteries have been successfully used as conduits for patients undergoing coronary artery bypass graft surgery without complication in patients with an abnormal Allen test.[16] Radial artery access is associated with lower complication rates as compared to femoral artery access. Diagnostic and interventional endovascular procedures through radial artery access for carotid, renal, subclavian, and iliac arteries have been reported.[17-19] When performing angiography or intervention from the radial artery, the operator must account for patient height and distance to the target vessel when planning equipment for the procedure. In many cases of renal and iliac intervention, interventional devices will require a 150-cm platform with guiding catheters and sheaths of appropriate length.

Bleeding Complications

Acute bleeding complications are a potentially fatal complication of vascular access for endovascular procedures, thus they must be promptly diagnosed and treated. We have adopted the practice of performing angiography through the sheath after obtaining vascular access prior to any other angiography or administration of anticoagulants. The angiographic evaluation of the access site as well as neighboring branch vessels allows the interventionalist to detect and treat bleeding before it might otherwise become clinically obvious. Prior to systemic anticoagulation, steps may be taken to achieve hemostasis, which will often allow the operator to proceed with the planned procedure. In some cases, the operator may choose to defer the planned procedure for a later date.

Procedural Hemorrhage

Despite the performance of angiography at the outset, intraprocedural hemorrhage may still occur. Hematoma at the sheath insertion site may be managed with manual compression, or insertion of the next larger sheath size. If the hematoma continues to expand despite these measures, a complete evaluation of anticoagulation status must be performed, including the measurement of *activated clotting time (ACT)* if heparin has been administered. Protamine sulfate should be administered to reverse heparin anticoagulation. Expanding hematoma may rapidly progress to shock,[20] thus fluid resuscitation including transfusion, if appropriate, is crucial. Interruption of the planned procedure to perform arteriography through the sheath should be performed as soon as is feasible. Digital subtraction angiography may be required to reveal smaller sources of bleeding.

The diagnosis of the source of bleeding will determine the next course of action. If the cause of bleeding is around the sheath itself, frequently caused by kinking at the point of entry, the interventionalist may replace the sheath for the next larger sheath. Repeat angiography should then be performed to confirm that hemostasis has been achieved. If bleeding continues from the sheath insertion site, the sheath should be removed and manual pressure applied to achieve hemostasis, and a decision regarding timing of the completion of the originally planned procedure must be made.

If hemorrhage continues, then contralateral access should be obtained and a 6-Fr cross-over (Cook) or 6-Fr 45-cm Pinnacle (Boston Scientific) sheath placed in the external iliac artery. In cases with difficult aortic bifurcations due to anatomy, post-iliac stenting or post-aortobifemoral grafting, it may be necessary to obtain brachial artery access. In these cases, a 6-Fr shuttle sheath (Cook) or 6-Fr 90-cm Pinnacle sheath (Boston Scientific) is positioned in the external iliac artery. Angiography localizes the source of bleeding, and an 0.035-in wire is placed in the superficial femoral artery. A 6- to 8-mm by 4-cm peripheral angioplasty balloon can then positioned across the bleeding source and inflated at low pressure to tamponade the bleeding from inside the vessel (Figure 16.1). Angiography should be performed through the sheath while the balloon is inflated to confirm that the balloon achieves hemostasis; if it is not hemostatic, the next larger balloon may be required. Reassessment of anticoagulation status and bleeding parameters should be performed to confirm that they have been corrected. Prolonged inflations of 3 to 5 minutes with interval angiography will stop bleeding in most patients. For those patients in whom hemostasis cannot be achieved with balloon tamponade, the placement of a covered stent (endoluminal graft) should be considered. The site of bleeding will determine whether a covered stent can be deployed, as major side branches preclude their use. The optimal location for a covered stent is in the external iliac, superficial femoral, or deep femoral arteries. The common femoral artery is suboptimal, secondary to the disadvantages of possibly covering the profunda femoris, graft

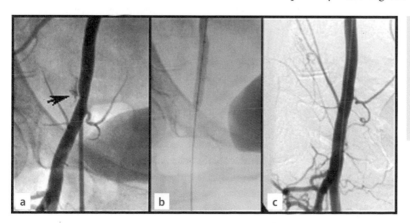

Figure 16.1 (a) Hemorrhage near the sheath insertion site. (b) After contralateral access is obtained, a balloon is positioned across the bleeding site and inflated. (c) After balloon tamponade of 5 minutes, hemostasis is achieved.

fracture at this flexion point, and loss of a site for vascular access for future procedures. Angiography prior to completion of the procedure must demonstrate that there is no ongoing bleeding. If hemostasis cannot be achieved, then surgical repair of the source of bleeding should follow immediately.

Laceration of a side branch artery, such as the inferior epigastric artery, is an important potential source of bleeding. In these cases, balloon tamponade will have to be performed within the branch artery at the site of laceration. This technique will require an 0.014-in wire and smaller balloons, 2 to 3 mm in diameter—typically coronary equipment (Figure 16.2). If bleeding persists despite prolonged balloon tamponade and reversal of any anticoagulation administered, then embolization of the side branch artery may be considered. The operator must be proficient in the deployment of microcoils or delivery of thrombin through a catheter due to the risk of thrombosis of the arterial supply to the lower extremity when this procedure is not performed with precision. After positioning a 0.014- or 0.018-in wire distally in the artery, a 2.5-Fr Transit catheter (Cordis Endovascular) is advanced distal to the site of bleeding. An appropriately sized microcoil is then advanced to the tip of the catheter. The

catheter is then positioned for final deployment of the microcoil. Angiography is performed prior to deployment to confirm that the coil will be deployed completely in the branch artery. It is not unusual for 2 or more microcoils to completely embolize an artery, so the interventionalist should plan appropriately to provide a sufficient landing zone to prevent deployment within the parent vessel. The microcoils are then deployed and final angiography performed to confirm embolization of the vessel and control of hemorrhage.

If microcoils are unavailable, then the operator may consider other means of embolization of the side branch. Silva et al[21] report the use of intra-arterial thrombin for the embolization of the inferior epigastric artery for the treatment of retroperitoneal hemorrhage. After positioning an over-the-wire catheter in the inferior epigastric artery near the ostium, the balloon is inflated. Angiography is performed through the crossover sheath with the balloon inflated as well as through the wire lumen of the balloon. These 2 injection angiograms are performed to confirm sealing of the vessel by the balloon to prevent reflux of thrombin into the femoral artery. Thrombin-JMI (Jones Pharma) is reconstituted and diluted in normal saline to a concentration of 50 IU/mL. Thrombin is

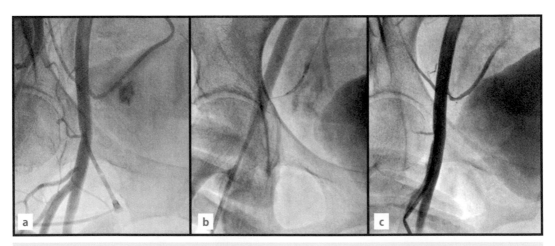

Figure 16.2 (a) The inferior epigastric artery is a cause of bleeding due to inadvertent puncture when obtaining vascular access. (b) A 0.014-in wire is advanced distal to the site of hemorrhage and an appropriately sized coronary balloon is inflated to tamponade the vessel. (c) Hemostasis is achieved.

then administered through the balloon catheter lumen in 100-IU doses, and angiography performed through the balloon lumen to determine embolization is complete with no further evidence of hemorrhage. Finally, angiography is performed through the crossover sheath to confirm that no thrombin has embolized to the femoral artery.

Postprocedure Hemorrhage

Patients recovering from femoral artery access must be monitored closely for evidence of bleeding. A routine of frequent vital signs, pulse, and access site examination should be established in the recovery area. Any evidence of overt bleeding or expanding hematoma requires applying pressure to the common femoral artery proximal to the puncture site. As described previously, anticoagulation status should be established and corrected promptly. If prolonged compression is required, a mechanical compression device can be applied. If hemorrhage cannot be controlled with compression, the patient should be brought back to the procedure room for angiography and treatment as described.

Hypotension following a procedure should be presumed to be secondary to bleeding until this diagnosis can be excluded. High arterial puncture site and postprocedural anticoagulation are important risk factors for retroperitoneal hemorrhage, which is a life-threatening complication of endovascular procedures; prompt diagnosis is crucial.[22] The reported incidence of retroperitoneal hematoma has been reported to occur in the range of 0.12% to 0.44% of percutaneous interventional procedures.[23] Kinnaird et al[24] reported that the incidence of retroperitoneal hemorrhage after percutaneous intervention in nearly 10,000 unselected patients was 0.27%. The majority of patients with retroperitoneal hemorrhage can be managed conservatively with bed rest, fluid resuscitation, analgesia, and transfusion, but this complication is potentially fatal.[22,25]

In patients with unexplained hypotension, ipsilateral fullness, guarding, and tenderness generally confirm the diagnosis of retroperi-

toneal bleeding. Hypotensive patients with these findings should not undergo noninvasive imaging such as computed tomography angiography or ultrasonography, as this strategy will only confirm the obvious and delay treatment. Unstable patients diagnosed with ongoing hemorrhage should undergo immediate angiography from the contralateral femoral or brachial artery. After identification of the cause of bleeding, corrective measures can taken as described. If digital subtraction angiography does not demonstrate bleeding, but ongoing hemorrhage is strongly suspected, surgical exploration should be considered to exclude venous laceration.

Persistent retroperitoneal hemorrhage has traditionally been treated by surgical repair of the artery.[22,25] Patients undergoing percutaneous interventional procedures have a high prevalence of significant atherosclerotic disease, as well as other comorbid conditions. These patients are at increased risk for surgery, with reports of morbidity associated with surgery, including myocardial infarction and wound infection, as high as 21% and mortality rates as high as 2% to 5%.[26,27] Endovascular treatment of bleeding complications is an attractive alternative treatment to avoid additional surgical morbidity and mortality.[21]

In summary, the potential for intraprocedure and postprocedure bleeding complications requires that the interventionalist maintains vigilance. In many patients who suffer a bleeding complication, it represents a self-limited event that can be conservatively managed with observation and fluid resuscitation. But in those who demonstrate hemodynamic instability, rapid assessment and treatment are mandatory.

Pseudoaneurysm

A *pseudoaneurysm* is a persistent defect in the arterial wall following a percutaneous procedure. Blood accumulates in a pocket in the surrounding tissue, and is in continuity with the lumen of the artery. The patient presents commonly with a painful swelling in the groin but may report numbness or paresthesias of the anteromedial aspect of the thigh from nerve compression, or ipsilateral lower-extremity swelling secondary to deep venous thrombosis. On examination, a pulsatile mass is found at the access site, and a bruit may be auscultated, although physical exam alone may be insufficient to distinguish pseudoaneurysm from hematoma.[26] Color-flow Doppler ultrasonography of the mass should be performed to identify whether it is a pseudoaneurysm. Puncture of the superficial femoral or profunda femoris artery is more likely to result in formation of pseudoaneurysm due to the small caliber of the vessel as well as difficulty with hemostasis due to lack of bony structures beneath these arteries.[9] The incidence of pseudoaneurysm after femoral arterial puncture is 0.1% to 1.5% after diagnostic procedures and as high as 7.7% after interventional procedures.[4,28-30]

Toursarkissian et al[31] reported on a series of 147 patients with pseudoaneurysm who had spontaneous resolution in 86% within 1 month. Others have reported that femoral artery pseudoaneurysm may rupture with life-threatening consequences.[32,33] Some authors recommend that asymptomatic patients with pseudoaneurysm be observed with ultrasound follow-up if the pseudoaneurysm is less than 3 cm.[34,35]

Treatment: Compression

Symptomatic patients can experience quite severe pain until closure of the pseudoaneurysm is achieved, which can be achieved in several ways. In 1991, Fellmeth et al[36] described ultrasound-guided compression repair. The ultrasonography probe identifies the defect in the femoral artery as it communicates with the blood collection. The transducer is positioned over this communication and used to compress this tract until flow has been eliminated. If the hole in the artery cannot be demonstrated, then the transducer compresses the body of the pseudoaneurysm itself. Pressure is applied for 20 to 30 minutes, and then released every 10 to 15 minutes to check if the pseudoaneurysm has been occluded. Once occlusion is obtained, a pressure dressing is applied and the patient is restricted to bed rest for 24 hours. Duplex ultrasonography is repeated at 24 hours to confirm occlusion. The patient nearly always requires sedation or analgesia to allow the degree and duration of compression needed to occlude the pseudoaneurysm. This method is labor intensive and time-consuming as well, with reported compression times up to 2.5 hours, and repeat attempts required in some cases.[37] The rate of successful closure of pseudoaneurysm is reported to be 55% to 98%,[20,32,38-51] avoiding or discontinuing anticoagulation increases the likelihood of success.[37]

Pseudoaneurysm Injection

Ultrasound-guided thrombin injection is an attractive alternative to ultrasound-guided compression repair. After the pseudoaneurysm and its "tract" or "neck" is identified, the skin over the pseudoaneurysm is prepared with Betadine. Thrombin (Thrombin JMI, Johnson & Johnson) is reconstituted with normal saline at a dilution of 1000 U/mL, and 1 mL is transferred to a tuberculin syringe. In most cases, a 1.5-in 19- to 22-gauge needle is then inserted into the pseudoaneurysm with ultrasound guidance. Blood return in the needle confirms puncture of the pseudoaneurysm, and the ultrasound ensures that the needle tip is not in the femoral artery, or near the tract of the pseudoaneurysm. An injection of saline may be performed to further ensure that the tip of the needle is positioned in the pseudoaneurysm. Thrombin is then slowly injected from the tuberculin syringe until thrombosis of the pseudoaneurysm is seen by color-flow duplex ultrasonography, usually after the injection of 0.1 to 0.3 mL (Figure 16.3). If more than 0.5 mL of thrombin is injected without thrombosis of the pseudoaneurysm, then the location of the injection should be reassessed; the needle may be in poor position, or the pseudoaneurysm may be more complex than initially appreciated. The minimum required dose is administered and directed away from the neck to reduce the risk of thrombus extension into the femoral artery.[52] The patient remains at bed rest for 2 hours, and follow-up duplex ultrasonography is performed at 24 hours to confirm occlusion. It is not mandatory for the patient to remain an inpatient before completion of the repeat imaging.

Liau et al[53] first reported thrombin injection for pseudoaneurysm in 1997 in 5 patients. Subsequently, several reports have confirmed that this procedure is safe and effective.[54-60] Ultrasound-guided injection of biodegradable collagen has also been reported to be a highly effective alternative to surgical therapy.[61] Mohler et al[62] report a multicenter experience using ultrasound-guided thrombin injection in 91 patients with pseudoaneurysm. Although the majority of patients were on antiplatelet or anticoagulant medication, the procedure was successful in 98% of cases. In a nonrandomized comparison of ultrasound-guided compression repair with thrombin injection for the treatment of iatrogenic pseudoaneurysms, Paulson

et al[63] report that the success rate of thrombin injection was significantly higher than compression repair, 96% versus 74% ($P = 0.013$). The mean time to thrombosis was 6 seconds for those undergoing thrombin injection as compared with 41.5 minutes for compression repair.

For patients who present after an endovascular procedure with complaints and physical findings suggestive of pseudoaneurysm, we recommend referral for Duplex ultrasonography. Those who have pseudoaneurysm and then undergo ultrasound-guided thrombin injection, for the reasons described: more rapid thrombosis and less discomfort for the patient.

At the time of a staged procedure, the interventionalist may recognize a pseudoaneurysm from the previous procedure. Angiographic guidance for injection of the pseudoaneurysm may be considered in these instances.[64,65] Contralateral access is obtained and angiography performed to confirm the presence of a pseudo-

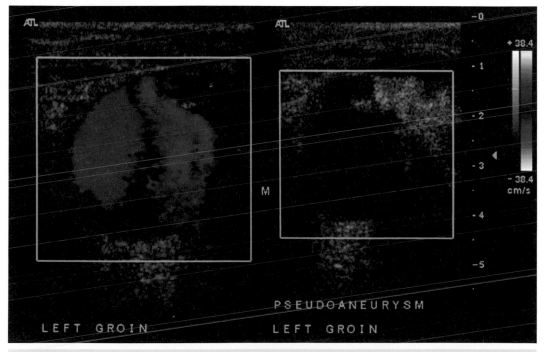

Figure 16.3 (a) Percutaneous intervention was performed through an 8-Fr sheath. Hemostasis was achieved with manual compression. The patient developed a painful pulsatile mass of the right groin. Duplex ultrasonography revealed a pseudoaneurysm, 3 x 3 cm. (b) After ultrasound-guided thrombin injection, rapid thrombosis of the pseudoaneurysm is achieved. (With kind assistance from Willi Chi, DO, of Oschner Medical Center.)

aneurysm. After positioning an angioplasty balloon across the stenosis, the balloon is inflated to occlude flow into the pseudoaneurysm and the distal vessel. An 18-gauge needle is inserted into the body of the pseudoaneurysm, and contrast is injected to confirm that no contrast escapes into the distal vessel. Thrombin, or fibrin adhesive (Beriplast P, Centeon) is then injected into the body of the pseudoaneurysm. Loose and Haslam[64] report success in all 13 patients using fibrin adhesive with an average balloon occlusion time of 10 minutes. Matson et al[66] reported success in 26 of 28 patients using fibrin adhesive. Samal et al[65] described the safe and effective use of thrombin for injection during balloon occlusion in 4 patients.

We recommend that symptomatic pseudoaneurysms be treated with ultrasound-guided thrombin injection, as this method has a high success rate with minimal time requirements for patients and personnel. This method also provides relief of symptoms with minimal patient discomfort. As stated, if the patient is undergoing another endovascular procedure, balloon occlusion during injection may be considered. Coil embolization has been employed for treatment of pseudoaneurysm, but this procedure is time-consuming.[67-69] Deployment of covered stents has been used to occlude pseudoaneurysm.[67,68,70] The bifurcation of the common femoral artery limits where a covered stent might be deployed. Endovascular access is no longer possible through the covered stent, and there may be an increased risk of stent thrombosis or late occlusion.[67,68] Coil embolization and covered stent deployment are less desirable alternatives to pseudoaneurysm injection.

Arteriovenous Fistulae

Most arteriovenous fistulae are small and require no therapy. They are a result of puncture of the superficial femoral artery or the profunda femoris. During the puncture the needle passes through the adjacent lateral circumflex vein, creating a communication. The natural history of arteriovenous fistulae is unclear; while most studies report spontaneous closure,[31,35] this is disputed.[34] Large arteriovenous fistulae are associated with ipsilateral edema and arterial ischemia. Chronic large arteriovenous fistulae may result in high-output heart failure. Percutaneous treatment of arteriovenous fistulae has been reported, using covered stents or coils, but the optimal management of the symptomatic patients is surgical ligation.

Ischemic Complications

Dissection

Retrograde dissection of the femoral or external iliac arteries is a potential complication when obtaining retrograde femoral artery access. This complication is often caused by advancing the guide wire against resistance, and is more likely to occur in tortuous or atherosclerotic arteries. If there is difficulty advancing the wire out of the distal end of the needle, the operator should not attempt to use fluoroscopy to guide it. The wire should be removed from the needle to confirm pulsatile flow, and the operator should adjust the needle position or angle to allow the wire to advance out of the needle tip without resistance. A hydrophilic or other coated wire should never be used to obtain access as the coating may be shorn off if the wire is removed from the needle. If a dissection occurs, the operator should perform angiography to determine its extent and the degree to which it occludes flow. Most retrograde dissections of the iliac are conservatively managed with removal of the catheters and wires. As the anterograde flow through the iliac will keep most of these dissection flaps open, they spontaneously heal. If the dissection is flow-limiting, then angioplasty or stenting may be employed to repair the dissection. Such an endovascular repair may be approached from the ipsilateral side, but if the dissection occurs in the common femoral artery, contralateral access may be required. An appropriately sized balloon is inflated across the dissection; stent placement is reserved for persistent flow-limiting dissection (Figure 16.4). If anterograde access is obtained, a resultant dissection flap is less likely to heal spontaneously. The operator should have a lower threshold to intervene on such a dissection.

Thromboembolic Complications

In early reports, the incidence of occlusive complications was as high as 5.7% after femoral artery access.[71] Thromboembolic complications occur less frequently now as the use of anticoagulation and the practice of flushing the sheath have increased. Emboli tend to become lodged in small branches and at bifurcation points potentially resulting in tissue loss due to ischemia.[72] Thrombotic occlusion is usually discovered after sheath removal, as the physical exam reveals loss of distal pulses. Depending on how well developed the collateral circulation is, the patient may or may not develop symptoms.

In the event of embolization, we recommend obtaining contralateral access to perform angiography and intervention. Once the location of the embolus is identified, a wire is positioned across the occlusion and an anticoagulant is administered. Initially thrombectomy is attempted with rheolytic or aspiration thrombectomy, which may be sufficient if flow is restored to the distal vessels (Figure 16.5). If a defect persists then angioplasty and stenting, if necessary, are performed.

If a large thrombus burden is still apparent on angiography after performing thrombectomy, then an infusion of intra-arterial thrombolytic may be necessary. Through a sheath in the contralateral groin, a multiholed infusion catheter such as a 5-Fr Mewissen (Boston Scientific) is positioned with its infusion holes within the thrombus. The thrombolytic is infused (tPA 0.05 mg/kg/hr) for 4 hours and repeat angiography is performed to assess the progress of lytic therapy. The procedure can be terminated if there is resolution of the thrombus, but may be continued overnight if residual thrombus is present. Although arteriotomy is a relative contraindication to thrombolytic therapy, in the urgent setting of embolization, targeted lytic

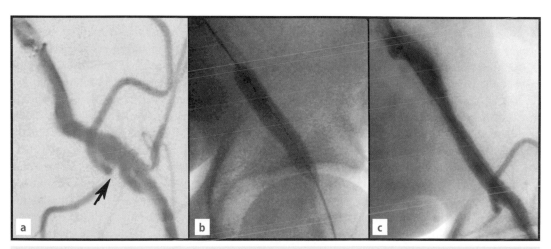

Figure 16.4 (a) After peripheral intervention was performed through the left common femoral artery (CFA) the patient returned with ischemic symptoms of the left leg. Ankle-brachial index of the left leg was 0.33 at rest. Angiography revealed stenosis, with possible dissection of the left CFA (arrow). (b) Several balloon inflations were performed, with (c) successful reduction of the stenosis.

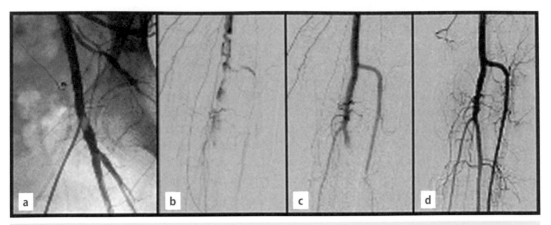

Figure 16.5 (a) A large filling defect at the sheath insertion site, consistent with thrombus. (b) Embolization of this thrombus to the distal popliteal and tibioperoneal trunk. After passing an AngioJet catheter, thrombus is removed and 3-vessel runoff is restored. (c) After passing an Angiojet catheter, thrombus is removed and (d) 3-vessel runoff is restored.

therapy may be limb- or lifesaving, and stenting may be required to achieve an acceptable angiographic result and restoration of flow to the distal extremity.

Complications Associated with Closure Devices

Manual compression after femoral access has been the traditional means to achieve hemostasis, however, this method is labor intensive and requires the patient to remain at bedrest for several hours. To provide for patient comfort, increase efficiency in the procedure room, and facilitate early discharge, vascular access closure devices have an increasing role in vascular management. EPIC, EPILOG, and IMPACT II investigators illuminated the importance of early sheath removal to reduce bleeding complications.[73-75] It is estimated that more than 1 million vascular closure devices are used each year in the United States.[76]

VasoSeal (Datascope) was approved by the FDA in 1995, with an indication for diagnostic and interventional procedures via a retrograde femoral access. A collagen plug is inserted adjacent to the artery, through the tract of the sheath, with the collagen acting as a hemostatic agent. There is no intra-arterial component to this device, and calcification is not a contraindication.

The Angio-Seal device (St. Jude Medical) applies a bovine collagen plug external to the vessel. As opposed to the VasoSeal, the Angio-Seal uses an absorbable, intra-arterial anchor consisting of a copolymer of polylactic and polyglycolic acids. An absorbable suture places traction on the collagen plug, holding it against the artery. The FDA approved this device in 1996. Femoral angiography is recommended prior to deployment; calcification, and deployment in the superficial femoral and profunda femoris arteries are relative contraindications. Deployment in the external iliac artery should also be avoided, as the inguinal ligament may prevent advancement of the collagen plug to the arteriotomy.

The Duett device (Vascular Solutions) utilizes the procoagulant effects of thrombin and collagen. A balloon catheter is inserted into the femoral sheath and inflated. The balloon is retracted to the arteriotomy. The combination of thrombin and collagen is injected through the side arm of the sheath, the inflated balloon preventing intra-arterial injection. The balloon is then deflated and removed, and manual pressure applied.

The Perclose (Abbott Laboratories) device provides suture-mediated closure of the arteriotomy and was approved by the FDA in 1997. Two needles place the suture through the arterial wall from the outside, capturing the suture, the knot slides down to the arteriotomy. The suture is bioabsorbable, monofilament polypropylene. Femoral angiography is recommended as heavy calcification may prevent proper deployment of the sutures. The StarClose (Abbott Laboratories) applies a nitinol clip to the outside of the arterial wall to achieve apposition of the arteriotomy. The SuperStitch (Sutura) is also capable of deploying a suture but is not indicated for blind vascular closure.

Newer Devices

The Boomerang device (Cardiva Medical) consists of a 0.037-in wire with a nitinol disk that is inserted through the femoral sheath. The disk is pulled against the arteriotomy to apply pressure. The disk is then removed and manual pressure applied. SoundSeal (Therus/Boston Scientific) applies ultrasound externally to thermally close the arteriotomy. Matrix VSG (AccessClosure) uses a polyethylene glycol sealant. A balloon catheter is used to prevent intra-arterial injection.

The majority of data on percutaneous vascular closure devices (PVCD) are based on single-center registries. Where randomized data exist, the trials have been designed to favor PVCDs over manual compression. Patients randomized to the manual compression arm of the trial were required to remain on bedrest for more than 4 hours, as is accepted practice. Those patients randomized to the PVCD arm were allowed to ambulate within 1 hour. These trials define time to ambulation as a measured end point, thus, per protocol, manual compression will be inferior to PVCD with respect to ambulation. Unless PVCDs resulted in a significantly larger number of bleeding or ischemic complications, manual compression would be found to be inferior.

In a meta-analysis of 30 studies (randomized, case-control, and cohort), 37,066 patients undergoing diagnostic or interventional procedures were included to determine the cumulative incidence of access site complication relative to manual compression. The overall analysis of favored compression over closure devices with an odds ratio (OR) of 1.34 (95% CI, 1.01–1.79). VasoSeal had an OR of 2.25 (CI 1.07–4.71) for interventional procedures. There were no differences in the rate of complications using Angio-Seal or Perclose for diagnostic or interventional procedures.[77] Another meta-analysis of 30 trials, with 4000 patients, examined the risk of groin hematoma, arteriovenous fistula, and pseudoaneurysm. In this analysis there was no difference in the incidence of any of these complications. When only trials with strict adherence to intention-to-treat principles were included, however, closure devices were associated with an increased risk of hematoma (RR 1.89, CI 1.13–3.15) and pseudoaneurysm (RR 5.4, CI 1.21–24.5).

Although the rates of occlusive and hemorrhagic complications are similar between devices and as compared to compression, several reports suggest that the severity of these complications may be more severe.[8,30,78] Sprouse et al[78] reported that after percutaneous closure devices, pseudoaneurysms tended to be larger (5.8 vs. 2.8 cm) and more resistant to ultrasound-guided compression than after compression (0% success vs. 66.6%).

When evaluating access site complications, the physician should identify which closure device, if any, was used and consider the mechanisms of complication and implication on therapy.[8,79] An intra-arterial component of a closure device might cause dissection, or embolize; unsuccessful deployment of a device may keep the arteriotomy open, making hemostasis more difficult. Some authors suggest that complications following use of an access closure device should be treated with a lower threshold for surgical therapy.[79]

The incidence of infectious complications following manual compression is extremely rare.[80-83] However, the incidence of infectious complications of PVCDs range from 0.0% to 5.1%.[84-90] In a review of the literature, Sohail et al[91] identified 90 cases of device-related infection, 52 of which listed infection as being the primary complication of the closure device. Among these 52 patients, 75% had cultures identifying *Staphylococcus aureus*, and 18% of those were due to oxacillin-resistant *S. aureus*. The median incubation period between the index procedure and presentation was 8 days. If infection is suspected, ultrasonography is performed to exclude hematoma, pseudoaneurysm, or abscess. The physician may attempt to treat a superficial skin infection with antibiotics alone.[79] If infection of the arterial wall is suspected, then immediate initiation of antibiotic therapy and prompt surgical treatment are of tantamount importance. At that time all foreign matter is removed as potential sources of infection.

We have found that most ischemic and hemorrhagic complications following the use of closure devices can be successfully treated percutaneously, using the techniques described (Figure 16.6). Physicians should keep in mind the potential for the intravascular portions of these devices to remain within the vascular system, compounding the management of the complication (Figure 16.7). For example, if the anchor of an Angio-Seal device were to embolize, it could appear as a filling defect and be mistaken for thrombus. Percutaneous thrombectomy will be unsuccessful aspirating such mechanical components of these devices. Occlusions at the access site may be secondary to a dissection plane being lifted by the device, which may subsequently suture, or otherwise adhere, the dissection plane to the anterior wall. The physician must ascertain that the true lumen has been visualized prior to attempting to dilate. There is no randomized data comparing percutaneous and surgical therapy for access site complications, so therapeutic decisions are dictated by the clinical scenario and the local expertise.

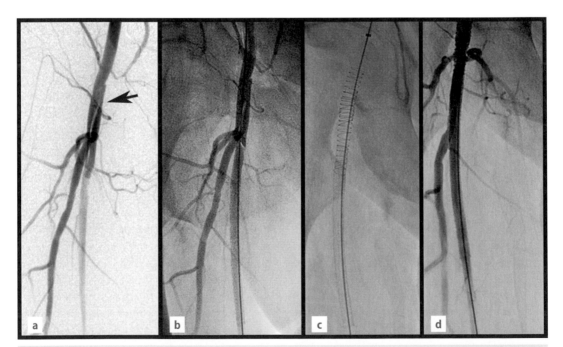

Figure 16.6 (a) A Duett device was deployed to successfully achieve hemostasis in the right common femoral artery (CFA) after angiography. The patient developed ischemic symptoms of the right leg on ambulation prior to discharge. Angiography revealed a linear filling defect beginning in the CFA (arrow) and extending through the superficial femoral artery. (b) The defect was improved but still present after balloon dilation. (c) 7 x 40 mm and 8 x 40 mm Intra-Coil self-expanding stents were deployed in the CFA, (d) reestablishing flow in the artery.

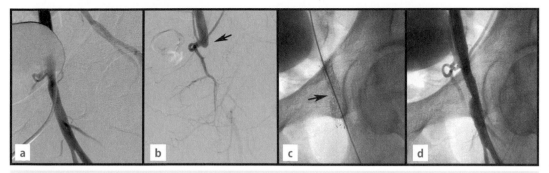

Figure 16.7 (a) Peripheral intervention was performed through the left common femoral artery (CFA) and hemostasis achieved with an Angio-Seal device. The patient developed ischemic symptoms of the left leg after ambulating. (b) Angiography revealed total occlusion of the CFA (arrow). (c) After balloon and stent, a persistent defect is seen in the stent (arrow), likely representing the anchor of the Angio-Seal. (d) Ischemic symptoms resolved with restoration of flow.

Summary

Endovascular procedures have been a mainstay for the diagnosis and treatment of PAD. As technology improves and awareness of PAD continues to grow, we can anticipate continued growth in the number of endovascular procedures performed. Although these procedures are safe, access site complications remain a cause of significant morbidity, prolonged hospitalization, and increased costs. Physicians performing these procedures must know how to avoid, recognize, and treat these potentially fatal complications.

References

1. Popma JJ, Satler LF, Pichard AD, et al. Vascular complications after balloon and new device angioplasty. *Circulation.* 1993;88(4 Pt 1):1569-1578.

2. Johnson LW, Esente P, Giambartolomei A, et al. Peripheral vascular complications of coronary angioplasty by the femoral and brachial techniques. *Cathet Cardiovasc Diagn.* 1994;31(3):165-172.

3. Waksman R, King SB III, Douglas JS, et al. Predictors of groin complications after balloon and new-device coronary intervention. *Am J Cardiol.* 1995;75(14):886-889.

4. Omoigui NA, Califf RM, Pieper K, et al. Peripheral vascular complications in the Coronary Angioplasty Versus Excisional Atherectomy Trial (CAVEAT-I). *J Am Coll Cardiol.* 1995;26(4):922-930.

5. Wyman RM, Safian RD, Portway V, Skillman JJ, McKay RG, Baim DS. Current complications of diagnostic and therapeutic cardiac catheterization. *J Am Coll Cardiol.* 1988;12(6):1400-1406.

6. Babu SC, Piccorelli GO, Shah PM, Stein JH, Clauss RH. Incidence and results of arterial complications among 16,350 patients undergoing cardiac catheterization. *J Vasc Surg.* 1989;10(2):113-116.

7. Oweida SW, Roubin GS, Smith RB III, Salam AA. Postcatheterization vascular complications associated with percutaneous transluminal coronary angioplasty. *J Vasc Surg.* 1990;12(3):310-315.

8. Eidt JF, Habibipour S, Saucedo JF, et al. Surgical complications from hemostatic puncture closure devices. *Am J Surg.* 1999;178(6):511-516.

9. Kim D, Orron DE, Skillman JJ, et al. Role of superficial femoral artery puncture in the development of pseudoaneurysm and arteriovenous fistula complicating percutaneous transfemoral cardiac catheterization. *Cathet Cardiovasc Diagn.* 1992;25(2):91-97.

10. Lilly MP, Reichman W, Sarazen AA Jr, Carney WI Jr. Anatomic and clinical factors associated with complications of transfemoral arteriography. *Ann Vasc Surg.* 1990;4(3):264-269.

11. Trigaux JP, Van Beers B, De Wispelaere JF. Anatomic relationship between the popliteal artery and vein: a guide to accurate angiographic puncture. *AJR Am J Roentgenol.* 1991;157(6):1259-1262.

12. Yilmaz S, Sindel T, Luleci E. Ultrasound-guided retrograde popliteal artery catheterization: experience in 174 consecutive patients. *J Endovasc Ther.* 2005;12(6):714-722.

13. Rao S, Ou MF-S, Wang T, et al. Trends in the prevalence and outcomes of radial and femoral approaches to percutaneous coronary intervention: a report from the National Cardiovascular Data Registry. *J Am Coll Cardio Interv.* 2008;1:379-386.

14. Slogoff S, Keats A, Arlund C. On the safety of radial artery cannulation. *Anesthesiology.* 1983;59(1):42-47.

15. Davis F, Stewart J. Radial artery cannulation. *Br J Anaesthesia.* 1980;52(1):41-47.

16. Hata M, Senzai A, Niino T, et al. Radial artery harvest using the sharp scissors method for patients with pathological findings on Allen's test. *Surg Today.* 2006;36(9):790-792.

17. Bakoyiannis C, Economopoulos KP, Georgopoulos S, et al. Transradial access for carotid artery stenting: a single-center experience. *Int Angiol.* 29(1):41-46.

18. Abdessalem S, Mjadlah S, Mourali S, Mechemeche R. Radial access for concomitant coronary, subclavian and renal artery angioplasty: one case report. *Tunis Med.* 2009;87(10):709-711.

19. Flachskampf FA, Wolf T, Daniel WG, Ludwig J. Transradial stenting of the iliac artery: a case report. *Catheter Cardiovasc Interv.* 2005;65(2):193-195.

20. Skillman JJ, Kim D, Baim DS. Vascular complications of percutaneous femoral cardiac interventions. Incidence and operative repair. *Arch Surg.* 1988;123(10):1207-1212.

21. Silva JA, Stant J, Ramee SR. Endovascular treatment of a massive retroperitoneal bleeding: successful balloon-catheter delivery of intra-arterial thrombin. *Catheter Cardiovasc Interv.* 2005;64(2):218-222.

22. Sreeram S, Lumsden AB, Miller JS, Salam AA, Dodson TF, Smith RB. Retroperitoneal hematoma following femoral arterial catheterization:

a serious and often fatal complication. *Am Surg.* 1993;59(2):94-98.

23. Wiley JM, White CJ, Uretsky BF. Noncoronary complications of coronary intervention. *Catheter Cardiovasc Interv.* 2002;57(2):257-265.

24. Kinnaird TD, Stabile E, Mintz GS, et al. Incidence, predictors, and prognostic implications of bleeding and blood transfusion following percutaneous coronary interventions. *Am J Cardiol.* 2003;92(8):930-935.

25. Kent KC, Moscucci M, Mansour KA, et al. Retroperitoneal hematoma after cardiac catheterization: prevalence, risk factors, and optimal management. *J Vasc Surg.* 1994;20(6):905-910; discussion 910-903.

26. Lumsden AB, Miller JM, Kosinski AS, et al. A prospective evaluation of surgically treated groin complications following percutaneous cardiac procedures. *Am Surg.* 1994;60(2):132-137.

27. Franco CD, Goldsmith J, Veith FJ, Calligaro KD, Gupta SK, Wengerter KR. Management of arterial injuries produced by percutaneous femoral procedures. *Surgery.* 1993;113(4):419-425.

28. Katzenschlager R, Ugurluoglu A, Ahmadi A, et al. Incidence of pseudoaneurysm after diagnostic and therapeutic angiography. *Radiology.* 1995;195(2):463-466.

29. Eichlisberger R, Frauchiger B, Schmitt H, Jager K. Aneurysma spurium following arterial catheterization: diagnosis and follow-up. *Ultraschall Med.* 1992;13(2):54-58.

30. Carey D, Martin JR, Moore CA, Valentine MC, Nygaard TW. Complications of femoral artery closure devices. *Catheter Cardiovasc Interv.* 2001;52(1):3-7; discussion 8.

31. Toursarkissian B, Allen BT, Petrinec D, et al. Spontaneous closure of selected iatrogenic pseudoaneurysms and arteriovenous fistulae. *J Vasc Surg.* 1997;25(5):803-808; discussion 808-809.

32. Graham AN, Wilson CM, Hood JM, Barros D'Sa AA. Risk of rupture of postangiographic femoral false aneurysm. *Br J Surg.* 1992;79(10):1022-1025.

33. Kazmers A, Meeker C, Nofz K, et al. Nonoperative therapy for postcatheterization

femoral artery pseudoaneurysms. *Am Surg.* 1997;63(2):199-204.

34. Kresowik TF, Khoury MD, Miller BV, et al. A prospective study of the incidence and natural history of femoral vascular complications after percutaneous transluminal coronary angioplasty. *J Vasc Surg.* 1991;13(2):328-333; discussion 333-325.

35. Johns JP, Pupa LE Jr, Bailey SR. Spontaneous thrombosis of iatrogenic femoral artery pseudoaneurysms: documentation with color Doppler and two-dimensional ultrasonography. *J Vasc Surg.* 1991;14(1):24-29.

36. Fellmeth BD, Baron SB, Brown PR, et al. Repair of postcatheterization femoral pseudoaneurysms by color flow ultrasound guided compression. *Am Heart J.* 1992;123(2):547-551.

37. Dean SM, Olin JW, Piedmonte M, Grubb M, Young JR. Ultrasound-guided compression closure of postcatheterization pseudoaneurysms during concurrent anticoagulation: a review of seventy-seven patients. *J Vasc Surg.* 1996;23(1):28-34; discussion 34-25.

38. Sorrell KA, Feinberg RL, Wheeler JR, et al. Color-flow duplex-directed manual occlusion of femoral false aneurysms. *J Vasc Surg.* 1993;17(3):571-577.

39. Schaub F, Theiss W, Heinz M, Zagel M, Schomig A. New aspects in ultrasound-guided compression repair of postcatheterization femoral artery injuries. *Circulation.* 1994;90(4):1861-1865.

40. Cox GS, Young JR, Gray BR, Grubb MW, Hertzer NR. Ultrasound-guided compression repair of postcatheterization pseudoaneurysms: results of treatment in one hundred cases. *J Vasc Surg.* 1994;19(4):683-686.

41. Sacks D, Robinson ML, Perlmutter GS. Femoral arterial injury following catheterization. Duplex evaluation. *J Ultrasound Med.* 1989;8(5):241-246.

42. Lacy JH, Box JM, Connors D, Penney L, Wright CB. Pseudoaneurysm: diagnosis with color Doppler ultrasound. *J Cardiovasc Surg.* (Torino). 1990;31(6):727-730.

43. Mills JL, Wiedeman JE, Robison JG, Hallett JW Jr. Minimizing mortality and morbidity from iatrogenic arterial injuries: the need for early recognition and prompt repair. *J Vasc Surg.* 1986;4(1):22-27.

44. Perler BA. Surgical treatment of femoral pseudoaneurysm following cardiac catheterization. *Cardiovasc Surg.* 1993;1(2):118-121.

45. Roberts SR, Main D, Pinkerton J. Surgical therapy of femoral artery pseudoaneurysm after angiography. *Am J Surg.* 1987;154(6):676-680.

46. Fellmeth BD, Roberts AC, Bookstein JJ, et al. Postangiographic femoral artery injuries: nonsurgical repair with US-guided compression. *Radiology.* 1991;178(3):671-675.

47. Chou YH, Tiu CM, Chiang BN, Chang T. Real-time and image-directed Doppler ultrasonography in deep femoral artery pseudoaneurysm: a new observation with graded compression of the femoral artery. *J Clin Ultrasound.* 1991;19(7):438-441.

48. Feld R, Patton GM, Carabasi RA, Alexander A, Merton D, Needleman L. Treatment of iatrogenic femoral artery injuries with ultrasound-guided compression. *J Vasc Surg.* 1992;16(6):832-840.

49. DiPrete DA, Cronan JJ. Compression ultrasonography. Treatment for acute femoral artery pseudoaneurysms in selected cases. *J Ultrasound Med.* 1992;11(9):489-492.

50. Schwend RB, Hambsch KP, Kwan KY, Boyajian RA, Otis SM. Color duplex sonographically guided obliteration of pseudoaneurysm. *J Ultrasound Med.* 1993;12(10):609-613.

51. McCann RL, Schwartz LB, Pieper KS. Vascular complications of cardiac catheterization. *J Vasc Surg.* 1991;14(3):375-381.

52. Dasyam AK, Middleton WD, Teefey SA. Development of nonobstructive intraarterial thrombi after injection of thrombin into pseudoaneurysms. *AJR Am J Roentgenol.* 2006;186(2):401-405.

53. Liau CS, Ho FM, Chen MF, Lee YT. Treatment of iatrogenic femoral artery pseudoaneurysm with percutaneous thrombin injection. *J Vasc Surg.* 1997;26(1):18-23.

54. Kang SS, Labropoulos N, Mansour MA, et al. Expanded indications for ultrasound-guided thrombin injection of pseudoaneurysms. *J Vasc Surg.* 2000;31(2):289-298.

55. Kang SS, Labropoulos N, Mansour MA, Baker

WH. Percutaneous ultrasound guided thrombin injection: a new method for treating post-catheterization femoral pseudoaneurysms. *J Vasc Surg.* 1998;27(6):1032-1038.

56. Brophy DP, Sheiman RG, Amatulle P, Akbari CM. Iatrogenic femoral pseudoaneurysms: thrombin injection after failed US-guided compression. *Radiology.* 2000;214(1):278-282.

57. Paulson EK, Nelson RC, Mayes CE, Sheafor DH, Sketch MH Jr, Kliewer MA. Sonographically guided thrombin injection of iatrogenic femoral pseudoaneurysms: further experience of a single institution. *AJR Am J Roentgenol.* 2001;177(2):309-316.

58. La Perna L, Olin JW, Goines D, Childs MB, Ouriel K. Ultrasound-guided thrombin injection for the treatment of postcatheterization pseudoaneurysms. *Circulation.* 2000;102(19):2391-2395.

59. McNeil NL, Clark TW. Sonographically guided percutaneous thrombin injection versus sonographically guided compression for femoral artery pseudoaneurysms. *AJR Am J Roentgenol.* 2001;176(2):459-462.

60. Pezzullo JA, Dupuy DE, Cronan JJ. Percutaneous injection of thrombin for the treatment of pseudoaneurysms after catheterization: an alternative to sonographically guided compression. *AJR Am J Roentgenol.* 2000;175(4):1035-1040.

61. Hamraoui K, Ernst SM, van Dessel PF, et al. Efficacy and safety of percutaneous treatment of iatrogenic femoral artery pseudoaneurysm by biodegradable collagen injection. *J Am Coll Cardiol.* 2002;39(8):1297-1304.

62. Mohler ER III, Mitchell ME, Carpenter JP, et al. Therapeutic thrombin injection of pseudoaneurysms: a multicenter experience. *Vasc Med.* 2001;6(4):241-244.

63. Paulson EK, Sheafor DH, Kliewer MA, et al. Treatment of iatrogenic femoral arterial pseudoaneurysms: comparison of US-guided thrombin injection with compression repair. *Radiology.* 2000;215(2):403-408.

64. Loose HW, Haslam PJ. The management of peripheral arterial aneurysms using percutaneous injection of fibrin adhesive. *Br J Radiol.* 1998;71(852):1255-1259.

65. Samal AK, White CJ, Collins TJ, Ramee SR, Jenkins JS. Treatment of femoral artery pseudoaneurysm with percutaneous thrombin injection. *Catheter Cardiovasc Interv.* 2001;53(2):259-263.

66. Matson MB, Morgan RA, Belli AM. Percutaneous treatment of pseudoaneurysms using fibrin adhesive. *Br J Radiol.* 2001;74(884):690-694.

67. Waigand J, Uhlich F, Gross CM, Thalhammer C, Dietz R. Percutaneous treatment of pseudoaneurysms and arteriovenous fistulas after invasive vascular procedures. *Catheter Cardiovasc Interv.* 1999;47(2):157-164.

68. Thalhammer C, Kirchherr AS, Uhlich F, Waigand J, Gross CM. Postcatheterization pseudoaneurysms and arteriovenous fistulas: repair with percutaneous implantation of endovascular covered stents. *Radiology.* 2000;214(1):127-131.

69. Lemaire JM, Dondelinger RF. Percutaneous coil embolization of iatrogenic femoral arteriovenous fistula or pseudo-aneurysm. *Eur J Radiol.* 1994;18(2):96-100.

70. Christensen L, Justesen P, Larsen KE. Percutaneous transluminal treatment of an iliac pseudoaneurysm with endoprosthesis implantation. A case report. *Acta Radiol.* 1996;37(4):542-544.

71. Kottke BA, Fairbairn JF, Davis GD. Complications of aortography. *Circulation.* 1964;30:843-847.

72. Greenberg RK, Ouriel K. *Arterial Thromboembolis.* 5th ed. Philadelphia: W.B. Saunders; 2000, p. 822-835.

73. Aguirre FV, Topol EJ, Ferguson JJ, et al. Bleeding complications with the chimeric antibody to platelet glycoprotein IIb/IIIa integrin in patients undergoing percutaneous coronary intervention. EPIC Investigators. *Circulation.* 1995;91(12):2882-2890.

74. Ellis SG, Lincoff AM, Miller D, et al. Reduction in complications of angioplasty with abciximab occurs largely independently of baseline lesion morphology. EPIC and EPILOG Investigators. Evaluation of 7E3 for the Prevention of Ischemic Complications. Evaluation of PTCA to Improve Long-term Outcome with abciximab GPIIb/IIIa Receptor Blockade. *J Am Coll Cardiol.* 1998;32(6):1619-1623.

75. Tcheng JE, Harrington RA, Kottke-Marchant K, et al. Multicenter, randomized, double-blind, placebo-controlled trial of the platelet integrin glycoprotein IIb/IIIa blocker Integrelin in elective coronary intervention. IMPACT Investigators. *Circulation.* 1995;91(8):2151-2157.

76. Turi Z. Overview of vacular closure devices. *Endovasc Today.* 2004:19-20.

77. Nikolsky E, Mehran R, Halkin A, et al. Vascular complications associated with arteriotomy closure devices in patients undergoing percutaneous coronary procedures: a meta-analysis. *J Am Coll Cardiol.* 2004;44(6):1200-1209.

78. Sprouse LR II, Botta DM Jr, Hamilton IN Jr. The management of peripheral vascular complications associated with the use of percutaneous suture-mediated closure devices. *J Vasc Surg.* 2001;33(4):688-693.

79. Kalapatapu VR, Ali AT, Masroor F, Moursi MM, Eidt JF. Techniques for managing complications of arterial closure devices. *Vasc Endovascular Surg.* 2006;40(5):399-408.

80. Evans BH, Goldstein EJ. Increased risk of infection after repeat percutaneous transluminal coronary angioplasty. *Am J Infect Control.* 1987;15(3):125-126.

81. Cleveland KO, Gelfand MS. Invasive staphylococcal infections complicating percutaneous transluminal coronary angioplasty: three cases and review. *Clin Infect Dis.* 1995;21(1):93-96.

82. Cowley MJ, Mullin SM, Kelsey SF, et al. Sex differences in early and long-term results of coronary angioplasty in the NHLBI PTCA Registry. *Circulation.* 1985;71(1):90-97.

83. Smith TP, Cruz CP, Moursi MM, Eidt JF. Infectious complications resulting from use of hemostatic puncture closure devices. *Am J Surg.* 2001;182(6):658-662.

84. Johanning JM, Franklin DP, Elmore JR, Han DC. Femoral artery infections associated with percutaneous arterial closure devices. *J Vasc Surg.* 2001;34(6):983-985.

85. Gerckens U, Cattelaens N, Lampe EG, Grube E. Management of arterial puncture site after catheterization procedures: evaluating a suture-mediated closure device. *Am J Cardiol.* 1999;83(12):1658-1663.

86. Cooper CL, Miller A. Infectious complications related to the use of the angio-seal hemostatic puncture closure device. *Catheter Cardiovasc Interv.* 1999;48(3):301-303.

87. Cherr GS, Travis JA, Ligush J Jr, et al. Infection is an unusual but serious complication of a femoral artery catheterization site closure device. *Ann Vasc Surg.* 2001;15(5):567-570.

88. Ward SR, Casale P, Raymond R, Kussmaul WG III, Simpfendorfer C. Efficacy and safety of a hemostatic puncture closure device with early ambulation after coronary angiography. Angio-Seal Investigators. *Am J Cardiol.* 1998;81(5):569-572.

89. Cura FA, Kapadia SR, L'Allier PL, et al. Safety of femoral closure devices after percutaneous coronary interventions in the era of glycoprotein IIb/IIIa platelet blockade. *Am J Cardiol.* 2000;86(7):780-782, A789.

90. von Hoch F, Neumann FJ, Theiss W, Kastrati A, Schomig A. Efficacy and safety of collagen implants for haemostasis of the vascular access site after coronary balloon angioplasty and coronary stent implantation. A randomized study. *Eur Heart J.* 1995;16(5):640-646.

91. Sohail MR, Khan AH, Holmes DR Jr, Wilson WR, Steckelberg JM, Baddour LM. Infectious complications of percutaneous vascular closure devices. *Mayo Clin Proc.* 2005;80(8):1011-1015.

Part 6

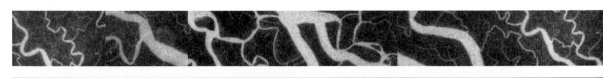

Nonatherosclerotic Artery Disease

17

Thromboangiitis Obliterans (Buerger's Disease)

Jeffrey W. Olin

Thromboangiitis obliterans (Buerger's disease) is a segmental, inflammatory disease that most commonly affects the small- and medium-sized arteries, veins, and nerves of the arms and legs.[1] The pathological findings are quite distinctive and are characterized by highly cellular and inflammatory occlusive thrombus with relative sparing of the blood vessel wall.[1,2] Patients are mostly young tobacco smokers who present with distal-extremity ischemic ulcers or gangrene.[3] The prevalence of disease has declined in North America and Asia over the last 30 years, attributed to the decline in smoking. However, Buerger's disease is still quite prevalent in the Middle East, Japan, Turkey, and India.[4,5]

Etiology

Thromboangiitis obliterans (TAO) is a vasculitis,[6] however, several important features of Buerger's disease distinguish it from other types of vasculitis.[7]

- Pathologically, the thrombus in TAO is highly cellular, the internal elastic lamina is preserved, and there is much less intense cellular activity in the wall of the blood vessel.

- Acute phase reactants such as erythrocyte sedimentation rate and C-reactive protein are usually normal unless gangrene or associated infection is present.

- Autoantibodies such as antinuclear antibody, rheumatoid factor, and complement levels are usually normal or negative.

There is a strong association between the use of tobacco and Buerger's disease. Despite an occasional poorly documented report suggesting that Buerger's disease may occur in nonsmokers,[8,9] there has never been a substantiated case in a patient who did not use tobacco in some form. Some of these misdiagnosed cases of TAO really represent a disease that occurs in older nonsmokers and is characterized by digital ischemia, eosinophilia, subcutaneous nodules, and steroid responsiveness (Kimura's disease).[10] Most patients with Buerger's disease are heavy cigarette smokers, but TAO has also been reported in cigar smokers and in users of smokeless tobacco such as chewing tobacco and snuff.[1,3,11] While tobacco use plays a central role

Vascular Disease: Diagnostic and Therapeutic Approaches. © 2011 Michael R. Jaff and Christopher J. White, editors. Cardiotext Publishing, ISBN: 978-1-935395-16-4.

in the pathogenesis, initiation, and continuation of the disease and is an absolute requirement for diagnosis, the exact etiology of Buerger's disease is still not well delineated.

Two interesting pathophysiologic observations have been reported in recent years. The first is increased levels of anti–endothelial cell antibodies in patients with active disease compared to those patients in remission.[12] If these findings are corroborated, assays that measure anti–endothelial cell antibody titers may prove to be useful in following disease activity of patients with Buerger's disease. The second observation is impairment of endothelium-dependent vasodilation, a marker of endothelial dysfunction, in angiographically normal limbs of patients with Buerger's disease.[13] In one report, even patients in clinical remission had a diminished capability of endothelium-dependent vasodilation and higher levels of some circulating markers of inflammation, such as leukocytes, C-reactive protein, intercellular adhesion molecule-1 (IL-1), and E-selectin. However, there were no significant differences in carotid artery intima-media thickness between patients with TAO and controls.[14] Other studies have demonstrated altered production of IL-6, IL-12, and IL-10 and increased apoptosis, as well as the elevated levels of circulating immune complexes, and suggested that this could be a reason for the persisting immune inflammation in TAO.[15]

Other etiologic factors such as genetic predisposition, immunologic mechanisms,[16-18] and abnormalities in coagulation may play a supporting role in some patients.

Clinical Presentation

Typically, Buerger's disease occurs in young smokers with the onset of symptoms before the age of 40 to 45 years. There are an increasing number of reports of Buerger's disease in women (especially from the Western countries), possibly due to the increased use of cigarettes among women in the twentieth century.[2,3,19-22]

This does not appear to be the case, however, in the Asian literature,[23,24] where there are some reports with no women patients.

The arterial involvement usually begins in the distal small arteries and veins. As the disease progresses, it may involve more proximal arteries. Large-artery involvement has been reported in TAO, but this is unusual and as a general rule does not occur in the absence of small-vessel occlusive disease.[25]

Patients may present with claudication of foot, legs, and occasionally arms and hands. Foot or arch claudication may be the presenting manifestation and is often mistaken for an orthopedic problem, resulting in a considerable delay before the correct diagnosis is made. Patients may develop ischemic ulcerations in the distal portion of the toes and/or fingers as the initial presentation of TAO (Figure 17.1).[2] The presence of superficial thrombophlebitis and ischemic ulceration in the same patient are highly suggestive of Buerger's disease (Table 17.1).

It is important to recognize that 2 or more limbs are always involved in Buerger's disease.[1,24] Because of the proclivity to involve more than one limb, it has been our practice to perform an imaging of both upper extremities and/or lower extremities in patients who clinically present with involvement of only one limb. It is quite common to see angiographic abnormalities consistent with Buerger's disease in limbs that are not yet clinically involved.

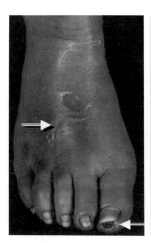

Figure 17.1 Ischemic ulceration on great toe (arrow) in a patient with Buerger's disease. Note the area of superficial thrombophlebitis on the dorsum of the foot (arrow). (From Olin JW, Lie JT. Thromboangiitis obliterans (Buerger's disease). In: Cooke JP, Frohlich ED, eds. *Current Management of Hypertension and Vascular Disease*. St. Louis, MO: Mosby Yearbook; 1992:265-271. With permission from Elsevier.)

Patients (n)	112
Mean age (years)	42
Men	86 (77%)
Women	26 (23%)
Intermittent claudication	70 (63%)
Rest pain	91 (81%)
Ischemic ulcers	85 (76%)
Upper extremity	24 (28%)
Lower extremity	39 (46%)
Both	22 (26%)
Thrombophlebitis	43 (38%)
Raynaud's phenomenon	49 (44%)
Sensory findings	77 (69%)
Abnormal Allen test	71 (63%)

Table 17.1. TAO: Demographic Characteristics and Presenting Signs and Symptoms (From Olin JW, Young JR, Graor RA, Ruschhaupt WF, Bartholomew JR. The changing clinical spectrum of thromboangiitis obliterans (Buerger's disease). *Circulation.* 1990;82(5 Suppl):IV3-IV8.)

Due to better noninvasive imaging such as gadolinium-enhanced magnetic resonance angiography (MRA) or multidetector computed tomography angiography (CTA), catheter angiography may not always be necessary in the evaluation of patients with TAO; however, to adequately visualize the blood vessels in the hands and feet, catheter angiography is usually required.

An Allen test should be performed in all patients with small-vessel occlusive disease to assess the circulation in the hands and fingers (Figure 17.2).[26] An abnormal Allen test in a young smoker with lower-extremity ulcerations is highly suggestive of TAO, since it demonstrates small-vessel involvement in both the upper and lower extremities.

Laboratory and Angiographic Evaluation

There are no specific laboratory tests to aid in the diagnosis of thromboangiitis obliterans. A complete serologic profile to exclude other diseases that may mimic TAO should be obtained.

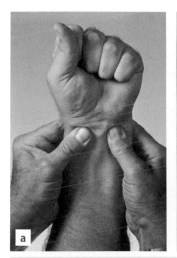
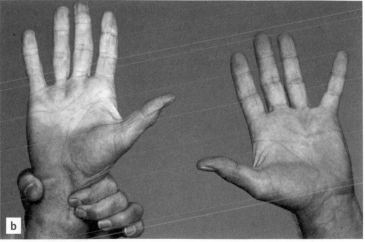

Figure 17.2 (a) Allen test with occlusion of the radial and ulnar pulse by compression. (b) The pressure on the ulnar pulse is released, while the radial is still compressed. The hand does not fill with blood; note the paleness of the hand on the right compared with the left, indicating occlusion of the ulnar artery. (Reproduced from Olin JW, Lie JT. Thromboangiitis obliterans (Buerger's disease). In: Cooke JP, Frohlich ED, eds. *Current Management of Hypertension and Vascular Disease.* St. Louis, MO: Mosby Yearbook; 1992:265-271. With permission from Elsevier.)

These include:

- complete blood count with differential;
- liver function, renal function, fasting blood sugar, urinalysis;
- acute phase reactants (erythrocyte sedimentation rate and C-reactive protein);
- antinuclear antibody;
- rheumatoid factor;
- complement measurements;
- cryoglobulins;
- serologic markers for CREST (anticentromere antibody) (calcinosis, Raynaud's, esophageal dysmotility, sclerodactyly, telangiectasias) syndrome;
- serologic markers for scleroderma (anticentromere antibody and SCL70);
- complete hypercoagulability screen to include antiphospholipid antibodies;
- toxicology screen for cocaine, amphetamines, and cannabis. These substances can mimic TAO.[27-32] The arteriographic findings in patients with cocaine or cannabis ingestion, including the presence of corkscrew collaterals, are virtually identical to those seen in Buerger's disease. Therefore, in patients who present with manifestations of Buerger's disease yet do not use tobacco, it is advisable to obtain a toxicology screen for cocaine, amphetamines, and cannabis. It is also important to obtain an eosinophil count and search for subcutaneous nodules to exclude Kimura's disease.[10]

To exclude a proximal source of emboli, the patient may need to undergo transthoracic and transesophageal echocardiography and arteriography.[1,33,34] While the arteriogram may be suggestive of TAO, there are no pathognomonic angiographic findings, since other small-vessel occlusive diseases can demonstrate identical findings as those seen in Buerger's disease.

Proximal arteries should be normal with no atherosclerosis, aneurysm, or other source of proximal emboli. The disease is confined most often to the distal circulation and is almost always infrapopliteal in the lower extremities and distal to the brachial artery in the upper extremities. There is small- and medium-sized vessel involvement such as the digital arteries in the fingers and toes, as well as the tibial, peroneal, radial, and ulnar arteries. Since TAO is a segmental disorder, there are diseased vessels interspersed with normal blood vessel segments. There is often evidence of multiple vascular occlusions with collateralization around the obstructions (corkscrew collaterals) (Figure 17.3). The arteriographic appearance (including the presence of corkscrew collaterals) may be identical to that seen in patients with lupus, mixed connective tissue disease, scleroderma, CREST syndrome, or any other small-vessel occlusive disease.

While there is some controversy over what criteria should be used to diagnose Buerger's

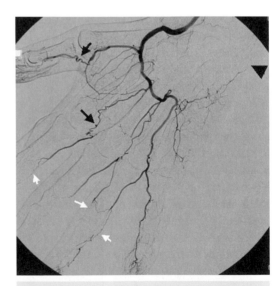

Figure 17.3 Angiogram of the hand showing a patent radial artery and deep palmer arch. The ulnar artery (arrowhead) is occluded at the level of the wrist. There are multiple areas of corkscrew collaterals (black arrows) and multiple digital artery occlusions (white arrows). The proximal arteries were normal. These angiographic findings are consistent with the diagnosis of Buerger's disease.

Tobacco user (this is an absolute requirement)
Distal extremity ischemic symptoms and signs • Claudication • Ischemic rest pain • Ischemic ulcerations • Gangrene
Document the distal nature of the disease • Segmental blood pressures and pulse volume recordings • MRA • CTA
Laboratory tests to exclude connective tissue diseases and hypercoagulable states
Exclude proximal source of emboli • MRA • CTA • Catheter-based angiogram • Echocardiography (transthoracic and transesophageal)
Consistent arteriographic findings

Treat for TAO; biopsy only indicated if there are unusual features
• Age > 45 at onset
• Disease in unusual location
  – Proximal disease
  – CNS disease
• Tobacco history is not consistent with diagnosis

Table 17.2 Criteria for Diagnosis of Thromboangiitis Obliterans (From Olin JW. Thromboangiitis obliterans [Buerger's disease]. In: Rutherford RB, ed. *Vascular Surgery.* 6th ed. Philadelphia: WB Saunders; 2005:404-419. With permission from Elsevier.)

disease, the criteria that we find most helpful are shown in Table 17.2.

Cases of typical Buerger's disease with the presence of elevated anticardiolipin antibodies have been encountered.[35-37] A pathological specimen would clearly differentiate these 2 entities since antiphospholipid antibody syndrome is in reality a vasculopathy (the presence of thrombus with no inflammatory components) as opposed to the typical pathological findings in Buerger's disease (inflammatory thrombus). The reason why some patients with Buerger's disease have increased levels of anticardiolipin antibodies is not known.

Histopathology

The acute phase is the most diagnostic of Buerger's disease, and biopsy of an acute superficial thrombophlebitis is most likely to show the characteristic acute-phase lesion. Acute inflammation involves all layers of the vessel wall in association with a highly cellular thrombosis. There are often polymorphonuclear leukocytes with karyorrhexis, the so-called microabscesses, in which one or more multinucleated giant cells may be present.[6,38] Progressive organization of the thrombus is present in the intermediate (or subacute) phase. There is still a prominent inflammatory cell infiltrate within the thrombus and less so in the vessel wall. The chronic phase or end stage is characterized by complete organization of the occlusive thrombus with extensive recanalization, prominent vascularization of the media, and adventitial and perivascular fibrosis. This phase is indistinguishable from the chronic phase of any disease process.

In all 3 stages, the normal architecture of the vessel wall, including the internal elastic lamina, remains intact. These findings distinguish Buerger's disease from atherosclerosis and other systemic vasculitides.[39]

Treatment

The cornerstone of therapy is the complete discontinuation of cigarette smoking or the use of tobacco in any form (Table 17.3). Complete abstinence from tobacco use is the only way to halt the progression of Buerger's disease and to avoid future amputations.[1,2] In the absence of gangrene, amputation does not occur in patients who discontinue cigarette smoking. In a series of 120 patients followed long term, 52 (43%) were able to discontinue smoking (Figure 17.4).[2,35] This observation has been confirmed in a more recent study.[40] Cooper and associates[41] have shown that patients with Buerger's disease were more likely to have made a serious attempt to stop smoking compared to patients with coronary artery disease. Patients can be reassured that if they are able to discontinue tobacco use, the disease will remit and amputation will not occur as long as gangrene and tissue loss has not already occurred. In all likelihood, however, the patient may continue to experience intermittent claudication and/or Raynaud's phenomenon.

Other than discontinuation of cigarette smoking, all other forms of therapy are palliative. Fiessinger and Schafer[42] conducted a prospective, randomized double-blind trial comparing a 6-hour daily infusion of iloprost (a prostaglandin analog) to aspirin. Iloprost was superior to aspirin at 28 days in causing total

relief of rest pain and complete healing of all trophic changes. In addition, at 6 months, 88% of the patients receiving Iloprost responded favorably to therapy compared with 21% of the aspirin group. Only 6% had amputations compared with 18% in the aspirin group. Bozkurt and colleagues[43] performed a randomized trial in 200 patients with TAO and rest pain or ischemic ulcerations to undergo lumbar sympathetomy (LS) or a 28-day intravenous infusion of iloprost. The primary end point was complete healing without pain or major amputation at 4 and 24 weeks. The comparison was carried out

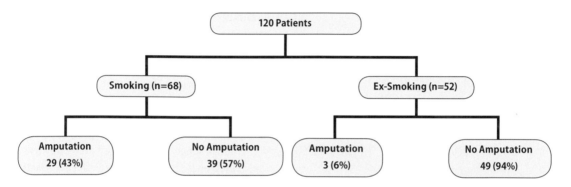

Figure 17.4 Smoking status related to amputation in 120 patients followed long term. (Adapted from Olin JW, Childs MB, Bartholomew JR, Calabrese LH, Young JR. Anticardiolipin antibodies and homocysteine levels in patients with thromboangiitis obliterans. *Arthritis Rheum.* 1996;39:S-47; and Olin JW, Young JR, Graor RA, Ruschhaupt WF, Bartholomew JR. The changing clinical spectrum of thromboangiitis obliterans [Buerger's disease]. *Circulation.* 1990;82[5 Suppl]:IV3-IV8.)

Discontinue smoking or tobacco use in any form
Avoid passive smoking as much as possible

Treat local ischemic ulcerations and pain:
• Foot care
  – Lubricate skin with moisturizer
  – Lamb's wool between toes
  – Avoid trauma (heel protectors, orthotics for shoes)
• If vasospasm is present, trial of dihydropyridine calcium channel blocker such as amlodipine or nifedipine
• Trial of cilostazol in attempt to heal ischemic ulcers
• Prostaglandin analogue (PGI or PGE)
• Revascularization (PTA or surgical) if anatomically feasible *and* patient has stopped smoking completely
• Sympathectomy
• Intermittent pneumatic compression pump
• Entry into a therapeutic angiogenesis trial if available
• As last resort prior to amputation: implantable spinal cord stimulator

Treat cellulitis with antibiotics and superficial phlebitis with nonsteroidal anti-inflammatory agents
Amputate if all else fails

Table 17.3 Treatment of TAO (Modified from Olin JW. Thromboangiitis obliterans (Buerger's disease). In: Rutherford RB, ed. *Vascular Surgery.* 6th ed. Philadelphia: WB Saunders; 2005:404-419. Copyright Elsevier.)

in 162 patients (iloprost: n = 84; LS: n = 78). Complete healing rate was 61.9% in the iloprost group, but 41% in the LS group at week 4 (P = 0.012); respective values for week 24 were 85.3%, 52.3%, P < 0.001. Analgesic requirement was lower in the iloprost group at weeks 4 and 24 (P = 0.01, and P = 0.098, respectively). The size of the ulcers decreased more in the iloprost group than in the LS group (P = 0.044 and P = 0.035 at weeks 4 and 24); 50% reduction in the ulcer size in the iloprost group was greater than in the LS group (P = 0.001 and P = 0.009 at weeks 4 and 24).

Good foot and hand care should be undertaken. If significant vasospasm is present, calcium channel blocking agents such as nifedipine, nicardipine, or amlodipine may be used.[1] There have been several reports of patients with ischemic ulcerations successfully treated with cilostazol when no other revascularization strategies were possible.[44,45]

The role of sympathectomy in preventing amputations or in treating pain is unclear. Despite the report by Bozkurt and associates[43] discussed previously, there have been several reports demonstrating that sympathectomy can be safely and effectively carried out laparoscopically in the lower[46,47] and upper extremities.[48,49]

An increasing number of reports exist on the use of an implantable spinal cord stimulator in patients with Buerger's disease.[50-52] In a series of 29 patients who underwent epidural spinal cord stimulator implantation, there was marked improvement in regional perfusion, especially in the 13 patients with trophic lesions.[53] The limb survival rate was 93.1%.

Surgical revascularization for Buerger's disease is not usually a viable alternative due to the diffuse segmental involvement and extreme distal nature of the disease. There is frequently not a distal blood vessel available for bypass surgery. In one report, surgical revascularization was undertaken in 19 patients.[54] The cumulative secondary patency rate was 57.9% for bypass grafts at a mean follow-up of 5.4 years. Seven major and 36 minor amputations were performed, with a limb salvage rate of 95.6%.

In a series of 216 patients receiving surgical therapy for Buerger's disease, Sayin and associates[55] noted that while the long-term patency of the bypass grafts was not good, the short-term patency was sufficient to allow healing of the ulcerations associated with TAO. Dilege and colleagues[56] reported on 27 of 36 (81%) patients with TAO who underwent revascularization procedures. During a 36-month follow-up, the patency rates at 12, 24, and 36 months were 59.2%, 48%, and 33.3%, respectively. However, the limb salvage rate was 92.5%. Although the patency rates are not very good, the limb salvage rate was quite satisfactory in this and other series.[56,57] It has been our experience that surgery is rarely needed if the patient is able to stop smoking.

Predictors of Outcome

Two studies have evaluated the long-term outcome in patients with Buerger's disease. Ohta and colleagues[40] followed 110 patients with Buerger's disease for a mean of 10.6 years. The cumulative survival rate was 84% up to 25 years after the initial consultation. Major amputation was necessary in only 5 of 35 limbs (14%) with failed grafts. Forty-seven patients (43%) underwent 108 amputation procedures, either major amputation (13 patients) or minor amputation (34 patients), of an upper or lower limb. No ischemic ulcers occurred or recurred in patients older than 60 years. Forty-one patients who stopped smoking did not undergo major amputation. Furthermore, of 69 patients who continued smoking, 13 patients (19%) underwent major amputation. There was a strong association between limb amputation and job loss (P < 0.0001).

Cooper and associates[19] followed 111 patients with Buerger's disease for a mean of 15.6 ± 10.1 years. The risk of major amputation was 11% at 5 years, 21% at 10 years, and 23% at 20 years. As in virtually every other study published, tobacco abstinence was associated with a good prognosis. This study showed 3 important findings: (1) the risk of amputation continues in ongoing smokers up to a median of 14.8 years (mean 15.6 years), (2) the risk of amputation in previous smokers was eliminated by 8 years after smoking cessation, and (3) there was an excessive late mortality in patients with TAO compared to the US population, a finding different from several other studies.[2,58]

Novel Therapies

The difficulty in studying rare diseases such as thromboangiitis obliterans is that there are no significant research dollars available. Therefore, little progress has been made in understanding the underlying pathogenesis of the disease in the last 100 years. There has been virtually nothing new in the pathological findings from those described in Leo Buerger's initial report.[59] Since the number of patients encountered in any given center is small, and the criteria for diagnosis are not consistent across centers, it is difficult to perform a randomized trial to determine if a given therapy is effective.

Several therapies are intriguing and may justify further study. Therapeutic angiogenesis has been used to treat the ischemic manifestations of TAO.[60] Ulcers that had not healed for more than 1 month before therapy completely healed in 3 of 5 limbs after the intramuscular *phVEGF165* gene therapy. Nocturnal rest pain was relieved in the remaining 2 patients, although both continued to have claudication. There was improved perfusion shown on magnetic resonance imaging in 7 of the 7 limbs, and newly visible collateral vessels shown with serial contrast angiography in 7 of the 7 limbs. A phase 1 clinical trial tested the safety of intramuscular gene transfer by using naked plasmid DNA encoding the gene for VEGF given by intramuscular injections in 7 patients with Buerger's disease.[61] Ischemic pain of the affected limb was relieved or improved markedly in 6 of 7 patients. Ischemic ulcers healed or improved in 4 of 6 patients. Cell-based therapy with autologous bone marrow mononuclear cell implantation has also been used with some degree of success.[62,63]

And most recently human leukocyte antigen-matched human umbilical cord blood–derived mesenchymal stem cells were transplanted into 4 men with Buerger's disease who had already received medical treatment and surgical therapies. After the stem cell transplantation, ischemic rest pain suddenly disappeared from their affected extremities. The necrotic skin lesions were healed within 4 weeks. In the follow-up angiography, digital capillaries were increased in number and size. In addition, vascular resistance in the affected extremities, compared with the preoperative examination, was markedly decreased due to improvement of the peripheral circulation.[64]

Another method of stimulating angiogenesis using a Kirschner wire placed in the medullary canal of the tibia was used in 6 patients with Buerger's disease.[65] In a mean follow-up of 19 months, there was significant improvement in clinical manifestations including reduced rest pain and increased claudication distance. Foot ulcers completely healed after Kirschner wire intervention.

A small pilot project demonstrated that the concentration of endothelin-I, a potent vasoconstrictor, is higher in patients with clinical exacerbations of Buerger's disease, suggesting that endothelin antagonists such as bosentan may be beneficial.[66]

Intermittent pneumatic compression has been shown to enhance calf inflow in patients with intermittent claudication or critical limb ischemia, and may serve a role as adjunctive therapy in Buerger's patients who are not candidates for revascularization. Application of intermittent pneumatic compression to the foot and calf augments popliteal artery flow through a sharp decrease in peripheral arterial resistance manifested by increases in peak systolic and end diastolic flow velocities on Doppler ultrasonography.[67] The Mayo Clinic group demonstrated the ability to completely heal ischemic ulcers in patients with small-vessel occlusive diseases such as scleroderma, CREST, and TAO.[68]

Summary

Thromboangiitis obliterans (Buerger's disease) is a vasculitis that mainly affects medium- and small-sized arteries and veins in the extremities. Rarely, larger vessels are involved such as the iliac, mesenteric, coronary, and cerebrovascular arteries. TAO is characterized by segmental inflammatory thrombotic occlusions and is clinically and histopathologically different from atherosclerosis or necrotizing vasculitis. It occurs most often in the infrapopliteal and infrabrachial arteries of young men and women who are heavy smokers. The only effective therapy is complete and permanent discontinuation of tobacco products, but therapeutic angiogenesis and stem cell transplantation are exciting new therapies on the horizon.

References

1. Olin JW. Thromboangiitis obliterans (Buerger's disease). *N Engl J Med.* 2000;343:864-869.

2. Olin JW, Young JR, Graor RA, Ruschhaupt WF, Bartholomew JR. The changing clinical spectrum of thromboangiitis obliterans (Buerger's disease). *Circulation.* 1990;82(5 Suppl):IV3-IV8.

3. Mills JL Sr. Buerger's disease in the 21st century: diagnosis, clinical features, and therapy. *Semin Vasc Surg.* 2003;16(3):179-189.

4. Laohapensang K, Rerkasem K, Kattipattanapong V. Seasonal variation of Buerger's disease in Northern part of Thailand. *Eur J Vasc Endovasc Surg.* 2004;28(4):418-420.

5. Ates A, Yekeler I, Ceviz M, et al. One of the most frequent vascular diseases in northeastern of Turkey: thromboangiitis obliterans or Buerger's disease (experience with 344 cases). *Int J Cardiol.* 2006;111(1):147-153.

6. Lie JT. Diagnostic histopathology of major systemic and pulmonary vasculitis syndromes. *Rheum Dis Clin North Am.* 1990;16:269-292.

7. Olin JW, Shih A. Thromboangiitis obliterans (Buerger's disease). *Curr Opin Rheumatol.* 2006;18(1):18-24.

8. Sasaki S, Sakuma M, Yasuda K. Current status of thromboangiitis obliterans (Buerger's disease) in Japan. *Int J Cardiol.* 2000;75(Suppl 1):S175-S181.

9. Heper G, Kose S, Akkoc O, Amasyali B, Kilic A. Two female nonsmoker Buerger's disease cases with anticardiolipin autoantibodies and a poor prognosis. *Int Heart J.* 2005;46(3):563-569.

10. Nagashima T, Kamimura T, Nara H, Iwamoto M, Okazaki H, Minota S. Images in cardiovascular medicine. Kimura's disease presenting as steroid-responsive thromboangiitis obliterans. *Circulation.* 2006;114(1):e10-e11.

11. Joyce JW. Buerger's disease (thromboangiitis obliterans). *Rheum Dis Clin North Am.* 1990;16(2):463-470.

12. Eichhorn J, Sima D, Lindschau C, et al. Anti-endothelial cell antibodies in thromboangiitis obliterans. *Am J Med Sci.* 1998;315(1):17-23.

13. Makita S, Nakamura M, Murakami H, Komoda K, Kawazoe K, Hiramori K. Impaired endothelium-dependent vasorelaxation in peripheral vasculature of patients with thromboangiitis obliterans (Buerger's disease). *Circulation.* 1996;94(9 Suppl):II211-II215.

14. Joras M, Poredos P, Fras Z. Endothelial dysfunction in Buerger's disease and its relation to markers of inflammation. *Eur J Clin Invest.* 2006;36(6):376-382.

15. Slavov ES, Stanilova SA, Petkov DP, Dobreva ZG. Cytokine production in thromboangiitis obliterans patients: new evidence for an immune-mediated inflammatory disorder. *Clin Exp Rheumatol.* 2005;23(2):219-226.

16. Adar R, Papa MZ, Halpern Z, et al. Cellular sensitivity to collagen in thromboangiitis obliterans. *N Engl J Med.* 1983;308(19):1113-1116.

17. Lee T, Seo JW, Sumpio BE, Kim SJ. Immunobiologic analysis of arterial tissue in Buerger's disease. *Eur J Vasc Endovasc Surg.* 2003;25(5):451-457.

18. Kobayashi M, Ito M, Nakagawa A, Nishikimi N, Nimura Y. Immunohistochemical analysis of arterial wall cellular infiltration in Buerger's disease (endarteritis obliterans). *J Vasc Surg.* 1999;29(3):451-458.

19. Cooper LT, Tse TS, Mikhail MA, McBane RD, Stanson AW, Ballman KV. Long-term survival and amputation risk in thromboangiitis obliterans (Buerger's disease). *J Am Coll Cardiol*. 2004;44(12):2410-2411.

20. Ehrenfeld M, Adar R. Rheumatic manifestations in patients with thromboangiitis obliterans (Buerger's disease). *J Rheumatol*. 2000;27(7):1818-1819.

21. Lie JT. Thromboangiitis obliterans (Buerger's disease) in women. *Medicine (Baltimore)*. 1987;66(1):65-72.

22. Mills JL, Taylor LM Jr, Porter JM. Buerger's disease in the modern era. *Am J Surg*. 1987;154(1):123-129.

23. Lau H, Cheng SW. Buerger's disease in Hong Kong: a review of 89 cases. *Aust N Z J Surg*. 1997;67(5):264-269.

24. Shionoya S. Buerger's disease (thromboangiitis obliterans). In: Rutherford RB, ed. *Vascular Surgery*. Philadelphia: W.B. Saunders; 1989:207-217.

25. Shionoya S, Ban I, Nakata Y, Matsubara J, Hirai M, Kawai S. Involvement of the iliac artery in Buerger's disease (pathogenesis and arterial reconstruction). J *Cardiovasc Surg*. (Torino) 1978;19(1):69-76.

26. Allen EV. Thromboangiitis obliterans. Methods of diagnosis of chronic occlusive arterial lesions distal to the wrist with illustrative cases. *Am J Med Sci*. 1929;178:237-244.

27. Combemale P, Consort T, Denis-Thelis L, Estival JL, Dupin M, Kanitakis J. Cannabis arteritis. *Br J Dermatol*. 2005;152(1):166-169.

28. Disdier P, Granel B, Serratrice J, et al. Cannabis arteritis revisited—ten new case reports. *Angiology*. 2001;52(1):1-5.

29. Marder VJ, Mellinghoff IK. Cocaine and Buerger disease: is there a pathogenetic association? *Arch Intern Med*. 2000;160(13):2057-2060.

30. Noel B. Cocaine and arsenic-induced Raynaud's phenomenon. *Clin Rheumatol*. 2002;21(4):343-344.

31. Noel B. Regarding "cannabis arteritis revisited—ten new case reports." *Angiology*. 2001;52(7):505-506.

32. Noel B. Vascular complications of cocaine use. *Stroke*. 2002;33(7):1747-1748.

33. McKusick VA, Harris WS, Ottsen OE, Goodman RM. The Buerger's syndrome in the United States. Arteriographic observations with special reference to involvement of the upper extremities and the differentiation from atherosclerosis and embolism. *Bull Johns Hopkins Hosp*. 1962;110:145-176.

34. McKusick VA, Harris WS, Ottsen OE. Buerger's disease: a distinct clinical and pathologic entity. *JAMA*. 1962;181:93-100.

35. Olin JW, Childs MB, Bartholomew JR, Calabrese LH, Young JR. Anticardiolipin antibodies and homocysteine levels in patients with thromboangiitis obliterans. *Arthritis Rheum*. 1996;39:S-47.

36. Olin JW. Are anticardiolipin antibodies really important in thromboangiitis obliterans (Buerger's disease)? *Vasc Med*. 2002;7(4):257-258.

37. Maslowski L, McBane R, Alexewicz P, Wysokinski WE. Antiphospholipid antibodies in thromboangiitis obliterans. *Vasc Med*. 2002;7(4):259-264.

38. Lie JT. Thromboangiitis obliterans (Buerger's disease) revisited. *Pathol Annu*. 1988;23(Pt 2):257-291.

39. Olin JW, Lie JT. Thromboangiitis obliterans (Buerger's disease). In: Cooke JP, Frohlich ED, eds. *Current Management of Hypertension and Vascular Disease*. St. Louis, MO: Mosby Yearbook; 1992:265-271.

40. Ohta T, Ishioashi H, Hosaka M, Sugimoto I. Clinical and social consequences of Buerger disease. *J Vasc Surg*. 2004;39(1):176-180.

41. Cooper LT, Henderson SS, Ballman KV, et al. A prospective, case-control study of tobacco dependence in thromboangiitis obliterans (Buerger's disease). *Angiology*. 2006;57(1):73-78.

42. Fiessinger JN, Schafer M. Trial of iloprost versus aspirin treatment for critical limb ischaemia of thromboangiitis obliterans. The TAO Study. *Lancet*. 1990;335(8689):555-557.

43. Bozkurt AK, Koksal C, Demirbas MY, et al. A randomized trial of intravenous iloprost (a stable prostacyclin analogue) versus lumbar sympathectomy in the management of Buerger's disease. *Int Angiol*. 2006;25(2):162-168.

44. Dean SM, Satiani B. Three cases of digital ischemia successfully treated with cilostazol. *Vasc Med*. 2001;6(4):245-248.

45. Dean SM, Vaccaro PS. Successful pharmacologic treatment of lower extremity ulcerations in 5 patients with chronic critical limb ischemia. *J Am Board Fam Pract*. 2002;15(1):55-62.

46. Watarida S, Shiraishi S, Fujimura M, et al. Laparoscopic lumbar sympathectomy for lower-limb disease. *Surg Endosc*. 2002;16(3):500-503.

47. Chander J, Singh L, Lal P, Jain A, Lal P, Ramteke VK. Retroperitoneoscopic lumbar sympathectomy for Buerger's disease: a novel technique. *JSLS*. 2004;8(3):291-296.

48. De Giacomo T, Rendina EA, Venuta F, et al. Thoracoscopic sympathectomy for symptomatic arterial obstruction of the upper extremities. *Ann Thorac Surg*. 2002;74(3):885-888.

49. Rizzo M, Balderson SS, Harpole DH, Levin LS. Thoracoscopic sympathectomy in the management of vasomotor disturbances and complex regional pain syndrome of the hand. *Orthopedics*. 2004;27(1):49-52.

50. Swigris JJ, Olin JW, Mekhail NA. Implantable spinal cord stimulator to treat the ischemic manifestations of thromboangiitis obliterans (Buerger's disease). *J Vasc Surg*. 1999;29(5):928-935.

51. Chierichetti F, Mambrini S, Bagliani A, Odero A. Treatment of Buerger's disease with electrical spinal cord stimulation—review of three cases. *Angiology*. 2002;53(3):341-347.

52. Pace AV, Saratzis N, Karokis D, Dalainas D, Kitas GD. Spinal cord stimulation in Buerger's disease. *Ann Rheum Dis*. 2002;61(12):1114.

53. Donas KP, Schulte S, Ktenidis K, Horsch S. The role of epidural spinal cord stimulation in the treatment of Buerger's disease. *J Vasc Surg*. 2005;41(5):830-836.

54. Bozkurt AK, Besirli K, Koksal C, et al. Surgical treatment of Buerger's disease. *Vascular*. 2004;12(3):192-197.

55. Sayin A, Bozkurt AK, Tuzun H, Vural FS, Erdog G, Ozer M. Surgical treatment of Buerger's disease: experience with 216 patients. *Cardiovasc Surg*. 1993;1(4):377-380.

56. Dilege S, Aksoy M, Kayabali M, Genc FA, Senturk M, Baktiroglu S. Vascular reconstruction in Buerger's disease: is it feasible? *Surg Today*. 2002;32(12):1042-1047.

57. Nishikimi N. Fate of limbs with failed vascular reconstruction in Buerger's disease patients. *Int J Cardiol*. 2000;75(Suppl 1):S183-S185.

58. Borner C, Heidrich H. Long-term follow-up of thromboangiitis obliterans. *Vasa*. 1998;27(2):80-86.

59. Buerger L. Thromboangiitis obliterans: a study of the vascular lesions leading to presenile spontaneous gangrene. *Am J Med Sci*. 1908;136(567):580.

60. Isner JM, Baumgartner I, Rauh G, et al. Treatment of thromboangiitis obliterans (Buerger's disease) by intramuscular gene transfer of vascular endothelial growth factor: preliminary clinical results. *J Vasc Surg*. 1998;28(6):964-973.

61. Kim HJ, Jang SY, Park JI, et al. Vascular endothelial growth factor-induced angiogenic gene therapy in patients with peripheral artery disease. *Exp Mol Med*. 2004;36(4):336-344.

62. Miyamoto M, Yasutake M, Takano H, et al. Therapeutic angiogenesis by autologous bone marrow cell implantation for refractory chronic peripheral arterial disease using assessment of neovascularization by 99mTc-tetrofosmin (TF) perfusion scintigraphy. *Cell Transplant*. 2004;13(4):429-437.

63. Durdu S, Akar AR, Arat M, Sancak T, Eren NT, Ozyurda U. Autologous bone-marrow mononuclear cell implantation for patients with Rutherford grade II-III thromboangiitis obliterans. *J Vasc Surg*. 2006;44(4):732-739.

64. Kim SW, Han H, Chae GT, et al. Successful stem cell therapy using umbilical cord blood-derived multipotent stem cells for Buerger's disease and ischemic limb disease animal model. *Stem Cells*. 2006;24(6):1620-1626.

65. Inan M, Alat I, Kutlu R, Harma A, Germen B. Successful treatment of Buerger's disease with intramedullary K-wire: the results of the first 11 extremities. *Eur J Vasc Endovasc Surg*. 2005;29(3):277-280.

66. Czarnacki M, Gacka M, Adamiec R. A role of endothelin 1 in the pathogenesis of thromboangiitis obliterans (initial news). *Przegl Lek*. 2004;61(12):1346-1350.

67. Labropoulos N, Watson WC, Mansour MA, Kang SS, Littooy FN, Baker WH. Acute effects of intermittent pneumatic compression on popliteal artery blood flow. *Arch Surg.* 1998;133(10):1072-1075.

68. Montori VM, Kavros SJ, Walsh EE, Rooke TW. Intermittent compression pump for nonhealing wounds in patients with limb ischemia. The Mayo Clinic experience (1998-2000). *Int Angiol.* 2002;21(4):360-366.

18

Systemic Vasculitides

Reena L. Pande and Joshua A. Beckman

Vasculitis is an inflammation of the vasculature affecting blood vessels of any size and type and involving any organ. As a result, the clinical manifestations are diverse, but ultimately result from stenosis and tissue ischemia or from aneurysm formation with embolization, thrombosis, or rupture and bleeding. The varied signs and symptoms, coupled with relatively similar histologic patterns of vessel inflammation, make the diagnosis of specific forms of vasculitis challenging. Determining the correct diagnosis has significant clinical implications since different forms of vasculitis have varying prognoses and respond differently to treatment.

Given the challenge of accurate identification of these disorders, creating an acceptable classification scheme was imperative. In 1990, the American College of Rheumatology (ACR) published the most widely adopted research criteria for the classification of the major vasculitic syndromes.[1-10] These criteria were designed to differentiate the vasculitides, particularly for research and classification purposes, but have been employed to make diagnoses in affected patients, although the criteria in many cases are too specific for use in individual patients. Notably lacking from the 1990 ACR classification scheme was *microscopic polyangiitis (MPA)* as a distinct disease entity and the presence of *antineutrophil cytoplasmic antibodies (ANCA)* as a diagnostic criterion. The 1990 ACR clinical criteria were followed by publication in 1994 of the classification from the Chapel Hill Consensus Conference.[11] This classification provided definitions of 10 forms of vasculitis, aiming to reach consensus on the names of the major vasculitides, including MPA.

The most widely accepted approach of vasculitis classification relies on the size and location of the vessels involved. Table 18.1 delineates the major categories of vasculitis according to vessel size. "Large vessel" refers to the aorta and its main branches (to the head, neck, and extremities); "medium vessel" refers to visceral arteries and branches thereof; and "small vessel" refers to arterioles, capillaries, and venules and on occasion may include the smallest muscular arteries. Despite the distinct differences, there is significant overlap among these disorders such that the size of vessel is a prominent feature but only one of many features that should be considered as a diagnosis is sought.

This chapter focuses on five of the most common and clinically important vasculitides,

Vascular Disease: Diagnostic and Therapeutic Approaches. © 2011 Michael R. Jaff and Christopher J. White, editors. Cardiotext Publishing, ISBN: 978-1-935395-16-4.

including both of the major large-vessel vasculitides (Takayasu's arteritis and giant cell arteritis), a medium-vessel vasculitis (polyarteritis nodosa), and one of each of the major categories of small-vessel vasculitis (Wegener's granulomatosis, an ANCA-associated vasculitis, and hypersensitivity vasculitis, an immune-complex vasculitis).

Large-Vessel Vasculitis
Takayasu's arteritis
Giant cell arteritis
Behçet's disease
Aortitis associated with spondyloarthropathies
Medium-Vessel Vasculitis
Polyarteritis nodosa (PAN)
Wegener's granulomatosis (Can also affect small vessels)
Microscopic polyangiitis
Churg-Strauss syndrome
Kawasaki's disease
Small-Vessel Vasculitis
Hypersensitivity vasculitis (including drug-induced immune-complex vasculitis and infection-induced immune-complex vasculitis)
Henoch-Schönlein purpura
Cryoglobulinemic vasculitis
Connective tissue disorders (systemic lupus erythematosus, rheumatoid arthritis, Sjögren's syndrome)
Hypocomplementemic urticarial vasculitis
Goodpasture's syndrome

Table 18.1 Major Categories of Vasculitis Based on Most Commonly Affected Vessel Size

Takayasu's Arteritis

Epidemiology

Takayasu's arteritis is a large-vessel vasculitis classically affecting the large elastic arteries, specifically the aorta and its major branches. The disease has a significant female predominance with the peak age of onset in the second and third decades of life. While the disease was initially described in Asia, and is more prevalent in this region, it does have a worldwide distribution, affecting people of all ethnicities. The annual estimated incidence rate in North America is nearly 2.6 cases per million people,[12] but the disease may be underappreciated in Europe and North America.[13]

Takayasu's arteritis, also referred to as *pulseless disease* or *occlusive thromboarthropathy,* is an idiopathic, chronic, granulomatous inflammation of large elastic arteries. The most common abnormality is arterial stenosis or occlusion resulting from panarteritis and luminal narrowing (Figure 18.1). In rarer cases, aortic aneurysms may be the predominant feature. In Asia, distinct patterns of vessel involvement have been noted in different countries. In one series of 80 Japanese and 102 Indian patients, patients from Japan had vascular lesions primarily involving the ascending aorta, aortic arch, and its branches, with disease extending into the abdominal aorta. In contrast, Indian patients tended to have lesions primarily in the abdominal aorta with involvement of the renal arteries and with disease extending upwards into the thoracic aorta.[14,15] In the largest North American experience, 60 patients with Takayasu's arteritis followed prospectively at the National Institutes of Health, 98% of affected individuals had stenotic lesions and 27% had aneurysms.[12] Aneurysms tend to involve the aortic root and can result in significant aortic insufficiency. Rarely, the pulmonary arteries and renal arteries can be involved, the latter causing renovascular hypertension.

Pathophysiology

The pathogenesis of Takayasu's arteritis remains incompletely understood, but recent progress in understanding the pathogenesis of giant cell arteritis has shed light on the mechanisms of Takayasu's given their underlying similarities. Takayasu's arteritis is a T-cell-mediated pan-

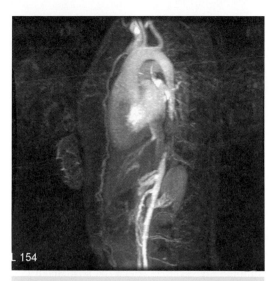

Figure 18.1 Takayasu's arteritis. A 21-year-old female presented with severe hypertension and bilateral lower-extremity claudication. MRA demonstrated long-segment narrowing and occlusion of the aorta at the thoracoabdominal junction. Multiple arterial collateral vessels reconstitute the abdominal aorta distal to the occlusion.

arteritis, affecting all layers of the vessel wall. During an initial acute phase, the most prominent inflammation is in the adventitial layer, specifically within the vasa vasorum. While the trigger for this inflammatory response remains unknown, the responsible antigen is likely recognized in the vasa vasorum by T cells activated by abnormally mature antigen-presenting cells (dendritic cells). The T cells undergo clonal expansion and release interferon gamma that stimulates local macrophages to produce the proinflammatory cytokines IL-1 and IL-6, eventually resulting in granuloma formation and vessel wall damage. The repair mechanisms that ensue involve production of platelet-derived growth factor (PDGF) and vascular endothelial growth factor (VEGF), leading to destruction of the elastic lamina and lumen occlusion. If this destructive process is more rapid than the reparative fibrotic process that naturally follows, then aneurysms may form.[16,17]

The specific antigens that provoke the inflammatory response in Takayasu's arteritis remain unknown. Infectious triggers may be important in the pathogenesis of Takayasu's.

Tuberculosis was first proposed as a potential trigger in light of its prevalence in affected individuals, albeit in patients from regions where tuberculosis is endemic. This association is supported by the strong expression in aortic tissue of a 65-kilodalton heat-shock protein, which is associated with tuberculosis.[18] Viral pathogens may also serve as triggers in Takayasu's, though none specifically has yet been identified. Others have postulated that Takayasu's arteritis is an autoimmune phenomenon.[19] This theory is supported by the link with specific human leukocyte antigen (HLA) alleles in certain populations[16] and by the association with several autoimmune disorders, including pyoderma gangrenosum, erythema nodosum, autoimmune thyroiditis, Crohn's disease, and ulcerative colitis.[12,20]

Clinical Manifestations

The clinical manifestations of Takayasu's arteritis generally appear in the organs affected by involved blood vessels. In a series of 60 subjects with the disease, Kerr et al[12] showed that all patients had vascular symptoms. Claudication was reported in the upper limbs in 62% and in the lower limbs in 32% of patients. Carotidynia was noted in one-third of patients. Central nervous system symptoms (lightheadedness, visual impairment or loss, stroke, or transient ischemic attack [TIA]) were present in 57% of patients. More than 50% had musculoskeletal symptoms while only 43% had constitutional symptoms including fever, sweats, weight loss, malaise, and anorexia. Cardiac findings (including aortic regurgitation, angina, palpitations, pericarditis, myocardial infarction, or congestive heart failure) were noted in 38% of patients studied. In an Indian series of 106 patients with Takayasu's arteritis, hypertension was the most common finding, seen in 77% of individuals,[21] but constitutional symptoms were rare, occurring in only 16% of subjects.[22]

Bruits are the most common finding on physical examination, present in nearly 80% of patients. Most commonly audible in the carotid arteries, many patients exhibit bruits in several vascular beds.[12,21,22] More than 50% of patients will have asymmetric or diminished pulses or asymmetric blood pressure measurements.[12] Aortic root involvement may be associated with aortic valvular regurgitation with a diastolic murmur noted on examination.

Diagnostic Evaluation

In 1990, the ACR selected 6 criteria for the classification of Takayasu's arteritis: (1) onset at age $\leq$ 40 years, (2) claudication of an extremity, (3) decreased brachial artery pulse, (4) > 10 mm Hg difference in systolic blood pressure between arms, (5) a bruit over the subclavian arteries or the aorta, and (6) arteriographic evidence of narrowing or occlusion of the entire aorta, its primary branches, or large arteries in the proximal upper or lower extremities (Table 18.2). The presence of 3 or more of these 6 criteria had a sensitivity and specificity of 90.5% and 97.8%, respectively. A classification tree using 5 of these criteria (excluding claudication of an extremity) had a sensitivity of 92.1% and a specificity of 97.0%.[1]

Laboratory testing includes C-reactive protein (CRP) and an erythrocyte sedimentation rate (ESR). These markers of inflammation are elevated in the acute phase in > 70% of patients but remain positive in nearly 50% of patients even when in clinical remission.[12] Angiography remains the gold standard for diagnosis and may demonstrate focal narrowing or occlusion of the aorta or its main branches, in both the proximal upper and lower extremities. Affected vessels appear smooth and tapered with long, segmental stenoses. Traditional angiography, however, only detects fixed changes in lumen diameter that may not occur until later stages of disease and, as such, may be unreliable for diagnostic purposes in the earliest phase of Takayasu's arteritis. Several groups have evaluated the role of noninvasive techniques—18-fluourodeoxyglucose positron emission tomography (18F-FDG-PET) and magnetic resonance angiography (MRA)—in identifying early disease activity. FDG-PET scanning detects areas of high metabolic activity, suggesting vascular inflammation. MRA can detect vessel wall thickening. Early identification of vessel wall inflammation or thickening may allow for diagnosis in the prestenotic phase of disease.[23] While several studies have suggested potential clinical utility of these noninvasive techniques,[23-28] larger clinical trials are needed before their widespread clinical use in diagnosis of large-vessel vasculitis.

Criterion	Definition
Age at disease onset ≤ 40 years	Development of symptoms or findings related to Takayasu's arteritis at age ≤ 40 years
Claudication of extremities	Development and worsening of fatigue and discomfort in muscles of one or more extremity while in use, especially the upper extremities
Decreased brachial artery pulse	Decreased pulsation of one or both brachial arteries
BP difference >10 mm Hg	Difference of > 10 mm Hg in systolic BP between arms
Bruit over subclavian arteries or aorta	Bruit audible on auscultation over one or both subclavian arteries or abdominal aorta
Arteriogram abnormality	Arteriographic narrowing or occlusion of the entire aorta, its primary branches, or large arteries in the proximal upper or lower extremities, not due to arteriosclerosis, fibromuscular dysplasia, or similar causes; changes usually focal or segmental

Table 18.2 ACR Criteria (1990) for the Classification of Takayasu's Arteritis
Note: For purposes of classification, a patient shall be said to have Takayasu's arteritis if at least 3 of these 6 criteria are present. The presence of any 3 or more criteria yields a sensitivity of 90.5% and a specificity of 97.8%.[1] BP = blood pressure.

Given the challenge of diagnosis, it is critical to rule out other causes of aortitis that may mimic Takayasu's arteritis. These include infections (tuberculosis, fungal infections, syphilis), inherited vascular disorders (Marfan's syndrome, Ehlers-Danlos), idiopathic inflammatory disorders (Kawasaki's disease, giant cell arteritis, sarcoidosis, and spondyloarthropathies with aortitis), and atherosclerotic disease.

Histopathology of affected blood vessels is helpful in confirming the diagnosis, but unfortunately, given the location of involvement, diagnostic biopsy is often difficult to obtain.

Treatment

The goals of treatment of Takayasu's arteritis are both suppression of inflammation and restoration of blood flow by revascularization. Several issues make management of Takayasu's arteritis particularly challenging: (1) by the time of diagnosis, most patients will have already developed fixed stenoses that are not reversible with medical therapy alone, and (2) disease progression occurs even when patients are felt to be in clinical remission on stable medical therapy. In one study with serial angiography, 61% of patients developed new lesions while in clinical remission.[12]

Corticosteroids

Anti-inflammatory therapy with corticosteroids constitutes the first line of treatment. In doses of 0.5 to 1.0 mg/kg/day, as many of 60% of patients will achieve remission over a median time period of 22 months.[12] However, relapses occur in nearly 50% of patients as steroids doses are tapered,[12] necessitating the initiation of other immunosuppressive and cytotoxic agents, both to halt disease progression and to limit steroid-related side effects.[12,29]

Methotrexate

Methotrexate has been used as a second-line agent in steroid-resistant Takayasu's arteritis.[29-32] Hoffman et al[29] prospectively evaluated the utility of weekly low-dose methotrexate with a starting dose of 0.3 mg/kg/week (up to 15 mg/week) titrated up to a maximum dose of 25 mg/week. Remission was achieved in 13 of 16 patients. Seven of these patients relapsed as steroid therapy was reduced or discontinued, but remission could again be achieved by reinstitution of the original regimen.

Azathioprine

The role of azathioprine (Imuran) was evaluated in 15 patients with newly diagnosed and clinically active Takayasu's arteritis who received a combination of azathioprine at 2 mg/kg/day and prednisolone at 1 mg/kg/day as a first-line regimen.[33] Treatment was administered for 6 weeks and then tapered to a dose of 10 mg/day by 12 weeks. All patients had improved systemic symptoms, no angiographically demonstrable progression of disease, and no new lesions. It is unclear to what extent the effect was due to azathioprine versus glucocorticoid therapy.

Cyclophosphamide

Chronic cyclophosphamide (Cytoxan) therapy in doses of 1 to 2 mg/kg/day has been recommended only for use in severe Takayasu's arteritis refractory to other immunosuppressive medications.[34] In one small study, 6 patients unresponsive to steroids alone were treated with cyclophosphamide (at a dose of 2 mg/kg/day) in addition to steroids, allowing for tapering of steroid doses and attenuation of disease progression in 4 patients.[35] Significant side effects of cyclophosphamide therapy, including hemorrhagic cystitis, are a major limitation of its use.

Antitumor necrosis factor agents

Recently, a greater understanding of the role of tumor necrosis factor-alpha (TNF-α) in inflammatory disorders and in granuloma formation has prompted research on the effectiveness of anti-TNF drugs, such as infliximab and etanercept, in the treatment of Takayasu's arteritis. In one such pilot study of these medications, 14 of 15 patients unresponsive to steroids alone achieved remission (with discontinuation of steroid therapy) or partial remission (allowing 50% reduction in steroid dose) sustained over an average of 1 to 3 years.[36] Nine of the

14 patients required sustained treatment with anti-TNF therapy or increasing doses to maintain remission.

The appropriate length of therapy remains uncertain. Most patients will require steroid therapy for at least 1 to 2 years; in the study by Kerr et al,[12] the median time to achieving remission on steroids alone was 22 months. Because more than 50% of patients ultimately relapse on steroid therapy, many patients require several more years of therapy with other immunosuppressive agents, and most will require long-term suppressive therapy to prevent disease progression.

Surgical revascularization

Revascularization in Takayasu's arteritis is reserved for patients with severe stenosis or occlusion who demonstrate symptoms of diminished perfusion. Because many patients present when arterial stenoses have already developed, medical therapy may be ineffective and revascularization is often required to alleviate symptoms. Clinical indications for revascularization include severe refractory hypertension associated with renal artery stenosis, claudication from peripheral arterial involvement, stroke or other evidence of cerebrovascular ischemia, and angina from coronary artery involvement.[12,34] Surgical revascularization has been evaluated in several nonrandomized prospective cohorts. In the series by Kerr et al,[12] 23 patients underwent 50 bypass procedures, most performed with Dacron or saphenous vein conduits. Bypassed vessels included the common carotid (12 cases), subclavian or axillary (10 cases), iliofemoral (7), renal (7), and coronary (6) arteries. Complications (predominantly restenosis) occurred in 30% of procedures, but the majority of restenosis occurred in synthetic grafts (36%) versus only 9% of autologous grafts. Bypass surgery for renal artery stenosis due to Takayasu's arteritis was evaluated in a study of 32 aortorenal bypass procedures in 32 patients.[37] Graft stenosis or occlusion occurred in 6 cases, and patency rate was 79% at 5 years. Renal revascularization resulted in a significant reduction in blood pressure, reduction in need for antihypertensive medica-

tions, improvement in glomerular filtration rate, and resolution of congestive heart failure.[37]

Graft failure from local inflammation is a concern that has led several authors to stress the importance of choosing regions for anastomoses that have no evidence of active vasculitis. While restenosis is the most common cause of graft failure, one study found a 12% rate of anastomotic aneurysms over 20 years of follow-up that was directly related to the presence of aneurysmal disease preoperatively, not to disease state or steroid therapy.[38] In general, revascularization should be performed when the disease is quiescent.

Percutaneous revascularization

Percutaneous angioplasty with and without stenting is a viable option depending on the type and location of stenoses. Results have been mixed, and studies suggest higher success rates for short-segment disease and higher restenosis rates for longer-segment lesions or total occlusions. Balloon angioplasty with or without stenting appears to be successful in the treatment of subclavian stenosis[12,39] and renal artery stenosis.[12,40-42] Patency rates for renal artery angioplasty were 86.5% at 1 year[40] and 33% at 5 years,[41] and for subclavian arteries, 78% over 3 to 120 months of follow-up.[39] Restenosis was more common than in patients who undergo angioplasty for atherosclerotic disease, although not statistically significant (21.7% vs. 10%, P = NS)[39] and in longer-segment stenoses and total occlusions.[34] On the forefront of treatment in Takayasu's arteritis is the percutaneous management of aortoiliac disease[43] and carotid disease.[44,45] The evolution of drug-eluting stents may revolutionize percutaneous treatment of inflammatory diseases as they limit restenosis related to vascular inflammation and improve long-term patency rates. For the present time, however, it appears that bypass surgery continues to have the most favorable long-term patency rates.

Natural History and Prognosis

Survival estimates vary significantly depending on the severity of disease and number of resultant complications. Ishikawa et al[46] followed 54 Japanese patients and found the overall 5-year survival rate to be 83.1%. However, those individuals with uncomplicated disease had a 100% survival rate, compared with a 70% survival in patients with one or more severe complications of the disease. A similar assessment of 88 patients in India found significantly lower 5-year survival in patients with a single severe complication or with multiple complications (59.7% compared with 97% in those with no complications).[18] Severe hypertension, severe functional disability, or cardiac involvement were the strongest predictors of death or a major nonfatal event.[18]

Giant Cell Arteritis

Epidemiology

Giant cell arteritis, also known as *temporal arteritis,* is a vasculitis of large- and medium-sized vessels. The disease can be widespread but has a tendency to involve the secondary and tertiary branches of the aorta, and vascular inflammation leads to stenosis or aneurysmal disease. Giant cell arteritis affects individuals older than 50 years, peaking between the ages of 70 and 80, with a female to male ratio of 3:2.[47] The prevalence in the United States is approximately 20 per 100,000 persons, determined primarily from epidemiologic studies in Olmstead County, Minnesota.[47,48] In Europe, incidence is lower in more southern European countries, and higher prevalence at more northern geographic latitudes or a genetic predisposition in individuals of northern European descent.[48,49]

Population studies have demonstrated an overlap between giant cell arteritis and *polymyalgia rheumatica (PMR).* Nearly 40% to 60% of patients with giant cell arteritis will have a concurrent diagnosis of PMR.[48] Conversely, 16% to 21% of patients with PMR have biopsy-proven giant cell arteritis.[48,49]

In giant cell arteritis, transmural inflammation affects the major branch vessels of the aorta with a characteristic involvement of the extracranial branches of the carotid artery. Temporal artery involvement is by far the most common, but the disease can also involve the ophthalmic arteries and the vessels that supply the tongue, jaw muscles, and pharynx. Nearly 10% to 15% of patients also develop disease of the aorta and its primary branches (eg, subclavian arteries).[50] Some have suggested that large-vessel involvement may be underappreciated.[51] While disease of the medium-sized vessels almost exclusively results in stenosis and occlusion, inflammation of the aorta results in aneurysms, dissection, and rupture (Figure 18.2, on the following page). In 96 patients with giant cell arteritis, Evans et al[52] found 11 thoracic aortic aneurysms (TAAs) and 5 abdominal aortic aneurysms (AAAs) with a frequency significantly higher than in the general population (RR 17.3 for TAA and 2.4 for AAA). The high morbidity and mortality of TAA in giant cell arteritis was demonstrated in a series of 41 such patients, in which 16 patients developed aortic dissection (with 8 deaths), 19 developed aortic insufficiency from aortic root disease, and 18 required surgical repair.[53]

Pathophysiology

Because of the easy accessibility of temporal artery biopsy specimens, much has been elucidated about the pathogenesis of giant cell arteritis.[17] As in other vasculitides, the specific antigen that triggers inflammation remains unknown. However, the clonal expansion of specific T-cell populations certainly suggests an antigen-driven process. In particular, cyclic fluctuation in the incidence of giant cell arteritis raises the suspicion of an infectious etiology.[48] The inflammatory response begins in the adventitial layer as the antigen triggers T-cell activation, clonal T-cell expansion, and production of interferon gamma. The interferon gamma–mediated activation of macrophages creates a chemical milieu that promotes both inflammation (via IL-1 and IL-6) and tissue destruction (via matrix metalloproteinases). The formation of granulomas has the beneficial effect of

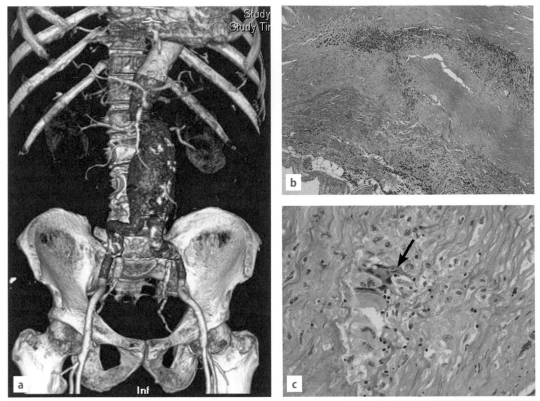

Figure 18.2 Giant cell aortitis. (a) 3D computed tomography reconstruction of a juxtarenal abdominal aortic aneurysm measuring 6.0 x 5.8 cm and suprarenal aortic aneurysm measuring 3.9 x 3.6 cm in a 75-year-old patient. There is also aneurysmal dilatation of both common iliac arteries. Incidental note is made of the common trunk of celiac and superior mesenteric arteries. (b) Pathologic specimen from the same patient taken at the time of aneurysm repair (10x). The aortic media contains multiple foci of a chronic inflammatory infiltrate consisting of giant cells, lymphocytes, and numerous plasma cells associated with areas of elastic lamellar disruption, fragmentation, and frank medial necrosis. There is mild scarring of the adventitia with chronic inflammation. (c) High-power image demonstrating lymphoplasmacytic infiltrate and a multinucleated giant cell (arrow). (Courtesy of Jey Chen, MD, Department of Pathology, Brigham and Women's Hospital, Boston, MA.)

walling off potential antigens, but simultaneously causes vessel wall damage. The inflammatory cell infiltrate in the arterial wall degrades the elastic lamina, promoting aneurysm formation, and results in intimal proliferation, promoting luminal occlusion.[54] These pathologic changes are nearly identical to those found in Takayasu's arteritis.

Clinical Manifestations

The clinical manifestations of giant cell arteritis are varied, ranging from vague and benign-appearing symptoms of headache and consti-tutional symptoms to life-threatening aortic dissection, stroke, and vision loss. One-half of patients describe constitutional symptoms such as fever, loss of appetite, sweats, fatigue, and weight loss. Headaches and scalp or temporal tenderness are present in at least 65% of patients and in up to 90% of patients with biopsy-proven disease.[55] Jaw claudication resulting from stenosis of vessels supplying the muscles of mastication affects nearly one-half of patients.[56] Approximately 20% of patients will develop visual symptoms including blurry vision, diplopia, amaurosis fugax, or permanent vision loss, starting as partial obscuration of the visual field and progressing to complete blindness.[57] These patients are at risk for contralateral vision loss if the disease is left untreated. Involvement of the vertebral arteries can result in posterior circulation stroke or transient ischemic attack, with symptoms including vertigo or dizziness. Neurologic symptoms, including stroke, TIA, or neuropathy, occur in 31% of patients.[57] Polymyalgia rheumatica, characterized by neck, shoulder, and pelvic muscle stiffness and myalgias, is present in nearly 50% of patients with giant cell arteritis.[48] Aortic aneurysms with dissection and rupture occur in 1% to 10% of affected individuals.[52,53]

Physical examination in giant cell arteritis may reveal thickened, nodular, and tender branches of the superficial temporal arteries with decreased or absent pulses. Funduscopic examination may show pallor and edema of the optic disk, scattered cotton-wool patches, and hemorrhages. In the 10% to 15% of patients with involvement of the subclavian or axillary arteries or other branches of the aorta, bruits may be present and pulses may be absent or diminished.[51] Concurrent polymyalgia rheumatica may be manifest by proximal muscle pain and stiffness.

Diagnostic Evaluation

The 5 diagnostic criteria proposed by the ACR in 1990 include (1) patient age $\geq$ 50 years, (2) new onset of a localized headache, (3) temporal artery tenderness or decreased pulse, (4) ESR above 50 mm per hour, and (5) an arterial biopsy specimen demonstrating necrotizing vasculitis (Table 18.3).[5] The presence of 3 or more criteria suggests a diagnosis of giant cell arteritis with a sensitivity of 93.5% and a specificity of 91.2%.[5] Temporal artery biopsy remains the gold standard with a diagnostic yield of approximately 80%. Yield is greatest for biopsy segments greater than 1 mm,[58] but longer segments (3–5 mm) should be obtained if no obvious region of active disease can be identified by palpation. Ideally biopsy should be performed before the initiation of treatment. Some report that diagnostic yield falls from approximately 80% to 60% after 1 week of steroid therapy, although biopsy specimens can demonstrate evidence of inflammation even 2 weeks after initiation of steroid therapy.[59] In 535 patients from the Mayo Clinic, the rate of positive biopsies was similar in patients who had received steroids prior to biopsy (35%, or 86/249) and those who had not (31%, or 89/286) even when controlling for differences in clinical and laboratory features at presentation.[59]

Criterion	Definition
Age at disease onset $\geq$ 50 years	Development of symptoms or findings beginning at age 50 or older
New headache	New onset of or new type of localized pain in the head
Temporal artery abnormality	Temporal artery tenderness to palpation or decreased pulsation, unrelated to arteriosclerosis of cervical arteries
Elevated erythrocyte sedimentation rate	Erythrocyte sedimentation rate $\geq$ 50 mm/hour by the Westergren method
Abnormal artery biopsy	Biopsy specimen with artery showing vasculitis characterized by a predominance of mononuclear cell infiltration or granulomatous inflammation, usually with multinucleated giant cells

Table 18.3 ACR Criteria (1990) for the Classification of Giant Cell (Temporal) Arteritis
Note: For purposes of classification, a patient shall be said to have giant cell (temporal) arteritis if at least 3 of these 5 criteria are present. The presence of any 3 or more criteria yields a sensitivity of 93.5% and a specificity of 91.2%.[5]

Noninvasive evaluation for giant cell arteritis begins with a measurement of ESR or CRP, though neither provides a definitive diagnosis. An ESR ≥ 50 mm per hour is 1 of the 5 major criteria for giant cell arteritis according to the ACR, but nearly 20% of patients present with a normal ESR.[60] Therefore, a negative ESR does not exclude the diagnosis. CRP may also be a helpful marker of inflammation, though there are no defined guidelines for its use as a diagnostic tool in giant cell arteritis.[61] Other laboratory studies may reveal nonspecific signs of ongoing inflammation, including anemia of chronic disease and liver function test abnormalities. ESR and CRP are often used to evaluate disease activity but as with other vasculitides, these inflammatory markers may remain elevated even with adequate therapy.

Imaging studies in giant cell arteritis include ultrasonography, MRA, CTA, and conventional angiography. As a diagnostic tool, ultrasonography can be used to identify luminal narrowing, wall thickening, and flow assessment (to identify stenosis) in temporal, carotid, and upper-extremity vessels.[62] In one report, the presence of a dark halo around the lumen of the affected temporal artery on ultrasonography identifies 73% of patients with giant cell arteritis, and the finding may disappear after treatment with steroids.[62] In a study of 69 patients evaluating the utility of a periluminal dark halo, positive predictive value was only 50% but negative predictive value was 96%, with a sensitivity and specificity of 86% and 78%, respectively.[63] Duplex ultrasonography is not presently part of routine clinical management of giant cell arteritis.

While invasive angiography used to be the gold standard for imaging in giant cell arteritis, MRA and CTA are now becoming more widely employed as a noninvasive means to evaluate stenosis or aneurysms in the aorta or its main branches.[64-66] As in Takayasu's arteritis, stenotic lesions appear long and smooth with "skip" lesions separated by angiographically normal-appearing regions.[56]

FDG-PET scanning is a novel tool that may be able to identify vascular inflammation due to enhanced glucose metabolism in the vessel wall,[67-69] but the role of this imaging modality in giant cell arteritis has yet to be fully established.

Treatment

Corticosteroids

The treatment of choice for patients with giant cell arteritis is corticosteroids. The typical initial dose used is 40 to 60 mg/day, although some data suggest that a starting dose of 30 to 40 mg/day is equally efficacious, allowing a lower cumulative steroid dose and fewer steroid-related side effects.[70] Daily dosing regimens are superior to alternate-day regimens.[71] Steroids are continued for several months, at the initial dose for 4 to 6 weeks, and then tapered by 10% every 1 to 2 weeks as disease activity subsides, based on clinical resolution of symptoms and fall in ESR. More rapid tapering may result in recurrence of symptoms. Steroids significantly reduce the systemic inflammatory symptoms but do not always reduce intravascular inflammation, and as a result, 30% to 50% of patients will develop new or worsening symptoms irrespective of steroid treatment.[56] Typically, the response to steroid treatment is fast and lack of response may suggest an incorrect diagnosis. Length of therapy has not been well defined but steroid treatment for up to 2 years is sometimes necessary.

Methotrexate

Conflicting reports exist regarding the value of methotrexate in the management of giant cell arteritis. Several randomized trials over the last decade have shown that methotrexate has no steroid-sparing effect and does not affect outcomes in giant cell arteritis.[72-74] In the largest and most recent of these trials, 98 patients with giant cell arteritis received prednisone (≤ 60 mg/day) and either methotrexate (0.15 mg/kg/week up to 15.0 mg/week) or placebo; the study showed no difference in morbidity, treatment toxicity, ESR levels, or cumulative corticosteroid doses between the 2 groups.[72] Another trial of 42 patients taking steroids, with or without weekly methotrexate, did demonstrate a significantly reduced rate of relapse, lower cumulative steroid dose, and no difference in adverse events in the methotrexate group.[75] The difference in results may be attributable in part to an alternate-day steroid regimen in the former study compared to a daily dosing regimen and to lack of statistical power to detect a difference, despite a trend toward fewer relapses in the methotrexate group (57% vs. 77%).[76] Little is known about the role of methotrexate as a single agent in steroid-resistant cases of giant cell arteritis.[77]

Aspirin

Aspirin has been proposed as a potential treatment in giant cell arteritis because of its ability to inhibit interferon gamma, an anti-inflammatory property that steroids lack,[78] and its antiplatelet effects. A retrospective study on the effect of low-dose aspirin (100 mg/day) in 175 patients found that aspirin therapy reduced the risk of cranial ischemic complications (acute vision loss or cerebrovascular accident) from 29% to 8% at time of diagnosis of giant cell arteritis and from 13% to 3% after initiation of steroid therapy.[79] The significant reduction in cranial ischemic complications was all the more impressive because the aspirin group had significantly higher risk factors for atherosclerosis.[79,80] These data support the initiation of low-dose aspirin along with steroids at the time of initial diagnosis.

Percutaneous revascularization

Percutaneous revascularization is reserved for patients with symptoms of arterial insufficiency and inadequate end-organ perfusion. One prospective study evaluated balloon angioplasty in 10 patients with giant cell arteritis (with 30 lesions collectively). Initial patency rate was 67% at 24 months of follow-up with secondary and tertiary patency rates of 88% and 90% with repeat procedures.[81] Lesions amenable to percutaneous intervention typically included brachial, axillary, and subclavian arteries.[81-83] There are case reports on the use of stents in conjunction with balloon angioplasty in medium-sized vessels and endovascular stent grafting for aortic aneurysmal disease.[84]

Surgical revascularization

Scant data exist on surgical revascularization for large-vessel involvement in giant cell arteritis, in part because most disease can be adequately managed with medical therapy alone. Lower-extremity revascularization has been used in a small series of patients with lower-extremity claudication.[85] Surgery is indicated for repair of ascending aortic aneurysms and aortic root disease in giant cell arteritis, but nearly 50% of patients develop additional aneurysms in other segments of the aorta, mandating rigorous postoperative surveillance.[86]

Natural History

The natural history of giant cell arteritis depends in large measure on the rapidity with which the diagnosis is made and treatment is initiated. Identified and treated early, the symptoms can dissipate within 1 to 2 weeks and vision loss can be prevented. However, while steroids can avert vision loss, they rarely reverse it once it has occurred. Most patients discontinue steroid therapy or reduce doses to physiologic levels after 1 to 2 years without recurrence of disease.[47,87] Overall, long-term mortality in patients with giant cell arteritis treated with steroids is low and parallels that of the general population.[80,90] However, patients with thoracic aortic aneurysms have markedly increased mortality in the absence of steroid therapy.[53,89]

Polyarteritis Nodosa

Definition and Epidemiology

Polyarteritis nodosa (PAN) is a systemic necrotizing vasculitis typically involving the small- and medium-sized muscular arteries. The entity that is recognized today as classic PAN was first recognized by Kussmaul and Maier in 1866 in the description of a case of a 27-year-old tailor. They initially coined the term *periarteritis nodosa*, but in the early 1900s the disease was given the name it bears today, *polyarteritis nodosa*, emphasizing the panarteritic nature of the vasculitis. The epidemiology of PAN is difficult to ascertain given the changing classification employed over the years. Early categorizations of the disease also included what was felt to be a microscopic form of PAN now known as a distinct clinical entity, *microscopic polyangiitis (MPA)*. This latter disorder is now recognized to have discrete clinicopathologic features, including (1) the involvement of capillaries, venules, and arterioles not present in classic PAN; (2) an association with antineutrophilic cytoplasmic antibodies (ANCA); and (3) the presence of glomerulonephritis. Due to the frequency of positive ANCA assays in patients with MPA, the disease is felt to be less related to PAN and more related to the pauci-immune small-vessel vasculitides, such as Wegener's granulomatosis and Churg-Strauss syndrome, which are also associated with ANCA. Unlike these other small-vessel vasculitides, PAN is not associated with ANCA and does not cause glomerulonephritis. While the 1990 ACR criteria did not distinguish PAN from MPA, the 1994 Chapel Hill Consensus Conference did clarify the definition of PAN as a necrotizing inflammation of small- and medium-sized arteries that spares the smallest blood vessels and that is not associated with glomerulonephritis.[11]

Given this more strict definition, PAN is actually felt to be quite rare, with prevalence estimates ranging from 2 to 33 cases per million with an annual incidence of 2 to 9 cases per million.[91-93] The highest incidence (77 per million) was reported in a group of Alaskan Eskimos in a region where hepatitis B was highly endemic.[94] The disorder is more prevalent in older adults with a peak in the sixth decade of life. PAN associated with the hepatitis B virus (HBV) appears to affect men twice as frequently as women.[95] However, men and women are affected with idiopathic PAN in similar proportions.[96,97]

Pathophysiology

PAN induces a necrotizing inflammation in the small- and medium-sized muscular arteries, characteristically involving the renal and visceral arteries. The disease spares the aorta, its major branches, the pulmonary arteries, and the smallest vessels (arterioles, capillaries, and venules). PAN has a predilection for arterial bifurcations and branch points. The causative factors are not well understood, but the disease has been associated with HBV and may be related to other infections that remain unidentified. Nearly one-third of PAN cases are associated with HBV.[95,98] The rates of HBV infection associated with PAN vary according to the prevalence of HBV in the population but have ranged from 10% to 50%.[98,99] With the advent of the HBV vaccine, hepatitis B now likely accounts for less than 10% of PAN cases.[96] The role of the hepatitis C virus (HCV) has also been evaluated;[100] one study found 5 HCV-positive patients out of 16 patients with isolated cutaneous PAN.[101] While other infectious agents have been implicated—antigens of streptococci, staphylococci, and mycobacteria have been shown in arterial lesions and in blood of patients[102]—none has been definitively proven as a causative factor.

The precise pathogenesis of PAN is unclear. The histology of arterial specimens in the disease shows panarteritis with degeneration of the arterial wall and breakdown of the internal and external elastic laminae. Fibrinoid necrosis and leukocytoclasia (nuclear fragmentation) result from degranulation of neutrophils. PAN classically results in aneurysmal dilatation of the involved small arteries, resulting from segmental noncircumferential destruction of the elastic lamina (Figure 18.3). In later stages, endothelial proliferation and thrombosis lead to luminal occlusion. Distinctly lacking is the presence of granulomas, and their presence should raise the suspicion of Wegener's granulomatosis, Churg-Strauss syndrome, or other granulomatous vasculitides. In HBV-associated PAN, immune complex deposition appears to mediate the inflammatory response.[103] This finding is supported by the presence of circulating immune complexes and hypocomplementemia and the successful response to treatments (such as plasma exchange) geared to removal of circulating immune complexes.[95] The immunogenic mechanism in idiopathic PAN remains unclear.

Clinical Manifestations

The clinical manifestations of PAN are nonspecific and develop in a subacute fashion over weeks to months.[96] Any organ except the lung can be affected. Typically, PAN involves peripheral nerves, skin, muscle, kidney, and the gastrointestinal tract. Constitutional symptoms are present in nearly 70% of patients and can include fever, weight loss, malaise, headache, and myalgias.[104,105] Arthralgias are common, but true synovitis is rare. Neurologic involvement can include peripheral neuropathy or stroke. Mononeuritis multiplex, which results from inflammation of the vasa nervorum, occurs in up to 60% of patients.[106] Along with peripheral neuropathy, gastrointestinal symptoms were found to be the most common symptoms at initial presentation in a series of 36 patients with PAN.[105] Involvement of the splanchnic arteries results in abdominal pain ("intestinal angina"), diarrhea, or nausea and vomiting. Renal insufficiency and renovascular hypertension from involvement of medium-sized arteries are present in up to 40% of patients, but true glomerulonephritis is absent. Cardiac involvement in PAN can present as pericarditis, cardiomyopathy, and coronary artery inflammation resulting in stenosis or

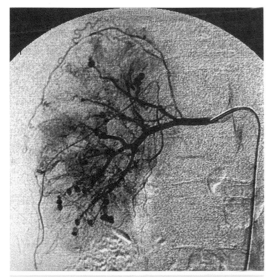

Figure 18.3 HBV-associated polyarteritis nodosa. Selective arteriography of the right kidney revealed multiple aneurysms with vessel narrowing and irregularity in medium-sized arteries. (From Chauveau D, Christophe JL. Renal aneurysms in hepatitis B-associated polyarteritis nodosa. *N Engl J Med*. 1995;332:1070. Reprinted with permission. Copyright © 1995 Massachusetts Medical Society.)

aneurysm development. Cutaneous manifestations include nonblanching livedo reticularis, nodules on the lower extremities (classically on the malleoli or calves), ulcerations, and digital ischemia. Despite the name, nodules are in fact the least frequent of these abnormalities.

Diagnostic Evaluation

Ten criteria are included in the ACR's 1990 classification for PAN, including (1) weight loss ≥ 4 kg, (2) livedo reticularis, (3) testicular pain or tenderness, (4) myalgias, (5) mononeuropathy or polyneuropathy, (6) diastolic blood pressure > 90 mm Hg, (7) elevated blood urea nitrogen or creatinine levels, (8) positive hepatitis B titers, (9) abnormality on arteriography, and (10) evidence of granulocytic or mixed leukocytic infiltrate on biopsy (Table 18.4).[2] The incidence of 3 or more of these criteria had an 82.2% sensitivity and 86.6% specificity for diagnosing PAN.[2] The 1994 Chapel Hill Consensus Conference further clarified the definition calling classic PAN a disease involving small- and medium-sized arteries without involvement of smaller vessels (arterioles, venules, capillaries), which differentiates PAN from MPA.[11] Laboratory evaluation is valuable in diagnosis of PAN and may reveal an elevated white blood cell count with neutrophilic predominance, as well as an elevated CRP or ESR. Patients with HBV-associated PAN will have positive hepatitis B surface antigen serologies and may have hypocomplementemia as a result of immune complex deposition. ANCA and eosinophilia are rarely found in PAN, and their presence should raise the suspicion of an alternative diagnosis, in particular Wegener's granulomatosis or Churg-Strauss syndrome, respectively. Angiography in PAN typically demonstrates microaneurysms that measure 1 to 5 mm in diameter. Biopsy of affected muscle or nerve will demonstrate the diagnostic pathological features. Definitive diagnosis depends upon the clinical history, evidence of involvement of small- and medium-sized arteries, and sparing of the aorta, pulmonary artery, and the smallest vessels. The presence of pulmonary hemorrhage or glomerulonephritis, the

Criterion	Definition
Weight loss ≥ 4 kg	Loss of 4 kg or more of body weight since illness began, not due to dieting or other factors
Livedo reticularis	Mottled reticular pattern over the skin of portions of the extremities or torso
Testicular pain or tenderness	Pain or tenderness of the testicles, not due to infection, trauma, or other causes
Myalgias, weakness, or leg tenderness	Diffuse myalgias (excluding shoulder and hip girdle) or weakness of muscles or tenderness of leg muscles
Mononeuropathy or polyneuropathy	Development of mononeuropathy, multiple mononeuropathies, or polyneuropathy
Diastolic BP > 90 mm Hg	Development of hypertension with the diastolic BP higher than 90 mm Hg
Elevated BUN or creatinine	Elevation of BUN > 40 mg/dL or creatinine > 1.5 mg/dL, not due to dehydration or obstruction
Hepatitis B virus	Presence of hepatitis B surface antigen or antibody in serum
Arteriographic abnormality	Arteriogram showing aneurysms or occlusions of the visceral arteries, not due to arteriosclerosis, fibromuscular dysplasia, or other noninflammatory causes
Biopsy of small- or medium-sized artery containing polymorphonuclear neutrophils	Histologic changes showing the presence of granulocytes or granulites and mononuclear leukocytes in the artery wall

Table 18.4 ACR Criteria (1990) for the Classification of PAN

Note: For purposes of classification, a patient shall be said to have PAN if at least 3 of these 10 criteria are present. The presence of any 3 or more criteria yields a sensitivity of 82.2% and a specificity of 86.6%.[2] BP = blood pressure; BUN = blood urea nitrogen.

presence of ANCA, and the presence of granulomas in most cases should be exclusion criteria for classic PAN.

Treatment

The choice of treatment of PAN is dictated by etiology and disease severity. Several guiding principles can be drawn from studies using combinations of steroids, cyclophosphamide, plasma exchange, and antiviral medications in the treatment of PAN. First, there is no standard first-line therapy; treatment should be guided by disease severity and disease etiology. Second, corticosteroids alone remain first-line therapy for initial management of patients with less severe forms of non-HBV-associated PAN. Immunosuppressants, such as cyclophosphamide, are used as first-line agents in the most severe cases. Plasma exchange can be used as a

second-line therapy in PAN refractory to other regimens. Lastly, the goals of treatment of HBV-associated PAN differ from idiopathic PAN and are geared toward limitation of viral replication and clearance of circulating immune complexes. Unlike idiopathic PAN, HBV-associated PAN can only be treated with steroids for short periods of time and immunosuppressant medications are potentially contraindicated because of increased viral replication and a tendency toward disease relapse.[107]

Two scores have been devised to evaluate disease severity and predict prognosis in PAN, and both may be useful in guiding selection of appropriate therapy. The five-factors score (FFS) is a prognostic score that incorporates 5 clinical parameters, each receiving one point: (1) renal insufficiency (serum creatinine > 1.58 mg/dL), (2) proteinuria (> 1 gm/day), (3) gastrointestinal tract involvement (defined as bleeding, perforation, infarction, and/or pancreatitis), (4) cardiomyopathy, and (5) central nervous system involvement.[104] When none of the 5 factors are present, 5-year mortality was shown to be 11.9%, with increasing mortality for patients with higher scores (46% mortality with 3 or more factors present).[104] Renal and gastrointestinal involvement were found to be the most serious prognostic variables. A second scoring system, the Birmingham Vasculitis Activity Score (BVAS), is a clinical index of disease activity based on symptoms and signs in 9 organ categories: (1) systemic signs, (2) skin, (3) mucous membranes and eyes, (4) ear-nose-throat, (5) chest, (6) heart and vessels, (7) GI tract, (8) kidney, and (9) nervous system. Each variable is counted only if felt to be attributable to active vasculitis. The weighted score (maximum of 63 points) correlates with disease activity and mortality and can be used to guide therapeutic response.[97,108]

Corticosteroids

For patients with less severe forms of idiopathic PAN, steroids alone are the initial treatment of choice. Therapy is initiated with pulse-dose methylprednisolone (15 mg/kg intravenous given daily for 1–3 days).[107] Prednisone is then given orally at a dose of 1 mg/kg/day either once or twice daily. Full-dose therapy is administered for 1 month, doses are then tapered and continued for up to 9 to 12 months. If used in combination with immunosuppressant medications, steroids can be tapered more rapidly. In patients with less severe disease and few poor prognostic variables, nearly 50% will achieve successful remission or cure with high-dose corticosteroids alone.[96,104] The 7-year survival for these patients is 79% despite a significant relapse rate.[109]

Cyclophosphamide

Cyclophosphamide should be used as a second-line agent in patients with mild disease in whom steroids alone are ineffective, or as a first line therapy in patients with more severe disease (FFS ≥1).[97,104] Pulse doses of intravenous cyclophosphamide can control disease activity more rapidly and produce fewer side effects than oral

cyclophosphamide.[107,110] Clinical trials of cyclophosphamide employed pulse doses of 0.6 g/m² given monthly for 1 year,[107] with careful adjustment in patients with renal insufficiency. This regimen can be followed by oral doses of cyclophosphamide if initial pulse therapy is unsuccessful in controlling disease.

Antiviral agents

The suppression of viral replication is one of the primary goals in the management of HBV-associated PAN. The utility of the antiviral strategy has been established in small studies of patients treated with a regimen of oral prednisone for 2 weeks, followed by an antiviral agent (vidarabine, interferon alpha, or lamivudine) for a maximum of 6 months along with concurrent plasma exchange.[111,112] Rates of seroconversion from HBeAg to anti-HBe antibodies range from 50% to 66% and > 50% of patients no longer show evidence of viral replication at the end of the study period.[98,112] However, antiviral agents should not be used alone, as seroconversion rates are lower and occur much later in course of treatment.[95]

Plasma exchange

Plasma exchange is an important component of the treatment regimen for HBV-associated PAN for the clearance of circulating immune complexes. In one study of 33 patients with HBV-associated PAN, all patients received 2 weeks of oral steroids followed by antiviral medications and plasma exchange, and 24 of 26 patients had complete recovery at 18 months.[112] While all recent studies of HBV-associated PAN have included plasma exchange in their treatment regimens, no randomized clinical trial of plasma exchange has been performed. In idiopathic PAN, no data support use of plasma exchange as a first-line treatment, although it can be employed as a second-line therapy in PAN refractory to other medications.[107]

Natural History and Prognosis

Survival in PAN is very low if the disease is left untreated (5-year survival, 10%–15%). The advent of corticosteroids has dramatically improved the prognosis of PAN, increasing 5-year survival to nearly 50%.[97] Survival can be predicted by disease severity at initial presentation. Using the FFS, 5-year mortality was 11.9% in the absence of any poor prognostic factors, 25.9% with 1 factor, and as high as 46% with 3 or more factors present, with proteinuria and gastrointestinal tract involvement found to be the most worrisome prognostic markers.[104] Prognosis in HBV-associated PAN is comparable to idiopathic PAN with mortality rates as high as 25% to 30% in treated patients.[95,98] Relapse rates for successfully treated PAN are low, ranging from 8% for HBV-associated PAN to 20% for idiopathic PAN.[97]

Wegener's Granulomatosis

Classification and Epidemiology

Wegener's granulomatosis is a small-vessel vasculitis associated with antineutrophilic cytoplasmic antibodies (ANCA) resulting in granulomatous inflammation involving the pulmonary and renal vasculature. The earliest descriptions of the disorder are from the late 1930s. Early recognition of distinct forms of vasculitis with necrotizing granulomatous inflammation occurred in the 1950s. A subcategory of necrotizing vasculitides was found to be associated with ANCA, to involve the smaller vessels, and to result in necrotizing inflammation of the respiratory tract and glomerulus. This group of disorders includes Wegener's granulomatosis, Churg-Strauss syndrome, and microscopic polyangiitis, all clinically similar and notably distinct from PAN.[113] Histologically, the 3 disorders are identical and all preferentially involve the venules, capillaries, and arterioles. Wegener's is distinguished from the other 2 by the presence of granulomatous inflammation and by the absence of asthma or eosinophilia.

The prevalence of ANCA-associated vasculitides is approximately 1 to 3 per 100,000 individuals, with an incidence of 8.5 to 20.0 per million.[114,115] Men and women are equally affected. The disease can present at any age, although typical age of onset is between ages 50 and 60. In the United States, the disorder appears more common in whites than blacks,[116] and in Europe it appears to be more common in northern than southern Europeans.[115]

The ACR criteria for the classification of Wegener's granulomatosis include (1) oral ulcers or nasal discharge, (2) abnormal chest imaging (nodules, cavities or infiltrates), (3) abnormal urinary sediment (microhematuria with > 5 red blood cells per high-power field, or presence of red cell casts in urine), and (4) biopsy showing granulomatous inflammation within the wall of an artery or in the perivascular or extravascular area (Table 18.5). The presence of 2 or more of these factors was associated with a sensitivity and specificity of 88.2% and 92.0%, respectively.

Pathophysiology

The precise pathogenesis of Wegener's granulomatosis remains unknown. Some have postulated that an antigen enters or is present in the airway and promotes a cell-mediated immune response. Putative etiologic factors include inorganic substances, such as silica or hydrocarbons, dust, or infectious agents such as *Staphylococcus aureus*.[117,118] The subsequent vascular response includes small-vessel inflammation and granuloma formation typically involving the respiratory tract and kidney. Pulmonary involvement is characterized by nodular cavitary infiltrates with evidence of necrotizing granulomatous vasculitis on lung biopsy. The renal disease seen with Wegener's is a focal and segmental glomerulonephritis that may evolve into a more rapidly progressive crescentic glomerulonephritis. Biopsy of these lesions does not reveal evidence of immune complex deposition, hence the label *pauci-immune*. At the vascular level, Wegener's produces granulomatous inflammation of medium-sized vessels, with fibrinoid necrosis and eventual destruction of the arterial wall and thrombus development.

Criterion	Definition
Nasal or oral inflammation	Development of painful or painless oral ulcers or purulent or bloody nasal discharge
Abnormal chest radiograph	Chest radiograph showing presence of nodules, fixed infiltrates, or cavities
Urinary sediment	Microhematuria (> 5 red blood cells per high power field) or red cell casts in urine sediment
Granulomatous inflammation on biopsy	Histologic changes showing granulomatous inflammation within the wall of an artery or in the perivascular or extravascular area (artery or arteriole)

Table 18.5 ACR Criteria (1990) for the Classification of Wegener's Granulomatosis
Note: For purposes of classification, a patient shall be said to have Wegener's granulomatosis if at least 2 of these 4 criteria are present. The presence of any 2 or more criteria yields a sensitivity of 88.2% and a specificity of 92.0%.[8]

Antineutrophilic Cytoplasmic Antibodies

Greater than 90% of patients with generalized Wegener's granulomatosis have immunologic studies positive for ANCA. These are autoantibodies that react against cytoplasmic proteins within polymorphonuclear leukocytes. The 2 kinds of ANCA have specificity for different cytoplasmic antigens within neutrophils. The first, c-ANCA, produces a characteristic *cytoplasmic* staining pattern resulting from reactivity with the target antigen proteinase-3. The c-ANCA is present in more than 90% of systemic Wegener's cases; however, the rate of ANCA positivity may be as low as 50% to 60% in patients with localized disease or those without renal involvement.[102,119,120] A second ANCA has been identified with a *perinuclear* fluorescence pattern and specificity for the antigen myeloperoxidase. This antibody, p-ANCA, is detected in microscopic polyangiitis and Churg-Strauss syndrome.

The role of ANCA in the pathogenesis of Wegener's granulomatosis is uncertain. One potential role may be to bind myeloperoxidase or proteinase-3, which becomes expressed on the surface of neutrophils activated by infections or inflammatory triggers. ANCA binding to the surface of neutrophils may promote degranulation and development of reactive oxygen species, which in turn cause vascular damage and inflammation.[121] On the other hand, data arguing against the direct role of ANCA in the pathogenesis of Wegener's granulomatosis include the number of patients with localized disease who are ANCA-negative (50% of patients with localized disease have negative ANCA titers),[120] the lack of definite correlation between antibody titers and disease activity, and the persistence of high ANCA titers despite clinical remission.[119]

Clinical Manifestations

The clinical manifestations of Wegener's granulomatosis result from tissue ischemia and destruction by granulomatous inflammation. Though any organ system can be affected, the disease has a predilection for the respiratory tract and the kidney. Nearly 90% of patients will have involvement of the upper or lower respiratory tract.[122,123] Symptoms include sinus pain, sinusitis, nasal mucosal ulceration, otitis media, necrosis of the nasal septum resulting in saddle nose deformity, and subglottic tracheal stenosis causing stridor. The most potentially morbid of the pulmonary manifestations include hemoptysis and pulmonary hemorrhage due to alveolar capillaritis. Almost 80% develop glomerulonephritis during the course of illness, usually over the first 2 years, but only 20% of patients have renal involvement at the time of initial presentation.[122,124] While pulmonary and renal diseases are most common, involvement of other organ systems produces a wide array of symptoms. Ocular manifestations, including diplopia, conjunctival hemorrhage, and proptosis, developed in 15% of patients in a prospective study of 158 patients.[122] Skin manifestations developed in 46%, musculoskeletal symptoms in 67%, and constitutional symptoms in nearly 50% at some point over the course of the illness.[122] Cardiovascular manifestations, including coronary vasculitis, pericarditis, and, rarely, cardiomyopathy occur in up to 6% to 8%.[122,123] Neurologic symptoms arise in nearly 25% of patients; mononeuritis multiplex occurs in 15% to 23% of patients and central nervous system symptoms of stroke and cranial nerve abnormalities in 8% of patients.[122,123]

Diagnostic Evaluation

The diagnosis of Wegener's granulomatosis is strongly suggested by the presence of characteristic pulmonary and renal involvement. Biopsy of the affected organ system is the most informative diagnostic tool, with the upper airways and kidneys being the most accessible sites. Supportive laboratory findings include c-ANCA, which is present in greater than 90% of patients with systemic Wegener's granulomatosis, though in only 50% of patients with localized disease.[119,120] Notably, the positive predictive value of a positive c-ANCA titer is only 40%,[125] in part due to elevated antibody levels in patients with disorders causing hypergammaglobulinemia as well as in the setting of infections and malignancies.[119] Erythrocyte sedimentation rate (ESR) is elevated to a mean rate of 71 mm/hour in 80% of patients with active disease (range, normal to 140 mm/hour).[122] Imaging of the chest with conventional CTA commonly shows pulmonary parenchymal abnormalities including nodules or masses, with or without cavitation, and ground-glass opacities and consolidation (Figure 18.4).[126] Tracheobronchial findings include bronchial wall thickening and bronchiectasis in fewer cases. Dedicated sinus CTA can show mucosal thickening with a nodular appearance and bony destruction of the na-

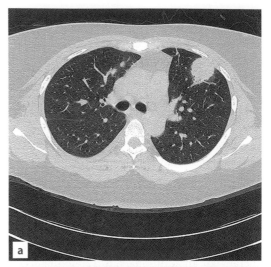

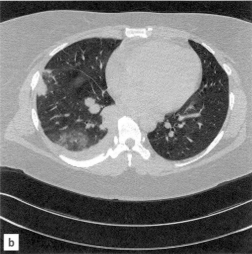

Figure 18.4 Wegener's granulomatosis. A 42-year-old female presented with persistent cough, wheezing, shortness of breath, and purulent nasal discharge. (a) and (b) Chest CTA showed multiple pulmonary nodules, the largest measuring 4 cm. (Courtesy of Christopher Fanta, MD, Pulmonary Division, Center for Chest Diseases, Brigham and Women's Hospital, Boston, MA.)

sal cavity and paranasal sinuses (predominantly involving midline structures).[127,128] Less specific laboratory findings include presence of mild hypergammaglobulinemia (IgA and IgG) and elevated rheumatoid factor.

Treatment

Wegener's granulomatosis can be fatal in the absence of treatment; therefore, prompt diagnosis and early initiation of the appropriate therapy is critical.

Induction of remission

Steroids alone are inadequate for induction of remission in active disease. Early studies established the role of a combination of high-dose steroids and cyclophosphamide as the first-line treatment for induction of remission.[129,130] Prednisolone orally in a dose of 1 mg/kg with cyclophosphamide, 2 mg/kg/day orally, induces remission in 93% of patients.[129] Steroids are continued at high dose for 1 to 2 months and then gradually tapered, while cyclophosphamide therapy is continued as maintenance therapy for an additional 6 to 12 months. Dose adjustment and steroid tapering are based on age, renal function, side effects, and clinical response. The median time to remission on this regimen is 12 months.[122]

Despite promising initial remission rates (75%), relapse rates are high (nearly 50%),[122] and maintenance therapy is universally required to prevent disease relapse. However, extended use of cyclophosphamide is limited by its side effects, including hemorrhagic cystitis, bladder cancer, and bone marrow suppression, increasing with cumulative cyclophosphamide doses.[107] Given the increased toxicity associated with long-term daily oral cyclophosphamide use, alternate regimens have been sought, both for induction of remission in active disease and for maintenance therapy.

Pulse-dose intravenous cyclophosphamide (0.5–0.7 gm/m² every 3–4 weeks) has been compared to oral therapy in initial therapy of active Wegener's. Pulse therapy results in comparable remission rates, lower mortality, and fewer initial side effects but is significantly less effective in the long-term maintenance of remission (59% compared with 13% with oral cyclophosphamide).[131,132] Pulse therapy is also less effective in patients with the most severe disease (involving more than 4 organ systems), those with very high ANCA titers,[133] or those who have failed oral cyclophosphamide.

Methotrexate is a proven alternative to cyclophosphamide in the initial management of patients with non-life-threatening forms of disease. Methotrexate (0.3 mg/kg/week) in combination with low-dose prednisone can induce rates of remission comparable to cyclophosphamide (60%–90%) with only minimal side effects.[134-136]

Maintenance therapy

Original regimens used oral cyclophosphamide as maintenance therapy for 1 year after remission was achieved, and steroids were discontinued. Excessive medication toxicity and high relapse rates make cyclophosphamide an inadequate choice for long-term maintenance therapy.

Methotrexate has been used with variable success in lieu of cyclophosphamide for maintenance therapy in patients with less severe forms of disease. Studies evaluating a regimen of initial therapy with steroids and cyclophosphamide, followed by methotrexate (0.3 mg/kg, not to exceed 15 mg, weekly) maintenance therapy, showed that the regimen is well tolerated but with relapse rates comparable to historical controls (one-third to one-half).[137-138]

Azathioprine has been successfully used for maintenance therapy. In a recent study, patients initially received standard therapy with cyclophosphamide and prednisolone, then low-dose prednisolone was continued along with either continued cyclophosphamide or azathioprine (2 mg/kg/day) for 12 months.[139] Relapse rates are comparable (13%–15%) in the 2 groups.[139] Substitution of azathioprine would allow shorter exposure to the more toxic cyclophosphamide therapy.

The tumor necrosis factor–alpha blocker, etanercept, was evaluated in the Wegener's Granulomatosis Etanercept Trial (WGET) in patients with severe or less severe forms of disease. Etanercept was initially given along with standard medication during initial therapy; all other drugs were eventually tapered and etanercept was continued as maintenance therapy. Etanercept was found to be no more effective as a maintenance therapy in preventing sustaining remission or preventing side effects.[140] Some have suggested, however, that the greatest benefit may not be in patients who have achieved remission already but rather in patients who are refractory to standard therapy.

Small series have evaluated mycophenolate mofetil for maintenance therapy, and while well tolerated, the drug has been associated with higher rates of relapse (43% in one series of 11 patients).[141]

Finally, because of the possibility that chronic nasal carriage of *S. aureus* may be related to the pathogenesis of Wegener's granulomatosis, some have suggested use trimethoprim-sulfamethoxazole (TMP-SMX) to prevent pulmonary relapse. Data on its use have been conflicting. One trial compared methotrexate and TMP-SMX, alone or in combination with prednisone; all patients in the TMP-SMX/prednisone group experienced disease relapse, while 92% of patients in the methotrexate/prednisone group remained in remission.[142] A second randomized trial showed that TMP-SMX used concurrently with steroid therapy was able to significantly reduce relapse rates, and the incidence of pulmonary tract infections compared to placebo, with 82% remaining in remission at 2 years.[143]

Management of Refractory Disease

Approximately 10% of cases do not respond to the standard regimen of steroids and cyclophosphamide to control disease activity.[144] Several options exist for the management of these most severe forms of the disease. The Methylprednisolone Versus Plasma Exchange (MEPEX) trial treated patients with severe renal manifestations of ANCA-associated vasculitis with cyclophosphamide; initial data suggested improved renal outcomes in the plasma exchange group. There have been reports of successful use of azathioprine in patients unresponsive to conventional therapies.[145] A small, nonrandomized trial of 10 patients suggested that the anti-CD20 antibody, rituximab, may have efficacy in treating refractory cases of Wegener's granulomatosis when used in conjunction with steroids.[146] Finally, conflicting data exist on the role of intravenous immunoglobulin in severe

cases, with one study showing improvement in all 26 patients and 50% achieving complete remission,[147] and another study demonstrating benefit in only 60% with no cases of complete remission.[148]

Natural History and Prognosis

Left untreated, the prognosis of Wegener's granulomatosis is poor, with < 10% survival rate within 2 years of diagnosis.[119] With the advent of combined immunosuppressive and cytotoxic therapy, more than 90% of patients achieve a significant improvement in symptoms, and survival rates now approach 75% to 95% at 5 years.[149,150] Poor prognostic variables include worse renal insufficiency, age > 60, and vasculitis limited to the kidneys.[150]

Hypersensitivity vasculitis

Classification

Hypersensitivity vasculitis is a small-vessel vasculitis that develops following exposure to an exogenous antigen. Offending agents may include drugs, toxins, serum, or infections.

Inappropriate consolidation of many disorders under one subheading has made characterization and nomenclature of this disorder challenging. In 1990, the ACR proposed 5 criteria for the classification of hypersensitivity vasculitis: (1) age > 16, (2) use of a medication at disease onset that may have been a precipitation factor, (3) palpable purpura, (4) maculopapular rash, and (5) skin biopsy showing neutrophilic infiltrate around an arteriole or venule (Table 18.6). The presence of 3 or more of these criteria has a sensitivity and specificity of 71.0% and 83.9%, respectively.[7] Despite these criteria, distinguishing hypersensitivity vasculitis from other disorders has been problematic because in many reported cases, no precipitating drug or antigen is found, and also the histopathologic features are similar to those seen in several other distinct disorders, including other sys-

Criterion	Definition
Age at disease onset > 16 years	Development of symptoms after age 16
Medication at disease onset	Medication was taken at the onset of symptoms, which may have been a precipitating factor
Palpable purpura	Slightly elevated purpuric rash over one or more areas of the skin; does not blanch with pressure and is not related to thrombocytopenia
Maculopapular rash	Flat and raised lesions of various sizes over one or more areas of the skin
Biopsy including arteriole and venule	Histologic changes showing granulocytes in a perivascular or extravascular location

Table 18.6 ACR Criteria (1990) for the Classification of Hypersensitivity Vasculitis
Note: For purposes of classification, a patient shall be said to have hypersensitivity vasculitis if at least 3 of these 5 criteria are present. The presence of any 3 or more criteria yields a sensitivity of 71.0% and a specificity of 83.9%.[7]

temic small-vessel vasculitides (Churg-Strauss syndrome, Wegener's granulomatosis, PAN, and microscopic polyangiitis), malignancies, connective tissue disorders (rheumatoid arthritis, systemic lupus erythematosus, and Sjögren's syndrome), Henoch-Schönlein purpura, and cryoglobulinemia.

Pathophysiology

The characteristic histopathologic finding in hypersensitivity vasculitis is leukocytoclastic vasculitis with inflammatory cell infiltration of the postcapillary venules and nuclear fragmentation. There may be a predominance of either neutrophils or mononuclear cells. In any given biopsy, all vasculitic lesions tend to be at the same stage of development.[151] Immunofluorescence may show complement and immunoglobulin deposition in the vessel wall,[152] supporting the theory of an immune-mediated phenomenon. There is also evidence for upregulation of various modulators, including adhesion molecules (ICAM-1 and E-selection) and interferon gamma, in cutaneous vasculitides.[153,154]

As previously noted, hypersensitivity vasculitis results from exposure to various exogenous antigens such as drugs, toxins, serum, or infections. A wide variety of drugs have been implicated and include antibiotics (penicillins, sulfonamides, cephalosporins, quinolones), allopurinol, phenytoin, retinoids, and propylthio-

uracil.[124] Newer biologic agents (interferons, granulocyte colony-stimulating factor) and vaccines have also been linked. Causality, however, is difficult to prove unambiguously given variability in reporting of adverse reactions and the rarity of reexposure, which might definitively determine causality. While drugs are the most common cause, hypersensitivity vasculitis can develop as a result of infection, such as hepatitis B, hepatitis C, endocarditis, and HIV, in decreasing order of frequency.

The mechanisms underlying drug-induced hypersensitivity vasculitis vary. Penicillins, for example, act as haptens, conjugating with serum proteins and inducing immune-complex formation akin to serum sickness. Drugs derived from foreign proteins (monoclonal antibodies, streptokinase, and cytokines) may cause direct immune-complex formation.

Clinical Manifestations

Cutaneous involvement is by far the most common manifestation of hypersensitivity vasculitis. Palpable purpura and maculopapular rash occur in at least 60% to 90% of patients (Figure 18.5).[151,155] Skin lesions typically involve the lower extremities.[155] Disease isolated to the skin occurs in up to 85% patients with biopsy-proven hypersensitivity vasculitis.[156] Joint symptoms, arthralgias, and true arthritis are present in nearly 40%.[151,157] Renal involvement (with elevated BUN and creatinine) develops in up to 40%.[151,157] Hepatic disease, central nervous system involvement, gastrointestinal symptoms, and cardiac disease (pericarditis and congestive heart failure) occur less commonly (< 25% of patients).[151]

The vasculitis develops within 1 to 3 weeks after exposure.[158] Onset can be even more delayed and chronic when idiopathic or associated with hepatitis B or C infection.

Differential diagnosis

Because the clinical syndrome and the histopathology are sometimes indistinguishable from other systemic disorders, a careful search for other systemic vasculitides and for disorders that mimic vasculitis (infections and malignancies) is imperative. *Henoch-Schönlein purpura (HSP)*, which may be challenging to distinguish from hypersensitivity vasculitis,[151,159] is characterized by purpura, abdominal pain, and glomerulonephritis. Diagnosis of HSP is suggested by the finding of IgA-dominant immune-complex deposition in skin lesions. It is far more common in individuals < 18 years old and typically presents after a respiratory tract infection. The diagnosis of *mixed cryoglobulinemia* is raised by the presence serum cryoglobulins, rheumatoid factor activity, and low complement levels. The cutaneous manifestations are similar, but cryoglobulinemia is more chronic and biopsy shows lesions at varying stages of development. The disorder is associated with infection (endocarditis or hepatitis B) or connective tissue diseases.[152] In both HSP and mixed cryoglobulinemia, morbidity arises mostly from the presence of renal disease, therefore, prompt recognition and treatment of the systemic vasculitis is critical. Cutaneous vasculitis mimicking hypersensitivity can also arise as a result of malignancy (usually lympho- or myeloproliferative disorders) and connective tissue disorders (rheumatoid arthritis, lupus, Sjögren's syndrome).[152]

Diagnostic evaluation

The laboratory evaluation in hypersensitivity is not diagnostic. Eosinophilia may be present in 79% of systemic cases but in only 22% of isolated cutaneous cases.[157] CRP and ESR are neither specific nor sensitive enough to make the diagnosis of hypersensitivity vasculitis. ESR may be elevated in 55% of skin-limited disease and in as many as 80% of patients with systemic manifestations.[159] ANCA should also be tested to ensure no alternative etiology of the small-vessel vasculitis. Biopsy of skin lesions or involved organs in systemic cases can provide a definitive diagnosis when used in concert with the clinical picture.

Treatment

Treatment of hypersensitivity vasculitis is dictated by the severity of disease and degree of systemic involvement. Disease localized to the

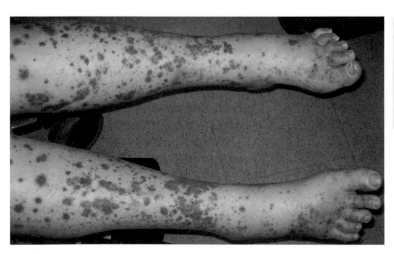

Figure 18.5 Hypersensitivity vasculitis. Multiple symmetric, violaceous, nonblanching papules favoring a dependent distribution. (Courtesy of Peter Lio, MD, Department of Dermatology, Beth Israel Deaconess Medical Center, Boston, MA.)

skin can most often be treated by discontinuation of the offending agent and use of nonsteroidal anti-inflammatory agents.[155] If these interventions prove unsuccessful or if severe cutaneous disease is present, oral corticosteroids can be used.[157] Steroids are generally reserved for more severe cases of cutaneous disease or cases with systemic involvement.[158] There are anecdotal reports of use of colchicine, dapsone, and cyclophosphamide.[155] When hypersensitivity vasculitis is the result of an infection or other disorder, treatment should be focused on the underlying cause.

Natural History and Prognosis

The overall prognosis in hypersensitivity vasculitis is excellent. In one study of 95 patients with the disease, 93% had complete resolution by 16 months.[155]

Summary

Vasculitis provides a distinct clinical challenge to the practitioner because of its diverse clinical manifestations. The clinical manifestations are diverse, but they ultimately result from stenosis and tissue ischemia or from aneurysm formation with embolization, thrombosis, or rupture and bleeding. The development of a widely adopted set of diagnostic criteria has allowed better disease definition, study, and development of treatment paradigms. Clinically, the approach to the patient with vasculitis should begin with an assessment of the size and location of the vessels involved. Significant overlap among these disorders occurs and may make diagnosis difficult. Despite this, early identification provides the best chance for successful therapy.

References

1. Arend WP, Michel BA, Bloch DA, et al. The American College of Rheumatology 1990 criteria for the classification of Takayasu arteritis. *Arthritis Rheum.* 1990;33(8):1129-1134.

2. Lightfoot RW Jr, Michel BA, Bloch DA, et al. The American College of Rheumatology 1990 criteria for the classification of polyarteritis nodosa. *Arthritis Rheum.* 1990;33(8):1088-1093.

3. Hunder GG, Arend WP, Bloch DA, et al. The American College of Rheumatology 1990 criteria for the classification of vasculitis. Introduction. *Arthritis Rheum.* 1990;33(8):1065-1067.

4. Fries JF, Hunder GG, Bloch DA, et al. The American College of Rheumatology 1990 criteria for the classification of vasculitis. Summary. *Arthritis Rheum.* 1990;33(8):1135-1136.

5. Hunder GG, Hunder GG, Bloch DA, et al. The American College of Rheumatology 1990 criteria for the classification of giant cell arteritis. *Arthritis Rheum.* 1990;33(8):1122-1128.

6. Mills JA, Michel BA, Bloch DA, et al. The American College of Rheumatology 1990 criteria for the classification of Henoch-Schonlein purpura. *Arthritis Rheum.* 1990;33(8):1114-1121.

7. Calabrese LH, Beat AM, Bloch DA, et al. The American College of Rheumatology 1990 criteria for the classification of hypersensitivity vasculitis. *Arthritis Rheum.* 1990;33(8):1108-1113.

8. Leavitt RY, Fauci AS, Bloch DA, et al. The American College of Rheumatology 1990 criteria for the classification of Wegener's granulomatosis. *Arthritis Rheum.* 1990;33(8):1101-1107.

9. Masi AT, Hunder GG, Lie JT, et al. The American College of Rheumatology 1990 criteria for the classification of Churg-Strauss syndrome (allergic granulomatosis and angiitis). *Arthritis Rheum.* 1990;33(8):1094-100.

10. Bloch DA, Michel BA, Hunder GG, et al. The American College of Rheumatology 1990 criteria for the classification of vasculitis. Patients and methods. *Arthritis Rheum.* 1990;33(8):1068-1073.

11. Jennette JC, Falk RJ, Andrassy K, et al. Nomenclature of systemic vasculitides. Proposal of an international consensus conference. *Arthritis Rheum.* 1994;37(2):187-192.

12. Kerr GS, Hallahan CW, Giordano J, et al. Takayasu arteritis. *Ann Intern Med.* 1994;120(11):919-929.

13. Sharma BK, Siveski-Iliskovic N, Singal PK. Takayasu arteritis may be underdiagnosed in North America. *Can J Cardiol*. 1995;11(4):311-316.

14. Hata A, Noda M, Moriwaki R, Numano F. Angiographic findings of Takayasu arteritis: new classification. *Int J Cardiol*. 1996;54 Suppl:S155-S163.

15. Yajima M, Numano F, Park YB, Sagar S. Comparative studies of patients with Takayasu arteritis in Japan, Korea and India—comparison of clinical manifestations, angiography and HLA-B antigen. *Jpn Circ J*. 1994;58(1):9-14.

16. Johnston SL, Lock RJ, Gompels MM. Takayasu arteritis: a review. *J Clin Pathol*. 2002;55(7):481-486.

17. Weyand CM, Goronzy JJ. Medium- and large-vessel vasculitis. *N Engl J Med*. 2003;349(2):160-169.

18. Subramanyan R, Joy J, Balakrishnan KG. Natural history of aortoarteritis (Takayasu's disease). *Circulation*. 1989;80(3):429-437.

19. Eichhorn J, Sima D, Thiele B, et al. Anti-endothelial cell antibodies in Takayasu arteritis. *Circulation*. 1996;94(10):2396-2401.

20. Ohta Y, Ohya Y, Fujii K, et al. Inflammatory diseases associated with Takayasu's arteritis. *Angiology*. 2003;54(3):339-344.

21. Jain S, Kumari S, Ganguly NK, et al. Current status of Takayasu arteritis in India. *Int J Cardiol*. 1996;54 Suppl:S111-S116.

22. Sharma BK, Sagar S, Singh AP, Suri S. Takayasu arteritis in India. *Heart Vessels Suppl*. 1992;7:37-43.

23. Andrews J, Al-Nahhas A, Pennell DJ, et al. Non-invasive imaging in the diagnosis and management of Takayasu's arteritis. *Ann Rheum Dis*. 2004;63(8):995-1000.

24. Belhocine T, Blockmans D, Hustinx R, et al. Imaging of large vessel vasculitis with (18)FDG PET: illusion or reality? A critical review of the literature data. *Eur J Nucl Med Mol Imaging*. 2003;30(9):1305-1313.

25. Meller J, Grabbe E, Becker W, Vosshenrich R. Value of F-18 FDG hybrid camera PET and MRI in early Takayasu aortitis. *Eur Radiol*. 2003;13(2):400-405.

26. Moreno D, Yuste JR, Rodríguez M, García-Velloso MJ, Prieto J. Positron emission tomography use in the diagnosis and follow up of Takayasu's arteritis. *Ann Rheum Dis*. 2005;64(7):1091-1093.

27. Walter MA, Melzer RA, Schindler C, et al. The value of [18F]FDG-PET in the diagnosis of large-vessel vasculitis and the assessment of activity and extent of disease. *Eur J Nucl Med Mol Imaging*. 2005;32(6):674-681.

28. Webb M, Chambers A, Al-Nahhas A, et al. The role of 18F-FDG PET in characterising disease activity in Takayasu arteritis. *Eur J Nucl Med Mol Imaging*. 2004;31(5):627-634.

29. Hoffman GS, Leavitt RY, Kerr GS, et al. Treatment of glucocorticoid-resistant or relapsing Takayasu arteritis with methotrexate. *Arthritis Rheum*. 1994;37(4):578-582.

30. Langford CA, Sneller MC, Hoffman GS. Methotrexate use in systemic vasculitis. *Rheum Dis Clin North Am*. 1997;23(4):841-853.

31. Mevorach D, Sneller MC, Hoffman GS. Induction of remission in a patient with Takayasu's arteritis by low dose pulses of methotrexate. *Ann Rheum Dis*. 1992;51(7):904-905.

32. Shetty AK, Stopa AR, Gedalia A. Low-dose methotrexate as a steroid-sparing agent in a child with Takayasu's arteritis. *Clin Exp Rheumatol*. 1998;16(3):335-336.

33. Valsakumar AK, Valappil UC, Jorapur V, et al. Role of immunosuppressive therapy on clinical, immunological, and angiographic outcome in active Takayasu's arteritis. *J Rheumatol*. 2003;30(8):1793-1798.

34. Liang P, Hoffman GS. Advances in the medical and surgical treatment of Takayasu arteritis. *Curr Opin Rheumatol*. 2005;17(1):16-24.

35. Shelhamer JH, Volkman DJ, Parrillo JE, et al. Takayasu's arteritis and its therapy. *Ann Intern Med*. 1985;103(1):121-126.

36. Hoffman GS, Merkel PA, Brasington RD, et al. Anti-tumor necrosis factor therapy in patients with difficult to treat Takayasu arteritis. *Arthritis Rheum*. 2004;50(7):2296-2304.

37. Weaver FA, Kumar SR, Yellin AE, et al. Renal revascularization in Takayasu arteritis-induced renal artery stenosis. *J Vasc Surg*. 2004;39(4):749-757.

38. Miyata T. Sato O, Deguchi J, et al. Anastomotic

aneurysms after surgical treatment of Takayasu's arteritis: a 40-year experience. *J Vasc Surg.* 1998;27(3):438-445.

39. Tyagi S, Verma PK, Gambhir DS, et al. Early and long-term results of subclavian angioplasty in aortoarteritis (Takayasu disease): comparison with atherosclerosis. *Cardiovasc Intervent Radiol.* 1998;21(3):219-224.

40. Tyagi S, Singh B, Kaul UA, et al. Balloon angioplasty for renovascular hypertension in Takayasu's arteritis. *Am Heart J.* 1993;125(5 Pt 1):1386-1393.

41. Fava MP, Foradori GB, García CB, et al. Percutaneous transluminal angioplasty in patients with Takayasu arteritis: five-year experience. *J Vasc Interv Radiol.* 1993;4(5):649-652.

42. Sharma S, Gupta H, Saxena A, et al. Results of renal angioplasty in nonspecific aortoarteritis (Takayasu disease). *J Vasc Interv Radiol.* 1998;9(3):429-435.

43. Bali HK, Bhargava M, Jain AK, Sharma BK. De novo stenting of descending thoracic aorta in Takayasu arteritis: intermediate-term follow-up results. *J Invasive Cardiol.* 2000;12(12):612-617.

44. Stoodley MA, Thompson RC, Mitchell RS, et al. Neurosurgical and neuroendovascular management of Takayasu's arteritis. *Neurosurgery.* 2000;46(4):841-851; discussion 851-852.

45. Sakaida H, Sakai N, Nagata I, et al. Stenting for the occlusive carotid and subclavian arteries in Takayasu arteritis. *No Shinkei Geka.* 2001;29(11):1033-1041.

46. Ishikawa K. Natural history and classification of occlusive thromboaortopathy (Takayasu's disease). *Circulation.* 1978;57(1):27-35.

47. Hunder GG. Epidemiology of giant-cell arteritis. *Cleve Clin J Med.* 2002;69(Suppl 2):SII79-SII82.

48. Salvarani C, Gabriel SE, O'Fallon WM, Hunder GG. The incidence of giant cell arteritis in Olmsted County, Minnesota: apparent fluctuations in a cyclic pattern. *Ann Intern Med.* 1995;123(3):192-194.

49. Salvarani C, Gabriel SE, O'Fallon WM, Hunder GG. Epidemiology of polymyalgia rheumatica in Olmsted County, Minnesota, 1970-1991. *Arthritis Rheum.* 1995;38(3):369-373.

50. Huston KA, Hunder GG, Lie JT, Kennedy RH,

Elveback LR. Temporal arteritis: a 25-year epidemiologic, clinical, and pathologic study. *Ann Intern Med.* 1978;88(2):162-167.

51. Klein RG, Hunder GG, Stanson AW, Sheps SG. Large artery involvement in giant cell (temporal) arteritis. *Ann Intern Med.* 1975;83(6):806-812.

52. Evans JM, O'Fallon WM, Hunder GG. Increased incidence of aortic aneurysm and dissection in giant cell (temporal) arteritis. A population-based study. *Ann Intern Med.* 1995;122(7):502-507.

53. Evans JM, Bowles CA, Bjornsson J, et al. Thoracic aortic aneurysm and rupture in giant cell arteritis. A descriptive study of 41 cases. *Arthritis Rheum.* 1994;37(10):1539-1547.

54. Weyand CM, Goronzy JJ. Arterial wall injury in giant cell arteritis. *Arthritis Rheum.* 1999;42(5):844-853.

55. Chmelewski WL, McKnight KM, Agudelo CA, Wise CM. Presenting features and outcomes in patients undergoing temporal artery biopsy. A review of 98 patients. *Arch Intern Med.* 1992;152(8):1690-1695.

56. Salvarani C, Cantini F, Hunder GG. Polymyalgia rheumatica and giant-cell arteritis. *N Engl J Med.* 2002;347(4):261-271.

57. Caselli RJ, Hunder GG, Whisnant JP. Neurologic disease in biopsy-proven giant cell (temporal) arteritis. *Neurology.* 1988;38(3):352-359.

58. Taylor-Gjevre R, Vo M, Shukla D, Resch L. Temporal artery biopsy for giant cell arteritis. *J Rheumatol.* 2005;32(7):1279-1282.

59. Achkar AA, Lie JT, Hunder GG, O'Fallon WM, Gabriel SE. How does previous corticosteroid treatment affect the biopsy findings in giant cell (temporal) arteritis? *Ann Intern Med.* 1994;120(12):987-992.

60. Salvarani C, Hunder GG. Giant cell arteritis with low erythrocyte sedimentation rate: frequency of occurrence in a population-based study. *Arthritis Rheum.* 2001;45(2):140-145.

61. Hayreh SS, Podhajsky PA, Raman R, Zimmerman B. Giant cell arteritis: validity and reliability of various diagnostic criteria. *Am J Ophthalmol.* 1997;123(3):285-296.

62. Schmidt WA, Kraft HE, Vorpahl K, Völker L, Gromnica-Ihle EJ. Color duplex ultrasonogra-

phy in the diagnosis of temporal arteritis. *N Engl J Med.* 1997;337(19):1336-1342.

63. Nesher G, Shemesh D, Mates M, Sonnenblick M, Abramowitz HB. The predictive value of the halo sign in color Doppler ultrasonography of the temporal arteries for diagnosing giant cell arteritis. *J Rheumatol.* 2002;29(6):1224-1226.

64. Mitomo T, Funyu T, Takahashi Y, Murakami K, Koyama K, Kamio K. Giant cell arteritis and magnetic resonance angiography. *Arthritis Rheum.* 1998;41(9):1702.

65. Schmidt WA. Use of imaging studies in the diagnosis of vasculitis. *Curr Rheumatol Rep.* 2004;6(3):203-211.

66. Schmidt WA, Gromnica-Ihle E. What is the best approach to diagnosing large-vessel vasculitis? *Best Pract Res Clin Rheumatol.* 2005;19(2):223-242.

67. Turlakow A, Yeung HW, Pui J, et al. Fludeoxyglucose positron emission tomography in the diagnosis of giant cell arteritis. *Arch Intern Med.* 2001;161(7):1003-1007.

68. Blockmans D, Maes A, Stroobants S, et al. New arguments for a vasculitic nature of polymyalgia rheumatica using positron emission tomography. *Rheumatology (Oxford).* 1999;38(5):444-447.

69. Blockmans D, Stroobants S, Maes A, Mortelmans L. Positron emission tomography in giant cell arteritis and polymyalgia rheumatica: evidence for inflammation of the aortic arch. *Am J Med.* 2000;108(3):246-249.

70. Nesher G, Rubinow A, Sonnenblick M, et al. Efficacy and adverse effects of different corticosteroid dose regimens in temporal arteritis: a retrospective study. *Clin Exp Rheumatol.* 1997;15(3): 303-306.

71. Hunder GG, Sheps SG, Allen GL, Joyce JW. Daily and alternate-day corticosteroid regimens in treatment of giant cell arteritis: comparison in a prospective study. *Ann Intern Med.,* 1975;82(5):613-618.

72. Hoffman GS, Cid MC, Hellmann DB, et al. A multicenter, randomized, double-blind, placebo-controlled trial of adjuvant methotrexate treatment for giant cell arteritis. *Arthritis Rheum.* 2002;46(5):1309-1318.

73. Spiera RF, Mitnick HJ, Kupersmith M, et al. A prospective, double-blind, randomized, placebo controlled trial of methotrexate in the treatment of giant cell arteritis (GCA). *Clin Exp Rheumatol.* 2001;19(5):495-501.

74. van der Veen MJ, Dinant HJ, van Booma-Frankfort C, et al. Can methotrexate be used as a steroid sparing agent in the treatment of polymyalgia rheumatica and giant cell arteritis? *Ann Rheum Dis.* 1996;55(4):218-223.

75. Jover JA, Hernández-García C, Morado IC, et al. Combined treatment of giant-cell arteritis with methotrexate and prednisone. a randomized, double-blind, placebo-controlled trial. *Ann Intern Med.* 2001;134(2):106-114.

76. Jover JA, Hernández-García C, Morado IC, et al. Disparate results in studies of methotrexate plus corticosteroids in the treatment of giant cell arteritis: comment on the article by Hoffman et al. *Arthritis Rheum.* 2003;48(4):1158-1159.

77. Wilke WS, Hoffman GS. Treatment of corticosteroid-resistant giant cell arteritis. *Rheum Dis Clin North Am.* 1995;21(1):59-71.

78. Weyand CM, Kaiser M, Yang H, Younge B, Goronzy JJ. Therapeutic effects of acetylsalicylic acid in giant cell arteritis. *Arthritis Rheum.* 2002;46(2):457-466.

79. Nesher G, Berkun Y, Mates M, Baras M, Rubinow A, Sonnenblick M. Low-dose aspirin and prevention of cranial ischemic complications in giant cell arteritis. *Arthritis Rheum.* 2004;50(4):1332-1337.

80. Hellmann DB. Low-dose aspirin in the treatment of giant cell arteritis. *Arthritis Rheum.* 2004;50(4):1026-1027.

81. Both M, Aries PM, Müller-Hülsbeck T, et al. Balloon angioplasty of arteries of the upper extremities in patients with extracranial giant cell arteritis. *Ann Rheum Dis.* 2006;65(9):1124-1130.

82. Both M, Jahnke T, Reinhold-Keller E, et al. Percutaneous management of occlusive arterial disease associated with vasculitis: a single center experience. *Cardiovasc Intervent Radiol.* 2003;26(1):19-26.

83. Dellaripa PF, Eisenhauer AC. Bilateral percutaneous balloon angioplasty of the axillary arteries in a patient with giant cell arteritis

and upper extremity ischemic symptoms not responsive to corticosteroids. *J Rheumatol.* 1998;25(7):1429-1433.

84. Engelke C, Sandhu C, Morgan RA, Belli AM. Endovascular repair of thoracic aortic aneurysm and intramural hematoma in giant cell arteritis. *J Vasc Interv Radiol.* 2002;13(6):625-629.

85. Le Hello C, Lévesque H, Jeanton M, et al. Lower limb giant cell arteritis and temporal arteritis: followup of 8 cases. *J Rheumatol.* 2001;28(6):1407-1412.

86. Zehr KJ, Mathur A, Orszulak TA, et al. Surgical treatment of ascending aortic aneurysms in patients with giant cell aortitis. *Ann Thorac Surg.* 2005;79(5):1512-1517.

87. Proven A, Gabriel SE, Orces C, O'Fallon WM, Hunder GG. Glucocorticoid therapy in giant cell arteritis: duration and adverse outcomes. *Arthritis Rheum.* 2003;49(5):703-708.

88. Matteson EL, Gold KN, Bloch DA, Hunder GG. Long-term survival of patients with giant cell arteritis in the American College of Rheumatology giant cell arteritis classification criteria cohort. *Am J Med.* 1996;100(2):193-196.

89. Nuenninghoff DM, Hunder GG, Christianson TJ, McClelland RL, Matteson EL. Mortality of large-artery complication (aortic aneurysm, aortic dissection, and/or large-artery stenosis) in patients with giant cell arteritis: a population-based study over 50 years. *Arthritis Rheum.* 2003;48(12):3532-3537.

90. Gonzalez-Gay MA, Blanco R, Abraira V, et al. Giant cell arteritis in Lugo, Spain, is associated with low longterm mortality. *J Rheumatol.* 1997;24(11):2171-2176.

91. Scott DG, Bacon PA, Elliott PJ, Tribe CR, Wallington TB. Systemic vasculitis in a district general hospital 1972-1980: clinical and laboratory features, classification and prognosis of 80 cases. *Q J Med.* 1982;51(203):292-311.

92. Sack M, Cassidy JT, Bole GG. Prognostic factors in polyarteritis. *J Rheumatol.* 1975;2(4):411-420.

93. Mahr A, Guillevin L, Poissonnet M, Aymé S. Prevalences of polyarteritis nodosa, microscopic polyangiitis, Wegener's granulomatosis, and Churg-Strauss syndrome in a French urban multiethnic population in 2000: a capture-recapture estimate. *Arthritis Rheum.* 2004;51(1):92-99.

94. McMahon BJ, Heyward WL, Templin DW, Clement D, Lanier AP. Hepatitis B-associated polyarteritis nodosa in Alaskan Eskimos: clinical and epidemiologic features and long-term follow-up. *Hepatology.* 1989;9(1):97-101.

95. Guillevin L, Mahr A, Callard P, et al. Hepatitis B virus-associated polyarteritis nodosa: clinical characteristics, outcome, and impact of treatment in 115 patients. *Medicine (Baltimore).* 2005;84(5):313-322.

96. Stone JH. Polyarteritis nodosa. *JAMA.* 2002;288(13):1632-1639.

97. Gayraud M, Guillevin L, le Toumelin P, et al. Long-term followup of polyarteritis nodosa, microscopic polyangiitis, and Churg-Strauss syndrome: analysis of four prospective trials including 278 patients. *Arthritis Rheum.* 2001;44(3):666-675.

98. Guillevin L, Lhote F, Cohen P, et al. Polyarteritis nodosa related to hepatitis B virus. A prospective study with long-term observation of 41 patients. *Medicine (Baltimore).* 1995;74(5):238-253.

99. Boki KA, Dafni U, Karpouzas GA, Papasteriades C, Drosos AA, Moutsopoulos HM. Necrotizing vasculitis in Greece: clinical, immunological and immunogenetic aspects. A study of 66 patients. *Br J Rheumatol.* 1997;36(10):1059-1066.

100. Quint L, Deny P, Guillevin L, et al. Hepatitis C virus in patients with polyarteritis nodosa. Prevalence in 38 patients. *Clin Exp Rheumatol.* 1991;9(3):253-257.

101. Soufir N, Descamps V, Crickx B, et al. Hepatitis C virus infection in cutaneous polyarteritis nodosa: a retrospective study of 16 cases. *Arch Dermatol.* 1999;135(8):1001-1002.

102. Ledford DK. Immunologic aspects of vasculitis and cardiovascular disease. *JAMA.* 1997;278(22):1962-1971.

103. Trepo CG, Zucherman AJ, Bird RC, Prince AM. The role of circulating hepatitis B antigen/antibody immune complexes in the pathogenesis of vascular and hepatic manifestations in polyarteritis nodosa. *J Clin Pathol.* 1974;27(11):863-868.

104. Guillevin L, Lhote F, Gayraud M, et al. Prognostic factors in polyarteritis nodosa and Churg-Strauss syndrome. A prospective study in 342 patients. *Medicine (Baltimore)*. 1996;75(1):17-28.

105. Agard C, Mouthon L, Mahr A, Guillevin L. Microscopic polyangiitis and polyarteritis nodosa: how and when do they start? *Arthritis Rheum*. 2003;49(5):709-715.

106. Griffin JW. Vasculitic neuropathies. *Rheum Dis Clin North Am*. 2001;27(4):751-760, vi.

107. Guillevin L, Pagnoux C. When should immunosuppressants be prescribed to treat systemic vasculitides? *Intern Med*. 2003;42(4):313-317.

108. Luqmani RA, Bacon PA, Moots RJ, et al. Birmingham Vasculitis Activity Score (BVAS) in systemic necrotizing vasculitis. *QJM*. 1994;87(11):671-678.

109. Guillevin L, Fain O, Lhote F, et al. Lack of superiority of steroids plus plasma exchange to steroids alone in the treatment of polyarteritis nodosa and Churg-Strauss syndrome. A prospective, randomized trial in 78 patients. *Arthritis Rheum*. 1992;35(2):208-215.

110. Gayraud M, Guillevin L, Cohen P, et al. Treatment of good-prognosis polyarteritis nodosa and Churg-Strauss syndrome: comparison of steroids and oral or pulse cyclophosphamide in 25 patients. French Cooperative Study Group for Vasculitides. *Br J Rheumatol*. 1997;36(12):1290-1297.

111. Guillevin L, Mahr A, Cohen P, et al. Short-term corticosteroids then lamivudine and plasma exchanges to treat hepatitis B virus-related polyarteritis nodosa. *Arthritis Rheum*. 2004;51(3):482-487.

112. Guillevin L, Lhote F, Leon A, Fauvelle F, Vivitski L, Trepo C. Treatment of polyarteritis nodosa related to hepatitis B virus with short term steroid therapy associated with antiviral agents and plasma exchanges. A prospective trial in 33 patients. *J Rheumatol*. 1993;20(2):289-298.

113. Godman GC, Churg J. Wegener's granulomatosis: pathology and review of the literature. *AMA Arch Pathol*. 1954;58(6):533-553.

114. Cotch MF, Hoffman GS, Yerg DE, et al. The epidemiology of Wegener's granulomatosis. Estimates of the five-year period prevalence, annual mortality, and geographic disease distribution from population-based data sources. *Arthritis Rheum*. 1996;39(1):87-92.

115. Watts RA, Scott DG. Epidemiology of the vasculitides. *Semin Respir Crit Care Med*. 2004;25(5):455-464.

116. Falk RJ, Hogan S, Carey TS, Jennette JC. Clinical course of anti-neutrophil cytoplasmic autoantibody-associated glomerulonephritis and systemic vasculitis. The Glomerular Disease Collaborative Network. *Ann Intern Med*. 1990;113(9):656-663.

117. Popa ER, Stegeman CA, Kallenberg CG, Tervaert JW. Staphylococcus aureus and Wegener's granulomatosis. *Arthritis Res*. 2002;4(2):77-79.

118. Capizzi SA, Specks U. Does infection play a role in the pathogenesis of pulmonary vasculitis? *Semin Respir Infect*. 2003;18(1):17-22.

119. Sneller MC. Wegener's granulomatosis. *JAMA*. 1995;273(16):1288-1291.

120. Lamprecht P, Gross WL. Wegener's granulomatosis. *Herz*. 2004;29(1):47-56.

121. Sarraf P, Sneller MC. Pathogenesis of Wegener's granulomatosis: current concepts. *Expert Rev Mol Med*. 2005;7(8):1-19.

122. Hoffman GS, Kerr GS, Leavitt RY, et al. Wegener granulomatosis: an analysis of 158 patients. *Ann Intern Med*. 1992;116(6):488-498.

123. Savage CO, Harper L, Cockwell P, Adu D, Howie AJ. ABC of arterial and vascular disease: vasculitis. *BMJ*. 2000;320(7245):1325-1328.

124. Jennette JC, Falk RJ. Small-vessel vasculitis. *N Engl J Med*. 1997;337(21):1512-1523.

125. Blockmans D, Stevens E, Mariën G, Bobbaers H. Clinical spectrum associated with positive ANCA titres in 94 consecutive patients: is there a relation with PR-3 negative c-ANCA and hypergammaglobulinaemia? *Ann Rheum Dis*. 1998;57(3):141-145.

126. Lohrmann C, Uhl M, Kotter E, Burger D, Ghanem N, Langer M. Pulmonary manifestations of Wegener granulomatosis: CT findings in 57 patients and a review of the literature. *Eur J Radiol*. 2005;53(3):471-477.

127. Lohrmann C, Uhl M, Warnatz K, Kotter E, Ghanem N, Langer M. Sinonasal computed tomography in patients with Wegener's

granulomatosis. *J Comput Assist Tomogr.* 2006;30(1):122-125.

128. Benoudiba F, Marsot-Dupuch K, Rabia MH, Cabanne J, Bobin S, Lasjaunias P. Sinonasal Wegener's granulomatosis: CT characteristics. *Neuroradiology.* 2003;45(2):95-99.

129. Fauci AS, Haynes BF, Katz P, Wolff SM. Wegener's granulomatosis: prospective clinical and therapeutic experience with 85 patients for 21 years. *Ann Intern Med.* 1983;98(1):76-85.

130. Fauci AS, Wolff SM. Wegener's granulomatosis: studies in eighteen patients and a review of the literature. *Medicine (Baltimore).* 1973;52(6):535-561.

131. Guillevin L, Cordier JF, Lhote F, et al. A prospective, multicenter, randomized trial comparing steroids and pulse cyclophosphamide versus steroids and oral cyclophosphamide in the treatment of generalized Wegener's granulomatosis. *Arthritis Rheum.* 1997.;40(12):2187-2198.

132. Hoffman GS, Leavitt RY, Fleisher TA, Minor JR, Fauci AS. Treatment of Wegener's granulomatosis with intermittent high-dose intravenous cyclophosphamide. *Am J Med.* 1990;89(4):403-410.

133. Reinhold Keller E, Kekow J, Schnabel A, et al. Influence of disease manifestation and anti-neutrophil cytoplasmic antibody titer on the response to pulse cyclophosphamide therapy in patients with Wegener's granulomatosis. *Arthritis Rheum.* 1994;37(6):919-924.

134. de Groot K, Mühler M, Reinhold-Keller E, Paulsen J, Gross WL. Induction of remission in Wegener's granulomatosis with low dose methotrexate. *J Rheumatol.* 1998;25(3):492-495.

135. De Groot K, Rasmussen N, Bacon PA, et al. Randomized trial of cyclophosphamide versus methotrexate for induction of remission in early systemic antineutrophil cytoplasmic antibody-associated vasculitis. *Arthritis Rheum.* 2005;52(8):2461-2469.

136. Sneller MC, Hoffman GS, Talar-Williams C, Kerr GS, Hallahan CW, Fauci AS. An analysis of forty-two Wegener's granulomatosis patients treated with methotrexate and prednisone. *Arthritis Rheum.* 1995;38(5):608-613.

137. Langford CA, Talar-Williams C, Barron KS, Sneller MC. Use of a cyclophosphamide-induction methotrexate-maintenance regimen for the treatment of Wegener's granulomatosis: extended follow-up and rate of relapse. *Am J Med.* 2003;114(6):463-469.

138. Reinhold-Keller E, Fink CO, Herlyn K, Gross WL, De Groot K. High rate of renal relapse in 71 patients with Wegener's granulomatosis under maintenance of remission with low-dose methotrexate. *Arthritis Rheum.* 2002;47(3):326-332.

139. Jayne D, Rasmussen N, Andrassy K, et al. A randomized trial of maintenance therapy for vasculitis associated with antineutrophil cytoplasmic autoantibodies. *N Engl J Med.* 2003;349(1):36-44.

140. The Wegener's Granulomatosis Etanercept Trial (WGET) Research Group. Etanercept plus standard therapy for Wegener's granulomatosis. *N Engl J Med.* 2005;352(4):351-361.

141. Langford CA, Talar-Williams C, Sneller MC. Mycophenolate mofetil for remission maintenance in the treatment of Wegener's granulomatosis. *Arthritis Rheum.* 2004;51(2):278-283.

142. de Groot K, Reinhold-Keller E, Tatsis E, et al. Therapy for the maintenance of remission in sixty-five patients with generalized Wegener's granulomatosis. Methotrexate versus trimethoprim/sulfamethoxazole. *Arthritis Rheum.* 1996;39(12):2052-2061.

143. Stegeman CA, Tervaert JW, de Jong PE, Kallenberg CG. Trimethoprim-sulfamethoxazole (co-trimoxazole) for the prevention of relapses of Wegener's granulomatosis. Dutch Co-Trimoxazole Wegener Study Group. *N Engl J Med.* 1996;335(1):16-20.

144. Hellmich B, Lamprecht P, Gross WL. Advances in the therapy of Wegener's granulomatosis. *Curr Opin Rheumatol.* 2006;18(1):25-32.

145. Aries PM, Hellmich B, Reinhold-Keller E, Gross WL. High-dose intravenous azathioprine pulse treatment in refractory Wegener's granulomatosis. *Rheumatology (Oxford).* 2004;43(10):1307-1308.

146. Keogh KA, Ytterberg SR, Fervenza FC, Carlson KA, Schroeder DR, Specks U. Rituximab for refractory Wegener's granulomatosis: report of

a prospective, open-label pilot trial. *Am J Respir Crit Care Med.* 2006;173(2):180-187.

147. Savage CO, Harper L, Adu D. Primary systemic vasculitis. *Lancet.* 1997;349(9051):553-558.

148. Richter C, Schnabel A, Csernok E, De Groot K, Reinhold-Keller E, Gross WL. Treatment of anti-neutrophil cytoplasmic antibody (ANCA)-associated systemic vasculitis with high-dose intravenous immunoglobulin. *Clin Exp Immunol.* 1995;101(1):2-7.

149. Lane SE, Watts RA, Shepstone L, Scott DG. Primary systemic vasculitis: clinical features and mortality. *QJM.* 2005;98(2):97-111.

150. Jayne DR. Conventional treatment and outcome of Wegener's granulomatosis and microscopic polyangiitis. *Cleve Clin J Med.* 2002;69(Suppl 2):SII110-115.

151. Michel BA, Hunder GG, Bloch DA, Calabrese LH. Hypersensitivity vasculitis and Henoch-Schonlein purpura: a comparison between the 2 disorders. *J Rheumatol.* 1992;19(5):721-728.

152. Calabrese LH. Differential diagnosis of hypersensitivity vasculitis. *Cleve Clin J Med.* 1990;57(6):506-507.

153. Burrows NP, Molina FA, Terenghi G, et al. Comparison of cell adhesion molecule expression in cutaneous leucocytoclastic and lymphocytic vasculitis. *J Clin Pathol.* 1994;47(10):939-944.

154. Shiohara T, Sagawa Y, Nagashima M. Systemic release of interferon-gamma in drug-induced cutaneous vasculitis. *Lancet.* 1992;339(8798):933.

155. Martinez-Taboada VM, Blanco R, Garcia-Fuentes M, Rodriguez-Valverde V. Clinical features and outcome of 95 patients with hypersensitivity vasculitis. *Am J Med.* 1997;102(2):186-191.

156. Garcia-Porrua C, Llorca J, González-Louzao C, González-Gay MA. Hypersensitivity vasculitis in adults: a benign disease usually limited to skin. *Clin Exp Rheumatol.* 200;19(1):85-88.

157. Merkel PA. Drug-induced vasculitis. *Rheum Dis Clin North Am.* 2001;27(4):849-862.

158. Calabrese LH, Duna GF. Drug-induced vasculitis. *Curr Opin Rheumatol.* 1996;8(1):34-40.

159. Garcia-Porrua C, Gonzalez-Gay MA. Comparative clinical and epidemiological study of hypersensitivity vasculitis versus Henoch-Schonlein purpura in adults. *Semin Arthritis Rheum.* 1999;28(6):404-412.

19

Vasospastic Diseases

Raghu Kolluri and John R. Bartholomew

The vasospastic diseases include Raynaud's phenomenon (RP), livedo reticularis (LR), and acrocyanosis. All 3 exist in primary and secondary forms, and it is important to distinguish between the 2. Primary forms are generally self-limiting and cause little or no tissue loss, whereas secondary forms are usually associated with an underlying disorder such as a connective tissue disorder or vasculitis, atherosclerosis, infections, or medications and may lead to digital ulceration, gangrene, or an amputation.

Raynaud's Phenomenon

Raynaud's phenomenon (RP) was initially described by the French physician Maurice Raynaud, who characterized the disorder as recurrent and episodic vasospasm of the fingers and/or toes associated with exposure to cold or stress. Although triphasic color changes are generally considered the hallmark for RP, these findings are not commonly seen. They include pallor due to ischemia, followed by cyanosis as a result of deoxygenation of blood, and rubor

seen upon rewarming as the vasospasm resolves (Figure 19.1).

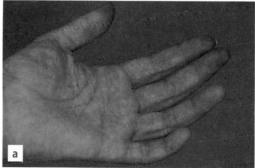

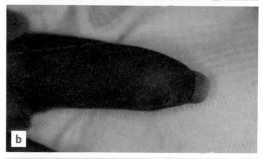

Figure 19.1 (a) Characteristic discoloration of the digits in a patient with PRP. (b) Digital ulceration and cyanosis seen in a patient with RP and limited scleroderma.

Vascular Disease: Diagnostic and Therapeutic Approaches. © 2011 Michael R. Jaff and Christopher J. White, editors. Cardiotext Publishing, ISBN: 978-1-935395-16-4.

Epidemiology

A Framingham Study offspring cohort prospective study looked at the incidence and the natural history of 641 women and 717 men with *primary Raynaud's phenomenon (PRP)*. This review collected data over a 7-year period and found that 2.2% of women and 1.5% of men had PRP.[1] In previous studies, however, the prevalence of PRP has varied from 3.2% to as high as 20.1% in colder climates.[2] Females are 4 times more likely to be affected than males, and there appears to be an increased prevalence of PRP in family members of affected individuals.

Pathophysiology

The clinical features of RP result from reversible, intermittent vasospasm due to cold or emotional stress, and although the exact cause remains unknown, multiple theories have been proposed.

According to a review by Herrick,[3] 3 mechanisms are largely responsible for the pathophysiology of RP: vascular, neural, and intravascular abnormalities.

Vascular abnormalities

The endothelium regulates vascular tone by secreting vasoactive substances that result in vasoconstriction or vasodilation; an imbalance in either of these mediators is thought to play a major role in the pathophysiology of RP. The vasoconstrictor substances include endothelin-1, angiotensin II, thromboxane A_2, and 5-hydroxytryptamine, while the vasodilator agonists consist of nitric oxide (NO), prostacyclin, leukotrienes, and prostaglandins.

The vasoconstrictor endothelin-1, an extremely potent agent produced by the endothelium, is thought to be "overexpressed" in patients with *secondary Raynaud's phenomenon (SRP)* (scleroderma) and has also been shown to rise in PRP patients exposed to cold temperatures.[4]

NO is produced by the endothelium by NO synthase and inhibits the production of endothelin-1, and as such it prevents vasoconstriction. In patients with RP an increase of endogenous inhibitor of endothelial NO synthase

(asymmetrical dimethylarginine [ADMA]) is noted. This results in a relative decrease in NO-induced vasodilation and an increase in endothelin-1-induced vasoconstriction.[5]

Neural abnormalities

Blood supply is regulated by smooth muscles in cutaneous vessels by the adrenergic receptors located in both the central and peripheral nervous systems. Alpha$_1$ and α_2 receptors regulate the peripheral vascular tone, inducing vasoconstriction. The α_2-adrenergic receptors are believed to be the more important of the 2 and the α_{2C} receptors have an additional function of thermoregulation.[6] In patients with SRP, α_{2C}-receptor reactivity has been shown to be increased.[7]

Sensory nerves innervating the capillaries of the digits release the most studied neurotransmitter in RP, *calcitonin gene-related peptide (CGRP)*, a potent vasodilator. Bunker et al[8] demonstrated that the cutaneous nerves of patients with PRP and SRP are CGRP deficient and also reported improved blood flow in small numbers of patients who received intravenous CGRP with both severe peripheral vascular insufficiency and RP. Other vasodilator substances believed to be released include substance P, neurokinin, and vasointestinal active peptide.

Although there is less evidence for central nervous system involvement in the pathophysiology of RP, several studies support its role. One theory suggests that a decrease in the central neural process of *habituation* (a phenomenon of acclimatization to repeated stimuli) occurs in patients with RP. In a study by Edwards et al,[9] initial responses to a sound stimulus (considered an emotional stress) were similar in patients with PRP and control subjects. When this stimulus was repeated, however, control subjects were habituated to the stimuli by day 5. However, the patients with PRP continued to demonstrate these responses, implying no habituation.

Intravascular or hematologic abnormalities

A number of intravascular or hematological abnormalities have been implicated in the pathogenesis of RP. These include platelet activation, impaired fibrinolysis, increased leucocyte activation, an excess of von Willebrand factor, and reduced red blood cell deformability. Platelet activation may lead to increased synthesis of thromboxane and serotonin, which results in vasoconstriction.

Fibrinolysis has been reported to be abnormal in patients with SRP. Elevated levels of tissue plasminogen activator inhibitor and tissue plasminogen antigen have been identified suggesting impaired fibrinolysis, which could result in fibrin deposition and vascular obstruction. Other hematological abnormalities include white blood cell activation and increased viscosity.

Genetic Basis

Genetics may play a role in the development of RP. Zhou et al[10] reported increased concordance of scleroderma and RP in monozygotic twins. Three potential candidate genes have been described and epidemiological studies have also shown clustering of RP.[11]

Natural History

The long-term prognosis of RP depends on whether it is primary or secondary. Tissue loss or the development of a connective tissue disorder in initially seronegative PRP patients is uncommon. In one long-term prospective study of 1039 RP patients followed over a 10-year period, only 2% to 9% of initially seronegative patients developed a connective tissue disorder. Individuals with SRP and a vasocclusive disorder, however, had a worse prognosis. The incidence of digital ulceration was 5% to 16% in PRP, compared with 48% to 56% in SRP, while digital amputations ranged from 1.4% to 1.6% in PRP, compared with 12% to 19% in SRP.[12]

Diagnostic Evaluation

Clinical features

The age of onset for most patients with PRP is between 11 and 45 years of age, and the va-

sospasm that occurs initially involves only the fingers, while involvement of the toes, generally covered with protective clothing and footwear, may only be apparent at a later stage or as the severity of the disease progresses. RP can also affect the nose, ears, tongue, and nipples. The classic triphasic color changes described earlier are rarely seen, and pallor may be the only presenting feature in RP. Throbbing pain, numbness, paresthesias, and cold sensation are often present during and/or following an attack, and superficial ulcerations involving the tips of digits may be seen in some individuals with PRP.

Although not often considered, RP can also affect the coronary and cerebral arteries, resulting in coronary vasospasm and migraine headaches.

Primary versus secondary Raynaud's phenomenon

Differentiating between PRP and SRP is extremely important in its management and prognosis. In 1932, Allen and Browne[13] established 5 clinical features required for the diagnosis of RRP:

1. presence of vasospasm precipitated by cold or emotional stress;
2. bilateral or symmetrical involvement of the extremities;
3. absence of gangrene, but if present ischemia limited to the fingertips;
4. absence of other conditions that can lead to vasospasm;
5. symptoms for at least 2 years.

These criteria remain valid today and continue to be used to differentiate PRP from SRP. More recently, the addition of negative serological testing to rule out a connective tissue disorder has strengthened these criteria. Some of the more common conditions associated with SRP are listed in Table 19.1 (on the following page).

History and Physical Examination

Evaluation of the patient should begin with a thorough history regarding onset of symptoms, color changes, and aggravating and relieving

Rheumatological/Connective Tissue Disorders
Scleroderma
Systemic lupus erythematosus
Rheumatoid arthritis
Dermatomyositis
Sjögren's syndrome
Mixed connective tissue disorders
Primary biliary cirrhosis
Giant cell arteritis or Takayasu's arteritis
Arterial Occlusive Disease
Atherosclerosis
Thromboangiitis obliterans/Buerger's disease
Atheroembolism
Distal embolization from grafts/aneurysms
Occupational/Environmental
Vibration-induced
Hypothenar hammer syndrome
Cold injury/frostbite
Arterial trauma
Endocrine
Pheochromocytoma
Hypothyroidism
Carcinoid syndrome
Hematological Abnormalities
Mixed cryoglobulinemia
Multiple myeloma
Cold agglutinin disease
Paraproteinemia
Polycythemia vera
Infections
Parvovirus B19
Helicobacter pylori
Hepatitis B and C antigenemia
Drugs/Chemicals
Amphetamines
Cocaine
Polyvinyl chloride
Cytotoxic drugs (vinblastine, bleomycin)
Beta-blockers
Ergot preparations
5-hydroxytryptamine receptor antagonist (sumatriptan)
Interferon alpha and beta
Lead poisoning
Arsenic poisoning
Oral contraceptives
Primary Pulmonary Hypertension
Large-Vessel Vasculitis
Takayasu's arteritis
Extracranial temporal arteritis
Miscellaneous
Thoracic outlet syndrome

Table 19.1 Disorders Associated with Secondary Raynaud's Phenomenon

factors. Specific questions must be asked in regard to additional signs and symptoms, including arthralgias, skin rashes, dryness of the eyes, difficulty swallowing, muscle aches, myalgias, or frontal headaches suggestive of a SRP. A previous or current history of smoking and an occupational history such as the use of vibratory tools or a prior history of frostbite related to occupation or recreation (paramedics/ice fishing/skiing) is important to elicit. The patient's medication list, including over-the-counter drugs and herbal remedies should be carefully reviewed.

The physical examination should include special attention to the skin for telangiectasias of the fingers or palms, thickening of the skin suggestive of sclerodactyly, splinter hemorrhages, digital ulcerations, or cyanosis. Palpation of all upper- and lower-extremity pulses is essential. Thoracic outlet maneuvers and an Allen test (to determine patency of the radial and ulnar arteries) should also be performed. The Allen test is normal in patients with PRP but is usually abnormal with SRP due to obstructed or sluggish flow in either of these arteries.

Nail fold capillary microscopy is a valuable tool that can be easily performed at bedside and may be helpful in distinguishing PRP from SRP. A drop of oil is placed on the skin near the nail fold bed and the capillary loops are examined using an ophthalmoscope. Normal capillaries are aligned parallel to the long axis of the digit and are regularly spaced with hairpin bends, favoring the diagnosis of PRP. In scleroderma, systemic lupus erythematosus (SLE), dermatomyositis, and other mixed connective tissue disorders an abnormal pattern is seen. Scleroderma patients demonstrate a decrease in the numbers of loops, enlarged and deformed capillaries, and avascular areas. Capillaries may be tortuous and end in prominent venous pools in SLE, and the presence of abnormal capillaries along with a positive antinuclear antibody (ANA) has both a high specificity and positive predictive value for SRP and an underlying connective tissue disorder.

Laboratory Evaluation

Initial testing should include a complete blood count (CBC), chemistry profile, check of sedimentation rate, urinalysis, ANA test, thyroid-stimulating hormone (TSH) level check, and chest x-ray looking for a cervical rib. Serum and urine immunoelectrophoresis, a rheumatoid factor, and complement levels may be indicated depending on the initial findings. If the ANA is positive or if any abnormality is found suggesting SRP, specific autoantibodies may be included (Table 19.2). If the patient's history suggests a vasculitis, C-ANCA and P-ANCA levels and a serum cryoglobulin level should be ordered.

Noninvasive laboratory evaluation

Digital and segmental blood pressure measurements and pulse volume recordings (PVRs) may be useful and help localize the level of disease in RP, for example, if there is large-vessel disease such as Takayasu's arteritis or fibromuscular dysplasia (FMD) (Figure 19.2; see pp. 376–77). These tests use changes in blood volume and/or detect pulsation in the fingertips. PVRs should also be performed in patients with a suspicion for thoracic outlet syndrome, where the waveforms may be blunted with appropriate (abduction) maneuvers.

Magnetic resonance angiography (MRA) or computed tomography angiography (CTA) of the aortic arch, the great vessels, and subclavian arteries may also be needed to rule out thoracic outlet syndrome, FMD, or Takayasu's arteritis. MRA may also be helpful to diagnose an ulnar artery occlusion in the hypothenar hammer syndrome.

Duplex ultrasonography is another useful noninvasive tool. It is capable of imaging the palmar arch and digital arteries for arterial patency and identify aneurysmal disease.

Other largely experimental noninvasive tests that have been used to evaluate the skin microcirculation include optical coherence tomography, laser Doppler fluxmetry, laser Doppler perfusion imaging, and photoplethysmography, however, these tests are not readily available and are largely used for research purposes.

Invasive evaluation.

Angiography is generally not needed for the diagnosis of PRP, however, it should be considered if occlusive arterial disease is suspected or if intervention or surgery is contemplated (Figure 19.3; see p. 377).

Therapeutic Options
Nonpharmacological therapy or behavioral techniques

The mainstay for the treatment of RP revolves around avoiding cold or stressful situations, wearing warm clothing, avoiding nicotine, behavioral therapy, and treatment of the underlying condition in SRP.

PRP does not disable the patient; however, lifestyle may be affected by symptoms. Patients must avoid all precipitating agents listed previously. Nonpharmacologic interventions or behavioral therapy should be used initially to control symptoms and include educating the patient about the condition and the possible triggering events. Patients should be advised to wear warm clothing to cover their entire body, including the head and neck if they go out in

Autoantibodies	Associated Condition
Rheumatoid factor (RF)/anti-CCP (citrulline-containing proteins)	Rheumatoid arthritis
Anti-centromere	Limited scleroderma/CREST
Anti-Smith (Sm)/anti-RNP	Systemic SLE
Anti-topoisomerase (Scl 70) and anti-mRNA polymerase	Scleroderma
Anti-Ro/SSA and anti-La/SSB	Sjögren's syndrome

Table 19.2 Autoantibodies and Associated Rheumatological Conditions

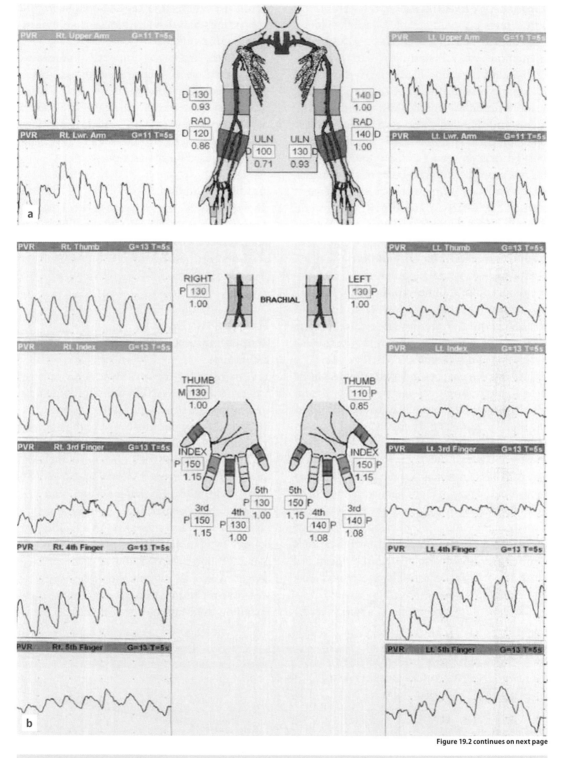

Figure 19.2 continues on next page

Figure 19.2 Patient with RP secondary to thoracic outlet syndrome. (a) Normal segmental blood pressures and PVRs at rest. (b) Decreased amplitude of PVRs in the left thumb, index, and third digits. (c) Decreased amplitude of PVRs in the left index finger with thoracic outlet maneuvers. Note normal waveforms in the right index finger.

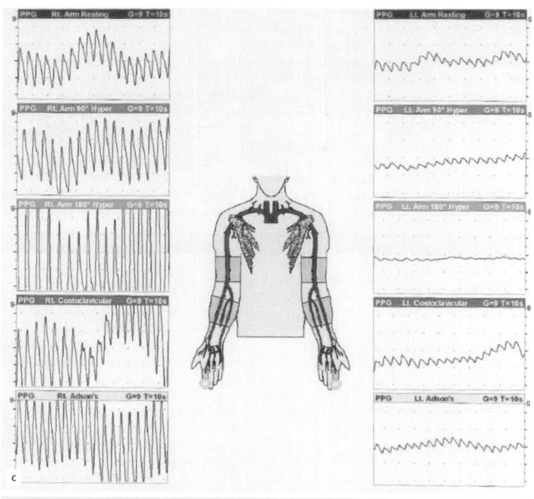

Figure 19.2 *Continued from previous page.*

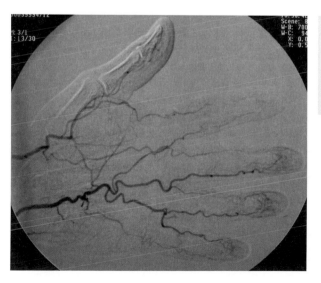

Figure 19.3 Angiogram of the hand in a patient with limited scleroderma. Note the ulnar artery supplying an incomplete superficial arch and absence of a deep palmar arch. All digital arteries are tortuous, irregular, and diminutive distally. Changes are most pronounced in the left index finger.

cold weather. Sudden temperature changes should be avoided. Education must also include useful techniques to help terminate attacks (exiting from a cold environment and warming the affected areas). Biofeedback may be beneficial in some patients.[14]

Pharmacological therapy

If nonpharmacological management fails, patients with PRP can be treated with drugs that have also been found useful for SRP. Calcium channel blockers (CCBs) are the mainstay of treatment, and numerous studies (including a meta-analysis) have demonstrated both a decrease in the number of attacks and their severity.[15] A long-acting CCB (dihydropyridine) is generally recommended. These agents should be titrated to the highest tolerated dose that provides relief from symptoms. The combination of a CCB and/or another indirect or direct vasodilator can also be used if symptoms are not well controlled. Aspirin or an alternative antiplatelet agent should be started unless there is a contraindication to its use. Table 19.3 lists a number of other medications that have been tried and proven useful for treating RP.

Drug Class	Drug
Direct Vasodilator Calcium channel blockers	Nifedipine Amlodipine
Others	Nitroglycerin Hydralazine Nitroprusside Niacin Minoxidil
Indirect Vasodilators Serotonin S_2 receptor uptake inhibitor	Ketanserin
Selective serotonin receptor uptake blocker	Fluoxetine
Angiotensin-converting enzyme inhibitors	Captopril
Angiotensin receptor blocker	Losartan
Phosphodiesterase inhibitor	Sildenafil
Endothelin-1 receptor inhibitor	Bosentan
Sympatholytics	Prazosin Reserpine Methyldopa
Prostaglandins	Alprostadil Beraprost Misoprostol Cicaprost Iloprost Prostacyclin Epoprostenol
Antithrombotics/Anticoagulation	Aspirin Dipyridamole Heparin LMWH
Miscellaneous Rheologic modifiers	Pentoxifylline Cilostazol
Neuropeptide—vasodilator	intravenous CGRP
NO release enhancer	L-arginine

Table 19.3 Pharmacotherapy for RP

The rheologic modifier pentoxifylline (Trental) and phosphodiesterase inhibitor cilostazol (Pletal) have shown benefits in several case reports of RP. In a placebo-controlled prospective study, an increase in the mean diameter of the radial artery, improved flow-mediated diameter, and improved nitroglycerin-mediated flow in both PRP and SRP patients were demonstrated using cilostazol, although these changes did not translate into improvement in the frequency or severity of attacks.[16] In refractory patients, the combination of cilostazol, a CCB, and aspirin have also been recommended if the patient is not responding to initial treatment.

Two other phosphodiesterase inhibitors (tadalafil and sildenafil) have recently received significant interest in the management of RP, and multiple case reports have demonstrated their benefits. Fries et al[17] performed a double-blinded, placebo-controlled, crossover study in 16 SRP patients using sildenafil and demonstrated a decrease in the mean frequency, cumulative attack duration, and increased capillary blood-flow velocity.

Bosentan, an endothelin-1 inhibitor, has been FDA approved for the treatment of pulmonary arterial hypertension, and although results from a randomized, multicenter, placebo-controlled study did not show any benefit in healing ischemic digital ulcers in scleroderma patients (RAPIDS-1), it prevented the development of new ulceration and improved hand function in patients with SRP who had systemic sclerosis and scleroderma.[18]

Anxiety plays a significant role in the aggravation of symptoms; therefore, patients may also benefit from anxiolytics. The selective serotonin reuptake inhibitor (SSRI) fluoxetine has been shown to improve symptoms in females with PRP,[19] however, long-term data on its use in this setting are lacking.

Several reports of novel biological therapies include the use of intravenous calcitonin gene receptor protein (CGRP) infusions, antioxidant therapy such as N-acetyl cysteine,[20] and L-arginine therapy.[21,22] These agents have shown some promise in the improvement of symptoms, however, larger prospective studies are needed to establish their efficacy.

Botulism toxin A has anticholinergic effects at both the neuromuscular junction level and sweat glands and has been shown to be beneficial in the treatment of hyperhidrosis of the palms. Sycha and colleagues[23] tested the effect of intradigital botulism toxin injections in 2 patients, 1 with PRP and the other with SRP, and found beneficial effects based on a visual analog scale for clinical symptoms and superficial skin blood flow as assessed with laser Doppler interferometry.

Endovascular therapy

If angiography reveals an underlying anatomical problem such as arterial occlusive disease or a thrombus or embolism, further therapy, including endovascular options, should be considered. These were addressed in Chapter 6.

Surgical therapy

Cervical and lumbar sympathectomy is an option that may be considered for patients who fail pharmacotherapy. Unfortunately, sympathectomy may only palliate symptoms for a short period of time, and many patients will relapse. It is also reported to be less effective in patients with SRP. Several approaches are utilized including endoscopic and surgical. Matsumoto et al[24] showed high initial success rates using an endoscopic approach in 26 patients. Ninety-two percent had complete resolution or significant improvement in their digital ischemia immediately, however, there was a recurrence rate of 82% in the patients within a mean period of 16 months. Although a less invasive procedure than an open thoracic sympathectomy, its availability may be a limiting factor. Most physicians recommend using sympathectomy for patients with refractory RP and/or digital ischemia and ulcerations.

Percutaneous computed tomography–guided thoracic sympathectomy using 5% phenol has been tested in patients with digital ischemia and RP. Although temporary improvement allowing wound healing has been noted, this technique has high recurrence rates after 6 months.

Spinal cord stimulation has been used in the management of RP for almost 2 decades with fairly good results, however, its availability may be the limiting factor.[25] It is usually considered in patients who fail medical therapy prior to sympathectomy.

Management of acute RP with digital ischemia

The management of acute RP with digital ischemia requires an aggressive approach. Patients generally require admission to the hospital, and initial measures should include bed rest, pain control, and a warm environment. CCBs should be initiated and titrated to the maximum tolerated dose. Pain control including intravenous narcotics and/or digital block (chemical sympathectomy) using lidocaine or bupivacaine may be necessary. If tissue ischemia is present, anticoagulation (heparin or low-molecular-weight heparin) should be initiated and continued until symptoms resolve. If the patient does not respond to CCBs, other drugs listed in Table 19.3 can be tried.

Initial studies using prostaglandins in the treatment of pulmonary hypertension in patients with scleroderma showed improvement in digital blood flow, suggesting a potential for its use in patients with RP. In one study, the cycling of intravenous iloprost and alprostadil in RP secondary to a connective tissue disorder decreased recurrence and ulceration and improved clinical outcomes.[26]

Prostaglandin infusions should be used in patients who are refractory to outpatient management and for individuals with significant pain. The procedures/surgeries described should also be considered for refractory RP while the underlying associated condition must be aggressively treated in patients with SRP.

If RP is secondary to vasoocclusive disease, a diagnostic workup and treatment should include identifying and removing the occlusion with endovascular or surgical procedures.

Livedo Reticularis

Livedo reticularis (LR) is a reticular, violet-blue mottling or fishnet pattern that is seen principally on the lower extremities and involves the cutaneous microvascular system (Figures 19.4 and 19.5). It has also been called cutis marmorata, livedo racemosa, or livedo annularis. *Primary livedo reticularis (PLR)* is generally benign and not associated with a secondary disorder, while a number of systemic syndromes, including connective tissue disorders, atheromatous embolization, and hyperviscosity syndromes, as well as drugs and infection, are associated with *secondary livedo reticularis (SLR)*.

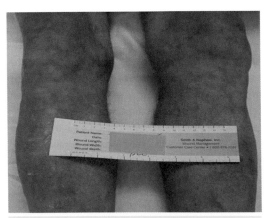

Figure 19.4 Patient with LR secondary to atheroembolism.

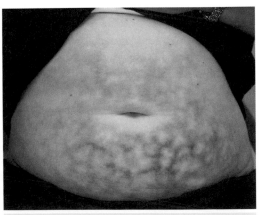

Figure 19.5 Patient with idiopathic LR on the abdomen that does not respond to warming.

Ischemia and digital ulcerations are seen only in the secondary form.

PLR is further subdivided into 3 types based on the patient's response to warming and the duration of the pattern: idiopathic, physiologic or cutis marmorata,[27] and primary.[28] Figure 19.6 outlines an algorithm for evaluating the 3 types, and Table 19.4 (on following page) lists conditions associated with SLR.

Conditions Associated with Secondary Livedo Reticularis

Antiphospholipid syndrome (APS) is frequently associated with SLR and is reported to occur in as many as 25% to 40% of patients with this condition. These individuals are at an increased risk for venous or arterial thrombosis, fetal loss, and thrombocytopenia. Anticardiolipin antibodies (ACAs) and a lupus anticoagulant profile should be checked in all LR patients with suspicion for this disorder. If present in an individual without evidence for current or prior thrombo-

sis, treatment with low-dose aspirin is generally adequate, whereas long-term anticoagulation is recommended for those with thrombotic manifestations of this syndrome.

LR can also be seen in patients with atheromatous embolization. In this population, LR often develops after a vascular or cardiovascular surgical procedure or following endovascular procedures, including percutaneous coronary intervention, percutaneous transluminal angioplasty, or stenting of the carotid, renal, or lower-extremity vessels. Patients generally have severe systemic atherosclerosis with underlying hypertension, hyperlipidemia, diabetes mellitus, and a strong smoking history. They are at increased risk for renal failure, stroke, or myocardial infarction as well as ischemic and gangrenous changes of the extremities.

Several additional yet rare conditions associated with SLR include Sneddon's syndrome, Moyamoya disease, and a cutaneous form of polyarteritis nodosa (PAN).

Sneddon's syndrome is associated with cerebral ischemic arterial events (stroke or

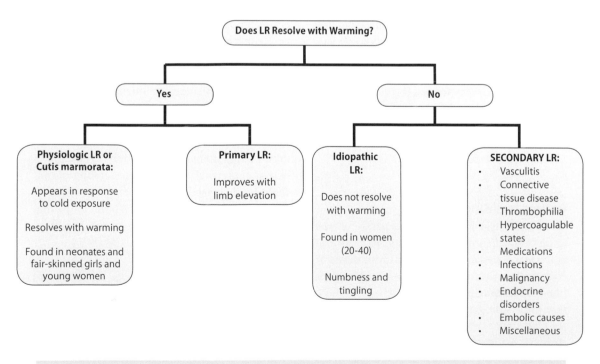

Figure 19.6 Algorithm for the evaluation of patients with livedo reticularis.

Hypercoagulable or hyperviscosity states: antiphospholipid syndrome, Sneddon's syndrome, proteins C and S, antithrombin deficiency, multiple myeloma, cryoglobulinemia, cryofibrinogenemia, cold agglutinin disease, DIC
Connective tissue disorders/autoimmune disorders
Vasculitis (cutaneous form of PAN), rheumatoid vasculitis, SLE, Sjögren's syndrome
Atheroembolism
Myeloproliferative disorders (polycythemia vera, essential thrombocytosis)
Septic embolism, atrial myxoma
Pernicious anemia
Medications: amantadine, Gemcitabine, interferon, minocycline, thrombolytic therapy, heparin
Infections: hepatitis C, mycoplasma pneumonia, tuberculosis, endocarditis
Cancer (renal cell carcinoma and inflammatory breast disease)
Neurologic: reflex sympathetic dystrophy, multiple sclerosis, Parkinson's disease, Moyamoya disease
Endocrine: hypothyroidism, pheochromocytoma, carcinoid syndrome, and hypercalcemia/calciphylaxis

Table 19.4 Conditions Associated with SLR[29-38]

transient ischemic attack). A significant percentage (incidence reported is variable) of patients have been found to have anticardiolipin antibodies, and LR is reported to precede vascular events by several years.

Moyamoya disease is seen primarily in children and is characterized by progressive stenosis of the Circle of Willis that may eventually lead to ischemic and/or hemorrhagic strokes. Fever, arthralgias, subcutaneous nodules, and LR characterize cutaneous PAN.

Pathophysiology

The pathophysiology of SLR depends on the underlying disorder. In patients with APS, it is unclear whether LR is due to thrombosis or endothelial dysfunction. The phospholipid-binding protein ß2-glycoprotein I, or ß2GPI, is a target antigen of anticardiolipin antibodies seen in the antiphospholipid antibody syndrome.[39] Antibodies to ß2GPI are often elevated in patients with LR,[40] and it is hypothesized that these lead to a hypercoagulable condition re-

sulting in microvascular thrombosis. Still others have suggested that the mechanism for LR is a result of endothelial dysfunction leading to vasoconstriction and leucocyte adhesion.

In connective tissue disorders, a biopsy from an area of LR often reveals a livedoid vasculitis. A segmental hyalinizing vasculitis is reported, and infarction of the skin is a result of obstructed arterioles. In a small study, anti–endothelial cell antibodies were found in one-third of all patients with Sneddon's syndrome.[41] In patients with atheromatous embolization, cholesterol crystals and other atheromatous material embolize from manipulation following surgery or endovascular procedures, resulting in the LR pattern.

Natural History

PLR is a benign condition that requires little or no treatment, whereas the prognosis for SLR depends largely on the underlying condition. A poorer prognosis is likely expected for those individuals with APS, atheroembolism, a connective tissue disorder, or malignancy, whereas patients with LR secondary to medications or an infectious process may expect complete resolution of symptoms once these factors are removed or treated.

Diagnostic Evaluation

Clinical evaluation

A thorough history and physical examination are essential to the diagnosis of LR. Attention should focus on past medical history, including all recent and past medical illnesses, recent surgical or endovascular procedures, and medications. A family history of thrombophilia or thrombosis is also important.

Physical examination

The physical examination is particularly important in LR and should pay particular attention to location as well as precipitating and alleviating factors. The pulse examination is expected to be normal in patients with PLR, with mottling found predominately on the lower extremities and occasionally on the trunk. In addition, most primary forms are aggravated by cold exposure and relieved by warming.

In patients with physiologic LR or cutis marmorata, the mottling discoloration resolves completely with warming. This form is most commonly found in neonates and fair-skinned young girls and women.

The idiopathic and primary forms of LR are generally diagnoses of exclusion. Elevation of the affected limb usually results in resolution of symptoms in the primary form, and it is generally independent of the ambient temperature and has more of a fluctuating course. The idiopathic form, however, is persistent, does not respond to warming, and is most commonly seen in young women (age 20–40) who may complain of numbness and tingling.

In patients with SLR, the pulses exam may be abnormal depending on the underlying condition, while purpuric macular lesions or cutaneous nodules that progress to ulceration may be observed.

Laboratory studies

No specific laboratory studies are recommended for PLR, whereas the underlying condition will dictate the need for more specific testing in SLR. Anticardiolipin antibodies, a LAC (Lupus Anticoagulant), and select thrombophilia screening tests (antithrombin, proteins C and S) may be warranted. A complete blood count and review of the peripheral blood smear may help to determine if there is an underlying myeloproliferative disorder, while appropriate cultures are indicated whether there is an infectious cause. Skin biopsies may help to determine whether there is vasculitis or vasculopathy.

Therapeutic Options

PLR without ulceration does not generally require treatment, unless the appearance is bothersome to the patient. Conservative measures including avoiding cold exposure or use of vasodilators, including the CCBs, can be tried and may be helpful.

The treatment of SLR should be directed toward the underlying cause. Antiplatelet therapy using low-dose aspirin should be considered in all symptomatic patients with LR and in those asymptomatic individuals with APS.

Acrocyanosis

Acrocyanosis is a symmetric persistent violaceous or bluish discoloration and coolness of the hands (and less commonly the feet). It was first described in 1896 and although it is seen in both cold and warm environments, is generally worsens with cold exposure.

Acrocyanosis can be primary (without tissue loss) or secondary and associated with an underlying connective tissue disorder, medication, toxin, malignancy, or infection. *Primary acrocyanosis* is generally seen in young women, while *secondary acrocyanosis* can be found in individuals with an underlying malignancy, infectious mononucleosis, or spinal cord injuries. Secondary acrocyanosis is also associated with certain drugs, including imipramine, butyl nitrite, and the fungicide blasticidin S. Other rare causes include ethyl malonic aciduria associated with encephalopathy, petechiae, and acrocyanosis, as well as diffuse palmoplantar keratoderma.[42-44] Patients with secondary acrocyanosis may develop digital ulceration, and some individuals report edema and excess sweating of the hands and feet.

Epidemiology

The incidence of acrocyanosis is unknown, but it is more prevalent in the second to fourth decades. There appears to be no sex predominance.

Pathophysiology

The pathophysiology of acrocyanosis is not clear, but proposed theories include vasospasm, decreased capillary blood flow,[45,46] blood viscosity abnormalities, and increased levels of and/or an exaggerated response of endothelin-1 to cold stimulation.[47,48]

Diagnostic Evaluation

A complete history and physical examination should be performed. Appropriate laboratory tests will help rule out some of the secondary causes.

Nail fold capillary microscopy has revealed dilated efferent capillary loops and venules and a decreased number of capillaries, and in patients with secondary acrocyanosis due to anorexia nervosa, the leucocyte count and eosinophil counts were low.[46]

Clinical evaluation

The physical examination, including the peripheral pulse exam, is generally unrevealing except for the characteristic appearance (Figure 19.7). Acrocyanosis may also involve the ears, nose, cheeks, lips, nipples, elbows, and knees.

Differential diagnosis

The differential diagnosis includes peripheral cyanosis, peripheral artery disease (PAD), RP, and erythromelalgia. Peripheral cyanosis can be identified by the presence of cyanosis on the mucus membranes and hypoxia on an arterial blood gas. PAD can be distinguished by the history and absent or decreased peripheral pulses, while acrocyanosis is distinguished from RP by its persistence in both warm and cool environments. Pain, tingling, warmth, and redness of the extremities with heat exposure characterize erythromelalgia.

Therapeutic Options

Initial nonpharmacological therapy should include avoidance of cold environments and other general measures outlined in RP. Pharmacotherapy is not needed in most patients, however, in individuals bothered by their

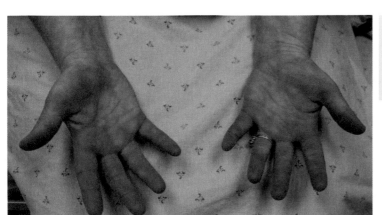

Figure 19.7 Patient with primary acrocyanosis. Note the characteristic violaceous discoloration, which is persistent and does not change with temperature changes.

physical appearance, drugs such as low doses of guanethidine or reserpine,[49] topical minoxidil, and bromocriptine[50] have been used. Radical procedures such as sympathectomy and spinal cord stimulation are generally not needed. Biofeedback and hypnosis may be beneficial in some patients.

Summary

Raynaud's phenomenon (RP), livedo reticularis (LR), and acrocyanosis are all vasospastic diseases. Episodic vasospasm upon exposure to cold temperature or stressful conditions is the hallmark of RP. Differentiating PRP from SRP is the key in the initial workup, as these 2 conditions differ in their natural history and prognosis. Vasospasm occurs as a result of vascular abnormalities, central and peripheral nervous system abnormalities, or hematologic components. Calcium channel blockers are the mainstay of treatment, while management of acute digital ischemia requires hospitalization and the use of intravenous medications. Several experimental treatment trials are underway and large-scale studies and long-term outcomes are awaited.

References

1. Suter LG, Murabito JM, Felson DT, Fraenkel L. The incidence and natural history of Raynaud's phenomenon in the community. *Arthritis Rheum*. 2005;52:1259-1263.

2. Maricq HR, Carpentier PH, Weinrich MC, et al. Geographic variation in the prevalence of Raynaud's phenomenon: Charleston, SC, USA, vs Tarentaise, Savoie, France. *J Rheumatol*. 1993;20:70-76.

3. Herrick AL. Pathogenesis of Raynaud's phenomenon. *Rheumatology (Oxford)*. 2005;44:587-596.

4. Vancheeswaran R, Azam A, Black C, Dashwood MR. Localization of endothelin-1 and its

binding sites in scleroderma skin. *J Rheumatol*. 1994;21:1268-1276.

5. Cooke JP, Marshall JM. Mechanisms of Raynaud's disease. *Vasc Med*. 2005;10:293-307.

6. Coffman JD, Cohen RA. Role of alpha-adrenoceptor subtypes mediating sympathetic vasoconstriction in human digits. *Eur J Clin Invest*. 1988;18:309-313.

7. Bailey SR, Mitra S, Flavahan S, Flavahan NA. Reactive oxygen species from smooth muscle mitochondria initiate cold-induced constriction of cutaneous arteries. *Am J Physiol Heart Circ Physiol*. 2005;289:H243-250.

8. Bunker CB, Reavley C, O'Shaughnessy DJ, Dowd PM. Calcitonin gene-related peptide in treatment of severe peripheral vascular insufficiency in Raynaud's phenomenon. *Lancet*. 1993;342:80-83.

9. Edwards CM, Marshall JM, Pugh M. Lack of habituation of the pattern of cardiovascular response evoked by sound in subjects with primary Raynaud's disease. *Clin Sci (Lond)*. 1998;95:249-260.

10. Zhou X, Tan FK, Xiong M, Arnett FC, Feghali-Bostwick CA. Monozygotic twins clinically discordant for scleroderma show concordance for fibroblast gene expression profiles. *Arthritis Rheum*. 2005;52:3305-3314.

11. Freedman RR, Mayes MD. Familial aggregation of primary Raynaud's disease. *Arthritis Rheum*. 1996;39:1189-1191.

12. Landry GJ, Edwards JM, McLafferty RB, Taylor LM Jr, Porter JM. Long-term outcome of Raynaud's syndrome in a prospectively analyzed patient cohort. *J Vasc Surg*. 1996;23:76-85; discussion 85-86.

13. Allen EV, Browne GE. Raynaud's disease: a critical review of minimal requisites for diagnosis. *Am J Med Sci*. 1932;183:187.

14. Ford MR. Biofeedback treatment for headaches, Raynaud's disease, essential hypertension, and irritable bowel syndrome: a review of the long-term follow-up literature. *Biofeedback Self Regul*. 1982;7:521-536.

15. Thompson AE, Pope JE. Calcium channel blockers for primary Raynaud's phenomenon: a meta-analysis. *Rheumatology (Oxford)*. 2005;44:145-150.

16. Rajagopalan S, Pfenninger D, Somers E, et al. Effects of cilostazol in patients with Raynaud's syndrome. *Am J Cardiol.* 2003;92:1310-1315.

17. Fries R, Shariat K, von Wilmowsky H, Bohm M. Sildenafil in the treatment of Raynaud's phenomenon resistant to vasodilatory therapy. *Circulation.* 2005;112:2980-2985.

18. Korn JH, Mayes M, Matucci Cerinic M, et al. Digital ulcers in systemic sclerosis: prevention by treatment with bosentan, an oral endothelin receptor antagonist. *Arthritis Rheum.* 2004;50:3985-3993.

19. Buecking A, Rougemont E, Fabio Zullino D. Treatment of Raynaud's phenomenon with escitalopram. *Int J Neuropsychopharmacol.* 2005;8:307-308.

20. Sambo P, Amico D, Giacomelli R, et al. Intravenous N-acetylcysteine for treatment of Raynaud's phenomenon secondary to systemic sclerosis: a pilot study. *J Rheumatol.* 2001;28:2257-2262.

21. Agostoni A, Marasini B, Biondi ML, et al. L-arginine therapy in Raynaud's phenomenon? *Int J Clin Lab Res.* 1991;21:202-203.

22. Rembold CM, Ayers CR. Oral L-arginine can reverse digital necrosis in Raynaud's phenomenon. *Mol Cell Biochem.* 2003;244:139-141.

23. Sycha T, Graninger M, Auff E, Schnider P. Botulinum toxin in the treatment of Raynaud's phenomenon: a pilot study. *Eur J Clin Invest.* 2004;34:312-313.

24. Matsumoto Y, Ueyama T, Endo M, et al. Endoscopic thoracic sympathicotomy for Raynaud's phenomenon. *J Vasc Surg.* 2002;36:57-61.

25. Francaviglia N, Silvestro C, Maiello M, Bragazzi R, Bernucci C. Spinal cord stimulation for the treatment of progressive systemic sclerosis and Raynaud's syndrome. *Br J Neurosurg.* 1994;8:567-571.

26. Marasini B, Massarotti M, Bottasso B, et al. Comparison between iloprost and alprostadil in the treatment of Raynaud's phenomenon. *Scand J Rheumatol.* 2004;33:253-256.

27. Gibbs MB, English JC III, Zirwas MJ. Livedo reticularis: an update. *J Am Acad Dermatol.* 2005;52:1009-1019.

28. Freeman R, Dover JS. Autonomic neurodermatology (Part I): erythromelalgia, reflex sympathetic dystrophy, and livedo reticularis. *Semin Neurol.* 1992;12:385-393.

29. Gross AS, Thompson FL, Arzubiaga MC, et al. Heparin-associated thrombocytopenia and thrombosis (HATT) presenting with livedo reticularis. *Int J Dermatol.* 1993;32:276-279.

30. Speight EL, Lawrence CM. Reticulate purpura, cryoglobulinaemia and livedo reticularis. *Br J Dermatol.* 1993;129:319-323.

31. Hasegawa H, Ozawa T, Tada N, et al. Multiple myeloma-associated systemic vasculopathy due to crystal globulin or polyarteritis nodosa. *Arthritis Rheum.* 1996;39:330-334.

32. Lauchli S, Widmer L, Lautenschlager S. Cold agglutinin disease—the importance of cutaneous signs. *Dermatology.* 2001;202:356-358.

33. Maroon M. Polycythemia rubra vera presenting as livedo reticularis. *J Am Acad Dermatol.* 1992;26:264-265.

34. Weir NU, Snowden JA, Greaves M, Davies-Jones GA. Livedo reticularis associated with hereditary protein C deficiency and recurrent thromboembolism. *Br J Dermatol.* 1995;132:283-285.

35. Donnet A, Khalil R, Terrier G, Koeppel MC, Njee BT, Aillaud MF. Cerebral infarction, livedo reticularis, and familial deficiency in antithrombin-III. *Stroke.* 1992;23:611-612.

36. Chaudhary K, Wall BM, Rasberry RD. Livedo reticularis: an underutilized diagnostic clue in cholesterol embolization syndrome. *Am J Med Sci.* 2001;321:348-351.

37. Howe SC, Murray JD, Reeves RT, Hemp JR, Carlisle JH. Calciphylaxis, a poorly understood clinical syndrome: three case reports and a review of the literature. *Ann Vasc Surg.* 2001;15:470-473.

38. Naldi L, Marchesi L, Locati F, Berti E, Cainelli T. Unusual manifestations of primary cutaneous amyloidosis in association with Raynaud's phenomenon and livedo reticularis. *Clin Exp Dermatol.* 1992;17:117-120.

39. Takeya H, Mori T, Gabazza EC, et al. Anti-beta2-glycoprotein I (beta2GPI) monoclonal antibodies with lupus anticoagulant-like activity enhance the beta2GPI binding to phospholipids. *J Clin Invest.* 1997;99:2260-2268.

40. Aubry F, Crickx B, Nicaise P, Labarre C, Viard JP, Belaich S. Anti-beta 2 glycoprotein 1 antibodies in idiopathic livedo reticularis. *Ann Dermatol Venereol.* 1995;122:667-670.

41. Frances C, Le Tonqueze M, Salohzin KV, et al. Prevalence of anti-endothelial cell antibodies in patients with Sneddon's syndrome. *J Am Acad Dermatol.* 1995;33:64-68.

42. Ohtake N, Sou K, Tsukamoto K, Furue M, Tamaki K. Diffuse palmoplantar keratoderma associated with acrocyanosis and livedo reticularis. Two sporadic cases. *Acta Derm Venereol.* 1995;75:331.

43. Nielsen PG. Diffuse palmoplantar keratoderma associated with acrocyanosis. A family study. *Acta Derm Venereol.* 1989;69:156-161.

44. Grosso S, Mostardini R, Farnetani MA, et al. Ethylmalonic encephalopathy: further clinical and neuroradiological characterization. *J Neurol.* 2002;249:1446-1450.

45. Martinez R, Saponaro A, Russo R, et al. Effects of sympathetic stimulation on microcirculatory dynamics in patients with essential acrocyanosis. A study using mental stress. *Panminerva Med.* 1993;35:9-11.

46. Klein-Weigel P, Rein P, Kronenberg F, et al. Microcirculatory assessment of vascular acrosyndrome in anorexia nervosa and analysis of manifestation factors. *J Psychosom Res.* 2004;56:145-148.

47. Mangiafico RA, Malatino LS, Spada RS, Santonocito M. Circulating endothelin-1 levels in patients with "a frigore" vascular acrosyndromes. *Panminerva Med.* 1996;38:229-233.

48. Mangiafico RA, Malatino LS, Santonocito M, Spada RS, Tamburino G. Plasma endothelin-1 concentrations during cold exposure in essential acrocyanosis. *Angiology.* 1996;47:1033-1038.

49. Coffman JD. Vasospastic phenomenon. *Peripheral Vascular Diseases.* 2nd ed. Philadelphia: Mosby; 1996:418.

50. Morrish DW, Crockford PM. Acrocyanosis treated with bromocriptine. *Lancet.* 1976;2:851.

20

Fibromuscular Dysplasia

Jeffrey W. Olin

Fibromuscular dysplasia (FMD) is a non-inflammatory, nonatherosclerotic vascular disease that has been observed in nearly every arterial bed.[1] The renal and internal carotid arteries are most frequently involved, and less often the vertebral, iliac, subclavian, visceral, and coronary arteries.

The clinical presentation may vary from asymptomatic to a multisystem disease mimicking necrotizing vasculitis,[2] depending on the arterial segment involved, the degree of stenosis, and the type of FMD. In 28% of patients, multiple vascular beds are involved[3,4] and in some situations multiorgan failure may occur, especially with the intimal type of FMD.[5,6] Although a variety of genetic, mechanical, and hormonal factors have been proposed, the etiology of FMD remains unknown.

Classification of Fibromuscular Dysplasia

Fibrous lesions of the renal artery are classified based upon the arterial layer—intima, media, or adventitia—in which the lesion predominates (Table 20.1).[7] Lesions involving the medial layer are further subdivided into *medial fibroplasia, perimedial fibroplasia,* and *medial hyperplasia.* Medial fibroplasia represents the most common type of FMD, accounting for approximately 80-90% of all lesions.[4,8] Angiographically, medial fibroplasia is characterized by the classic "string of beads" appearance (Figure 20.1). Typically, the beading is larger than the normal caliber of the artery. Perimedial fibroplasia (smaller and less numerous beads) (Figure 20.2), intimal fibroplasia (concentric band or long smooth narrowing) (Figure 20.3), and periarterial hyperplasia are distinct angiographically from medial fibroplasia.

Fibromuscular Dysplasia of the Renal Arteries

The renal arteries are involved in 60% to 75% of FMD patients[3] and are bilateral in 35% of patients.[4] FMD is most commonly diagnosed in women between the ages of 15 and 50.[1] Recently

Vascular Disease: Diagnostic and Therapeutic Approaches. © 2011 Michael R. Jaff and Christopher J. White, editors. Cardiotext Publishing, ISBN: 978-1-935395-16-4.

Classification	Frequency	Pathology	Angiographic Appearance
Medial Dysplasia			
Medial fibroplasia	80%–90%	Alternating areas of thinned media and thickened fibromuscular ridges containing collagen Internal elastic membrane may be lost in some areas	"String of beads" appearance where the diameter of the "beading" is larger than the diameter of the artery
Perimedial fibroplasia	1%–2%	Extensive collagen deposition in the outer half of the media	"Beading" in which the "beads" are smaller than the diameter of the artery
Medial hyperplasia	1%–2%	True smooth muscle cell hyperplasia without fibrosis	Concentric smooth stenosis (similar to intimal disease)
Intimal Fibroplasia			
	10%	Circumferential or eccentric deposition of collagen in the intima No lipid or inflammatory component Internal elastic lamina fragmented or duplicated	Concentric focal band Long smooth narrowing
Adventitial (Periarterial) Fibroplasia			
	< 1%	Dense collagen replaces the fibrous tissue of the adventitia and may extend into surrounding tissue	Sharply localized, tubular areas of stenosis (based on limited angiographic data)

Table 20.1   Classification of Fibromuscular Dysplasia (Adapted with permission from Begelman S, Olin JW. Fibromuscular dysplasia. *Curr Opin Rheumatol.* 2000;12:41-47.)

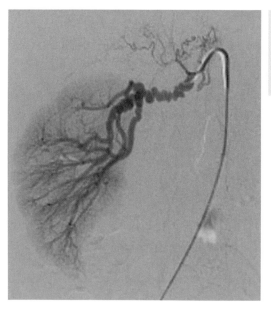

Figure 20.1   Renal artery angiogram showing typical "string of beads" appearance diagnostic of medial fibroplasia. Note that the beading is larger than the normal caliber of the artery. (From Slovut DP, Olin JW. Fibromuscular dysplasia. *N Engl J Med.* 2004; 350(18):1862-1871. Copyright © 2004. Massachusetts Medical Society. All rights reserved.)

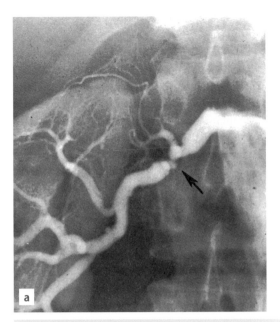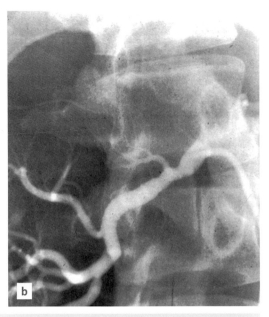

Figure 20.2 Perimedial fibroplasia (a) before and (b) after percutaneous angioplasty. Small beads are present, which are less numerous than encountered in medial fibroplasia. Note the collateral vessel around the area of beading. This is characteristic of perimedial fibroplasia. (From Slovut DP, Olin JW. Fibromuscular dysplasia. *N Engl J Med.* 2004; 350(18):1862-1871. Copyright © 2004. Massachusetts Medical Society. All rights reserved.)

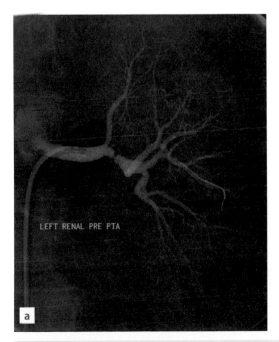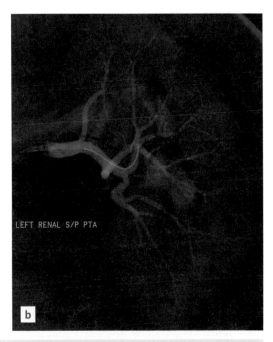

Figure 20.3 Intimal fibroplasia of the renal artery (a) before and (b) after angioplasty. Note the concentric bandlike stenosis present. (Courtesy of J. Michael Bacharach, MD.)

there have been cases of FMD first discovered in patients > 70 years old, suggesting that these individuals may be asymptomatic for many years and the FMD was discovered incidentally while investigating for some other reason or that the symptoms appeared later in life.[9] FMD accounts for < 10% of all patients with renal artery stenosis while atherosclerosis represents > 90%.[10] Angiographic evaluation has demonstrated that FMD is present in 3.8% to 10.1% of prospective renal donors.[11,12]

Clinical Presentation

Fibromuscular dysplasia of the renal arteries usually presents with hypertension in a young woman. A decrease in renal perfusion activates the rennin-angiotensin-aldosterone system, causing vasoconstriction, salt and water retention, and effects on sympathetic nerve activity and intrarenal prostaglandin and nitric oxide production. These effects ultimately lead to the development of renovascular hypertension.

Renal artery FMD presents most commonly in women with

- a long systolic or systolic and diastolic epigastric bruit;
- the onset of hypertension under the age of 35 years;
- severe or resistant hypertension;
- a sudden rise in previously stable hypertension;
- elevated serum creatinine after the administration an angiotensin-converting enzyme inhibitor or angiotensin-receptor blocker;
- elevated creatinine without a clear-cut cause.

It is not difficult to differentiate atherosclerosis from FMD. Typically, atherosclerotic lesions occur at the origin or proximal portion of the renal artery, while FMD occurs in the mid- or distal segments and the branches. Patients with atherosclerosis are older and have typical cardiovascular risk factors such as hypertension, dyslipidemia, and diabetes mellitus, whereas subjects with FMD are more often younger and have fewer cardiovascular risk factors. At times, it may be difficult to distinguish FMD from vasculitis, particularly in patients with multivessel intimal disease.[5] Unlike vasculitis, FMD is a noninflammatory process and is not associated with anemia, thrombocytopenia, or abnormalities of acute phase reactants except when it occurs in the presence of acute infarction. In some cases, intravascular ultrasonography may help distinguish FMD from vasculitis.[13]

Duplex Ultrasonography of Renal Arteries

While a variety of indirect tests, such as captopril renography and renal vein sampling, have been used to detect renal artery stenosis, direct imaging studies such as renal artery duplex ultrasonography and computed tomography angiography (CTA) have emerged as the best methods for diagnosis.[14]

Renal artery duplex ultrasonography can accurately detect elevated blood-flow velocities not only in the proximal portion of the renal artery but also the mid- and distal portions of the artery, the most common locations for FMD.[14,15] Therefore, it is important that the patient be imaged not only from the anterior approach but also from the oblique or flank approach to adequately visualize the distal portions of the renal artery. Since atherosclerosis rarely occurs in these segments, velocity elevations that begin in the mid- to distal portions of the renal artery are most often due to FMD.

Some investigators have demonstrated that intrarenal velocimetric indices improve after renal artery angioplasty in patients with FMD. For example, Marana and colleagues[16] used noninvasive Doppler to examine 29 arteries with FMD prior to and within 5 days of renal artery angioplasty. Successful renal artery revascularization was associated with an increase in acceleration, resistive index, and pulsatility index, as well as a decrease in acceleration time; the postintervention values were equal to those in the contralateral normal renal artery. In the normal arteries, all of the indices remained unchanged. In patients with atherosclerotic renal artery stenosis, a high level of resistance within the renal circulation detected by duplex ultrasonography may identify patients more likely to have an unfavorable clinical response to renal artery revascularization.[17] Other investigators have failed to show a correlation between resistive index and blood pressure or renal function improvement.[18,19] It is uncertain data can be extrapolated to patients with FMD. Renal duplex scanning also may be used to assess the adequacy of intervention (Figure 20.4). In successfully treated patients, the ratio of renal artery peak systolic velocity to aortic peak systolic velocity (ie, renal-aortic ratio, RAR) decreases to less than 3.5, a value that classifies the diameter stenosis as < 60%.[20]

Multidetector CTA offers more rapid image acquisition, variable section thickness, 3D rendering, diminished helical artifacts, and smaller contrast requirements; it has assumed an increased role in the diagnosis and follow-up of renal artery FMD.[21-23] The role of magnetic resonance angiography (MRA) for evaluating renal

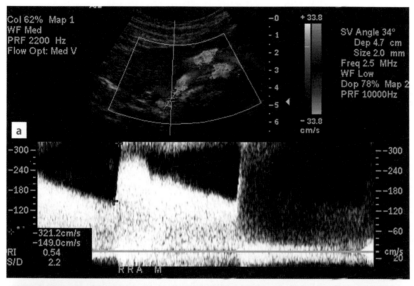

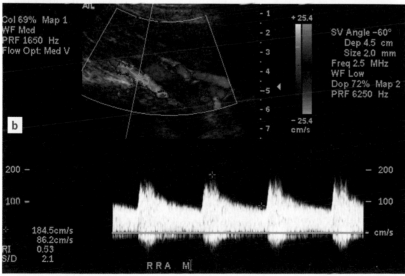

Figure 20.4 Duplex ultrasonography of the renal artery in the mid- to distal portion of the artery. (a) Note the marked increase in velocity (peak systolic velocity = 321 cm/sec, end diastolic velocity = 149 cm/sec) before angioplasty. (b) Postangioplasty duplex demonstrating normal velocities.

artery FMD remains uncertain. Even with better equipment and the use of gadolinium contrast, however, the spatial resolution of MRA (~ 1 mm) in the distal main renal arteries and its branches is inferior to catheter angiography (200–300 μm).[24] In addition, MRA may give the appearance of beading when none exists. This artifact most commonly arises due to patient movement and poor spatial resolution. However, some studies have suggested that MRA can accurately diagnose patients with FMD.[25] Fifty renal arteries were evaluated and showed a sensitivity and specificity of contrast-enhanced MRA (compared with contrast angiography) of 97% and 93%, respectively. The sensitivity was 68%, 95%, and 100% for the diagnosis of stenosis, string of beads, and aneurysm, respectively.[25] If noninvasive tests are inconclusive and the clinical suspicion for FMD is high, the patient should undergo catheter angiography for definitive diagnosis.[1]

Natural History

The natural history of renal FMD has been described in several studies.[26-29] Anatomic disease progression is difficult to ascertain because it is often impossible to determine whether the stenosis is worse in patients with medial fibroplasia who have multiple beads.[27] Angiographic disease progression, defined as a new focal lesion, worsening arterial stenosis, or enlargement of a mural aneurysm, occurs in up to 37% of renal FMD patients.[27,28]

A change in renal parenchyma may provide a better means of monitoring disease progression. Mournier-Vehier and colleagues[30] used CTA to compare mean cortical thickness and renal length in 20 patients with essential hypertension and 20 patients with hypertension and unilateral renal artery FMD. Compared to those with essential hypertension, patients with unilateral renal FMD had significantly decreased mean cortical thickness and reduced renal length. In the contralateral, unaffected kidney, cortical thickness was also markedly decreased, although renal length was preserved. Ultimately, progression of FMD is reflected by

loss of renal mass, which occurred in up to 63% of patients with FMD in one study.[31] The atrophic changes in the renal parenchyma persist even after revascularization.[31] For reasons that are not entirely clear, patients with renal artery FMD rarely progress to renal failure.

Perhaps the most accurate way to assess natural history in patients with FMD is to follow clinical parameters such as blood pressure control, and level of renal function.

Treatment of Renal Artery FMD

The aim of therapy is to achieve normal blood pressure levels based on the guidelines of the Joint National Committee on Prevention, Detection, Evaluation, and Treatment of High Blood Pressure.[32] The mainstay of therapy is percutaneous transluminal angioplasty (PTA) of the renal artery with a goal of normalizing blood pressure without the use of medications.[1]

Medical therapy

Since the underlying pathogenesis of the hypertension includes activation of the renin-angiotensin-aldosterone system and sodium retention, the initial drug class of choice in FMD is an angiotensin-converting enzyme inhibitor (ACE inhibitor) or angiotensin-receptor blocker (ARB).[33] If blood pressure is not at goal after a first-line agent, a thiazide diuretic is a good second agent to consider. If blood pressure control remains suboptimal, other agents should be added as recommended by the Joint National Committee on Prevention, Detection, Evaluation, and Treatment of High Blood Pressure.[32]

The major potential complication of this regimen is a hemodynamically mediated decline in glomerular filtration rate (GFR), especially if the stenotic lesions are severe and bilateral. The normal autoregulatory response to maintain GFR in the setting of reduced renal perfusion involves an angiotensin II–mediated preferential increase in resistance at the efferent (postcapillary) arteriole. This is blunted by blocking angiotensin II formation with an ACE inhibitor, and the effect is more pronounced with diuretic-induced volume depletion.[34] These abnormalities are virtually always reversible.

There are 2 important limitations of pursuing medical therapy alone:

- The degree of stenosis may progress and kidney function may worsen over time despite excellent blood pressure control. This is most commonly seen in patients with intimal or perimedial fibroplasia. As a result, every patient with FMD should have periodic measurement of serum creatinine along with imaging studies.
- FMD occurs most commonly in young women. Even though the blood pressure may be easily controlled with 1 or 2 antihypertensive medications, these young patients will require medications for the rest of their lives. Percutaneous revascularization may result in a cure of blood pressure, thus allowing the patients to remain medication-free.

Renal artery revascularization

The principal rationale for renal artery revascularization, either by surgery or PTA, is control of hypertension. There is also the possibility of delaying or preventing loss of renal mass, particularly in patients with intimal or perimedial disease, although this is not well established.

Hypertension is cured or improved (better blood pressure control on fewer antihypertensive agents) following renal artery revascularization (either PTA or surgery) in a large proportion of patients with FMD (Table 20.2). The reported hypertension cure rate ranges from 20% to 85%, and most remaining patients are improved.[3,45] The rate of cure of hypertension may be lower if FMD affects multiple vascular beds, or if the intrarenal vessels are involved. In one report, hypertension was cured following angioplasty in 62% versus 28% of patients with unilateral, isolated renal FMD versus systemic FMD, respectively.[3]

Data regarding preservation of kidney function are less clear. Although revascularization does not reverse cortical thinning and lost renal mass, renal function appears to be stabilized.[31]

Study	Year	No. of Patients	Technical Success (%)	BP Cure (%)	BP improved (%)	Mean F/U (mo)
Sos et al[35]	1983	31	87	59	34	16
Baert et al[36]	1990	22	83	58	21	26
Tegtmeyer et al[37]	1991	66	100	39	59	39
Bonelli et al[38]	1995	105	89	22	63	43
Jensen et al[39]	1995	30	97	39	47	12
Davidson et al[40]	1996	23	100	52	22	NR
Klow et al[41]	1998	49	98	26	44	9
Birrer et al[42]	2002	27	100	(74)		10
Surowiec et al[43]	2003	14	95	(79)		NR
de Fraissinette et al[44]	2003	70	94	14	74	39

Table 20.2 Angioplasty for Renal Artery FMD (Source: Slovut DP, Olin JW. Fibromuscular dysplasia. *N Engl J Med.* 2004;350:1862-1871. Copyright © 2004. Massachusetts Medical Society. All rights reserved.)

Virtually all patients with renal artery FMD can be successfully treated with percutaneous balloon angioplasty. Surgery is rarely necessary in the absence of a macroaneurysm. The most commonly accepted indications for angioplasty include:

- Patients with recent onset hypertension, especially young patients less likely to have concomitant atherosclerosis. In this instance the goal is cure of hypertension or at least a reduction in the number of blood pressure medications.
- Patients whose blood pressure cannot be normalized despite compliance with an appropriate medical regimen.
- Patients who are unable to tolerate antihypertensive medications or are noncompliant with their medication regimen.
- Patients with loss of parenchymal mass from ischemic nephropathy. This most commonly occurs in patients with intimal or perimedial fibroplasia.

There are reports of elderly patients diagnosed with FMD[9] or patients who have both atherosclerosis and FMD.[46] In these instances the patients often have had hypertension for many years and thus are less likely to experience a cure after angioplasty. It is reasonable to continue to treat these patients medically if the blood pressure is well controlled and the renal function is stable.

PTA has largely supplanted surgery for managing renal artery stenosis in FMD, primarily related to similar technical success rates and lower risk of the procedure. The reported technical (angiographic) success rates for PTA range from 83% to nearly 100%.[41,42] Hypertension is usually cured (22%–59%) or improved (22%–74%), but a significant proportion fail to improve (2%–30%)[35-44] (Table 20.2).

The rate of restenosis following PTA for FMD ranges from 12% to 25% over follow-up intervals of 6 months to 2 years.[39,40,41,43,44,47] Restenosis, however, is not necessarily associated with recurrent hypertension. Immediate technical success with PTA is usually determined by visual inspection during the procedure. It may be difficult to determine whether balloon dilation has been adequate when multiple sequential stenoses are present. The postangioplasty artery may look similar to the preangioplasty artery. Some angiographers will measure pressure gradients, or use intravascular ultrasonography to determine whether the PTA was adequate from an anatomic standpoint.[13] The best approach is to compare preangioplasty duplex ultrasonography to a postangioplasty duplex. If the velocities have returned to normal after angioplasty, then one can be certain that the patient was adequately dilated.[45,48]

Advances in guide wires, catheters, and balloons, as well as an improvement in operator skill, have made it possible to perform PTA for even the most complex renal artery lesions. Angioplasty is generally sufficient, as long-term renal artery patency following PTA is ~ 80%. Stenting is usually performed only for bailout in cases of a suboptimal balloon result or flow-limiting dissection.[49] Stenting in the renal artery is associated with a restenosis rate of up to 20%. Should surgical revascularization become necessary (eg, for in-stent restenosis that has recurred despite repeat stenting), patients may require more complex branch repair to bypass the occluded stent. Drug-eluting stents have not been evaluated in the treatment of renal artery stenosis due to FMD.

If the patient either has no improvement in blood pressure or an initial improvement followed by recurrence of hypertension a few weeks after PTA, a repeat angiogram and PTA should be performed. In this case, "restenosis" may actually represent inadequate angioplasty during the first procedure. Hypertension that persists despite technically successful PTA, particularly if confirmed using intravascular ultrasonography or a pressure guide wire, suggests that the cause of hypertension is unrelated to FMD.

Complications of PTA are mostly related to vascular access. In rare cases, renal artery perforation, dissection, or segmental renal infarction may occur.[37] The rate of complications has decreased, a trend attributed in part to use of more flexible guiding catheters and lower heparin doses. In a series of 268 patients who underwent 320 procedures, the complication rate decreased from 16% in 1998 to 3% in 2001.[50,51]

Patients who undergo percutaneous revascularization should undergo periodic duplex ultrasonography examinations to detect disease progression, restenosis, or loss of kidney volume.[52] One protocol is to image soon after renal artery angioplasty, and repeating this at 6 months and every 6 months thereafter or whenever there is recurrence or worsening of hypertension, or unexplained increase in the serum creatinine.

Surgical revascularization

Before the advent of PTA, surgical revascularization was the primary therapeutic alternative for patients with suboptimally controlled hypertension. In contemporary surgical series, technical success rates are > 88%, long-term blood pressure was cured in 33% to 63%, and improved in 24% to 57%.[54,55] Improvement or stabilization of renal function was seen in up to 92% of patients. Surgical cure rates are lower in older patients and those with hypertension of longer duration, a greater degree of concomitant atherosclerotic disease, and more complex disease necessitating branch vessel repair.[55]

Occasionally, renal artery aneurysms may be identified in patients with FMD (Figure 20.5). Aneurysms may rupture or lead to infarction from embolization. Renal artery aneurysms may be treated percutaneously using a covered stent graft or repaired surgically with minimal morbidity or mortality.[56-58]

Although both surgery and PTA lead to similar technical success rates, surgery is associated with a higher morbidity and mortality.[59] Thus, surgical revascularization is usually reserved for patients who have failed PTA or

whose arterial anatomy is not amenable to PTA.[49] This includes patients who have disease in secondary branch vessels, long stenotic segment, or aneurysms, and thus might need complex, sometimes *ex vivo* reconstructions. Given the morbidity associated with surgery, this modality is considered only in patients in whom medical therapy alone is insufficient to control blood pressure and/or there is evidence of significant loss of renal parenchymal mass.

Given that surgical revascularization is usually limited to complex cases, reported success and complication rates are probably higher than if simpler cases were included. In one series of 26 patients, 6 of whom had failed PTA and 20 who were unsuitable for PTA, there were 2 bypass occlusions resulting in renal loss, and 5 significant nonrenal complications during a median follow-up of 2.4 years.[60] Cumulative patency at 1 and 3 years was 89% and 82%, respectively.

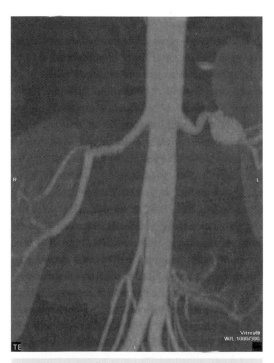

Figure 20.5 CTA demonstrating medial fibroplasia bilaterally. There is a large aneurysm in the left renal artery. This 32-year-old patient underwent angioplasty of the right renal artery and an aortorenal bypass of the left renal artery with exclusion of the aneurysm.

Cerebrovascular Fibromuscular Dysplasia

Extracranial cerebrovascular involvement occurs in approximately 70% of patients (unpublished data). Often, there is bilateral involvement of the internal carotid arteries, as well as coexisting vertebral artery disease. FMD is described less commonly in the external carotid, middle cerebral, anterior cerebral, basilar, and anterior communicating arteries.[61] Cerebrovascular FMD occurs more frequently in women, with mean age at diagnosis of 50 years.[61,62]

Cerebrovascular FMD may be asymptomatic or associated with a variety of nonspecific symptoms including headache, mental distress, lightheadedness, or syncope.[61,64-65] Tinnitus, or a "swishing" sound synchronous with the pulse, is a frequent complaint.[66] FMD may be discovered during the evaluation of a patient who presents with a cervical bruit or when an imaging study is performed for unrelated reasons.[1,8,67]

FMD of the carotid or vertebral arteries may result in transient ischemic attack, amaurosis fugax, stroke, Horner's syndrome, or cranial nerve palsies.[61,64-65]

In one series, 18 of 32 (56%) female patients with cerebrovascular FMD presented with a sudden, focal neurologic deficit.[62] Symptoms may be related to critical stenosis or occlusions of major arteries, to rupture of intracranial aneurysms, or from intravascular thrombi in stenotic regions embolizing to the cerebral circulation.

The prevalence of intracranial aneurysms in patients with FMD has been reported to be as high as 51%.[61,68] This value, however, may be overestimated because of selection bias.[68] When patients who presented with subarachnoid hemorrhage are excluded from the prevalence estimates, the prevalence of incidental, asymptomatic cerebral aneurysms in patients with internal carotid or vertebral artery fibromuscular dysplasia is 7.3%.[68] Patients with extracranial FMD should undergo MRA of the head to exclude intracranial aneurysm.[45]

Several imaging modalities may be used to detect cerebrovascular FMD. Duplex ultrasonography of the carotid arteries may demonstrate irregular patterns of stenosis and aneurysm, but compared to angiography, color-coded duplex ultrasonography has a lower sensitivity for detecting cerebrovascular FMD.[69,70] Since FMD affects the middle and distal portion of the carotid and vertebral arteries at the level of the first and second cervical vertebrae, it is important to image the carotid arteries as distally as possible. CTA, MRA, and catheter-based angiography are useful for diagnosing cerebrovascular FMD (Figure 20.6).

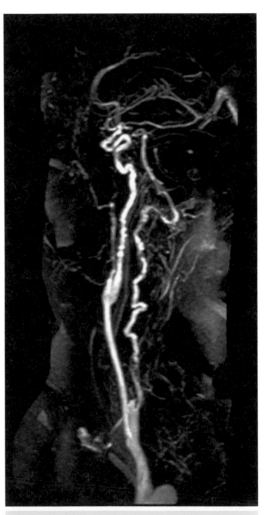

Figure 20.6 MRA showing the typical appearance (string of beads) in the carotid and vertebral arteries.

Treatment of Cerebrovascular FMD

The natural history of cerebrovascular FMD of the medial type is generally benign.[62,71] In one study of 49 patients who had involvement of 88 internal carotid arteries, all patients who were initially asymptomatic remained so during follow-up.[71] Therefore, it is reasonable to treat asymptomatic patients or patients with nonspecific symptoms (headache, tinnitus, lightheadedness) with antiplatelet therapy, such as aspirin, for stroke prevention.[1,66] However, patients presenting with amaurosis fugax, hemispheric TIA, Horner's syndrome, cranial nerve palsies, or stroke should be treated with angioplasty or surgery.

Surgical therapy

Before the advent of angioplasty, surgery was the mainstay of therapy for patients with symptomatic cerebrovascular FMD. The surgical technique depended upon the type of lesion and its location, but the most widely used procedure was graduated intraluminal dilatation alone,[67,72-74] or in combination with other procedures such as resection of the diseased segment and primary anastomosis, autogenous saphenous vein grafting, aneurysm resection, and carotid endarterectomy.[73,75,76] Operative balloon angioplasty has also been used,[77] and polytetrafluoroethylene-(PTFE)-covered endografts have been deployed through a transverse incision in the neck and open puncture of the common carotid artery.[78]

Surgery is the recommended treatment if there are associated aneurysms in patients with cerebrovascular FMD.[79,80] The short- and long-term results following surgical repair are excellent.[47,67,73,79,80]

Endovascular therapy

While there have been no randomized, controlled trials comparing surgery and angioplasty, percutaneous angioplasty has become the preferred treatment for symptomatic cerebrovascular FMD.[1,81,82] It is usually not necessary to insert a stent for fibromuscular dysplasia of the carotid or vertebral arteries. However, if there is a suboptimal result with angioplasty alone, or if there is an associated dissection of the carotid artery, then stent implantation may be necessary.

Fibromuscular Dysplasia in Other Vascular Territories

In the lower extremities, FMD occurs most often in the iliac arteries, although it has been described in the femoral, popliteal, and peroneal arteries as well (Figure 20.7). Patients with lower-extremity FMD may present with intermittent claudication, critical limb ischemia, or embolization presenting as painful, cyanotic, or gangrenous toes.[83] In the upper extremities,

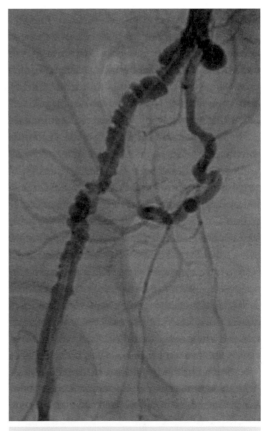

Figure 20.7 Medial fibroplasia in the external iliac artery. (Courtesy of J. Michael Bacharach, MD.)

FMD may occur in the subclavian, axillary, or brachial arteries. For symptomatic upper- and lower-extremity FMD, angiographic evaluation and percutaneous balloon angioplasty are warranted.[83-85]

FMD in the visceral arteries typically involves the celiac, superior mesenteric, inferior mesenteric, hepatic, and splenic arteries. Intestinal angina occurs when at least 2 of the major mesenteric arteries are obstructed. Patients may present with the classic triad of postprandial abdominal pain, weight loss, and an epigastric bruit. In rare cases, the stenosis progresses to total occlusion leading to acute intestinal ischemia.[86,87] Treatment options include percutaneous revascularization or surgical bypass. FMD has also been rarely reported in the coronary arteries.

treatment. FMD should be considered under the following circumstances:

1. A young person with a cervical bruit. It is important for the vascular laboratory to image the mid and distal portion of the carotid (or renal) artery.
2. A patient describing a "swishing" (swooshing, whooshing) sound or pulisitile tinnitus in the ear(s).
3. Any patient (especially those under 60 years) presenting with a TIA or stroke.
4. Any patient with a dissection of any artery (other than the aorta).
5. Onset of hypertension in individuals 35 years old or younger or difficult to control hypertension in anyone under the age of 55.

Summary

Fibromuscular dysplasia (FMD) is a non atherosclerotic non inflammatory vascular disease that primarily affects women from age 20-60 but may also occur in infants and children, men and the elderly. It most commonly affects the renal and carotid arteries but has been observed in almost every artery in the body.

When there is renal artery involvement, the most common presentation is hypertension. When there is FMD in the carotid or vertebral arteries, the patient may present with TIA/stroke or dissection. An increasing number of patients are asymptomatic and only discovered incidentally when imaging is performed for some other reason or by the detection of an asymptomatic bruit. Treatment consists of antiplatelet therapy for asymptomatic individuals and percutaneous balloon angioplasty for patients with indications for intervention. Patients with aneurysms should be treated with either a covered stent or open surgical repair.

There are a large number of patients with FMD who are either not diagnosed or for whom there is a significant delay in diagnosis and thus

References

1. Slovut DP, Olin JW. Fibromuscular dysplasia. *N Engl J Med.* 2004;350(18):1862-1871.
2. Olin JW. Syndromes that mimic vasculitis. *Curr Opin Cardiol.* 1991;6:768-774.
3. Luscher TF, Keller HM, Imhof HG, et al. Fibromuscular hyperplasia: extension of the disease and therapeutic outcome. Results of the University Hospital Zurich Cooperative Study on Fibromuscular Hyperplasia. *Nephron.* 1986;44(Suppl 1):109-114.
4. Stanley JC, Gewertz BL, Bove EL, Sottiurai V, Fry WJ. Arterial fibrodysplasia. Histopathologic character and current etiologic concepts. *Arch Surg.* 1975;110(5):561-566.
5. Stokes JB, Bonsib SM, McBride JW. Diffuse intimal fibromuscular dysplasia with multiorgan failure. *Arch Intern Med.* 1996;156(22):2611-2614.
6. Kojima A, Shindo S, Kubota K, et al. Successful surgical treatment of a patient with multiple visceral artery aneurysms due to fibromuscular dysplasia. *Cardiovasc Surg.* 2002;10(2): 157-160.

7. Begelman SM, Olin JW. Fibromuscular dysplasia. *Curr Opin Rheumatol.* 2000;12(1):41-47.

8. Harrison EG Jr, McCormack LJ. Pathologic classification of renal arterial disease in renovascular hypertension. *Mayo Clin Proc.* 1971;46(3):161-167.

9. Pascual A, Bush HS, Copley JB. Renal fibromuscular dysplasia in elderly persons. *Am J Kidney Dis.* 2005;45(4):e63-e66.

10. Safian RD, Textor SC. Renal-artery stenosis. *N Engl J Med.* 2001;344(6):431-442.

11. Andreoni KA, Weeks SM, Gerber DA, et al. Incidence of donor renal fibromuscular dysplasia: does it justify routine angiography? *Transplantation.* 2002;73(7):1112-1116.

12. Neymark E, LaBerge JM, Hirose R, et al. Arteriographic detection of renovascular disease in potential renal donors: incidence and effect on donor surgery. *Radiology.* 2000;214(3):755-760.

13. Gowda MS, Loeb AL, Crouse LJ, Kramer PH. Complementary roles of color-flow duplex imaging and intravascular ultrasound in the diagnosis of renal artery fibromuscular dysplasia: should renal arteriography serve as the "gold standard"? *J Am Coll Cardiol.* 2003;41(8):1305-1311.

14. Carman TL, Olin JW, Czum J, Noninvasive imaging of the renal arteries. *Urol Clin North Am.* 2001;28(4):815-826.

15. Olin JW, Piedmonte MR, Young JR, DeAnna S, Grubb M, Childs MB. The utility of duplex ultrasound scanning of the renal arteries for diagnosing significant renal artery stenosis. *Ann Intern Med.* 1995;122(11):833-838.

16. Marana I, Airoldi F, Burdick L, et al. Effects of balloon angioplasty and stent implantation on intrarenal echo-Doppler velocimetric indices. *Kidney Int.* 1998;53(6):1795-1800.

17. Radermacher J, Weinkove R, Haller H. Techniques for predicting a favourable response to renal angioplasty in patients with renovascular disease. *Curr Opin Nephrol Hypertens.* 2001;10(6):799-805.

18. Garcia-Criado A, Gilabert R, Nicolau C, et al. Value of Doppler sonography for predicting clinical outcome after renal artery revascularization in atherosclerotic renal artery stenosis. *J Ultrasound Med.* 2005;24(12):1641-1647.

19. Zeller T, Muller C, Frank U, et al. Stent angioplasty of severe atherosclerotic ostial renal artery stenosis in patients with diabetes mellitus and nephrosclerosis. *Catheter Cardiovasc Interv.* 2003;58(4):510-515.

20. Edwards JM, Zaccardi MJ, Strandness DE Jr. A preliminary study of the role of duplex scanning in defining the adequacy of treatment of patients with renal artery fibromuscular dysplasia. *J Vasc Surg.* 1992;15(4):604-609.

21. Funabashi N, Komiyama N, Komuro I. Fibromuscular dysplasia in renovascular hypertension demonstrated by multislice CT: comparison with conventional angiogram and intravascular ultrasound. *Heart.* 2003;89(6):639.

22. Rubin GD. MDCT imaging of the aorta and peripheral vessels. *Eur J Radiol.* 2003;45 (Suppl 1):S42-S49.

23. Sabharwal R, Vladica P, Coleman P. Multidetector spiral CT renal angiography in the diagnosis of renal artery fibromuscular dysplasia. *Eur J Radiol.* 2007;61(3):520-527.

24. Marcos HB, Choyke PL. Magnetic resonance angiography of the kidney. *Semin Nephrol.* 2000;20(5):450-455.

25. Willoteaux S, Faivre-Pierret M, Moranne O, et al. Fibromuscular dysplasia of the main renal arteries: comparison of contrast-enhanced MR angiography with digital subtraction angiography. *Radiology.* 2006;241(3): 922-929.

26. Cragg AH, Smith TP, Thompson BH, et al. Incidental fibromuscular dysplasia in potential renal donors: long-term clinical follow-up. *Radiology.* 1989;172(1):145-147.

27. Goncharenko V, Gerlock AJ Jr, Shaff MI, Hollifield JW. Progression of renal artery fibromuscular dysplasia in 42 patients as seen on angiography. *Radiology.* 1981;139(1):45-51.

28. Kincaid OW, Davis GD, Hallermann FJ, Hunt JC. Fibromuscular dysplasia of the renal arteries. Arteriographic features, classification, and observations on natural history of the disease. *Am J Roentgenol Radium Ther Nucl Med.* 1968;104(2):271-282.

29. Schreiber MJ, Pohl MA, Novick AC. The natural history of atherosclerotic and fibrous

renal artery disease. *Urol Clin North Am.* 1984;11(3):383-392.

30. Mounier-Vehier C, Lions C, Jaboureck O, et al. Parenchymal consequences of fibromuscular dysplasia renal artery stenosis. *Am J Kidney Dis.* 2002;40(6):1138-1145.

31. Mounier-Vehier C, Haulon S, Devos P, et al. Renal atrophy outcome after revascularization in fibromuscular dysplasia disease. *J Endovasc Ther.* 2002;9(5):605-613.

32. Chobanian AV, Bakris GL, Black HR, et al. The Seventh Report of the Joint National Committee on Prevention, Detection, Evaluation, and Treatment of High Blood Pressure: The JNC 7 Report. *JAMA.* 2003;289(19):2560-2571.

33. Tullis MJ, Caps MT, Zierler RE, et al. Blood pressure, antihypertensive medication, and atherosclerotic renal artery stenosis. *Am J Kidney Dis.* 1999;33(4):675-681.

34. Hricik DE, Dunn MJ. Angiotensin-converting enzyme inhibitor-induced renal failure: causes, consequences, and diagnostic uses. *J Am Soc Nephrol.* 1990;1(6):845-858.

35. Sos TA, Pickering TG, Sniderman K, et al. Percutaneous transluminal renal angioplasty in renovascular hypertension due to atheroma or fibromuscular dysplasia. *N Engl J Med.* 1983;309:274-279.

36. Baert AL, Wilms G, Amery A, Vermylen J, Suy R. Percutaneous transluminal renal angioplasty: initial results and long-term follow-up in 202 patients. *Cardiovasc Intervent Radiol.* 1990;13:22-28.

37. Tegtmeyer CJ, Selby JB, Hartwell GD, Ayers C, Tegtmeyer V. Results and complications of angioplasty in fibromuscular disease. *Circulation.* 1991;83:Suppl I:I-155–I-161.

38. Bonelli FS, McKusick MA, Textor SC, et al. Renal artery angioplasty: technical results and clinical outcome in 320 patients. *Mayo Clin Proc.* 1995;70:1041-1052.

39. Jensen G, Zachrisson BF, Delin K, Volkmann R, Aurell M. Treatment of renovascular hypertension: one year results of renal angioplasty. *Kidney Int.* 1995;48:1936-1945.

40. Davidson RA, Barri Y, Wilcox CS. Predictors of cure of hypertension in fibromuscular reno-

vascular disease. *Am J Kidney Dis.* 1996;28:334-338.

41. Klow NE, Paulsen D, Vatne K, Rokstad B, Lien B, Fauchald P. Percutaneous transluminal renal artery angioplasty using the coaxial technique: ten years of experience from 591 procedures in 419 patients. *Acta Radiol.* 1998;39:594-603.

42. Birrer M, Do DD, Mahler F, Triller J, Baumgartner I. Treatment of renal artery fibromuscular dysplasia with balloon angioplasty: a prospective follow-up study. *Eur J Vasc Endovasc Surg.* 2002;23:146-52.

43. Surowiec SM, Sivamurthy N, Rhodes JM, et al. Percutaneous therapy for renal artery fibromuscular dysplasia. *Ann Vasc Surg.* 2003;17:650-5.

44. de Fraissinette B, Garcier JM, Dieu V, et al. Percutaneous transluminal angioplasty of dysplastic stenoses of the renal artery: results on 70 adults. *Cardiovasc Intervent Radiol.* 2003;26:46-51.

45. Slovut DP, Olin JW. Fibromuscular dysplasia. *Curr Treat Options Cardiovasc Med.* 2005;7(2):159-169.

46. Aqel R, Gupta R, Zoghbi G. Coexistent fibromuscular dysplasia and atherosclerotic renal artery stenosis. *J Invasive Cardiol.* 2005;17(10):572-573.

47. Oertle M, Do DD, Baumgartner I, Triller J, Mahler F. Discrepancy of clinical and angiographic results in the follow-up of percutaneous transluminal renal angioplasty (PTRA). *Vasa.* 1998;27(3):154-157.

48. Edwards JM, Zaccardi MJ, Strandness DE Jr. A preliminary study of the role of duplex scanning in defining the adequacy of treatment of patients with renal artery fibromuscular dysplasia. *J Vasc Surg.* 1992;15(4):604-609.

49. Hirsch AT, Haskal ZJ, Hertzer NR, et al. ACC/AHA Guidelines for the management of patients with peripheral arterial disease (lower extremity, renal, mesenteric, and abdominal aortic): a collaborative report from the American Association of Vascular Surgery/Society for Vascular Surgery, Society for Cardiovascular Angiography and Interventions, Society for Interventional Radiology, Society for Vascular Medicine and Biology and the American Col-

lege of Cardiology/American Heart Association Task Force on Practice Guidelines. *Circulation*. 2006.

50. Zeller T. Percutaneous endovascular therapy of renal artery stenosis: technical and clinical developments in the past decade. *J Endovasc Ther*. 2004;11(Suppl 2):II96-106.

51. Zeller T, Frank U, Muller C, et al. Technological advances in the design of catheters and devices used in renal artery interventions: impact on complications. *J Endovasc Ther*. 2003;10(5):1006-1014.

52. Olin JW, Kaufman JA, Bluemke DA, et al. Atherosclerotic Vascular Disease Conference. American Heart Association, Imaging, Writing Group IV. *Circulation*. 2004;109:2626-2623.

53. Reiher L, Pfeiffer T, Sandmann W. Long-term results after surgical reconstruction for renal artery fibromuscular dysplasia. *Eur J Vasc Endovasc Surg*. 2000;20(6):556-559.

54. Marekovic Z, Mokos I, Krhen I, Goreta NR, Roncevic T. Long-term outcome after surgical kidney revascularization for fibromuscular dysplasia and atherosclerotic renal artery stenosis. *J Urol*. 2004;171(3):1043-1045.

55. Novick AC, Ziegelbaum M, Vidt DG, Gifford RW Jr, Pohl MA, Goormastic M. Trends in surgical revascularization for renal artery disease. Ten years' experience. *JAMA*. 1987;257(4):498-501.

56. Bisschops RH, Popma JJ, Meyerovitz MF. Treatment of fibromuscular dysplasia and renal artery aneurysm with use of a stent-graft. *J Vasc Interv Radiol*. 2001;12(6):757-760.

57. English WP, Pearce JD, Craven TE, et al. Surgical management of renal artery aneurysms. *J Vasc Surg*. 2004;40(1):53-60.

58. Pfeiffer T, Reiher L, Grabitz K, et al. Reconstruction for renal artery aneurysm: operative techniques and long-term results. *J Vasc Surg*. 2003;37(2):293-300.

59. Mackrell PJ, Langan EM III, Sullivan TM, et al. Management of renal artery stenosis: effects of a shift from surgical to percutaneous therapy on indications and outcomes. *Ann Vasc Surg*. 2003;17(1):54-59.

60. Carmo M, Bower TC, Mozes G, et al. Surgical management of renal fibromuscular dysplasia: challenges in the endovascular era. *Ann Vasc Surg*. 2005;19(2):208-217.

61. Schievink WI, Bjornsson J. Fibromuscular dysplasia of the internal carotid artery: a clinicopathological study. *Clin Neuropathol*. 1996;15(1):2-6.

62. Wesen CA, Elliott BM. Fibromuscular dysplasia of the carotid arteries. *Am J Surg*. 1986;151(4):448-451.

63. Mettinger KL, Ericson K. Fibromuscular dysplasia and the brain. I. Observations on angiographic, clinical and genetic characteristics. *Stroke*. 1982;13(1):46-52.

64. Mettinger KL. Fibromuscular dysplasia and the brain. II. Current concept of the disease. *Stroke*. 1982;13(1):53-58.

65. Wells RP, Smith RR. Fibromuscular dysplasia of the internal carotid artery: a long term follow-up. *Neurosurgery*. 1982;10(1):39-43.

66. Leary MC, Finley A, Caplan LR. Cerebrovascular complications of fibromuscular dysplasia. *Curr Treat Options Cardiovasc Med*. 2004;6(3):237-248.

67. Chiche L, Bahnini A, Koskas F, Kieffer E. Occlusive fibromuscular disease of arteries supplying the brain: results of surgical treatment. *Ann Vasc Surg*. 1997;11(5):496-504.

68. Rinkel GJ, Djibuti M, Algra A, Van Gijn J. Prevalence and risk of rupture of intracranial aneurysms: a systematic review. *Stroke*. 1998;29(1):251-256.

69. Arning C. Nonatherosclerotic disease of the cervical arteries: role of ultrasonography for diagnosis. *Vasa*. 2001;30(3):160-167.

70. Furie DM, Tien RD. Fibromuscular dysplasia of arteries of the head and neck: imaging findings. *AJR Am J Roentgenol*. 1994;162(5):1205-1209.

71. Stewart MT, Moritz MW, Smith RB III, Fulenwider JT, Perdue GD. The natural history of carotid fibromuscular dysplasia. *J Vasc Surg*. 1986;3(2):305-310.

72. Collins GJ Jr, Rich NM, Clagett GP, Spebar MJ, Salander JM. Fibromuscular dysplasia of the internal carotid arteries. Clinical experience and follow-up. *Ann Surg*. 1981;194(1):89-96.

73. Effeney DJ, Krupski WC, Stoney RJ, Ehrenfeld WK. Fibromuscular dysplasia of the carotid artery. *Aust N Z J Surg*. 1983;53(6):527-531.

74. Starr DS, Lawrie GM, Morris GC Jr. Fibro-muscular disease of carotid arteries: long term results of graduated internal dilatation. *Stroke.* 1981;12(2):196-199.

75. Moreau P, Albat B, Thevenet A. Fibromus-cular dysplasia of the internal carotid artery: long-term surgical results. *J Cardiovasc Surg.* (Torino) 1993;34(6):465-472.

76. Martin EC, Diamond NG, Casarella WJ. Percutaneous transluminal angioplasty in non-atherosclerotic disease. *Radiology.* 1980;135(1):27-33.

77. Smith LL, Smith DC, Killeen JD, Hasso AN. Operative balloon angioplasty in the treatment of internal carotid artery fibromuscular dyspla-sia. *J Vasc Surg.* 1987;6(5):482-487.

78. Finsterer J, Strassegger J, Haymerle A, Hag-muller G. Bilateral stenting of symptomatic and asymptomatic internal carotid artery stenosis due to fibromuscular dysplasia. *J Neurol Neuro-surg Psychiatry.* 2000;69(5):683-686.

79. Faggioli GL, Freyrie A, Stella A, et al. Extracra-nial internal carotid artery aneurysms: results of a surgical series with long-term follow-up. *J Vasc Surg.* 1996;23(4):587-594.

80. Bour P, Taghavi I, Bracard S, Frisch N, Fieve G. Aneurysms of the extracranial internal carotid artery due to fibromuscular dysplasia: results of surgical management. *Ann Vasc Surg.* 1992;6(3):205-208.

81. Van Damme H, Sakalihasan N, Limet R. Fibromuscular dysplasia of the internal carotid artery. Personal experience with 13 cases and literature review. *Acta Chir Belg.* 1999;99(4):163-168.

82. Brown MM. Balloon angioplasty for cere-brovascular disease. *Neurol Res.* 1992;14(2 Suppl):159-163.

83. Sauer L, Reilly LM, Goldstone J, Ehrenfeld WK, Hutton JE, Stoney RJ. Clinical spec-trum of symptomatic external iliac fibro-muscular dysplasia. *J Vasc Surg.* 1990;12(4): 488-495.

84. Yoshida T, Ohashi I, Suzuki S, Iwai T. Fibro-muscular disease of the brachial artery with digital emboli treated effectively by translumi-nal angioplasty. *Cardiovasc Intervent Radiol.* 1994;17(2):99-101.

85. Mandke JV, Sharma S, Phatak AM, Sanzgiri VP, Loya YS, Desai DM. Catheter atherectomy of intimal fibroplasia of the common iliac artery. *Cathet Cardiovasc Diagn.* 1993;30(1): 30-32.

86. Hamed RM, Ghandour K. Abdominal angina and intestinal gangrene—a catastrophic presen-tation of arterial fibromuscular dysplasia: case report and review of the literature. *J Pediatr Surg.* 1997;32(9):1379-1380.

87. Horie T, Seino Y, Miyauchi Y, et al. Unusual petal-like fibromuscular dysplasia as a cause of acute abdomen and circulatory shock. *Jpn Heart J.* 2002;43(3):301-305.

Part 7

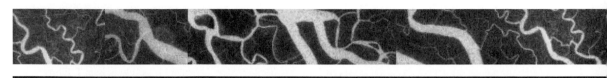

Venous Disease

21

Deep Venous Thrombosis and Pulmonary Embolism

John A. O'Dea, Thomas J. Kiernan, and Michael R. Jaff

Venous thromboembolism (VTE) represents one of the most common cardiovascular disorders facing the clinician in modern medicine today. The risk factors for the development of *deep venous thrombosis (DVT)* and *pulmonary embolism (PE)* are common, and many patients hospitalized have several, including advanced age, obesity, and major medical comorbidities (congestive heart failure, chronic lung disease, malignancy). Prevention of VTE is critical in patients who possess risk factors, and a myriad of strategies exist, largely based on the severity of risk. The symptoms and signs of these disorders are nonspecific and require a high index of suspicion by the clinician, who may then use a wide array of accurate diagnostic tests to confirm or refute the presence of VTE. Once the diagnosis of acute VTE is confirmed, standard anticoagulation is commonly employed, using a variety of anticoagulant agents administered both parenterally and orally. Recent interest in thrombus removal has focused attention on thrombolytic agents and catheter-based mechanical thrombectomy devices. The duration and intensity of anticoagulation depends on the underlying medical illnesses and frequency of recurrent events. Cardiovascular specialists must possess an in-depth knowledge of this evolving field to offer the most appropriate therapy to their patients.

Etiology and Clinical Presentation

VTE includes DVT and PE. It is a major cause of morbidity and mortality in the United States, where an estimated 2 million people develop DVT annually. DVT progresses to PE in 600,000 of these patients and is fatal in 60,000 cases.[1,2] Apart from the significant mortality risk, the morbidity of the debilitating postthrombotic syndrome can arise in up to one-third of patients, striking in particular those with extensive DVT and recurrent disease.[3]

Venous thrombi typically form along the valve cusps within the soleal sinuses of the calf as a result of platelet aggregation and altered venous flow dynamics. The propensity of the thrombus to embolize is greatest in the early phase (first 7 days), when the thrombus is composed of red blood cells, white blood cells, and platelets within a fibrin mesh. The thrombus ultimately becomes adherent to the vessel wall.

The risk of developing VTE is directly related to 3 factors first described by Rudolph Virchow in the nineteenth century and now known as *Virchow's triad:* venous endothelial damage, localized or systemic hypercoagulability, and stasis of venous blood.

Risk factors for VTE are increasingly common as the population ages and becomes more overweight, and the prevalence of malignancy continues to rise. Virtually any patient admitted to a hospital for care of an underlying illness is at risk of VTE.[4]

Given the need to identify risk for VTE in patients prospectively, investigators have reported the use of electronic alerts. In a large prospective randomized study of hospitalized patients at risk of VTE, an electronic alert system notified admitting physicians of the need for prophylaxis against VTE.[5] The physicians for the "control patients" did not receive an alert. After 90 days, there was a statistically significant reduction in documented VTE rates among the patients whose physicians were alerted.

Diagnosis of Acute Pulmonary Embolus

Chest Radiography

Most patients with PE have an abnormal but nonspecific chest radiograph. Common radiographic findings include atelectasis, pleural effusion, pulmonary infiltrates, and elevation of a hemidiaphragm. Classic findings of pulmonary infarction such as a pleural-based, wedge-shaped opacity at the costophrenic angle indicating pulmonary infarction (Hampton's hump) or decreased vascularity in a segment of lung distal to a pulmonary embolus (Westermark's sign) may suggest the diagnosis, but they are infrequent. A normal chest radiograph in the setting of severe dyspnea and hypoxemia without evidence of bronchospasm or anatomic

cardiac shunt is strongly suggestive of PE. The chest radiograph cannot be used to conclusively diagnose or exclude PE. Other processes such as pneumonia, congestive heart failure, pneumothorax, or rib fracture may cause symptoms similar to acute PE and should be considered. The confirmed presence of musculoskeletal or cardiopulmonary diseases does not necessarily exclude the possibility of acute PE. In the Prospective Investigation of Pulmonary Embolism Detection (PIOPED) study,[4] the chest radiograph was abnormal in 98 of 117 (84%) patients, with the most common abnormalities being atelectasis and/or parenchymal abnormalities occurring in 79 of 117 (68%) individuals. The findings of dyspnea, tachypnea, pleuritic pain, atelectasis, or a parenchymal abnormality on the chest radiograph was present in 115 of 117 (98%) patients with PE.

Electrocardiography

The electrocardiogram cannot be relied upon for the diagnosis of acute PE. Findings in acute PE are generally nonspecific and include T-wave changes, ST-segment abnormalities, and left or right axis deviation. Even with massive or submassive PE, manifestations such as the S1Q3T3 pattern, right bundle branch block, "P pulmonale," or right axis deviation occurred only in 26% of patients. The low frequency of specific electrocardiographic changes associated with PE was confirmed in the PIOPED study.[4] Nonspecific ST-segment or T-wave changes were the most common electrocardiographic abnormalities and were noted in 44 of 89 (49%) patients.

Arterial Blood Gas Analysis

Hypoxemia is common in acute PE. In the PIOPED subset of patients suspected of PE without preexisting cardiopulmonary disease, the PaO_2 and A-a gradient values were compared.[5] Interestingly, patients with and without PE could not be distinguished based upon either of these values. Although the A-a gradient is usually elevated in PE, it may rarely be normal in patients without preexisting cardiopulmonary disease.

D-dimer Testing

D-dimer represents a specific derivative of cross-linked fibrin and has been extensively evaluated in the setting of suspected acute DVT and PE. A normal *enzyme-linked immunosorbent assay (ELISA)* appears sensitive in excluding PE. When a positive D-dimer level is considered to be ≥ 500 µg/L, the sensitivity and specificity for PE have been shown to be 98% and 39%, respectively.[6] However, many clinical conditions in addition to acute thromboembolism are associated with an elevated D-dimer level. While the sensitivity of the D-dimer appears high, the specificity is not high enough to be diagnostic.

A negative D-dimer assay together with a respiratory rate < 20 breaths per minute, and a pO_2 > 80 mm Hg, has proven to be very sensitive in excluding acute PE.[7] Symptoms, signs, radiographic findings, electrocardiography, and the plasma D-dimer assay cannot be considered diagnostic of PE or DVT. When these entities are suspected, further evaluation with noninvasive or invasive testing is necessary.

Formal clinical prediction rules have since been created and validated that can help even the novice clinician determine the pretest probability for DVT and PE. In one prospective clinical trial, the SimpliRED assay was used together with a scoring system utilizing parameters that were readily available in the emergency department.[8]

Cardiac Troponin

Patients with PE may have elevated troponin levels. Elevated troponin is specific for cardiac myocyte damage, and the right ventricle appears to be the source of the enzyme elevation in acute PE. Cardiac troponin T and troponin I levels have been found to be elevated in acute PE. Several studies have suggested that troponin levels may be elevated in acute PE,[9] and one study suggested that an elevated level might be of

prognostic value.[10] Troponin levels are not sensitive enough to exclude PE when clinical suspicion is low without additional diagnostic testing.

Ventilation/Perfusion Scanning and Pulmonary Arteriography

Based on well-designed, prospective clinical trials, when the *ventilation/perfusion scan (V/Q scan)* is nondiagnostic, it should be interpreted together with the index of clinical suspicion.[11] In the PIOPED study, the utility of V/Q scanning combined with clinical assessment of patients with suspected PE was prospectively evaluated.[12] Patients with confirmed PE had scans that were high, intermediate, or low probability, as did most patients without PE. Although the specificity of high-probability scans was 97%, the sensitivity was only 41%. If the clinical scenario suggests PE, the diagnosis of this condition should be rigorously pursued even when the lung scan is low or intermediate probability. When the V/Q scan is normal, PE is essentially excluded. A nondiagnostic scan requires further evaluation.

In the setting of a nondiagnostic V/Q scan, performance of lower-extremity venous duplex ultrasonography is a reasonable strategy. If this is positive for DVT, treatment can be instituted and no additional studies are needed. When the ultrasound is negative, PE cannot, however, be definitively excluded, since ultrasonography is not adequately sensitive when there are no symptoms or signs of DVT on examination.

Spiral (Helical) Computerized Tomographic Pulmonary Arteriography

The use of computed tomography (CT) scanning has become the initial confirmatory diagnostic test for suspected PE in modern clinical practice. Administration of iodinated contrast via a peripheral vein is required for vascular imaging of the pulmonary vessels. Spiral CT may reveal emboli in the main, lobar, or segmental pulmonary arteries with > 90% sensitivity and specificity. Three-dimensional reconstruction techniques (multiplanar re-formation) can be applied to the opacified pulmonary vasculature to better define vessels located within the plane that has been sectioned. Goodman and colleagues[13] have strongly endorsed the incorporation of CT scanning into diagnostic algorithms for PE. Studies evaluating spiral CT to determine sensitivity and specificity for acute PE have revealed a range of 53% to 100% and 81% to 97%, respectively, for these parameters.[14] Different study designs, patient exclusion criteria, levels of experience, and reading protocols have accounted for some of the differences.

The sensitivity for PE in smaller (subsegmental) vessels remains suboptimal, and the importance of such small emboli also is controversial.

An important advantage of spiral CT over V/Q scanning in suspected PE is the ability to define nonvascular etiologies for symptoms, including pneumonia, aortic dissection, and pneumothorax. The most common relative contraindications to performing contrast-enhanced spiral CT scanning are renal insufficiency and contrast allergy. The cost-effectiveness of utilizing spiral CT scanning for suspected PE has been studied. Because of the frequency of nondiagnostic V/Q scans, spiral CT scanning may prove to reduce cost in the evaluation of patients with suspected PE.[15]

Some investigators have suggested that a single contrast injection will provide adequate imaging of the pulmonary vasculature and peripheral venous segments of the lower extremities. CT venography is also very helpful in determining the presence of extrinsic compression on pelvic veins, increasing the propensity for iliac venous thrombosis. Previous studies have suggested the potential for diagnosing DVT, PE, or both with one contrast injection.[16] Nonetheless, algorithms for the diagnosis of PE include clinical probabilities, laboratory testing, and imaging.[17]

Magnetic Resonance Angiography

Magnetic resonance angiography (MRA) has been utilized to evaluate clinically suspected PE.[18] In view of relatively frequent contraindications to CT scanning such as renal insufficiency, further evaluation of MRA for PE diagnosis is appropriate. Many patients with preexisting azotemia are not candidates for iodine contrast-based examinations, therefore providing an opportunity for MRA of the pulmonary vasculature, including scanning with ventilation and perfusion phases.[19]

Echocardiography

Other diagnostic techniques can sometimes prove useful, particularly in the setting of massive PE. Echocardiography, which can often be obtained more rapidly than either V/Q lung scanning, spiral CT, or pulmonary arteriography may reveal findings that strongly support hemodynamically significant PE. Direct visualization of massive PE may occasionally be noted, particularly if transesophageal echocardiography is performed. Echocardiography is sometimes used to gauge the extent of right ventricular dysfunction in the setting of proven acute PE.[20] Intravascular ultrasonography (IVUS) has been used to visualize acute PE directly at the bedside.[21]

Diagnostic Testing for Acute Deep Venous Thrombosis

Compression Duplex Ultrasonography

Evidence from multiple prospective randomized clinical trials indicates that compression ultrasonography is highly sensitive and specific for symptomatic, proximal acute DVT, but insensitive for asymptomatic acute DVT, as well as isolated calf DVT. The diagnosis of DVT by ultrasonography relies on the lack of compressibility of thrombosed venous segments. More than a decade ago, the sensitivity and specificity of compression ultrasonography for symptomatic proximal DVT was demonstrated to be well above 90%.[22-24] Limitations were also recognized, including the insensitivity for asymptomatic DVT, operator dependence, difficulty in accurately distinguishing acute from remote DVT in symptomatic patients, and insensitivity for calf vein thrombosis. Ultrasonography is inexpensive and is the preferred diagnostic modality for suspected symptomatic proximal DVT. In those cases in which there is a high clinical suspicion for DVT in the face of a negative venous duplex ultrasonography examination, serial ultrasonography is a reasonable strategy.[25]

Ascending Contrast Venography

Contrast venography remains the gold standard for the diagnosis of DVT, but it is considered a second-line test for the modern diagnosis of DVT. It is utilized when noninvasive testing is nondiagnostic, or if a patient may undergo invasive treatment for proximal DVT. Although generally safe and accurate, venography is an uncomfortable, invasive procedure that may result in superficial phlebitis, DVT, contrast-induced renal insufficiency, or hypersensitivity reactions.[26]

Magnetic Resonance and Computed Tomography Venography

MR venography is being used increasingly to diagnose DVT and may be an accurate noninvasive alternative to contrast venography. A major advantage of this technique is excellent resolution of the inferior vena cava and pelvic veins. It appears to be at least as accurate as contrast venography or ultrasonography for imaging of the proximal deep veins and perhaps more sensitive for pelvic vein thrombosis. MR venography offers the opportunity for simultaneous bilateral lower-extremity imaging and it may accurately distinguish acute from chronic DVT. Newer techniques have improved the accuracy of MR venography for the diagnosis of DVT.[27] Spiral CT scanning has also been studied for suspected acute DVT. These techniques may fit into diagnostic algorithms for DVT and PE but at present these algorithms are institution-specific depending upon resources and expertise with certain techniques.

Risk Factors for Venous Thromboemboli

Risk factors for DVT and PE are many.[28]

- Surgery
- Trauma (major or lower extremity)
- Immobility, paresis
- Malignancy
- Cancer therapy (hormonal, chemotherapy, or radiotherapy)
- Previous VTE
- Increasing age
- Pregnancy and the postpartum period
- Estrogen-containing oral contraception or hormone replacement therapy
- Selective estrogen receptor modulators
- Acute medical illness
- Heart or respiratory failure
- Inflammatory bowel disease
- Nephrotic syndrome
- Myeloproliferative disorders
- Paroxysmal nocturnal hemoglobinuria
- Obesity
- Smoking
- Varicose veins
- Central venous catheterization
- Inherited or acquired thrombophilia

These risk factors are commonly considered as demographic factors (age, weight, activity level), associated medical comorbidity (malignancy, congestive heart failure, stroke with paresis, inflammatory bowel disease), acquired surgical (long-bone fracture, need for total joint replacement, spinal cord trauma, radical abdominal/pelvic surgery), or associated with acquired hypercoagulability states (systemic lupus erythematosus with antiphospholipid syndrome, protein C/S/antithrombin

III deficiency, Factor V Leiden or prothrombin gene 20210A mutations).

Increasingly, anatomic factors are recognized as playing a role in iliofemoral DVT. May-Thurner syndrome (MTS) is the most common example of this condition. MTS is a congenital anomaly in which the muscular right common iliac artery overlies the left common iliac vein. It is postulated that a combination of extrinsic arterial compression on the overlying vein and repetitive left common iliac vein may lead to endothelial damage and ultimately, thrombus formation. The overall incidence of MTS in the general population is unknown, with one study reporting 37% of 24 patients with isolated left lower-extremity edema having left iliac vein compression as identified by MR venography.[29] Patients with MTS tend to be young women, in the second to fourth decade of life, who have experienced periods of prolonged immobilization or pregnancy. In 1992, Kim et al[30] described 3 clinical stages of the disease associated with iliac vein compression: stage I, asymptomatic; stage II, development of a venous "spur"; and stage III, thrombosis of the left common iliac vein.

Prevention

Options for prevention of DVT range from early mobilization to mechanical (graduated compression stockings, intermittent pneumatic compression devices) and pharmacologic prophylaxis (subcutaneous adjusted-dose unfractionated heparin, low-molecular-weight heparin, adjusted-dose warfarin). The decision as to which method to use depends on the level of risk of DVT and the potential hazards of prophylaxis. For example, patients preparing to undergo total knee arthroplasty are advised to receive perioperative low-molecular-weight heparins (LMWH), fondaparinux, or adjusted-dose warfarin. However, in younger patients undergoing laparoscopic cholecystectomy, early ambulation and mobilization are all that are required.[4]

In a retrospective review of the medical records of 3778 Medicare patients (mean age 66 years) from 38 US medical centers over a 3-year period, only 85% of patients following orthopedic total joint replacement received appropriate prophylaxis. More frighteningly, among patients with newly established VTE, < 50% of them maintained parenteral therapy with LMWH or unfractionated heparin until the International Normalized Ratio (INR) was ≥ 2 on warfarin.[31] It is this modern data that underscores the need for a complete understanding of the risks of failing to provide adequate prophylaxis and inadequate therapy among patients at risk for VTE.

Pharmacological Management of Venous Thromboembolic Disease

Anticoagulant Therapy

Anticoagulant therapy is the cornerstone of treatment for acute VTE. It offers 2 important therapeutic components. First, rapid initiation of anticoagulation prevents thrombus extension and fatal pulmonary embolus, and second, extended anticoagulation reduces the risk of recurrent VTE. It is no surprise that treatment regimens for DVT and PE are similar as the 2 conditions are manifestations of the same disease process.

Unfractionated Heparin

Heparin, an acidic glycosaminoglycan, is the longstanding agent used in the initial treatment of VTE. Despite its efficacy, unfractionated heparin, either via continuous intravenous or intermittent subcutaneous injection, requires careful monitoring and dose adjustment when used to treat acute events. It catalyzes the effect of the plasma inhibitor antithrombin III and by doing so inactivates thrombin (factor IIa), factor

Xa, and factor IXa. Indirectly heparin inhibits activation of factors V and VIII. The clearance of the drug is not affected by renal or hepatic impairment.

The benefit of heparin in the treatment of DVT and PE is well established.[32] Indeed, an early trial prior to the advent of perfusion scanning or pulmonary angiography included a group with PE on no active treatment. The mortality (25%) seen in the untreated group with autopsy-proven PE attests to the benefit of heparin.[33] Randomized clinical trials have also proven the benefit of continuous intravenous unfractionated heparin in treating acute DVT.[34-40] A minimum level of heparin anticoagulation is required to maintain an effective antithrombotic state,[41-43] and failure to achieve this will result in higher rates of recurrent thromboembolism. A plasma level between 0.2I U/mL and 0.4I U/mL is necessary to prevent thrombus progression.[44-47] Recurrent VTE is minimized by maintaining a continuous IV heparin infusion targeting an activated partial thromboplastin time (aPTT) > 1.5 times the control value.[48] This corresponds to a blood heparin level of 0.2I U/mL. Other studies suggest a low risk of VTE recurrence with a dose of approximately 1,250 U/hour.[49] During the initiation of anticoagulation with heparin a weak association exists between a supratherapeutic aPTT and bleeding, while a clear association exists between a subtherapeutic aPTT and recurrent VTE.[49] Nomograms have been devised to direct physicians in adjusting the rate of heparin infused to achieve therapeutic anticoagulation by checking the aPTT regularly in the first few days of therapy. Heparin is best given for 5 to 7 days for patients with VTE, although therapy may be extended for extensive iliofemoral disease. Current practice most commonly involves the initiation of heparin and an oral anticoagulant simultaneously at the time of diagnosis and the discontinuation of heparin when the oral agent, most commonly warfarin, yields a therapeutic international normalized ratio (INR) of ≥ 2 for 2 consecutive days at a minimum.

Low-Molecular-Weight Heparin

Low-molecular-weight heparin (LMWH), as its name implies, has a lower mean weight in contrast to unfractionated heparin, with a mean molecular weight of 15,000 daltons (Da).[50] LMWH has excellent bioavailability and plasma half-life, facilitating its use in a once- or twice-daily injection. The predictable anticoagulant effect allows it to be given without regular monitoring. If needed, monitoring can be performed by measuring the anti-Xa level. Clearance is achieved through the kidney and dose adjustment is advised when the glomerular filtration rate (GFR) < 30mL/min. Monitoring may also be required in pregnant women, as increased clearance of the drug arises as a result.[51] LMWH has a number of advantages. Ease of administration without the need for monitoring, low risk of heparin-induced thrombocytopenia, and the ability to be administered in the outpatient setting make it an attractive and potentially cost-effective therapeutic strategy. Indeed most studies show an efficacy benefit when compared to intravenous heparin.[52-54] Meta-analyses suggest a benefit in terms of recurrence of DVT and bleeding when compared to heparin.[55,56] The use of LMWH in oncology patients with VTE may confer a small survival benefit over long-term warfarin.[57,58] LMWH has replaced intravenous unfractionated heparin in daily practice for initial treatment of VTE.

Vitamin K Antagonists

Derived from 4-hydroxycoumarin, vitamin K antagonists are absorbed in the gut, plasma protein bound and metabolized in the liver. Their mechanism of action is via the inhibition of vitamin K–dependent coagulation factors II, VII, IX, and X. The onset of action is delayed commonly for ≥ 96 hours while normal coagulation factor levels are reduced in plasma. The lag period varies according to the plasma clearance rates of the various vitamin K–dependent factors.

The anticoagulant vitamin K–dependent proteins C and S have clearance kinetics similar to factor VII. Therefore, through a loading dose of warfarin the hemostatic balance can be tipped toward coagulation and thrombosis rather than anticoagulation in the first 24 to 48 hours of therapy. This provides the rationale for overlapping therapy with intravenous heparin or LMWH when treating acute VTE.[57-59] Multiple studies have demonstrated that similar to heparin, a certain threshold must be reached to achieve therapeutic anticoagulation. This is represented by an INR of ≥ 2.[60] The desired range of anticoagulation intensity for acute VTE is commonly 2 to 3. This therapeutic range minimizes bleeding and prevents recurrent thromboembolism.

The duration of therapy should be tailored to individual patients. Patients with modifiable risk factors such as transient immobility should do well with 3 to 6 months of therapy. Longer duration of anticoagulation (6–12 months) benefits those with idiopathic thrombosis by preventing recurrence. Long-term anticoagulation is warranted in cases of VTE and cancer, antiphospholipid syndrome, major hypercoagulable syndromes, or recurrent idiopathic venous thromboembolism.

Complications

The primary complication associated with anticoagulation is that of hemorrhage. The risk of bleeding increases with higher INR levels. Targeting the lowest effective INR of 2 to 3 minimizes this risk.[61,62] Minor bleeding is generally managed by withholding warfarin for short periods. More significant bleeding is treated with administration of vitamin K and/or fresh frozen plasma.

Healthy patients have a 2% annual bleeding incidence, while debilitated and severely ill patients have a 25% annual risk of bleeding. Aspirin is known to increase the hemorrhagic risk when combined with heparin but has been administered commonly without serious bleeding.[63,64]

Bleeding with unfractionated heparin (UFH) can be managed by close observation, as the half-life is only 90 minutes. If hemodynamic compromise is developing, reversal of heparin effects with intravenous protamine sulfate is helpful. The standard dose is 1 mg of Protamine for every 100 U of unfractionated heparin administered. Protamine sulfate administration must be closely monitored, as serious side effects, including anaphylaxis, hypotension, and possibly bleeding, can occur. It is advised to administer a test dose prior to full-dose therapy.

A serious adverse effect with all forms of heparin is heparin-induced thrombocytopenia (HIT) and heparin-induced thrombosis–thrombocytopenia syndrome (HITTS). HITTS is the paradoxical development of thrombocytopenia, arterial, and/or venous thromboembolic in the face of heparin administration. The incidence of HITTS is 3.5% with unfractionated heparin and 0.6% with LMWH. Although HITT Scan occur acutely with the first administration of heparin, it classically develops after at least 5 days of heparin administration. The diagnosis of HITTS requires ≥ 50% reduction in the platelet count when compared to pretreatment platelet counts, or an absolute reduction to 100,000/mm^3. This is an antigen-antibody reaction between heparin and platelet factor 4.[65] HIT has a frequency of 1%, typically if unfractionated intravenous heparin is given for more than 5 to 7 days.[66] Platelet counts should be checked routinely between days 3 and 5. If the infusion is prolonged, it should be checked again on day 7 and day 14. HIT is rare after 2 weeks of IV heparin.[66] A precipitous fall (> 50%) or platelet count of < 100,000/μL should mark a cessation in the heparin infusion and assay for antibody-mediated HIT.

Alternative anticoagulants to heparin include recombinant hirudin and danaparoid. These agents are approved for documented cases of HIT either without or with thrombosis and should be commenced as a temporary bridge to warfarin therapy.[66]

Other side effects of unfractionated heparin therapy include the risk of osteopenia associated with long-term high-dose heparin administration, hyperkalemia in patients with hypoaldosteronism,[67] and alopecia.

Warfarin-induced skin necrosis is a catastrophic complication of oral vitamin K antagonists and arises during the first weeks of therapy. This complication is rarely anticipated and is associated with protein C deficiency or malignancy, which results in thrombosis of the dermal blood vessels causing full thickness skin necrosis (Figure 21.1). Warfarin crosses the placenta and can cause spontaneous abortion and fetal anomalies, particularly if administered during the first trimester. The long-term alternative is the protracted use of LMWH, which is preferable to unfractionated heparin. Warfarin can be administered safely during the postpartum period, even to nursing mothers, as its metabolite excreted in breast milk is not an anticoagulant.[68,69] Those affected by VTE during pregnancy should receive anticoagulation for at least 6 weeks postpartum.[49]

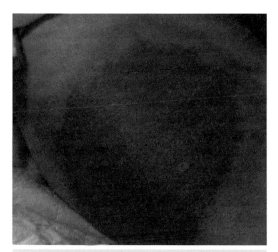

Figure 21.1 Classic appearance of warfarin-induced skin necrosis on the anterior thigh of a patient receiving warfarin.

Factor Xa Inhibitors (Pentasaccharides)

Fondaparinux is a synthetic analogue of a unique pentasaccharide sequence that mediates the interaction of heparin with antithrombin. Fondaparinux has been approved by the FDA for the treatment of DVT and PE. It inhibits both free and platelet bound factor Xa. It binds antithrombin with high affinity and is highly bioavailable, with a plasma half-life of 17 hours, which permits once-daily administration.

Despite the potential advantage of a prolonged half-life, the lack of reversibility in the face of fondaparinux-induced hemorrhage has significantly limited the widespread use of this agent. The drug is excreted unchanged in urine and is contraindicated in patients with severe renal impairment (Creatinine clearance < 30 mL/min). It does not bind platelet factor 4 antibody (PF4) and therefore should not cause HIT.

Another group of drugs that can be used to treat VTE include the direct thrombin inhibitors (DTIs). Presently, no DTI is FDA approved for VTE treatment alone. The only oral DTI that has completed phase III clinical trials is ximelagatran. It has a plasma half-life of 4 to 5 hours and is given twice daily in fixed doses. It does not have drug and food interactions, as does warfarin, and is renally cleared. Ximelagatran was rejected by the FDA in 2004 due to concerns about increased hepatotoxicity and the potential for adverse cardiac events. Other oral DTIs and oral heparin are in development and are the subject of multiple clinical trials.

Newer anticoagulants target individual components of the coagulation cascade and include heparinoids, oral SNAC/SNAD heparins, tissue factor pathway inhibitors, nematode anticoagulant peptide C2, and other investigational agents. These agents are at various stages of research and clinical trials, and have the potential to change the paradigm of therapy for acute VTE.

Thrombolytic Therapy

Thrombolytic agents promote the activation of plasminogen to plasmin, which in turn degrades fibrin to soluble peptides, thereby facilitating thrombus breakdown.[70] Streptokinase, urokinase, and tissue plasminogen activator (tPA) are the agents currently approved for use in VTE (Table 21.1).

All agents have similar capacity to act as a thrombolytic agent as judged by angiographic resolution (3 times that of heparin) and improvement in pulmonary vascular resistance (35% reduction at 24 hours, compared with 4% with heparin). Numerous studies have proven

Agent	Dose
Streptokinase	250,000IU loading dose + 100,000IU/hr x 24hrs
Urokinase	4,400IU/kg loading dose + 2,200IU/kg/hr x 12hrs
tPA	100mg infusion over 2hrs
Reteplase	2 doses of 10 Units each 30mins apart

Table 21.1 Dosing Regimen for Thrombolytic Agents for Treatment of PE

that PE when promptly identified and treated conservatively carries a mortality of 2%.[71,72] Given the small but measurable risk of intracranial hemorrhage attributed to thrombolysis (~1%–2%), it is understandable that this aggressive treatment is reserved for those with acute massive PE who are hemodynamically unstable and not predisposed to bleeding. It is also reserved for younger patients with massive iliofemoral thrombosis. Subselecting those patients at risk of developing chronic thromboembolic pulmonary hypertension is also a target for therapy in the future.

Thrombolysis for PE differs from that for myocardial infarction in that partial resolution is more commonly achieved because venous thromboemboli are older, larger, and more organized.[73-75] More recently, technical advances are being directed toward invasive catheter-based procedures to mechanically macerate the thromboembolic material and, it is hoped, improve results.

New Anticoagulants for Treatment of Thromboembolism

Newer, longer-acting parenteral and oral anticoagulants have the benefit of rapid onset of action without the need for regular monitoring, and there is rapid development of these agents. The new agents under development for VTE target factor Xa or thrombin for their mechanism of action. Most agents are in phase III of clinical trials.

Idraparinux is a second-generation penta-saccharide and is a hypermethylated derivative of fondaparinux. It binds antithrombin with high affinity to the extent that its plasma half-life is 80 hours,[76] which facilitates its administration as a once-weekly subcutaneous injection without coagulation monitoring. Its downside is that it does not have an antidote and accumulates in patients with renal impairment. It should be avoided in patients with a GFR of < 30mL/min.

SSR 126517 is a biotinylated version of idraparinux that was developed to address this shortcoming of reversal. The addition of the biotin moiety permits the rapid reversal of the anticoagulant effects by injection of avidin.[77] Avidin is derived from egg whites and permits the rapid clearance of the drug via the kidney.

Dabigatran etexilate is an oral direct thrombin inhibitor. This prodrug is metabolized to an active metabolite dabigatran once absorbed from the gastrointestinal tract. Twenty percent is excreted via the biliary system. It is not metabolized by the cytochrome P450 system, therefore, drug-drug interactions are uncommon.

The bioavailability of the drug is low (~6%) such that high doses are required to achieve adequate plasma concentrations. Absorption is optimized in an acidic environment such that proton pump inhibitors are identified as agents that curtail absorption by 20% to 25%. Peak plasma concentrations are obtained at 2 hours following administration. The half-life is 8 hours after a single dose and 14 to 17 hours after multiple doses. Eighty percent of the drug is cleared unchanged via the kidneys. Plasma concentrations therefore increase in patients with renal impairment. Dabigatran etexilate prolongs the aPTT. It has minimal effects on the prothrombin time (PT).

The RE-NOVATE trial was a multicenter, randomized, double-blind noninferiority study designed to compare the efficacy and safety of 2 doses of dabigatran etexilate (220 mg or 150 mg) with LMWH given for 1 month to reduce the risk of thromboembolism after hip surgery.[78] When given for a median of 33 days dabigatran was noninferior to LMWH, with similar bleeding rates (1%–2%). Extended-duration thromboprophylaxis with dabigatran led to a 50% reduction in asymptomatic DVT, while the rate of symptomatic venous thromboembolism during treatment was also low (0.4%–0.9%). These encouraging results may see a shift in the burden of thromboprophylaxis from an in-hospital setting to an outpatient setting, as this drug proves easy to manage and does not require monitoring.

Vena Cava Filters

The primary indications for inferior vena cava (IVC) filter placement include absolute contraindications to anticoagulation or recurrent thromboembolism while receiving therapeutic doses of anticoagulation. Filters can also be placed in the setting of massive PE when it is believed that any further pulmonary emboli might be lethal. Although effective in reducing the risk of recurrent pulmonary embolus, IVC filters do not afford protection from further DVT. In fact, IVC filters result in an increased risk for secondary DVT. Décousus et al[79] randomly assigned 400 patients to anticoagulation with or without filter placement. Follow-up at 2 years reported a 20.8% incidence of recurrent DVT compared with 11.6% for those on an IVC filter. Billett et al[80] retrospectively assessed outcome in 1628 patients after VTE and found no difference in the rate of secondary PE between those with or without a filter (HR at 90 days was 1.02 and at 5 years, 0.96).

IVC filter placement is usually undertaken in the angiography or surgical suite with fluoroscopy and intravenous contrast. Newer techniques of bedside duplex ultrasonography–guided and intravascular ultrasonography (IVUS)–guided insertion have proven safe, cost-effective, and convenient particularly for immobilized trauma patients. Those with spinal cord trauma, closed head injury, or multiple orthopedic injuries who have duplex ultrasonography–guided insertion of IVC filter avoid the need for transfer from intensive care and do not require administration of iodinated, nephrotoxic contrast agents. Pregnant women with DVT benefit from avoiding radiation exposure through this technique.[81]

Successful imaging of the IVC is achieved in 90% of cases of duplex ultrasonography–guided filter placement. Challenging cases arise due to body habitus, soft tissue edema in trauma patients, and small-bowel ileus in spinal cord injuries. For such individuals the option of IVUS-guided IVC filter insertion exists at the bedside as described by Matsumura et al.[82]

IVC filters are either designed as permanent or optionally retrievable. Optionally retrievable filters are approved for permanent placement but are designed to facilitate percutaneous retrieval once the risk of PE has passed.

Currently, there are 11 permanent or optionally retrievable filters with FDA approval in the United States. Percutaneous transjugular or transfemoral insertion is most commonly adopted. Smaller delivery sheaths and lower device profile have also allowed for delivery via the brachial vein. The choice of filter depends on the IVC size and required duration of insertion prior to safely starting anticoagulation. The popularity of IVC filters has increased dramatically over the last 20 years from 2000 to 49,000 per year.[83] This is accounted for by expanding indications for insertion, particularly primary prevention[83] (Table 21.2) and the increasing utilization of retrievable filters.

Manufacturer-recommended retrieval time varies from 14 days to several months, but retrieval after much longer indwelling times have been reported.[83] Data from 4 trials including 269 patients have demonstrated PE and IVC thrombosis rates of 1.5% and 6.5%, respectively, at follow-up.

Complications of IVC filters in general terms are categorized as procedure-related (from insertion or retrieval), device-related, and thrombosis-related such as IVC thrombosis or recurrent VTE. Device-related complications include malpositioning, tilting, failure of complete deployment, migration, fracture, and IVC perforation. These device-related complications affect the efficacy of the filter

Absolute indications in patients with documented VTE
Contraindications to anticoagulation
Perioperative management
Thrombocytopenia
Active bleeding or increased risk for bleeding
Complication of anticoagulation requiring cessation of therapy
Recurrent VTE despite documented therapeutic anticoagulation
Inability to manage anticoagulation despite patient compliance
Relative indications in patients with underlying VTE
Difficulty managing anticoagulation or poor compliance
Massive pulmonary embolism
Poor cardiopulmonary reserve
Increased risk for complications of anticoagulation
Before thromboendarterectomy for chronic thromboembolic disease
Before thrombolysis
Free-floating proximal deep venous thrombosis
Iliocaval thrombus
Prophylactic (no VTE, but primary pharmacologic or mechanical prophylaxis is not an option)
Trauma patients
Multiple fractures or pelvic injury
Spinal cord or head trauma
Surgical patient with high risk for VTE
Medical patient with high risk for VTE
VTE—venous thromboembolism

Table 21.2 Commonly Applied Indications for Inferior Vena Cava Filter Placement

in secondary PE prevention. Thankfully they are most commonly detected incidentally in asymptomatic individuals. Thrombotic complications include insertion-site thrombosis, postthrombotic chronic venous insufficiency, and IVC thrombosis. The severity of some of

these complications underlie the importance of appropriate case selection with absolute indications for filter placement.

Catheter-Directed Thrombolysis

Catheter-directed thrombolysis (CDT), which delivers thrombolytic agent locally into the thrombus using infusion catheters placed within the thrombus, has emerged as the superior method of thrombolysis. CDT addresses many limitations imposed by systemic thrombolysis, such as the high risk for hemorrhagic complication.[84] Intrathrombus delivery protects thrombolytic agents from neutralization by circulating antiplasmins such as plasminogen activator inhibitor (PAI-1) and allows dissolution of thrombus in smaller distal vessels that are otherwise not accessible to systemic thrombolysis.[85] This technique has the potential to accelerate thrombolysis, reduce the overall dose and duration of plasminogen activator infusion, and thus increase the likelihood of a successful outcome with a reduction in bleeding complications.

One of the earlier studies of CDT for the treatment of DVT in a series of patients with iliofemoral DVT resulted in complete thrombolysis in 72% and partial in 20% of patients with no major complications.[86] CDT using urokinase infusions for DVT reported by Bjarnason and colleagues[87] found secondary patency rates of 78% for iliac veins and 51% for femoral veins. A further series of 24 patients with iliofemoral DVT treated with CDT using recombinant tissue plasminogen activator (rt-PA) resulted in 79% of cases having successful restoration of patency, albeit with a puncture site bleeding complication rate of 25%.[88]

The largest published experience with CDT came from the National Venous Thrombolysis Registry, which reported a collective multicenter experience of 287 patients, in whom 71% involved the iliofemoral segments, treated with urokinase.[89] Complete lysis was achieved in 31% of cases and partial lysis in an additional 52% at 1 year of follow-up. DVT in the iliofemoral segment responded better, with a 64% 1-year patency rate compared with 47% in the femoropopliteal segment. One-year primary patency was maintained in 60% of patients. The grade of lysis predicted 1-year patency rates of 79%, 58%, and 32% for complete, partial, and no lysis, respectively. Preservation of valvular competence was demonstrated in 72% of patients with complete thrombolysis. In this registry, major bleeding requiring blood transfusion occurred in 11% of patients, with the majority being access site hematomas. The rate of intracranial hemorrhage was 0.2%. A further subsequent analysis involving a subset of this registry demonstrated better functioning and quality of life in patients treated with CDT than in those treated with anticoagulation alone.[90]

AbuRahma et al[91] published a 10-year experience in patients with iliofemoral DVT treated with anticoagulation versus CDT. At 5 years of follow-up, the group with CDT demonstrated 69% venous patency with only 22% suffering from postthrombotic chronic venous insufficiency, compared with an 18% patency rate and a 70% postthrombotic syndrome rate in the anticoagulation group. The only randomized trial of CDT versus anticoagulation in iliofemoral DVT showed that the CDT group had 72% patency and 11% venous reflux rates compared with 12% patency and 42% reflux rates in the anticoagulation group.[92]

A review by Baldwin et al[93] of more than 600 patients treated with CDT demonstrated diminished postthrombotic syndrome, improved quality of life, and evidence for reduced incidence of recurrent DVT. The pooled risk of intracranial hemorrhage was noted to be 0.2%. A potential complication of CDT included PE, which occurs in about 1% of cases. Routine prophylactic placement of an IVC filter before CDT is usually not recommended. However, the advent of retrievable filters may change clinical practice.

Percutaneous Mechanical Thrombectomy

Percutaneous mechanical thrombectomy has emerged as an important tool in the armamentarium for the management of DVT, particu-larly when a mechanical thrombectomy device can be used in conjunction with pharmacologic thrombolytic therapy. Many thrombectomy devices have been recently developed using various mechanisms such as rheolytic or mechanical aspiration or ultrasonic thrombolysis.

One of the thrombectomy systems that has been shown to be effective in the management of acute DVT is the AngioJet Rheolytic Thrombectomy system (MEDRAD). The principal mechanism of action of this device is based on the Venturi effect, which creates rapidly flowing saline jets that are directed backward from the tip of the device to outflow channels in a coaxial fashion. This generates a vacuum force that macerates and draws surrounding thrombus into the catheter. One major advantage of this percutaneous treatment modality is that the thrombectomy catheter can be delivered through a small-bore introducer sheath, which reduces access site trauma and avoids operative venous exposure required with conventional Fogarty thrombo-embolectomy. A clinical study using the AngioJet system for extensive DVT demonstrated that it is effective in thrombus removal, venous patency restoration, and symptom relief with > 50% thrombus extraction in 59% of patients and symptomatic improvement in 82% at 12 months of follow-up.[94]

Combining percutaneous mechanical thrombectomy with CDT, also known as *pharmaco-mechanical thrombectomy (PMT),* has the potential to achieve more complete clot removal as well as decrease the dose and duration of thrombolytic therapy than either therapy alone. Some interventionists employ the AngioJet system using the power-pulsed-spray technique. The AngioJet catheter is advanced over a guide wire and through the thrombosed vein segment. At this point, adjunctive thrombolytic agent is added to the infusion solution. Lytic agent is delivered under high pressure into the thrombus, which in theory leads to maximum thrombus penetration and fosters maximal drug exposure and resultant thrombolysis. After a dwell time of 20 to 30 minutes to allow for localized thrombolysis, the AngioJet catheter is reintroduced to perform mechanical thrombectomy, aspirating the thrombolytic agent and loose thrombus fragments. This sequence may be repeated if significant residual thrombus remains on subsequent venograms. A study of 24 patients with DVT treated with the power-pulsed-sprayed technique showed complete thrombus removal (> 90%) in 50% of patients and substantial thrombus removal (50%–99%) in 29% of patients.[95] All 24 patients had clinical resolution of their presenting symptoms postintervention.

Another device is the Trellis (Covidien) hybrid catheter, which isolates the thrombosed vein segment between 2 occluding balloons. The thrombolytic agent is infused into the thrombus between the occluding balloons. A dispersion wire is inserted into the catheter, resulting in the catheter shaft assuming a spiral configuration that, when activated, spins at 1500 rpm. After 20 minutes of dwell time, the liquefied and particulate thrombus is then aspirated. The proximal occluding balloon is designed to prevent PE. Isolation of thrombolytic agent to the thrombosed segment has the theoretical advantage of reducing the systemic effect of thrombolysis and hence the risk of bleeding.

To date, there have been no controlled studies comparing the efficacy of pharmacomechanical thrombectomy to CDT or anticoagulation treatment alone. In an observational study, Lin et al[96] compared the outcome in patients with symptomatic DVT who underwent either CDT or PMT with the Angio-Jet system. In the CDT group, complete and partial thrombus removal was accomplished in 70% and 30% cases, respectively. In the PMT group, complete and partial thrombus removal was accomplished in 75% and 25% cases, respectively. Immediate (< 24 hours) improvement in clinical symptoms in CDT and PMT groups were achieved in 72% and 81% of cases, respectively. Patency rates at 1 year of CDT and PMT groups were 64% and 68%, respectively. Bush et al[97] reported similar results using the AngioJet device in combination with CDT for the treatment of extensive DVT.[97] Complete thrombus removal was obtained in 65% and partial resolution in the remaining 35% of patients.

None of these studies using PMT reported clinically significant PE. However, in a study of patients with extensive ileofemoral thromboses where IVC filters were placed before PMT, evidence of captured thrombus in the cava filter was seen in 28% of patients.[97] Prophylactic IVC filter insertion prior to PMT is not routine.

The primary objective of PMT in pulmonary embolism is the fragmentation of central pulmonary thrombi to migrate distally, thereby allowing better pulmonary perfusion and unloading of the right ventricle. A small case series (13 patients) published by Eid-Lidt et al[98] used an 8-Fr aspiration device (Aspirex, Straub Medical) designed specifically for PE. This catheter consists of a spiral that rotates at 40,000 rpm within the body of the catheter, creating a negative pressure that macerates thrombus and subsequently aspirates the material. The catheter is deployed over a 0.018-in guide wire to the site of occlusive embolus before being activated. Prior to aspiration of thrombus, fragmentation of clot is achieved by use of a pigtail catheter. Hemodynamic improvement criteria were used to guide cessation of invasive therapy. Following PMT the hemodynamic results were encouraging. Mean systolic blood pressure increased from 74.3 ± 7.5 mm Hg to 89.4 ± 7.3 mm Hg. There was a significant reduction in the shock index (1.23 ± 0.22 vs. 0.74 ± 0.23).[88] In clinical terms this translated to a success in 88% of patients. One patient died due to PE and one patient recovered from a hemorrhagic cerebrovascular accident as a consequence of thrombolysis. PMT is currently the only alternative treatment to thrombolysis or surgical embolectomy in patients with massive PE, RV dysfunction and contraindications to thrombolysis, high bleeding risk, failed thrombolysis, or lack of availability or technical expertise to perform surgical pulmonary embolectomy. Further experience of this technology is required to establish its safety and where it lies in the treatment algorithm for PE in the future.

Pulmonary Embolectomy

Pulmonary embolectomy is performed in emergent cases of massive PE, hemodynamic instability despite resuscitative efforts, and failed thrombolysis. Case series have seen a mortality rate ranging from 10% to 75% following surgical pulmonary embolectomy despite availability of cardiopulmonary bypass.[99,100] In cases of cardiac arrest resuscitated and operated upon, the mortality rate can be between 50% and 94%.[101] Postoperative complications such as acute respiratory distress syndrome, mediastinitis, acute renal failure, and neurological deficit make this a very challenging subgroup of patients.

More recent efforts to broaden the indication for pulmonary embolectomy have been proposed by Aklog et al[101] from a single-center experience. Massive PE with associated right ventricular dilatation and dysfunction portends a progression to hemodynamic compromise and death. This formed the basis for intervening surgically on patients with anatomically extensive PE and right ventricle dysfunction despite preserved hemodynamic status. Over a 25-month period 29 patients underwent surgery. PE was confirmed by computerized tomographic pulmonary arteriogram (CTPA). Right ventricle dysfunction was confirmed on echo in 26 cases. Surgical technique was designed to minimize morbidity and mortality. Surgery was undertaken without cross clamp, cardioplegia, or circulatory arrest on a warm beating heart. Extraction was limited to directly visible thrombus to avoid trauma to the pulmonary arteries. Right ventricle thrombus was removed based on perioperative transcsophageal echocardiography (TEE) findings and an IVC filter placed for secondary prevention. The outcome was encouraging with 89% survival at 1 month postoperatively.

Summary

Current management of acute symptomatic DVT requires timely diagnosis and prompt intervention. Anticoagulation therapy remains the standard of care. However, the rationale for an aggressive pharmaco-mechanical approach in the treatment of acute DVT by means of mechanical thrombectomy or thrombolytic therapy is to achieve rapid alleviation of clinical symptoms, restoring venous patency and reducing the future risk of postthrombotic syndrome. Catheter-directed thrombolytic therapy with or without mechanical thrombectomy has been shown to be more effective and appears to be safer than systemic infusion. The use of thrombolysis is associated with an increased risk of bleeding and needs to be considered on a case-by-case basis. Although current guidelines do not advocate the routine use of thrombolysis or thrombectomy in the treatment of acute DVT, new techniques for patients with massive iliofemoral DVT at risk of phlegmasia cerulea dolens (venous gangrene), or in young patients who have significant occlusive symptomatic proximal DVT with acceptably low bleeding risk, have improved the safety and acceptability of this treatment.

Current management of PE includes more sophisticated diagnostic algorithms with advanced and readily available imaging, safe and effective anticoagulation agents, and more aggressive intervention for the cases of massive PE with hemodynamic compromise. Thrombolytic therapy, mechanical thrombectomy, and more aggressive surgical intervention with pulmonary embolectomy offer hope for the future.

References

1. Lilienfeld DE, Chan E, Ehland J, Godbold JH, Landrigan PJ, Marsh G. Mortality from pulmonary embolism in the United States: 1962 to 1984. *Chest.* 1990;98:1067-1072.

2. Lilienfeld DE. Decreasing mortality from pulmonary embolism in the United States, 1979-1996. *Int J Epidemiol.* 2000;29:465-469.

3. Kahn SR, Ginsberg JS. Relationship between deep venous thrombosis and the postthrombotic syndrome. *Arch Intern Med.* 2004;164: 17-26.

4. Geerts WH, Pineo GF, Heit JA, et al. Prevention of venous thromboembolism. The Seventh ACCP Conference on Antithrombotic and Thrombolytic Therapy. *Chest*. 2004;126:338S-400S.

5. Kucher N, Koo S, Quiroz R, et al. Electronic alerts to prevent venous thromboembolism among hospitalized patients. *N Engl J Med*. 2005;352:969-977.

6. Bounameaux H, Cirafici P, DeMoerloose P, et al. Measurement of D-dimer in plasma as diagnostic aid in suspected pulmonary embolism. *Lancet*. 1991;337:196.

7. Egermayer P, Town GI, Turner JG, et al. Usefulness of D-dimer, blood gas, and respiratory rate measurements for excluding pulmonary embolism. *Thorax*. 1998; 53:830-834.

8. Stein PD, Hull RD, Kalpesh CP, et al. D-dimer for the exclusion of acute venous thrombosis and pulmonary embolism: a systematic review. *Ann Intern Med*. 2004;140:589-607.

9. Mehta NJ, Jani K, Khan IA. Clinical usefulness and prognostic value of elevated cardiac troponin I in acute pulmonary embolism. *Am Heart J*. 2003;145:821-825.

10. Douketis JD, Crowther MA, Stanton EB, Ginsberg JS. Elevated cardiac troponin levels in patients with submassive pulmonary embolism. *Arch Intern Med*. 2002;162:79-81.

11. Remy-Jardin MJ, Remy J, Deschildre F, et al. Diagnosis of acute pulmonary embolism with spiral CT: comparison with pulmonary angiography and scintigraphy. *Radiology*. 1996;200:699-706.

12. Sostman HD, Layish DT, Tapson VF, et al. Prospective comparison of helical CT and MR imaging in patients with clinically suspected pulmonary embolism. *JMRI*. 1996;6:275-278.

13. Goodman LR, Curtin JJ, Mewissen MW, et al. Detection of pulmonary embolism in patients with unresolved clinical and scintigraphic diagnosis: helical CT versus angiography. *AJR Am J Roentgenol*. 1995;164:1369-1374.

14. Mayo JR, Remy-Jardin M, Muller NL, et al. Pulmonary embolism: prospective comparison of spiral CT with ventilation-perfusion scintigraphy. *Radiology*. 1997;205:447-452.

15. Perrier A, Howarth N, Didier D, et al. Performance of helical computed tomography in unselected outpatients with suspected pulmonary embolism. *Ann Intern Med*. 2001;135:88-97.

16. Ferretti GR, Bosson JL, Buffaz PD, et al. Acute pulmonary embolism: role of helical CT in 164 patients with intermediate probability at ventilation-perfusion scintigraphy and normal results at duplex US of the legs. *Radiology*. 1997;205:453-458.

17. van Belle A, Buller HR, Huisman PM, et al. Effectiveness of managing suspected pulmonary embolism using an algorithm combining clinical probability, D-dimer testing, and computed tomography. *JAMA*. 2006;295:172-179.

18. Meaney JFM, Weg JG, Chenevert TL, et al. Diagnosis of pulmonary embolism with magnetic resonance angiography. *N Engl J Med*. 1997;336:1422-1427.

19. Altes TA, Mai VM, Munger TM, et al. Pulmonary embolism: comprehensive evaluation with MR ventilation and perfusion scanning with hyperpolarized helium-3, arterial spin tagging, and contrast-enhanced MRA. *J Vasc Interv Radiol*. 2005;16:999-1005.

20. Evans AJ, Tapson VF, Sostman HD, et al. The diagnosis of deep venous thrombosis: a prospective comparison of venography and magnetic resonance imaging. *Chest*. 1992;102:120S.

21. Come PC. Echocardiographic evaluation of pulmonary embolism and its response to therapeutic interventions. *Chest*. 1992;101:151S-62S.

22. Tapson VF, Witty LA. Massive pulmonary embolism: diagnostic and therapeutic strategies. *Clin Chest Med*. 1996;16:329.

23. Tick LW, Ton E, van Voorthuizen T, et al. Practical diagnostic management of patients with clinically suspected deep vein thrombosis by clinical probability test, compression ultrasonography, and D-dimer test. *Am J Med*. 2002;113(8):630-635.

24. Weinmann EE, Salzman EW. Deep-vein thrombosis. *N Engl J Med*. 1994;331:1630-1641.

25. Prandoni P, Cogo A, Bernardi E, et al. A simple ultrasound approach for detection of recurrent proximal vein thrombosis. *Circulation*. 1993;88:1730-1735.

26. Aitkon AGF, Godden DJ. Real-time ultrasound

diagnosis of deep vein thrombosis: a comparison with venography. *Clin Radiol.* 1987;38:309-313.

27. Fraser DG, Moody AR, Davidson IR, et al. Deep venous thrombosis: diagnosis by using venous enhanced subtracted peak arterial MR venography versus conventional venography. *Radiology.* 2003;226:812-820.

28. Geerts WH, Heit JA, Clagett GP, et al. Prevention of venous thromboembolism. *Chest.* 2001;119:132S-175S.

29. Wolpert LM, Rahmani O, Stein B, Gallagher JJ, Drezner AD. Magnetic resonance venography in the diagnosis and management of May-Thurner syndrome. *Vasc Endovasc Surg.* 2002;36:51-57.

30. Kim D, Orron E, Porter DH. Venographic anatomy, technique and interpretation. In: Kim D, Orron DE, eds. *Peripheral Vascular Imaging and Intervention.* St. Louis: Mosby-Year Book; 1992):269-349.

31. Tapson VF, Myers TM, Waldo AL, et al. Antithrombotic therapy practices in US hospitals in an era of practice guidelines. *Arch Intern Med.* 2005;165:1458-1464.

32. Barritt DW, Jordan SC. Anticoagulant drugs in the treatment of pulmonary embolism: a controlled clinical trial. *Lancet.* 1960;1:1309-1312.

33. Kanis JA. Heparin in the treatment of pulmonary thromboembolism. *Thromb Haemost.* 1974;32:517-527.

34. Hull RD, Raskob GE, Hirsh J, et al. Continuous intravenous heparin compared with intermittent subcutaneous heparin in the initial treatment of proximal-vein thrombosis. *N Engl J Med.* 1986;315:1109-1214.

35. Brandjes DPM, Heijboer H, Büller HR, et al. Acenocoumarol and heparin compared with acenocoumarol alone in the initial treatment of proximal vein thrombosis. *N Engl J Med.* 1992;327:1485-1489.

36. Levine M, Jent M, Hirsh J, et al. A comparison of low-molecular-weight heparin administered primarily at home with unfractionated heparin administered in the hospital for proximal deep-vein thrombosis. *N Engl J Med.* 1996;334:677-668.

37. Koopman MMW, Prandoni P, Piovella F, et al.

Treatment of venous thrombosis with intravenous unfractionated heparin administered in the hospital as compared with subcutaneous low-molecular-weight heparin administered at home. *N Engl J Med.* 1996;334,682-668.

38. The Columbus Investigators. Low-molecular-weight heparin in the treatment of patients with venous thromboembolism. *N Engl J Med.* 1997;337:657-666.

39. Simonneau G, Sors H, Charbonnier B, et al. A comparison of low-molecular-weight heparin with unfractionated heparin for acute pulmonary embolism. *N Engl J Med.* 1997;337:663-669.

40. Hull RD, Raskob GE, Brandt RF, et al. Low-molecular-weight heparin vs heparin in the treatment of patients with pulmonary embolism. *Arch Intern Med.* 2000;160:229-236.

41. Basu D, Gallus A, Hirsh J, et al. A prospective study of the value of monitoring heparin treatment with the activated partial thromboplastin time. *N Engl J Med.* 1972;287:325-327.

42. Coon WW, Willis PW III, Symons MJ. Assessment of anticoagulant therapy of pulmonary thromboembolism. *Ann Surg* 1969;197.559-568.

43. The Urokinase Pulmonary Embolism Trial. A national cooperative study. *Circulation.* 1973;47(Suppl):1-100.

44. Gitel SN, Wessler S. The antithrombotic effects of warfarin and heparin following infusions of tissue thromboplastin in rabbits: clinical implication. *J Lab Clin Med.* 1979;94:481-484.

45. Wessler S, Reimer L, Freiman R, et al. Serum-induced thrombosis: studies of its induction and evolution under controlled conditions in vivo. *Circulation.* 1959;20:264-274.

46. Chui HM, Hirsh J, Yung WL, et al. Relationship between the anticoagulant and antithrombotic effects of heparin in experimental venous thrombosis. *Blood.* 1977;49:171-184.

47. Morris TA, Marsh JJ, Konopka RG, et al. Antibodies against the fibrin B-chain amino terminus detect active canine venous thrombi. *Circulation.* 1997;96:3173-3179.

48. Hull RD, Raskob GE, Brant RF, et al. Relation between the time to achieve the lower limit of the APTT therapeutic range and recurrent

venous thromboembolism during heparin treatment for deep vein thrombosis. *Arch Intern Med*. 1997;157:2562-2568.

49. Büller HR, Agnelli G, Hull RD, Hyers TM, Prins MH, Raskob GE. Antithrombotic therapy for venous thromboembolic disease: the Seventh ACCP Conference on Antithrombotic and Thrombolytic Therapy. *Chest*. 2004;126:401S-428S.

50. Salzman EW. Low molecular weight heparin: is small beautiful? *N Engl J Med*. 1986;315:957-959.

51. Casele HL, Laifer SA, Woelkers DA, et al. Changes in the pharmacokinetics of the low-molecular-weight heparin enoxaparin sodium during pregnancy. *Am J Obstet Gynecol*. 1999;181:1113-1117.

52. Prandoni P, Lensing AWA, Büller HR, et al. Comparison of subcutaneous low molecular weight heparin with intravenous standard heparin in proximal vein thrombosis. *Lancet*. 1992;339:441-445.

53. Hull RD, Raskob GE, Pineo GF, et al. Subcutaneous low-molecular-weight heparin compared with continuous intravenous heparin in the initial treatment of proximal-vein thrombosis. *N Engl J Med*. 1992;326:975-982.

54. Lindmarker P, Holmstrom M, Granqvist S, et al. Comparison of once-daily subcutaneous Fragmin with continuous intravenous unfractionated heparin in the treatment of deep vein thrombosis. *Thromb Haemost*. 1994;72:186-190.

55. Siragusa S, Cosmi B, Piovella F, et al. Low-molecular-weight heparins and unfractionated heparin in the treatment of patients with acute venous thromboembolism: results of a meta-analysis. *Am J Med*. 1996;100:269-270.

56. Gould MK, Dembitzer AD, Doyle RL, et al. Low-molecular-weight heparins compared with unfractionated heparin for treatment of acute deep venous thrombosis. *Ann Intern Med*. 1999;130:800-809.

57. Khamashta MA, Cuadrado MJ, Mujic R, et al. The management of thrombosis in the antiphospholipid-antibody syndrome. *N Engl J Med*. 1995;332:993-997.

58. O'Reilly RA, Aggler PM. Studies on coumarin anticoagulant drugs: initiation of warfarin therapy without a loading dose. *Circulation*. 1968;38:169-177.

59. Wessler S, Gitel SN. Warfarin: from bedside to bench. *N Engl J Med*. 1984;311(10):645-652.

60. Hull RD, Hirsh J, Jay R, et al. Different intensities of oral anticoagulant therapy in the treatment of proximal vein thrombosis. *N Engl J Med*. 1982;307:1676-1681.

61. Holmgren K, Anderson G, Fagrell B, et al. One month versus six month therapy with oral anticoagulants after symptomatic deep vein thrombosis. *Acta Med Scand*. 1985;218:279-284.

62. Bynum LJ, Wilson JE. Low-dose heparin therapy in the long-term management of venous thromboembolism. *Am J Med*. 1979;67:553-556.

63. Nieuwenhuis HK, Albada J, Banga JD, et al. Identification of risk factors for bleeding during treatment of acute venous thromboembolism with heparin or low molecular weight heparin. *Blood*. 1991;78:2337-2343.

64. Landefeld CS, Beyth RJ. Anticoagulant-related bleeding: clinical epidemiology, prediction, and prevention. *Am J Med*. 1993;95:315-328.

65. Warkentin TE, Levine MN, Hirsh J, et al. Heparin-induced thrombocytopenia in patients treated with low-molecular-weight heparin or unfractionated heparin. *N Engl J Med*. 1995;332:1330-1335.

66. Warkentin TE, Elavathil LJ, Hayward CPM. The pathogenesis of venous limb gangrene associated with heparin-induced thrombocytopenia. *Ann Intern Med*. 1997;127:804-812.

67. Edes TE, Sunderrajan EV. Heparin-induced hyperkalemia. *Arch Intern Med*. 1985;145:1070-1072.

68. Coon WW, Willis PW III. Hemorrhagic complications of anticoagulant therapy. *Arch Intern Med*. 1974;133:386-383.

69. O'Sullivan EF, Hirsh J. Duration of anticoagulation therapy in venous thromboembolism. *Med J Aust*. 1972;2:1104-1107.

70. Research Committee of the British Thoracic Society. Optimum duration of anticoagulation for deep-vein thrombosis and pulmonary embolism. *Lancet*. 1992;340:873-876.

71. Urokinase Pulmonary Embolism Trial phase I results. *JAMA*. 1970;214:2163-2172.

72. Urokinase Streptokinase Pulmonary Embolism Trial phase II results. *JAMA*. 1974;229:1606-1613.

73. Kearon C, Gent M, Hirsh J, et al. Extended anticoagulation prevented recurrence after a first episode of idiopathic venous thromboembolism. *N Engl J Med*. 1999;340:901-909.

74. Khamashta MA, Cuadrado MJ, Mujic R, et al. The management of thrombosis in the antiphospholipid-antibody syndrome. *N Engl J Med*. 1995;332:993-997.

75. Moll S, Ortel TL. Monitoring warfarin therapy in patients with lupus anticoagulants. *Ann Intern Med*. 1997;127:177-185.

76. Walenga JM, Jeske WP, Fareed J. Short- and long-acting synthetic pentasaccharides as antithrombotic agents. *Expert Opin Investig Drugs*. 2005;14:847-858.

77. Gross PL, Weitz JI. New anticoagulants for treatment of venous thromboembolism. *Arterioscler Thromb Vasc Biol*. 2008;28:380-386.

78. Eriksson BI, Dahl OE, Rosencher N, et al. Dabigatran etexilate versus enoxaparin for prevention of venous thromboembolism after total hip replacement: a randomised, double-blind, non-inferiority trial. *Lancet*. 2007;370(9591):915-917.

79. Décousus H, Leizorovicz A, Parent F, et al. A clinical trial of vena caval filters in the prevention of pulmonary embolism in patients with proximal deep vein thrombosis. Prevention du Risque d'Embolie Pulmonaire par Interruption Cave Study Group. *N Engl J Med*. 1998;338:409-415.

80. Billett HH, Jacobs LG, Madsen EM, et al. Efficacy of inferior vena cava filters in anticoagulated patients. *J Thromb Haemost*. 2007;5:1848-1853.

81. Conners MS, Becker S, Guzman RJ, et al. Duplex scan-directed placement of inferior vena cava filters: a five-year institutional experience Michael S. Conners III, MD et al. *J Vasc Surg*. 2002;35(2):286-291.

82. Matsumura JS, Morasch MD. Filter placement by ultrasound technique at the bedside. *Semin Vasc Surg*. 2000;13:199-203.

83. Carmen TL. Update on IVC filters. *Curr Treat Options Cardiovas Med*. 2008;10:101-111.

84. Janssen M, Wollersheim H, Schultze-Kool L, Thien T. Local and systemic thrombolytic therapy for acute deep vein thrombosis. *Neth J Med*. 2005;63:81-90.

85. Comerota A, Paolini D. Treatment of acute iliofemoral deep venous thrombosis: a strategy of thrombus removal. *Eur J Vasc Endovasc Surg*. 2007;33:351.

86. Semba CP, Dake MD. Iliofemoral deep venous thrombosis: aggressive therapy with catheter-directed thrombolysis. *Radiology*. 1994;191:487.

87. Bjarnason H, Kruse JR, Asinger DA, et al. Iliofemoral deep venous thrombosis: safety and efficacy outcome during 5 years of catheter-directed thrombolytic therapy. *J Vasc Interv Radiol*. 1997;8:405.

88. Verhaeghe R, Stockx L, Lacroix H, Vermylen J, Baert AL. Catheter-directed lysis of iliofemoral vein thrombosis with use of rt-PA. *Eur Radiol*. 1997;7:996.

89. Mewissen MW, Seabrook GR, Meissner MH, Cynamon J, Labropoulos N, Haughton SH. Catheter-directed thrombolysis for lower extremity deep venous thrombosis: report of a national multicenter registry. *Radiology*. 1999;211(1):39.

90. Comerota AJ, Throm RC, Mathias SD, Haughton S, Mewissen M. Catheter-directed thrombolysis for iliofemoral deep venous thrombosis improves health-related quality of life. *J Vasc Surg*. 2000;32:130.

91. AbuRahma AF, Perkins SE, Wulu JT, Ng HK. Iliofemoral deep vein thrombosis: conventional therapy versus lysis and percutaneous transluminal angioplasty and stenting. *Ann Surg*. 2001;233:752.

92. Elsharawy M, Elzayat E. Early results of thrombolysis vs anticoagulation in iliofemoral venous thrombosis. A randomised clinical trial. *Eur J Vasc Endovasc Surg*. 2002;24:209.

93. Baldwin ZK, Comerota AJ, Schwartz LB. Catheter-directed thrombolysis for deep venous thrombosis. *Vasc Endovasc Surg*. 2004;38:1.

94. Kasirajan K, Gray B, Ouriel K. Percutaneous AngioJet thrombectomy in the management of extensive deep venous thrombosis. *J Vasc Interv Radiol*. 2001;12:179.

95. Cynamon J, Stein EG, Dym RJ, Jagust MB,

Binkert CA, Baum RA. A new method for aggressive management of deep vein thrombosis: retrospective study of the power pulse technique. *J Vasc Interv Radiol*. 2006;17(6):1043.

96. Lin PH, Zhou W, Dardik A, et al. Catheter-direct thrombolysis versus pharmaco-mechanical thrombectomy for treatment of symptomatic lower extremity deep venous thrombosis. *Am J Surg*. 2006;192(6):782.

97. Bush R, Lin P, Bates J, Maureebe L, Zhou W, Lumsden A. Pharmacomechanical thrombectomy for treatment of symptomatic lower extremity deep venous thrombosis: safety and feasibility study. *J Vasc Surg*. 2004;40:965.

98. Eid-Lidt G, Gaspar J, Sandoval J, et al. Combined clot fragmentation and aspiration in patients with acute pulmonary embolism. *Chest*. 2008;134(1):54-60.

99. Meyer G, Tamisier D, Sors H, et al. Pulmonary embolectomy: a 20 year experience at one center. *Ann Thorac Surg*. 1991;51:232-236.

100. Gray HH, Morgan JM, Paneth M, et al. Pulmonary embolectomy for acute massive pulmonary embolism: an analysis of 71 cases. *Br Heart J*. 1988;60:196-200.

101. Aklog L, Williams CS, Byrne JG, Goldhaber SZ. Acute pulmonary embolectomy: a contemporary approach. *Circulation*. 2002;105:1416-1419.

22

Contemporary Management of Superior Vena Cava Syndrome

Andrew C. Eisenhauer

Superior vena cava (SVC) syndrome results from the obstruction of the blood flow in the superior vena cava.[1] Though malignancy with tumor infiltration or compression has historically been the most common etiology,[2] SVC syndrome can be caused by a variety of other conditions, including fibrosis and *in situ* venous thrombosis resulting from pacemaker/defibrillator leads or central venous catheters.[3] Given its association with advanced malignancy, previous therapy for SVC syndrome was primarily supportive. However, the widespread use of permanent central venous access catheters, coupled with the improved success of chemotherapy and the increasing use of multilead implantable cardiac rhythm management devices, has increased the incidence of SVC syndrome not caused by direct tumor infiltration ("nonmalignant" SVC syndrome). Further, with the increasing acceptance of percutaneous and minimally invasive therapy, the treatment of SVC syndrome with balloon dilatation and stenting has also become more common.

Etiology and Clinical Presentation

SVC syndrome is most frequently associated with malignancy (Table 22.1) leading to compression and/or infiltration of the vena cava by tumor.[1] Lung tumors are the most common, followed by lymphoma, teratoma, and others. The development of SVC syndrome in a patient with malignancy is a sign of a very poor prognosis. Rice and colleagues[4] in a series of 78 patients collected over 5 years found that malignancy was the etiology in 60% of the cases of SVC syndrome, and lung cancer was the most common malignancy. Small cell and non–small cell lung tumors accounted for 22% and 24% of cases, respectively. But of patients with lung cancer, a higher percentage of patients with small–cell lung cancer developed the syndrome (6% vs. 1%). Lymphoma and germ cell tumors were other significant malignant causes (8% and 3% of cases, respectively). Despite advances in cancer therapy, palliation remains the mainstay of malignant SVC syndrome therapy. As the survival for patients with neoplastic diseases has

Vascular Disease: Diagnostic and Therapeutic Approaches. © 2011 Michael R. Jaff and Christopher J. White, editors. Cardiotext Publishing, ISBN: 978-1-935395-16-4.

improved—largely because of improvements in chemotherapy—patients with cancer may also develop nonmalignant SVC syndrome due to the indwelling catheters and sclerosing properties of administered chemotherapy. Unlike the patients with SVC syndrome associated with direct tumor infiltration, many of those with nonmalignant SVC obstruction can look forward to decades of survival. Thus treatment of SVC obstruction in this group must be durable as well as effective.

Once an important cause of caval obstruction, infection leading to SVC syndrome has dramatically decreased in frequency in the antibiotic era.[5] An exception, however, is SVC syndrome in developing countries and SVC syndrome from septic thrombosis or thrombophlebitis associated with intravenous drug abuse.

Malignancy 95%
• Lung cancer (80%)
Small cell lung cancer
Non–small cell lung cancer
• Lymphoma (almost invariably non-Hodgkin's lymphoma)
• Thymoma
• Mediastinal germ cell neoplasms
• Solid tumors with mediastinal metastases (breast cancer most frequently)
Other 5%
• *Iatrogenic* Pacemaker and defibrillator leads, indwelling central venous catheters, postradiation vascular fibrosis
• *Infectious disease* Fibrosing mediastinitis secondary to tuberculosis, syphilis, histoplasmosis, actinomycosis, aspergillosis, blastomycosis, filariasis, direct spread of nocardiosis
• *Other* Fibrosing mediastinitis, sarcoidosis, sclerosing cholangitis, goiter, aortic aneurysm

Table 22.1 Historical Etiology of SVC Syndrome

More than 15,000 patients are diagnosed with SVC syndrome every year in the United States.[3] The diagnosis is usually made at the bedside and in up to 59% of the patients, SVC syndrome may be the first presentation of another underlying disease.[6] Whether patients present acutely or with the gradual onset of symptoms depends on the acuity of the pathological process and the development of collateral circulation. For example, in those with a rapidly invading malignancy, SVC obstruction will occur before the development of any collaterals and thus symptoms will present acutely and will often be severely limiting. Patients frequently delay in seeking medical attention and may observe symptoms for 2 to 4 weeks before the diagnosis is made.[2] Facial fullness, cough, shortness of breath, hoarseness, nasal congestion, epistaxis, hemoptysis, and dysphagia are all common presenting symptoms.[1] Venous distention and edema of the upper thorax, neck, face, and upper extremities are the most frequent signs on presentation. Upper-body cyanosis, facial plethora, and conjunctival injection may also be present. Severe SVC syndrome may cause life-threatening airway obstruction or a decline in mental status leading to coma due to cerebral venous hypertension.[7]

The clinical diagnosis of SVC syndrome is confirmed by an imaging study, usually computed tomography, which also helps to evaluate the underlying disease and severity of thrombosis in the SVC. Magnetic resonance imaging and/or gadolinium-enhanced magnetic resonance venography can also be used in diagnosing this condition but is not useful patients with a pacemaker or defibrillator in place.

SVC Syndrome of Nonmalignant Etiology

In the developed world, SVC syndrome of nonmalignant etiology ("benign" SVC syndrome) is usually iatrogenic in origin, most frequently due to indwelling intravenous catheters and pacing leads (Table 22.1). Complications of pacemaker lead placement, such as venous thrombosis or stenosis, occur in up to 30% of patients. Only a few patients, however, become symptomatic.[8] The presence of multiple leads, retention of severed lead(s), and previous lead infection may increase the risk of SVC syndrome.[9] Malignancy is the most common cause of SVC syndrome. In a series of 78 patients, Rice and colleagues[4] also found that the incidence of SVC syndrome arising from benign etiologies is increasing. An intravascular device was the most common etiology in benign cases (22 of 31 cases; 71%), with fibrosing mediastinitis the second most common benign etiology (6 cases). The most frequent signs and symptoms were face or neck swelling (82%), upper-extremity swelling (68%), dyspnea (66%), cough (50%), and dilated chest vein collaterals (38%). Dyspnea at rest, cough, and chest pain were more frequent in the patients with malignancy.

The largest series of percutaneous therapy in benign SVC syndrome included 16 patients. Ten patients had SVC syndrome due to indwelling catheter(s), 2 due to the pacemaker lead(s), and 1 each due to goiter, fibrous mediastinitis, heart-lung transplant, and spontaneous thrombosis. The patency rate in 13 patients who where followed for a mean of 17 months was 85%.[10] Rosenblum and colleagues[11] reported excellent results in their series of 6 patients with SVC syndrome due to central lines. All patients were successfully treated and 5 patients followed for up to 2 years with 100% patency. Schifferdecker and colleagues[12] treated 7 patients, all of whom underwent endovascular SVC stenting between 1996 and 2003. The cause of the SVC occlusion was related to central venous infusion catheters in 4 cases, and pacemaker/defibrillator leads in 3. The average follow-up was 36 months with all patients surviving and having achieved symptom resolution.[12]

Pieri et al[13] reported experience with the percutaneous treatment of nonmalignant SVC syndrome in a total of 14 patients. Central venous catheters were believed to be the cause in 11 patients, indwelling pacing leads in 1 case, and in 2 other cases, the cause was attributed to postradiation mediastinal fibrosis. All patients were initially treated using percutaneous techniques and technical success was achieved in 13 patients (92.8%); in one case the obstruction could not be negotiated with the guide wire, so the patient was referred for surgery. No complications related to the successful procedures were reported and symptoms resolved within 2 weeks.

Stenting Technique

Traditionally, access has been obtained through the femoral vein, though internal jugular, subclavian, and basilic vein access have been reported to be a safe alternatives.[14] In patients with bilateral innominate vein involvement, femoral access is preferable since bilateral stenting may be necessary. The area of stenosis is traversed with a guide wire that is used in an "over-the-wire" fashion. Contrast injections into the proximal and distal vein segment in at least 2 projections using rapid filming are necessary for accurate evaluation of the lesion. Pressure gradient measurements across the stenosis are useful in patients whose symptoms are not fully consistent with SVC syndrome, or can be explained by alternative medical conditions,[15] and to confirm resolution of hemodynamic obstruction after stenting. In patients with apparent ingrowth of the tumor into the lumen of the SVC, the use of a directional atherectomy device has been described to obtain tissue for histological diagnosis of underlying malignancy.[16]

The presence of extensive thrombus may prompt use of thrombolytics. After placing the tip of the infusion catheter inside the thrombus, the thrombolytic agent (most frequently, tissue plasminogen activator at a rate of 0.02 mg/kg/hour) is infused and venograms are repeated at 4- to 6-hour intervals. The catheter is then advanced into the remaining thrombus. Pulse-spray injection of thrombolytic agents significantly decreases lysis times.[17] Complications of intraprocedural thrombolytic use are identical to those seen with thrombolytic therapy for other indications. Massive intracerebral hemorrhage,[18] severe gastrointestinal bleeding, and the development of large hematoma have complicated its use in the treatment of SVC syndrome.[10] Thrombus removal with devices such as the Amplatz aspiration thrombectomy catheter[19] or AngioJet (MEDRAD) may be an adjunct or alternative to lengthy intralesional thrombolysis.

Predilatation of the stenosis is necessary in most cases since radial force with stent deployment may not be sufficient for lesion dilatation. The stenosis, however, should only be predilated to approximately 80% of the reference segment to prevent stent migration. Currently, the most frequently used stents in SVC stenting are self-expanding Wallstent (Meditech-Boston Scientific) composed of woven stainless steel mesh, S.M.A.R.T. Control Stent (Johnson and Johnson/Cordis), and other similar self-expanding nitinol stents. A variety of large balloon-expandable stents are available from a number a manufacturers such as Johnson and Johnson/Cordis or eV3. The Gianturco Z-stent (Cook), built from stainless steel wire bent in a zigzag pattern, is uncommonly used today, though it was popular as one of the first self-expanding stent designs.

The recommended diameter of self-expanding stents is 1.2 to 1.5 times venous diameter. Some self-expanding stents foreshorten by up to 30% of their total length. This process may continue beyond the period immediately after stent deployment, especially when the stent is not sufficiently postdilated. Length oversizing of such self-expanding stents is therefore crucial.[20] Due to continuous radial expanding force, self-expanding stents may also migrate if deployed into a tight stenosis. The stent becomes cone-shaped and the terminal prongs across the stenosis may worsen the obstruction and increase the risk of acute SVC thrombosis.[21] Two stents placed together forming a double stent may prevent migration. Such a stent segment, however, is more rigid and the low radial expanding force at the junction may result in poor stenosis dilatation or restenosis in the junction area.[22] Fixation barbs on the stent have also been employed as a strategy to prevent self-expanding stent migration.[23] The tight weave design of the

Wallstent may prevent tumor ingrowth even in patients with total encasement of SVC by tumor.[24] The open design of the older Gianturco stent, on the other hand, was believed to carry a lower risk of thrombosis and may remain useful in cases where critical side branches are covered by the stent.[25]

Balloon-expandable stents allow precise positioning, and their diameter can be adjusted with postdilatation. These stents can also be placed within self-expanding stents to treat short, resistant segments of a longer stenosis. Side branches covered by the original Palmaz stent usually remain patent.[26] The original Palmaz stent is rigid and therefore useful only in relatively straight vascular segments. Subsequent generations of balloon-expandable stents are more flexible. The final deployed diameter of balloon-expandable stents should not be oversized by postdilatation by more than 20% since the associated trauma may engender acute thrombosis or late restenosis secondary to more vigorous intimal hyperplasia.[27]

Most operators use heparin during the procedure but the use of long-term anticoagulation is controversial in SVC syndrome not associated with thrombus and nearly universal in SVC syndrome that is associated with thrombus. Some of the authors recommend warfarin to prevent abrupt stent closure after cessation of the procedural anticoagulation, while others use warfarin only in patients with a documented high burden of thrombus in SVC obstruction.[22] A trend toward use of antiplatelet agents such as aspirin, clopidogrel, or ticlopidine instead of long-term anticoagulation after stenting has occurred. Such a strategy, when associated with stenting, does not seem to increase the risk of SVC syndrome recurrence.[28]

Complications

The most frequently reported complication of SVC stenting is stent thrombosis (0.0%–21.4%).[29] Despite lack of randomized data or expert consensus, vigorous heparin anticoagulation is used routinely during the procedure. Stent migration has been reported with stents found in the heart[30] or pulmonary artery.[10] Avoidance of excessive predilation (> 80% of reference diameter) and length oversizing of self-expanding stents may help to prevent this complication. However, self-expanding stents may "extrude" out of a resistant severe stenosis (Figures 22.1 through 22.7). Pulmonary edema may develop after SVC stenting due to increased venous return and can be managed with diuretics, oxygen, and inotropes.[31] Infection of the stent has been described but is very rare due to early stent endothelization.[32] Antibiotic prophylaxis is considered on a case-by-case basis in high-risk patients. Transient hemidiaphragm elevation has occurred after stent placement, likely secondary to compression of phrenic nerve against tumor.[22] As is also true in stenting of the thoracic aorta, patients often report a pleuritic type of chest discomfort likely related to distention of the superior vena cava. This discomfort usually wanes within 48 hours. Some degree of pulmonary embolization may occur

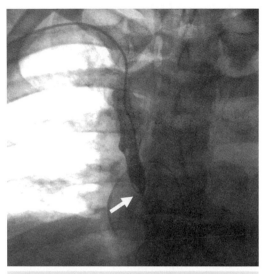

Figure 22.1 A frame from a cine angiogram of a superior vena cava injection in a patient who had developed severe SVC syndrome following placement of a permanent pacing system. The pacing system leads had been removed and a severe stenosis, indicated by the arrow, remains. The pigtail catheter used to perform this angiogram had been inserted from the right brachial approach.

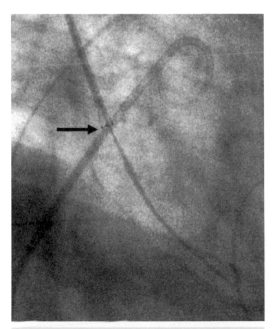

Figure 22.2 The same patient following balloon dilatation of this stenosis, and a 14-mm self-expanding stent placed across the lesion. The stent is just beginning to be deployed and is flaring (arrow) with its most proximal end at the cavo-atrial junction. A pigtail catheter that had been passed from below can be seen in the right atrium.

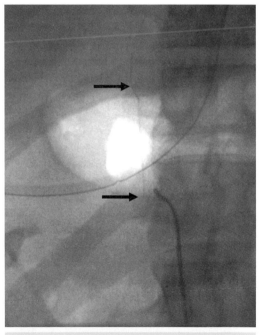

Figure 22.3 The self-expanding stent first shown in Figure 22.2 had been deployed and was "extruded" into the right atrium. In this figure, the stent has been snared and is being removed by being pulled into the inferior vena cava and out through a 16-Fr sheath that had been placed in the right femoral vein.

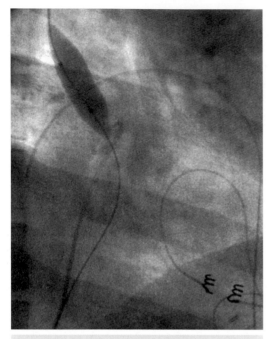

Figure 22.4 The subsequent placement of a balloon-expandable stent from below to salvage this procedure.

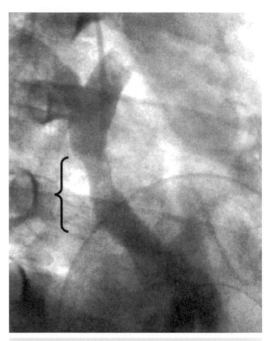

Figure 22.5 A final superior vena cava injection shows renewed patency of the SVC.

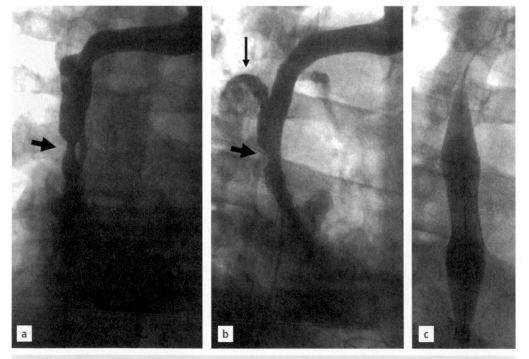

Figure 22.6 (a) The patient, whose initial procedure was outlined in Figures 22.1 through 22.5, returned 6 months later with recurrent, but less-severe, symptoms of facial and upper-extremity swelling. (b) Venography demonstrated in-stent restenosis (thick arrow) with evidence of retrograde flow into the azygos vein (thin arrow). (c) A second larger, balloon-expandable stent was placed and vigorously postdilated.

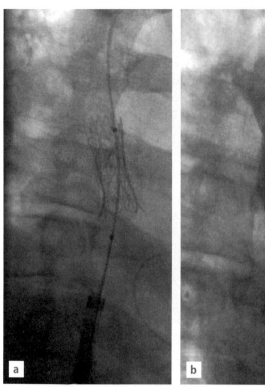
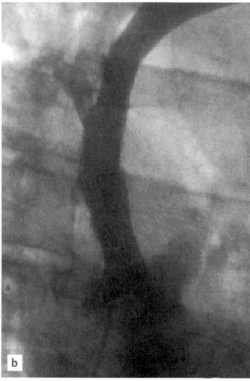

Figure 22.7 (a) The newly placed stent and (b) final venography shows wide patency of the superior vena cava with no retrograde flow in the azygos.

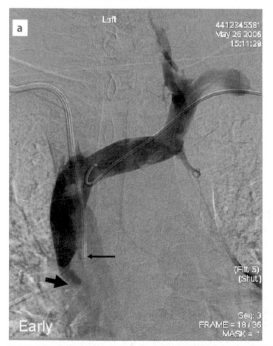
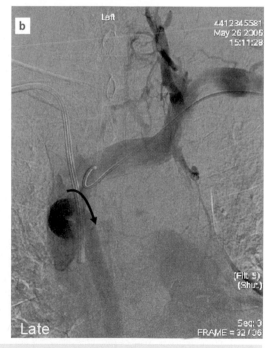

Figure 22.8 Venography of the superior vena cava in a patient with metastatic gastric carcinoma to the mediastinum in association with an indwelling chemotherapy catheter. (a) The tip of this catheter, which had been placed from the right subclavian approach, is indicated by the thin arrow. The thick arrow shows the area of severe stenosis, in part related to thrombus associated with the indwelling catheter, and in part related to metastatic compression from tumor. (b) In a late frame in this venogram, retrograde flow in the azygos vein can be seen.

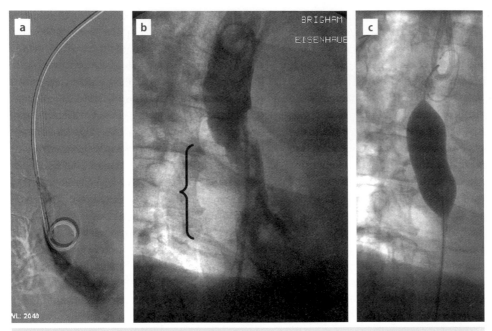

Figure 22.9 (a) A pigtail catheter tip in the right atrium with a local injection outlining the area of stenosis. (b) Following overnight infusion of t-PA, there is renewed patency of the vena cava, but complex filling defects related to thrombus and tumor. (c) Balloon dilatation with a large-diameter balloon was accomplished.

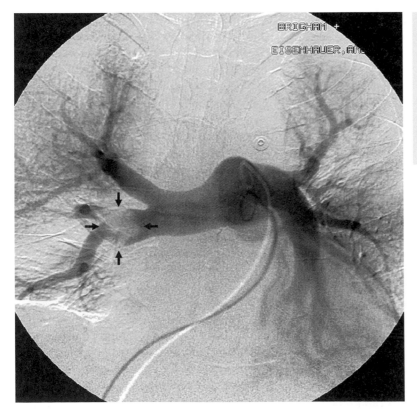

Figure 22.10 The patient described in Figures 22.8 and 22.9 developed moderate dyspnea after this balloon dilation, and pulmonary angiography using digital subtraction technique showed a large filling defect (arrows) in the right inferior division of the pulmonary artery.

from debris in many, if not most, cases involving residual thrombus; large-volume pulmonary embolus creating hemodynamic compromise is uncommon but may occur in patients with significant residual, friable thrombus after initial lysis (Figures 22.8 through 22.10). While complications *directly* related to the procedure are unusual, those associated with the underlying illness in the case of treatment of malignant SVC syndrome are not. Patients with SVC syndrome secondary to the thrombophilic state created by disseminated malignancy carry a poor prognosis even if the SVC syndrome is treated successfully.

Indications for Stenting Therapy

Opinion about the role of stenting in SVC syndrome is evolving. Its efficacy and safety are now established, and the procedure represents only a small increase in the overall cost of care of the patient.[18] SVC stenting is a low-risk procedure that provides fast and durable symptomatic relief. Debate about which therapy is better is not substantiated. Radiation and/or chemotherapy may be limited by side effects but may prolong a patient's life by also addressing the tumor burden. However, radiation and chemotherapy can be combined with SVC stenting, as needed, to provide patients with the benefit of life prolongation, together with effective symptom control. Stenting is indicated in SVC syndrome patients with moderate to severe or rapidly worsening symptoms, in those who have failed to respond to (or recurred after) radiation and/or chemotherapy, in those who have reached a dose limit of radiation or chemotherapy, and in patients who have a nonmalignant obstruction.

Stent therapy should not be used routinely in patients with mild symptoms who will undergo further radiation and/or chemotherapy that alone may be sufficient for relief. Patients, however, should be observed carefully and instructed to return if their symptoms do not improve, or continue to worsen, despite such a treatment. In patients with terminal disease with expected survival of only days to weeks, a generalized recommendation cannot be given.

Here, the benefit of SVC stenting has to be judged on a case-by-case basis considering the burden of symptoms related to SVC syndrome and the overall clinical picture. In patients with SVC syndrome of nonmalignant etiology, based on midterm follow-up results, stenting is the treatment of choice when mechanical relief of obstruction is needed. Surgical therapy should be reserved for patients with benign SVC syndrome refractory to percutaneous therapy, and few patients are likely to become truly refractory. The majority of patients with recurrent SVC syndrome can be treated successfully with repeated percutaneous intervention.[33]

Summary

SVC syndrome is an important clinical entity and, increasingly, is associated with nonmalignant etiologies and longer-term potential patient survival. Endovascular stenting provides sustained effectiveness as primary therapy in SVC syndrome of nonmalignant etiology. It provides immediate, pronounced, and durable symptom relief, and does not interfere with diagnostic evaluation and therapy of the underlying disease. It is minimally invasive, requires minimal hospital stay, and is well tolerated. Though there are potential complications, based on current evidence, SVC stenting should be used as the treatment of choice in the majority of patients with SVC syndrome whose symptoms warrant therapy.

References

1. Markman M. Diagnosis and management of superior vena cava syndrome. *Cleve Clin J Med.* 1999;66:59-61.
2. Stewart IE. Superior vena cava syndrome: an oncologic complication. *Semin Oncol Nurs.* 1996;12:312-317.
3. Schindler N, Vogelzang RL. Superior vena cava syndrome. Experience with endovascular stents

and surgical therapy. *Surg Clin North Am.* 1999;79:683-694, xi.

4. Rice TW, Rodriguez RM, Light RW. The superior vena cava syndrome: clinical characteristics and evolving etiology. *Medicine (Baltimore).* 2006;85:37-42.

5. Lanciego C, Chacon JL, Julian A, et al. Stenting as first option for endovascular treatment of malignant superior vena cava syndrome. *AJR Am J Roentgenol.* 2001;177:585-593.

6. Schraufnagel DE, Hill R, Leech JA, Pare JA. Superior vena caval obstruction. Is it a medical emergency? *Am J Med.* 1981;70:1169-1174.

7. Perez CA, Presant CA, Van Amburg AL III. Management of superior vena cava syndrome. *Semin Oncol.* 1978;5:123-134.

8. Imparato AM, Kim GE. Electrode complications in patients with permanent cardiac pacemakers. Ten years' experience. *Arch Surg.* 1972;105:705-710.

9. Goudevenos JA, Reid PG, Adams PC, Holden MP, Williams DO. Pacemaker-induced superior vena cava syndrome: report of four cases and review of the literature. *Pacing Clin Electrophysiol.* 1989;12:1890-1895.

10. Kee ST, Kinoshita L, Razavi MK, Nyman UR, Semba CP, Dake MD. Superior vena cava syndrome: treatment with catheter-directed thrombolysis and endovascular stent placement. *Radiology.* 1998;206:187-193.

11. Rosenblum J, Leef J, Messersmith R, Tomiak M, Bech F. Intravascular stents in the management of acute superior vena cava obstruction of benign etiology. *JPEN J Parenter Enteral Nutr.* 1994;18:362-366.

12. Schifferdecker B, Shaw JA, Piemonte TC, Eisenhauer AC. Nonmalignant superior vena cava syndrome: pathophysiology and management. *Catheter Cardiovasc Interv.* 2005;65:416-423.

13. Pieri S, Agresti P, Carnabuci A, Pizzarelli S, Ianniello S, De' Medici L. Endovascular treatment of benign superior vena cava syndrome: venographic patterns and implications for treatment. *Radiol Med.* (Torino) 2005;110:359-369.

14. Miller JH, McBride K, Little F, Price A. Malignant superior vena cava obstruction: stent placement via the subclavian route. *Cardiovasc Intervent Radiol.* 2000;23:155-158.

15. Kishi K, Sonomura T, Mitsuzane K, et al. Self-expandable metallic stent therapy for superior vena cava syndrome: clinical observations. *Radiology.* 1993;189:531-535.

16. Dake MD, Zemel G, Dolmatch BL, Katzen BT. The cause of superior vena cava syndrome: diagnosis with percutaneous atherectomy. *Radiology.* 1990;174:957-959.

17. Valji K, Roberts AC, Davis GB, Bookstein JJ. Pulsed-spray thrombolysis of arterial and bypass graft occlusions. *AJR Am J Roentgenol.* 1991;156:617-621.

18. Dyet JF, Nicholson AA, Cook AM. The use of the Wallstent endovascular prosthesis in the treatment of malignant obstruction of the superior vena cava. *Clin Radiol.* 1993;48:381-385.

19. Edwards RD, Jackson JE. Case report: superior vena caval obstruction treated by thrombolysis, mechanical thrombectomy and metallic stents. *Clin Radiol.* 1993;48:215-217.

20. Entwisle KG, Watkinson AF, Reidy J. Case report: migration and shortening of a self-expanding metallic stent complicating the treatment of malignant superior vena cava stenosis. *Clin Radiol.* 1996;51:593-595.

21. Gaines PA, Belli AM, Anderson PB, McBride K, Hemingway AP. Superior vena caval obstruction managed by the Gianturco Z Stent. *Clin Radiol.* 1994;49:202-206; discussion 207-208.

22. Irving JD, Dondelinger RF, Reidy JF, et al. Gianturco self-expanding stents: clinical experience in the vena cava and large veins. *Cardiovasc Intervent Radiol.* 1992;15:328-333.

23. Charnsangavej C, Carrasco CH, Wallace S, et al. Stenosis of the vena cava: preliminary assessment of treatment with expandable metallic stents. *Radiology.* 1986;161:295-298.

24. Jackson JE, Brooks DM. Stenting of superior vena caval obstruction. *Thorax.* 1995;50 (Suppl 1):S31-S36.

25. Oudkerk M, Kuijpers TJ, Schmitz PI, Loosveld O, de Wit R. Self-expanding metal stents for palliative treatment of superior vena

caval syndrome. *Cardiovasc Intervent Radiol.* 1996;19:146-151.

26. Wright KC, Wallace S, Charnsangavej C, Carrasco CH, Gianturco C. Percutaneous endovascular stents: an experimental evaluation. *Radiology.* 1985;156:69-72.

27. Antonucci F, Salomonowitz E, Stuckmann G, Stiefel M, Largiader J, Zollikofer CL. Placement of venous stents: clinical experience with a self-expanding prosthesis. *Radiology.* 1992;183:493-497.

28. Gross CM, Kramer J, Waigand J, et al. Stent implantation in patients with superior vena cava syndrome. *AJR Am J Roentgenol.* 1997;169:429-432.

29. Stock KW, Jacob AL, Proske M, Bolliger CT, Rochlitz C, Steinbrich W. Treatment of malignant obstruction of the superior vena cava with the self-expanding Wallstent. *Thorax.* 1995;50:1151-1156.

30. Furui S, Sawada S, Kuramoto K, et al. Gianturco stent placement in malignant caval obstruction: analysis of factors for predicting the outcome. *Radiology.* 1995;195:147-152.

31. Marcy PY, Magne N, Bentolila F, Drouillard J, Bruneton JN, Descamps B. Superior vena cava obstruction: is stenting necessary? *Support Care Cancer.* 2001;9:103-107.

32. Therasse E, Soulez G, Cartier P, et al. Infection with fatal outcome after endovascular metallic stent placement. *Radiology.* 1994;192:363-365.

33. Crowe MT, Davies CH, Gaines PA. Percutaneous management of superior vena cava occlusions. *Cardiovasc Intervent Radiol.* 1995;18:367-372.

23

Uncommon Venous Disorders

Jessica Nevins Morse and Bruce H. Gray

Deep venous thrombosis of the lower extremities and chronic venous insufficiency are the most common venous disorders. In this chapter we review lesser-known venous disorders, divided between congenital and acquired etiologies.

Congenital Venous Disorders

Congenital venous disorders affect 1% of the population. The pathology of these disorders ranges from agenesis to hyperplasia; most are subclinical and infrequently recognized. Several disorders present with characteristic signs and symptoms that warrant specific mention, including Klippel-Trenaunay syndrome, Parkes-Weber syndrome, Kasabach-Merritt syndrome, and cutis marmorata telangiectatica congenita.

Klippel-Trenaunay Syndrome

History, prevalence, and pathogenesis
Klippel-Trenaunay syndrome (KTS), also known as *nevus vasculosus hypertrophicus*, is the pro-

totypical congenital venous malformation. Initially described in 1900 by French physicians Maurice Klippel and Paul Trénaunay, the syndrome consists of the classic triad: (1) port-wine stain or capillary malformations, (2) soft tissue and bony hypertrophy, and (3) varicose veins.[1] Other frequent findings include lymphatic malformations and deep venous malformations (such as aplasia, hypoplasia, or deep venous reflux). Despite the spectrum of venous abnormalities associated with the syndrome, KTS is further characterized by the absence of hemodynamically significant arteriovenous fistulae. This characteristic distinguishes Klippel-Trenaunay-Weber or Parkes-Weber syndrome from KTS.[2,3]

KTS is a rare disorder with an estimated occurrence of 1 in 20,000 to 1 in 40,000 live births.[4] This is a congenital and not an inherited disorder, since all patients with KTS have a negative family history for KTS. Much of the knowledge gained about the syndrome since its initial description consists of retrospective case reviews. The Mayo Clinic provided a review of 252 KTS patients assessed over a 40-year period. From these data, no sexual predominance was noted. The majority of the patients were Caucasian with over 90% having evidence of KTS at birth. One or both lower extremities were involved in 88%. Figure 23.1 provides the distribution of anatomic site involvement in these patients.[5]

The etiology of KTS remains obscure. Initially, physicians Klippel and Trénaunay theorized that a spinal cord abnormality explained their findings. Later, physician M. Servelle attributed the syndrome to atresia of the deep leg veins; however, contemporary review of lower-extremity phlebography showed that KTS is predominantly associated with changes in the superficial veins.[6,7] In the 1970s several researchers hypothesized that a mesodermal defect involving angiogenesis could explain the syndrome and the multiple associated abnormalities.[2,3] More recently, this hypothesis has been supported by genetic research. Two separate mutations involving the potent angiogenic factor VG5Q have been implicated as increasing the fetus's susceptibility to KTS.[8] One such involves a 5;11 chromosomal translocation that results in increased VG5Q transcription, while the second is a functional mutation in the E133K gene that upregulates the activity of VG5Q.[8-10] Other mutations are also being studied. These genetic variations allow for the phenotypic heterogeneity that is characteristic of KTS. Further research is needed to determine whether this sporadic syndrome is due to mosaicism or incomplete penetrance.

Diagnostic evaluation

The diagnosis of KTS is based on the physical examination (Figures 23.2 and 23.3) and the presence of the classic triad (port-wine stain, soft tissue hypertrophy, and varicose veins).[11] Typically, the infant's appearance at birth will define the full extent of the syndrome with the presence of at least 2 characteristics. Sixty percent will manifest all 3 features at birth.[5]

The *port-wine stain,* or capillary malformation, histologically consists of vascular malformations with ectatic capillaries or venules in the upper dermis. Typically, this lesion is found on the extremity affected by venous disease but can be seen on the contralateral extremity or trunk.[5] If the central trunk is involved, the lesion rarely crosses the midline (exception seen in Figure 23.2). In most cases, the degree of capillary malformation is fully known at birth. Because these lesions are nonproliferative, they do not regress, however, the color intensity may vary with age.[4,5] *Nevus flammeus* differs from port-wine staining in that it usually occurs on the face and neck and regresses with time. Some patients may acquire nodular lesions either in conjunction with the initial capillary malformation or on previously unaffected areas of skin. These are ectatic venous channels and can be quite friable, leading to spontaneous bleeding with minor trauma. This fragile skin predisposes to infection, skin breakdown, and ulceration.[11] The confirmation of the port-wine stain is on clinical grounds—biopsy is not necessary. Capillary malformations on the trunk could warrant further evaluation for the exclusion of vascular malformations involving the underlying viscera.[12]

Limb and *soft tissue hypertrophy* is the most variable of the 3 cardinal features. It will be present in at least some degree at birth. Most often, the hypertrophy involves the limb with varicose veins. The more extensive the soft tissue hyper-

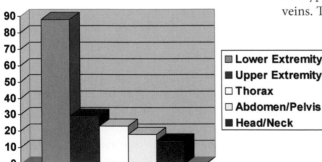

Figure 23.1 Percent site involvement of Klippel-Trenaunay syndrome in 252 patients.

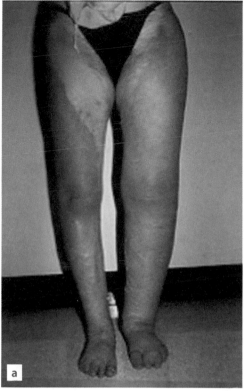

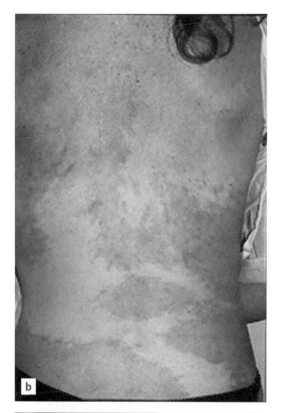

trophy, the greater the likelihood of associative lymphatic disease. Individuals with limb girth discrepancy greater than 4 cm will typically have more extensive lymphatic involvement.[4,5,9] Lymphoscintigraphy can determine the extent of involvement but rarely alters treatment.

Limb length discrepancies (unusual in KTS but common in Parkes-Weber syndrome) should be evaluated serially with growth charting, plain x-rays, or CTA. These objective measures should continue until growth plate closure (puberty) and stabilization of the discrepancy.[5,13]

Varicose veins, or venous malformations, constitute the third cardinal feature of KTS. Varicose veins are the most common and benign of the pathologies seen. The varicosities of KTS frequently involve the lateral aspect of the thigh. They are consistent with persistent embryonic veins, such as the lateral vein of the thigh or sciatic vein (Figure 23.3). While the venous malformations of KTS are characteristically superficial, deep and perforating vein

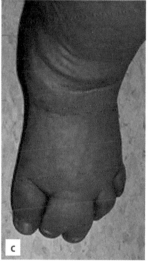

Figure 23.2
(a, above left) Klippel-Trenaunay syndrome involving both lower extremities. (b, above) Same patient viewed from the back. (c, left) Magnified view of the left foot; note the soft tissue hypertrophy and syndactyly.

incompetence, duplication, atresia, hypoplasia, or aneurysmal dilation can occur. Patency and valvular competence of the venous system can be evaluated with supine and standing Duplex ultrasonography. Duplex ultrasonography is often the most useful test to rule out superficial or deep vein thrombosis, which does occur in

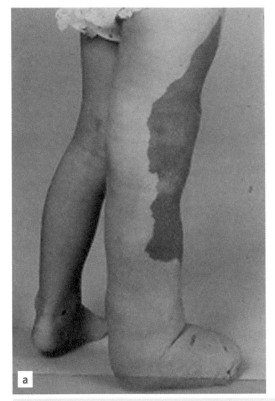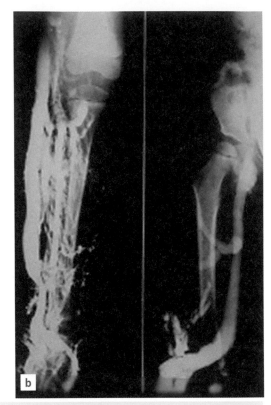

Figure 23.3 (a) Four-year-old with KTS with involvement of the right leg. (b) Venogram of the right leg demonstrating dysgenesis of the deep femoral vein and persistence of the lateral limb bud vein.

these patients (Figure 23.4). Occasionally, impedance plethysmography can be used to evaluate outflow obstruction, but it is not available in many laboratories. MRA can be used to evaluate not only venous anatomy but the soft tissue as well. Invasive ascending and descending venography of both the superficial and deep veins is unnecessary unless venous ablative or limb reduction surgery is considered.[13-16]

Management

The management of KTS is typically prophylactic in nature. The avoidance of trauma, infection, thrombosis, and unwarranted venous ablative procedures are the important outpatient treatment issues (Figure 23.5).

The capillary malformations do not require further management other than routine local skin care. Cosmetically, laser therapy can be attempted to lessen the lesions' intensity, but this has had varying success to date.[17] If the capillary malformation does lead to recur-

rent cellulitis, use of prophylactic antibiotics is necessary. Rarely is ligation, resection, or amputation necessary for persistent infection or bleeding.

Limb length discrepancy can require intervention. Typically, if the length discrepancy is < 2 cm, prosthetic lifts will alleviate symptoms and minimize scoliosis. A length discrepancy > 2 cm warrants orthopedic consultation for potential epiphysiodesis. This possibility needs to be considered in early adolescence before growth plate closure.

Debulking of soft tissue hypertrophy has been used infrequently for the treatment of limb girth discrepancy. The soft tissue can be removed with replacement of the skin over the muscle and fascia layers. This disfiguring surgery should be reserved for extreme cases of elephantiasis (huge, heavy limbs) that limit ambulatory ability. Otherwise, compression stockings or pneumatic compression can be used to minimize fluid (lymphedema) accumulation during the

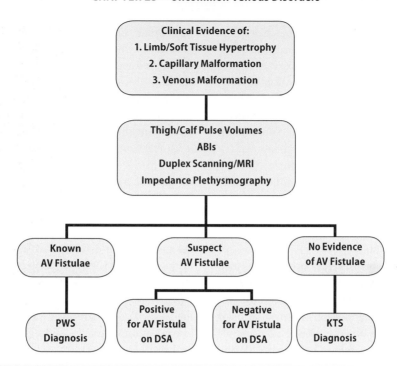

Figure 23.4 Diagnostic flowchart for Klippel-Trenaunay syndrome and Parkes-Weber syndrome.

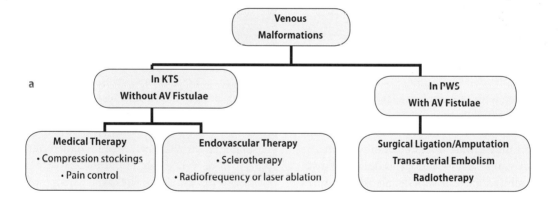

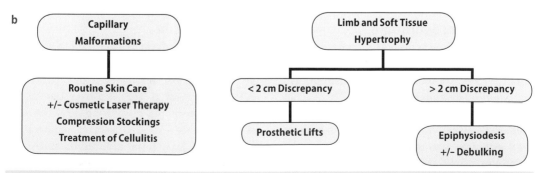

Figure 23.5 (a) Management of venous malformations in the Klippel-Trenaunay syndrome versus Parkes-Weber syndrome. (b) Management of the nonvenous aspects of Klippel-Trenaunay syndrome and Parkes-Weber syndrome.

day and maintain ambulatory status. Compression stockings also augment venous function.

Management of venous varicosities is perhaps the most common intervention in KTS patients. Chronic symptoms such as edema, pain, and fatigue of the limb are most common. The treatment options range from compression stockings to surgical ligation and stripping.

Superficial venous thrombosis can be managed with nonsteroidal anti-inflammatory medication if remote (> 10 cm) from the deep venous system. Otherwise, anticoagulation is preferred. Deep venous thrombosis requires the use of anticoagulation.

More extensive surgical procedures such as reconstruction or bypass have been infrequently used. Intimate knowledge of the venous anatomy via venography is essential prior to considering any intervention. This principle is also important to follow before considering even the removal or ablation (ultrasonic or laser light) of superficial varicosities. In patients with dysgenesis of the deep system, the lateral limb vein persists. This prominent thigh vein, as well as others, may provide the only significant outflow from the affected extremity. Removal of it could result in catastrophic venous insufficiency.[3,14,15]

Even with removal of unsightly superficial veins, the development of other varicosities is common (up to 50%). Injection sclerotherapy has been used with caution in these patients.[16]

Possible complications associated with intervention include worsening edema, ulcer formation, thrombophlebitis, cellulitis, and bleeding.[3,15]

Parkes-Weber Syndrome

History, prevalence, and pathogenesis

Parkes-Weber syndrome (PWS), also known as *Klippel-Trenaunay-Weber syndrome*, has evolved as a sister syndrome to KTS. In 1918, Frederick Parkes Weber denoted a subset of KTS patients who presented with hemodynamically significant arteriovenous fistulae. The natural history of this subset differs due to the presence of the AV fistulae, which are mul-

tiple, small, and confined to the affected limb. Fistulae are high flow and alter growth rates, and increase cardiac output and venous drainage from the affected limb.[18]

The gene *RASA1* has been associated with PWS. It is theorized that mutations in this gene are responsible for capillary and arteriovenous malformations that define the syndrome.[19,20]

Diagnostic evaluation

The diagnosis of PWS is based upon the objective confirmation of multiple arteriovenous fistulae. Auscultation of the affected limb can raise the suspicion for fistulae when systolic-diastolic bruits are heard. Further objective evaluation with Duplex ultrasonography, contrast arteriography, or MRA/CTA should be done[21,22] (see Figure 23.4). The demonstration of microscopic arteriovenous fistulae is pathognomonic for this syndrome (Figure 23.6).

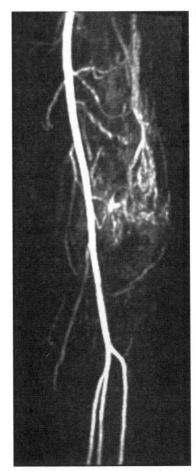

Figure 23.6 MRA demonstrating multiple small AV fistulae in the left thigh of a patient with Parkes-Weber syndrome.

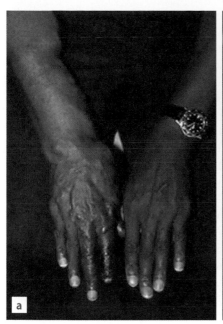
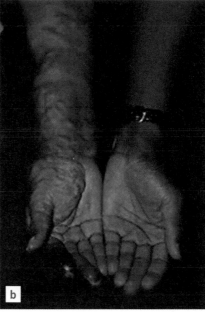

Figure 23.7
(a) Dorsal side and (b) palmar side of arms in a patient with large arteriovenous malformation of the right forearm. The index finger demonstrates necrosis. Noninvasive studies demonstrate nonpulsatile flow into the fingers at rest, but become pulsatile when a blood pressure cuff is inflated to 50 mm Hg on the right forearm.

Management

PWS management parallels that of KTS, with emphasis on prophylaxis against trauma, edema, and thrombosis (see Figure 23.5). Arteriovenous fistulae may need to be treated, particularly if cutaneous ulceration or distal steal phenomenon develops (Figure 23.7). The increased blood volume can lead to excessive limb growth. Early treatment of the arteriovenous fistula can decrease limb length discrepancy.[11] The older literature described surgical removal and/or ligation. Contemporary treatment uses percutaneous catheter-based embolization of the arterial inflow. Not infrequently, the embolization process is performed in a staged, stepwise fashion to avoid soft tissue necrosis and venous thrombosis. Radiotherapy has been described in the ablation of AV fistulae with variable success.[22,23]

Kasabach-Merritt Syndrome

History, prevalence, and pathogenesis

Kasabach-Merritt syndrome (KMS) was described in 1940 as the presence of a rapidly enlarging capillary hemangioma with thrombocytopenia. This consumptive thrombocytopenia is severe, with platelet counts dropping below 20,000/μL. Platelet half-life is also shortened to less than 24 hours. Early recognition is important since mortality rates reach 40% in infants. Ten percent of newborns have cutaneous hemangiomas, whereas only 0.3% of these develop KMS. KMS is not limited to cutaneous hemangioma but can also occur with visceral hemangioma, making diagnosis difficult. The size and site of the original hemangioma is not predictive of who will acquire KMS.[23] KMS can occur as an isolated syndrome or in conjunction with other syndromes associated with hemangiomas, such as Klippel-Trenaunay syndrome and Parkes-Weber syndrome.[11] Infrequently this syndrome can occur in adults, especially in women with gynecologic disorders or pregnancy.

The pathogenesis KMS is unknown. Histologically, KMS hemangiomas fall into 1 of 2 categories: *kaposiform hemangioendothelioma (KHE)*, a low-grade malignant tumor with sheets of infiltrating endothelial cells, or *tufted angioma (TA)*, a benign growth of vascular tufts. Both have evidence of microthrombi and hemosiderin deposits.[24] It has also been noted that patients with KMS have elevated urine levels of basic fibroblast growth factor (bFGF) and proangiogenic factor. Also, those who respond clinically to treatment have a correlative drop in their bFGF levels.[25] Therefore, downregulation of angiogenesis leads to involution of these cutaneous hemangiomas, decreasing the potential development of the syndrome.

Diagnostic evaluation

The diagnosis of KMS should be suspected in an infant with a rapidly evolving cutaneous hemangioma with or without thrombocytopenia. It should also be included in the differential diagnosis in patients with unexplained profound thrombocytopenia. Useful laboratory values are found in Table 23.1. Imaging studies, hematologic evaluation, and tissue/fluid culture may be helpful to exclude other causes of thrombocytopenia. A biopsy can differentiate benign from malignant tumors but should be done in the absence of coagulopathy.[23]

CBC
Reticulocyte count
Peripheral smear
Prothrombin time
Partial thromboplastin time
Fibrinogen
Fibrin degradation products
D-dimer

Table 23.1 Useful Laboratory Data in Suspected Kasabach-Merritt Syndrome

Management

The goals of treatment are to stop the consumptive coagulopathy and maintain hemostasis, and to stop the growth or progression of the vascular tumor.

The thrombocytopenia, when profound, requires platelet transfusions. Additional blood products, such as fresh-frozen plasma, cryoprecipitate, or factor VII concentrate, can also be of benefit in reestablishing hemostasis. Corticosteroids and interferon-α have both been shown to help, with a 50% to 60% response rate. Response time for prednisolone at a dose of 2 to 5 mg/kg/day is typically 1 week, while interferon-α produces response within the first month.[26,27] Risks of corticosteroid use are typical of any high-dose protocol, while interferon carries a risk of spastic diplegia with long-term use. This limits the use of interferon to 6 months or less.[28,29] Other medications that may have unsubstanti-

ated clinical benefit include chemotherapeutic agents and anticoagulants.

Direct treatment of the hemangioma includes elastic compression, catheter-based embolization, and surgical excision. Intervention should be aggressively pursued when the eyes, airway, or other vital organ is compromised by the hemangioma.[23,30,31] More benign lesions should be managed medically since these therapies are not definitive and recurrence rates are high.[23]

Cutis Marmorata Telangiectatica Congenita

History, prevalence, and pathogenesis

Cutis marmorata telangiectatica congenita (CMTC) was first described by Van Lohuizen[32] in 1922 as a fixed reticulated vascular pattern on the skin, similar to physiologic cutis marmorata, but nonreversible on skin warming. The reticular pattern is seen on the extremity in a localized or diffuse pattern. Other manifestations include skin atrophy, ulcerations, and hypoplasia of the affected limb. These skin changes are present at birth, regress during the first 2 years of life, and then stabilize.[33]

Little is known concerning the pathogenesis of this rare disorder.[34] Histologic specimens show nonspecific findings yielding little information. The prevalence is also unknown and, because CMTC has a relatively benign course, it is infrequently reported in the literature.

CMTC can be seen in patients with Adams-Oliver syndrome and CMTC-macrocephaly syndrome.[33] These syndromes have anomalies that help to distinguish them from CMTC. Table 23.2 lists the differential diagnosis of congenital reticular rashes.

Physiologic cutis marmorata
Cutis marmorata associated with genetic syndromes
Reticulated capillary malformations
Bockenheimer syndrome
Neonatal lupus erythematosus
CMTC syndromes

Table 23.2 Differential Diagnosis of Disease States Associated with Cutis Marmorata Telangiectatica Congenita

Diagnostic evaluation

CMTC remains a clinical diagnosis based on a reticular rash that is more often localized on an extremity. These patients may also have a capillary malformation (port-wine stain) but do not have arteriovenous malformations. Limb asymmetry is the most common associated finding with CMTC. Glaucoma is independently associated with CMTC as are multiple neurologic deficiencies ranging from psychomotor retardation to cerebral atrophy. These children should also be screened for cardiac anomalies and hypothyroidism.[33] Overall, the clinical course is benign, but attention should be focused on the associative conditions seen in CMTC.

Management

No therapy is necessary for the reticulated skin lesion. Laser therapy has been used for cosmetic reasons in case reports with varying success.[35]

Acquired Venous Disorders

In this section we review lesser-known disorders of venous thrombosis, including cerebral venous sinus thrombosis, mesenteric venous thrombosis, portal/hepatic vein thrombosis, suppurative internal jugular vein thrombosis, and thoracoepigastric superficial vein thrombosis.

Cerebral Venous Sinus Thrombosis

History, prevalence, and pathogenesis

Cerebral venous sinus thrombosis (CVST) is an uncommon disorder in which larger cerebral sinuses (ie, superior sagittal or cavernous sinus) thrombose.[36] CVST has been noted in all ages and patient demographics. However, there is a slight predilection toward young women, particularly those on oral contraceptives.[37] A predisposing factor is identified in 80% of patients. The most common thrombophilias are deficiencies in protein C or S and Factor V Leiden.[38,39] In general, sinus occlusion is a gradual process allowing for collateralization, but acute occlusion can occur.

Diagnostic evaluation

The presenting symptoms of CVST vary widely from ophthalmoplegia to stroke. The headache typically is insidious and chronic over several days to weeks. Thunderclap headache with neck stiffness seen with subarachnoid hemorrhage has been described. The triad of chemosis, proptosis, and painful ophthalmoplegia is the classic description for cavernous sinus thrombosis but is only present in 3% of cases. In patients with bilateral or alternating neurologic deficits, superior sagittal sinus thrombosis should be considered. Seizures are nonspecific, with postictal (Todd's) paralysis in some patients. Overall, the signs and symptoms are nonspecific and the classic ophthalmologic clues are less common than expected.[36,40]

The diagnosis is based on imaging the cerebral veins (Figures 23.8 and 23.9 on following page). The test of choice for specifically diagnosing CVST is MRI, with magnetic resonance venogram (MRV) having replaced cerebral angiography, although caveats remain. For example, a normal anatomic variant of anterior superior sagittal sinus hypoplasia can mistakenly be read as CVST. The accuracy of standard CTA is low. The flow void in a thrombosed superior sagittal sinus is seen in only 20%, with just as many patients having an entirely normal CTA. Attempts at combining CTA with venography are underway as a diagnostic option.[41] Central nervous system fluid analysis is often part of the diagnostic workup and helps to rule out infectious causes for the neurologic symptoms. The findings of a high opening pressure, elevated protein levels, and red blood cells are nonspecific. The patients should also undergo a thrombophilia workup to include a cancer screen in the absence of a hematologic abnormality. Approximately 20% will not have an identifiable cause for their thrombosis.[36]

Management

The treatment of CVST is systemic anticoagulation. During hospitalization, aqueous heparin sodium or low-molecular-weight heparin is given. Warfarin sodium is then given for a minimum of 6 months. Those with nonreversible risk factors may benefit from life-long therapy.[42]

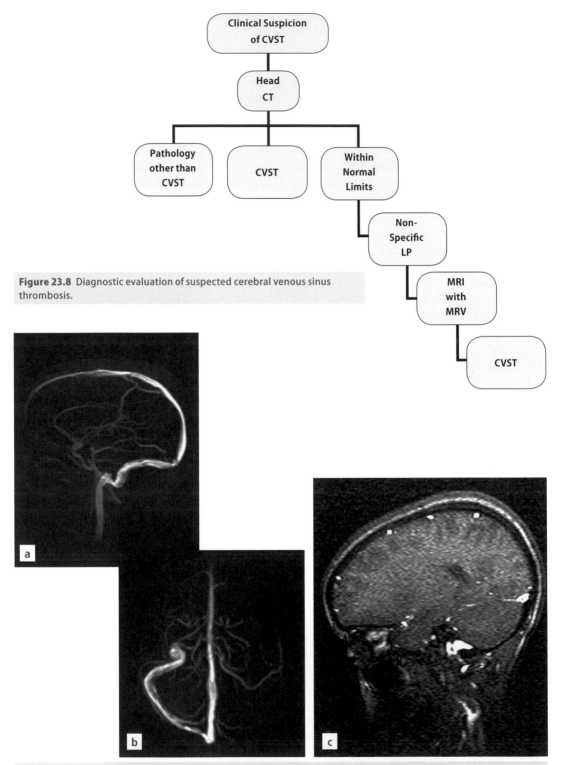

Figure 23.8 Diagnostic evaluation of suspected cerebral venous sinus thrombosis.

Figure 23.9 MRV of cerebral sinus thrombosis in a 12-year-old who presented with fever of unknown origin and altered mental status. The superior sagittal sinus is (a) patent with (b) thrombosis of the left transverse and (c) straight sinus. (Study courtesy of A. Ronald Cowley, MD, Greenville Hospital System University Medical Center, Greenville, SC)

In retrospective analyses of over 100 cases of CVST, the benefits of heparin therapy were noted even for those with evidence of hemorrhage at the time of presentation. Patients with worsening symptoms despite anticoagulation may benefit from catheter-directed thrombolysis or catheter thrombectomy. While initial data are favorable, thrombolysis is not considered first-line therapy, as the risk to benefit ratio is quite difficult to determine.[43] Antiepileptic and antibiotic therapy as dictated by individual clinical presentation may be helpful.

The prognosis of CVST is good, with 80% regaining their full functional status. Mortality is currently reported at 5% to 18%. The severity and duration of presenting symptoms is not a reliable predictor of mortality, although extremes of age, severe neurologic deficit, and extensive comorbidities are poor prognostic factors. Long-term follow-up is important since 12% of CVST patients have recurrence and 14% will develop a remote venous thrombosis.[44]

Mesenteric Venous Thrombosis

History, prevalence, and pathogenesis

First described in 1935 by Warren and Eberhard,[45] *mesenteric venous thrombosis (MVT)* comprises 5% to 15% of mesenteric ischemia. While generally considered an uncommon disorder, MVT ranks third in site behind the limb and lung. MVT can be characterized as either primary (idiopathic, 20%) or secondary (80%) in origin (Figure 23.10).[46,47] The most common thrombophilias in the general population are the most frequently seen with MVT. Those include Factor V Leiden, the prothrombin mutation G20210A, and the MTHFR TT677 genotypes.[48] Fifty percent of MVT patients have a personal or family history of deep venous thrombosis or pulmonary embolism.[49]

The etiology of MVT may impact the extent of thrombosis and the clinical presentation and course. When a thrombophilia is identified, both proximal and distal superior mesenteric vein thrombosis is seen. The thrombosis is usually isolated to the superior mesenteric vein without involvement of the splenic or portal veins. These patients typically present with acute symptoms and have more extensive bowel necrosis. In contrast, when intra-abdominal causes are found as the etiology, proximal thrombosis predominates with less-significant distal thrombosis, however, splenic or portal vein thrombosis are more common. These patients have a less acute course and less need for surgical intervention.[46,50]

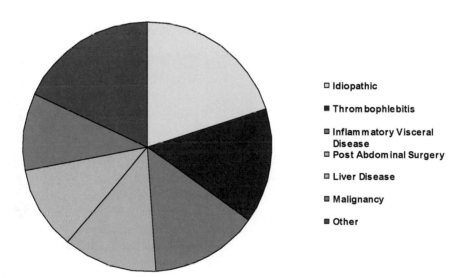

□ Idiopathic

■ Thrombophlebitis

▨ Inflammatory Visceral Disease

□ Post Abdominal Surgery

▨ Liver Disease

▨ Malignancy

■ Other

Figure 23.10 The etiology of mesenteric vein thrombosis in a review of 372 patients.

Diagnostic evaluation

The clinical presentation varies from acute abdominal pain with hypotension and peritonitis to chronic, persistent abdominal pain over the course of several weeks. The pain is typically out of proportion to the physical examination, raising the suspicion for mesenteric ischemia. Other nonspecific symptoms include nausea, emesis, diarrhea, and melena. Patients with subacute or chronic MVT are felt to be at a lesser risk of infarction and peritonitis due to compensation through collateralization. Unexplained ascites in a patient with a family history of venous thrombosis should raise suspicion for MVT.[51,52]

CTA is considered the test of choice for suspected cases of MVT and allows for diagnosis in 90% of cases. The thrombosis itself appears as a central lucency with a sharply defined rim of increased density (Figure 23.11). The vein is often enlarged as a result of the thrombosis. Associated findings include bowel-wall enhancement, pneumatosis intestinalis, and portal vein gas, which can be seen as late complications of infarction. CTA will also allow for detection of collateral flow associated with chronic MVT. CTA loses diagnostic accuracy when only small mesenteric veins are involved. Duplex ultrasonography can yield a diagnosis of MVT but with much less sensitivity than CTA (< 50%). MRA, although less available and more time consuming than CTA, has excellent sensitivity and specificity of MVT.[46,53] Mesenteric angiography should be reserved for those difficult to diagnose cases wherein small-vessel MVT is suspected.[54] Laboratory testing, barium enema, endoscopic studies, and paracentesis are nonspecific and nondiagnostic for MVT.[46,48]

Management

Patients with an acute or subacute presentation of MVT warrant systemic anticoagulation. This should be started without delay and is even warranted in patients presenting with melena in the absence of bowel infarction. Peritonitis, bowel infarction, and perforation are indications for emergent surgery.[46,51] Bowel resection is usually limited to a short segment. Second-look laparotomy is common. Postoperative anticoagulation is recommended to minimize the risk of subsequent venous thrombosis. Arterial dilators, such as papaverine, counteract the arterial vasospasm and can resuscitate reversibly ischemic bowel and minimize loss of bowel.[46]

Thrombolytic therapy has been used. The drugs (urokinase, tissue plasminogen activator, etc.) can be delivered via a selective catheter in the superior mesenteric artery or via transhepatic *transjugular intrahepatic portosystemic shunting (TIPS)*. Those patients without peritoneal signs, a short duration of symptoms, and no melena may be considered for thrombolysis.[55] Long-term anticoagulation would still be necessary in these patients.[46,51]

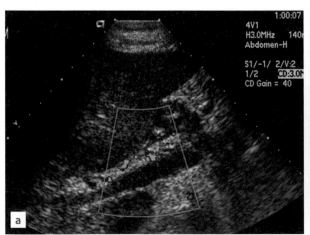
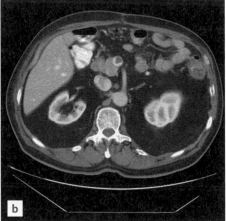

Figure 23.11 (a) Duplex ultrasonography and (b) CTA demonstrating thrombosis of the superior mesenteric vein. (Study courtesy of Thom W. Rooke, MD, Mayo Clinic, Rochester, MN)

Despite aggressive anticoagulation with or without surgical intervention, acute MVT carries a 20% to 50% mortality rate. This is certainly influenced by comorbidities and conditions predisposing the patient to developing MVT. Sixty percent of patients treated with surgical resection have subsequent thrombosis of veins adjacent to the anastomotic site, indicating that too little bowel was originally resected or propagation of residual thrombus.[46,47,51]

Budd-Chiari Syndrome

History, prevalence, and pathogenesis

Budd-Chiari syndrome (BCS) was first described in 1845 by George Budd, a British internist, and later in 1899 by Hans Chiari, an Austrian pathologist.[56] BCS is often used interchangeably with *hepatic vein thrombosis;* however, the syndrome is actually a heterogeneous group of disorders resulting in hepatic outflow tract obstruction. The actual obstruction can be present in the hepatic venules or hepatic veins, as well as the intrahepatic or suprahepatic inferior vena cava (IVC). Regardless of the level of obstruction, increased sinusoidal pressure and portal hypertension ensues. This decrease in portal vein perfusion provides a setup for potential portal vein thrombosis and causes hypoxic damage to the parenchymal liver cells. The end result is centrilobular necrosis, nodular regenerative hyperplasia, and eventual development of cirrhosis.[57]

Large retrospective studies have shown a female predilection (67%), with a median onset at 35 years of age. BCS develops from hepatic vein obstruction in > 60% of cases, with IVC obstruction causing < 10% of cases. An underlying cause is found in 75% of patients. The most prevalent cause is a myeloproliferative disorder, notably polycythemia rubra vera, which is reported in 10% to 40% of cases. Also, a majority of idiopathic cases may later develop a myeloproliferative disorder, suggesting that a subclinical myeloproliferative disorder was causative. Thrombophilias associated with BCS include deficiencies in protein C, protein S, or antithrombin III. Oral contraceptive therapy results in a relative risk of 2.37 for BCS. This is equivalent to the risk posed for stroke, myocardial infarction, and deep venous thrombosis with oral contraceptive pill use.[57-59]

Diagnostic evaluation

The clinical presentation of BCS can vary significantly based on the acuity of the disease. The syndrome can present in an acute, sometimes fulminant course, subacutely with symptoms of several weeks duration, or chronically, with symptoms > 6 months. Acute disease makes up ~ 20% of all BCS cases. Initial symptoms include the acute onset of right-upper-quadrant pain and hepatomegaly with rapid progression to jaundice and ascites. The symptoms are accompanied by liver function test abnormalities, including transaminases elevated to 5 times normal.[57,60]

Subacute and chronic BCS present insidiously. Over time collateral veins decompress the liver and can develop into varicosities. The caudate lobe of the liver can also hypertrophy and is seen in a subset of patients. This causes compression of the IVC producing leg edema. Long-term congestion results in cirrhosis with its subsequent problems. Hematologic studies show mild elevation in bilirubin and alkaline phosphatase levels. Ascitic fluid analysis shows a nonspecific finding of low serum-ascites albumin gradient.[60]

Given these clinical scenarios and information obtained from the history, physical examination, and laboratory values, further imaging is needed to make the diagnosis of BCS. Duplex ultrasonography yields a diagnosis of BCS in 85% of cases. Once suspected, CTA or MRA/MRV can provide details of the viscera and venous anatomy. Venography can be used at the time of catheterization to measure portal vein and caval pressures. This can be useful when considering other therapeutic options. It also provides access for transjugular liver biopsy in those who present with chronic disease.[56,57,60]

Management

Treatment modalities for BCS are based on the presentation of the disease and the evidence of hepatic damage (Figure 23.12). The goals of treatment are to prevent clot propagation, to decompress the congested liver, and to prevent fluid retention. Medical management consists of anticoagulation, sodium restriction (90 mmol/day), and diuretics. Thrombolytic therapy can be considered for patients with acute onset of symptoms and significant liver congestion. Catheter-directed infusion by accessing the hepatic veins from the internal jugular approach is preferred. Systemic infusion is not useful. After successful thrombolysis, long-term anticoagulation is required.[56,57,60] Concomitant angioplasty and stenting of hepatic or caval webs may also be necessary. Due to the high rate of restenosis, serial duplex ultrasonography is necessary to ensure continued patency. Failed thrombolytic or angioplasty patients are often candidates for TIPS, which decompresses congestion via creation of an alternative outflow tract. TIPS requires a portacaval venous pressure gradient of less than 10 mm Hg to function successfully. TIPS is not without its own complications, including the ability to shunt only small amounts of blood and a high thrombosis rate. TIPS remains a possible bridge to liver transplantation, which is reserved for refractory cases.[56-58,60-62]

Various surgical procedures exist for the management of BCS patients. First, surgical shunt placement can serve as a successful method of liver decompression. The ideal pa-

tient is an individual with a subacute presentation and documented ongoing hepatic necrosis via biopsy but an overall low grade of cirrhosis, that is, Child Pugh class A. In the case of surgical shunting, best results are seen with a portacaval venous pressure gradient of greater than 10 mm Hg. A poor prognostic factor is compression of the IVC by the hypertrophied caudate lobe of the liver. With a patent IVC, various shunts can be placed, including side-to-side portacaval, splenorenal, and mesocaval shunts. With an occluded IVC, a mesoatrial shunt connecting the portal-mesenteric system to the right atrium can be performed. This shunt, requiring graft material, is at a higher risk of occlusion. As with stenting, any patient undergoing surgical shunting should do so after consultation with the liver transplant team. Postoperatively, these patients require lifelong anticoagulation and are followed with serial duplex ultrasonography. Liver transplantation is an option for those with decompensated cirrhosis. Long-term success of transplantation depends upon the patient's initial predisposition to the thrombosis. Those with a protein deficiency such as protein S, protein C, or antithrombin III may be cured after the transplantation as the new liver would produce normal amounts of these enzymes.[60-62]

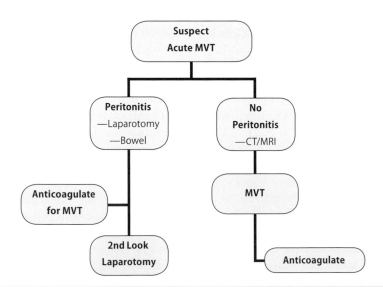

Figure 23.12 Diagnosis and treatment of acute mesenteric vein thrombosis.

Portal Vein Thrombosis

History, prevalence, and pathogenesis

Portal vein thrombosis (PVT) affects a wide variety of patient populations. PVT can be seen in the very young, the middle-aged female, or the cirrhotic patient. While the condition is rare in the young, it is present in 0.69% to 25.0% of all cirrhotic patients. The reported incidence in acquiring PVT for cirrhotic patients is only 1% per year. In patients with portal hypertension, PVT was the etiology in 8%.[63-65] There is also a notable association with hepatocellular carcinoma and PVT.[65] Noncirrhotic cases are often associated with a thrombophilic state. Studies have thus far implicated prothrombin G20210A and proteins C and S deficiencies.[66,67]

Diagnostic evaluation

PVT is thought to occur in either an acute or chronic manner. Acute PVT is usually due to infectious causes, such as pancreatitis. The inflammation around the portal vein leads to thrombosis. The impact of the thrombosis may be transient and reversible upon resolution of the underlying infection.

Chronic PVT is more commonly associated with a thrombophilia or liver disease such as cirrhosis. The portal vein thrombosis leads

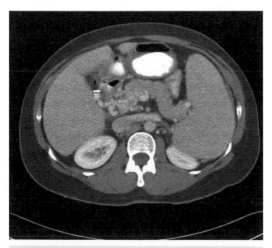

Figure 23.13 CTA demonstrating portal vein thrombosis. Note the enlarged spleen (secondary to splenic vein thrombosis) with compression of the left kidney.

to portal hypertension and the development of varicosities. Variceal bleeding is the presenting symptom in 70% of chronic PVT patients. Esophageal varices are more common than gastric varices (90% vs. 30%). Recurrent bleeding episodes are common.[63]

Clinical manifestations also include splenomegaly (50%), ascites (10%), jaundice, and the stigmata of chronic liver disease. Progression to liver failure in noncirrhotic PVT is negligible.[63]

Objective testing with duplex ultrasonography, contrast-enhanced CTA, or MRA/MRV establishes the diagnosis (Figure 23.13). Venography is the gold standard; however, it has a poor sensitivity unless the portal vein is directly imaged via transhepatic catheterization. Upper endoscopy is needed to evaluate the extent of varices and should be performed serially in follow-up. Liver biopsy is helpful to evaluate liver disease. Laboratory studies for thrombophilia, hepatitis, and coagulation state should also be performed.[68]

Management

Treatment of acute PVT caused by an infection is a short course of anticoagulation. The PVT usually resolves with little long-term ramifications. Long-term anticoagulation is required if an underlying thrombophilia is identified. Acute PVT may also be responsive to thrombolytic therapy. Delivery of the drug via the transhepatic route or through the superior mesenteric artery has been successful. The efficacy is dependent on the age of the thrombus and underlying etiology. Those patients without signs of chronicity (ie, varices, retracted portal vein) can be considered for this more aggressive approach. Once the signs of chronicity are present, the benefit of thrombolysis is offset by the risks.[63-68]

Subacute PVT can be treated with heparinization and at least 4 months of oral anticoagulation. Caveats to this treatment include the fact that there is not an established time frame that constitutes a subacute presentation and that anticoagulation can increase the risk of variceal bleeds. At present, this therapy should be selected for patients without underlying liver disease, recent short-term symptoms, and evidence of collateralization.[68]

Chronic PVT treatment is more controversial. Overall, there is little role for anticoagulation in the patient with evidence of collateralization unless the etiology of the PVT is felt to be noncirrhotic and irreversible. Anticoagulation minimizes thrombus propagation and involvement of adjacent veins and also the risk of remote DVT. Anticoagulation should be used with caution due to the potential risk of bleeding from varices. Beta-blockers have long been used for patients with varices. Endoscopic banding, sclerosis, and direct variceal treatment are necessary in symptomatic patients. When endoscopic therapies fail, surgical shunting should be considered since TIPS has a less-favorable outcome.[63-68]

Other Notable Acquired Venous Disorders

Traumatic arteriovenous fistula

Traumatic arteriovenous fistulae (AVF) result from a tangential arterial injury that juxtaposes a venous structure. The realm of traumatic AVF disease is as vast as the initial insults that can induce the arterial injury, be it external trauma or iatrogenic. Diagnosis is suggested by the presence of a pulsatile mass accompanied on auscultation by a machinelike murmur at the site of a prior penetrating wound. Imaging modalities such as duplex ultrasonography, CTA/MRA, and catheter arteriography can provide details as to the extent of the fistula (Figure 23.14).[69]

Once diagnosed and evaluated radiographically, large AV fistulae rarely resolve without intervention.[70] The distribution of the arterial segment involved is important and helps to determine the best treatment. Embolization is preferred when the arterial segment can be sacrificed. Surgical ligation of the fistula or direct repair itself can maintain distal perfusion. Bypass is infrequently needed.[69]

Lemierre's syndrome

Lemierre's syndrome is pharyngotonsillitis associated with *Fusobacterium necrophorum* (human necrobacillosis) and results in septic thrombophlebitis of the internal jugular vein. Andre Lemierre first described the syndrome in 1936, referring to it as "anaerobic postanginal septicemias."[71] Affected individuals develop pharyngotonsillitis that progresses to swelling and tenderness along the sternocleidomastoid muscle. Constitutional symptoms of high fever, rigors, and sepsis follow. Other infectious sources include the ear, mastoids, and soft tissue of the face. The syndrome can be further complicated by embolic seeding of other organs from the internal jugular venous thrombosis.[72]

Lemierre's syndrome comprises up to 80% of all documented human necrobacillosis yet it remains a rare disorder with an incidence as low as one per million per year. Judicious and effective use of antibiotics probably accounts for this low incidence. However, recent concerns over antibiotic overuse and development of antibiotic resistance have correlated with a slight increase in Lemierre's cases.[73]

Clinical suspicion is the key to diagnosis and must be made quickly given the fulminant course of the disease. It should be considered in any patient with severe sepsis and pulmonary symptoms presenting after an acute pharyngotonsillar infection. There is a male predominance of up to 3:1.[73] The internal jugular thrombophlebitis can readily be confirmed with duplex ultrasonograph, CTA, or MRA.[74]

Treatment is centered on antibiotic therapy. Current recommendations include either clindamycin as a sole agent or combination therapy with high-dose penicillin and metronidazole. Prolonged therapy is required (6 weeks). Systemic anticoagulation is not necessary unless the thrombophlebitis propagates into the cavernous sinus or subclavian/innominate vein. Historically, internal jugular ligation was employed to prevent septic embolization; however, this is rarely needed with appropriate antibiotic therapy. Surgery can be indicated for the sequelae of the septic emboli, such as empy-

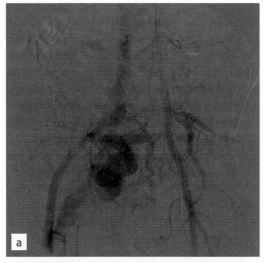
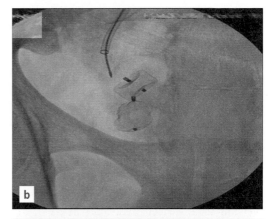
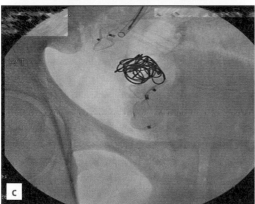
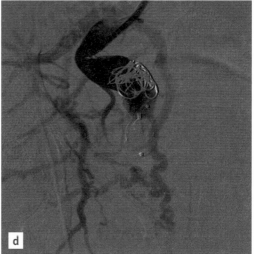

Figure 23.14 A 28-year-old was stabbed in the buttock 3 years prior and complained of pain with prolonged sitting. (a) Arteriogram of the right internal iliac artery demonstrating a fistula into the pelvic veins. (b) Vascular plugs placed into the proximal internal iliac artery, (c) followed by coils. (d) Completion arteriogram of the right internal iliac artery shows occlusion. On follow-up the patient remains asymptomatic.

ema formation, and is required for septic mediastinitis. Despite current treatment modalities, mortality can be as high as 17%.[74,75]

Mondor's disease

Mondor's disease, another rare venous condition, consists of superficial thrombophlebitis of the thoraco-epigastric veins. This disease of unknown etiology typically affects middle-aged women who present with lateral chest wall pain. The involved vein is tender, red, and cordlike to palpation. Predisposing conditions include trauma, surgery, infection, breast cancer, and tight clothing or banding.[76,77]

Diagnosis is based on clinical grounds, and treatment consists of nonsteroidal anti-inflammatory medication and hot compresses. Surgical intervention is indicated when Mondor's is associated with an underlying malignancy.

Summary

Congenital and acquired venous disorders, other than deep venous thrombosis and varicose veins, are a diagnostic challenge to the practitioner because they are uncommon and diverse in presentation. The description of each disorder provides a reference and starting point for the evaluation of these complex patients since most diagnoses are based on clinical features. As our understanding of the genetic predilection unfolds, specific genetic tests will be used to complement the clinical evaluation.

References

1. Klippel M, Trenaunay P. Du noevus variqueux osteohypertrophique. *Arch Gen Med*. 1900;185:641-672.

2. Baskerville PA, Ackroyd JS, Browse NL. The etiology of the Klippel-Trenaunay syndrome. *Ann Surg*. 1985;202:624-627.

3. Gloviczki P, Noel AA, Cherry KJ, et al. Surgical treatment of venous malformations in Klippel-Trenaunay syndrome. *J Vasc Surg*. 2000;32:840-847.

4. Lee A, Driscoll D, Gloviczki P, et al. Evaluation and management of pain in patients with Klippel-Trenaunay syndrome: a review. *Pediatrics*. 2005;115:744-749.

5. Jacob AG, Driscoll DJ, Shaughnessy WJ, et al. Klippel-Trenaunay syndrome: spectrum and management. *Mayo Clin Proc*. 1998;37:28-36.

6. Servelle M. La phlebographie va-t-elle nous permettre de démembrer le syndrome de Klippel et Trenaunay et l'hemangiectasie hypertrophique de Parkes-Weber? *Presse Med*. 1945;53:353-362.

7. Servelle M, Babillot J. Les malformations des veines profondes dans le syndrome de Klippel et Trenaunay. *Phlebologie*. 1980;33:31-36.

8. Whelan AJ, Watson MS, Porter FD, Steiner RD. Klippel Trenaunay Weber syndrome associated with a 5:11 balanced translocation. *Am J Med Genet*. 1995;59:492-494.

9. Berry SA, Peterson C, Mize W, et al. Klippel-Trenaunay syndrome. *Am J Med Genet*. 1998;79:319-326.

10. Tian X, Rajkumar K, You S, et al. Identification of an angiogenic factor that when mutated cause susceptibility to Klippel-Trenaunay syndrome. *Nature*. 2004;427:640-645.

11. Moodie D, Driscoll D, Salvatore D. Peripheral vascular disease in children. In: Young J, Olin J, Bartholomow J. *Peripheral Vascular Diseases*. 2nd ed. St. Louis: Mosby Yearbook Publishers; 1996:541-552.

12. Richards KA, Garden JM. The pulsed dye laser for cutaneous vascular and nonvascular lesions. *Semin Cut Med Surg*. 2000;19:276-286.

13. Kuo PH, Chang YC, Liou JH, Lee JM. Mediastinal cavernous haemangioma in a patient with Klippel-Trenaunay syndrome. *Thorax*. 2003;58:183-184.

14. Baskerville PA, Ackroyd JS, Thomas ML, Browse NL. The Klippel-Trenaunay syndrome: clinical, radiological and haemodynamic features and management. *Br J Surg*. 1985;72:232-236.

15. Young A, Ackroyd J, Baskerville P. Combined vascular malformations. In: Mulliken JB, Young AE, eds. *Vascular Birthmarks: Hemangiomas and Malformations*. Philadelphia: Saunders; 1988:246-274.

16. Gloviczki P, Stanson AW, Stickler GB, et al. Klippel-Trenaunay syndrome: the risks and benefits of vascular interventions. *Surgery*. 1991;100:469-479.

17. Lee BB, Do YS, Byun HS, et al. Advanced management of venous malformation with ethanol sclerotherapy: mid term results. *J Vasc Surg*. 2003;37:533-538.

18. Brandenburg VM, Graf J, Schubert H, Kock KC. Klippel-Trenaunay-Weber syndrome. *Circulation*. 2005;111:e23.

19. Boon LM, Mulliken JB, Vikkula M. RASA1: variable phenotype with capillary and arteriovenous malformations. *Curr Opin Genet Dev*. 2005;15:265-269.

20. Eerola I, Boon LM, Mulliken JB, et al. Capillary malformation-arteriovenous malformation and genetic disorder caused by RASA1 mutations. *Am J Hum Genet*. 2003;73:1240-1249.

21. Ziyeh S, Spreer J, Rossler J, et al. Parkes Weber or Klippel-Trenaunay syndrome? Non-invasive diagnosis with MR projection angiography. *Eur Radiol*. 2004;14:2025-2029.

22. Yildiz F, Yilmaz M, Cengiz M, et al. Radiotherapy in the management of Klippel-Trenaunay-Weber syndrome: report of two cases. *Ann Vasc Surg*. 2005;19:566-571.

23. Hall GW. Kasabach-Merritt syndrome: pathogenesis and management. *Br J Haematology*. 2001;112:851-862.

24. Enjolras O, Mulliken JB, Wassef M, et al. Residual lesions after Kasabach-Merritt phenomenon in 41 patients. *J Am Acad Derm*. 2000;42:225-235.

25. Chang E, Boyd A, Nelson CC, et al. Successful treatment of infantile hemangiomas with interferon-a-2b. *J Ped Hem Onc*. 1997;19:237-244.

26. Wananukul S, Nuchprayoon I, Seksarn P. Treatment of Kasabach-Merritt syndrome: a stepwise regimen of prednisolone, dipyridamole, and interferon. *Inter J Derm*. 2003;42:741-748.

27. Enjolras O, Riche MC, Merland JJ, Escande JP. Management of alarming hemangiomas in infancy: a review of 25 cases. *Pediatrics*. 1990;85:491-498.

28. Biban P. Kasabach-Merritt syndrome and interferon alpha: still a controversial issue. *Arch Dis Child*. 2003;88:645-646.

29. Barlow CF, Mulliken JB, Barnes PD, et al. Spastic diplegia as a complication of interferon alfa-2a treatment of hemangiomas of infancy. *J Pediatr*. 1998;132:527-530.

30. Drolet BA, Scott LA, Esterly NB, Gosain AK. Early surgical intervention in a patient with Kasabach-Merritt phenomenon. *J Pediatr*. 2001;138:756-758.

31. Barlow RJ, Walker NPJ, Markey AC. Treatment of proliferative haemangiomata with the 585nm pulsed dye laser. *Br J Derm*. 1996;134:700-704.

32. Van Lohuizen CHJ. Uber eine seltene angeborene Hautanomalie (cutis mormorata telangiectatica congenita). *Acta Derm Venereol*. 1922;93:202-211.

33. Garzon MC, Schweiger E. Cutis marmorata telangiectatica congenita. *Sem Cut Med Surg*. 2004;23:99-106.

34. Mazereeuw-Hautier J, Carel-Caneppele S, Bonafe JL. Cutis marmorata telangiectatica congenita: report of two persistent cases. *Pediatr Derm*. 2002;19:506-509.

35. Amitai DB, Fichman S, Merlob P, et al. Cutis marmorata telangiectatica congenita: clinical findings in 85 patients. *Pediatr Derm*. 2000;17:100-104.

36. Allroggen H, Abbott, RJ. Cerebral venous sinus thrombosis. *Postgrad Med J*. 2000;76:12-15.

37. Vandenbroucke JP. Cerebra sinus thrombosis and oral contraceptives. *BMJ*. 1998;317:483-484.

38. Bousser MG, Russell RR. *Cerebral Venous Thrombosis*. London: WB Saunders, 1997, 65.

39. Deschiens MA, Conard J, Horellou MH, et al. Coagulation studies, Factor V Leiden and anticardiolipin antibodies in 40 cases of cerebral venous thrombosis. *Stroke*. 1996;27:1724-1730.

40. de Bruijn SF, Stam J, Kapelle LF. Thunderclap headache as first symptom of cerebral venous sinus thrombosis. CVST Study Group. *Lancet*. 1996;348:1623-1625.

41. Provenzale JM, Joseph GJ, Barboriak DP. Dural sinus thrombosis: findings on CT and MRI imaging and diagnostic pitfalls. *AJR Am J Roentgenol*. 1998;170:777-783.

42. Einhaupl KM, Villringer A, Meister W, et al. Heparin treatment in sinus venous thrombosis. *Lancet*. 1991;338:597-600.

43. Bousser MG. Cerebral venous thrombosis: nothing, heparin, or local thrombolysis? *Stroke*. 1999;30:481-483.

44. Preter M, Tzourio C, Ameri A, Bousser MG. Long-term prognosis in cerebral venous thrombosis: follow-up of 77 patients. *Stroke*. 1996;27:243-246.

45. Warren S, Eberhard TP. Mesenteric venous thrombosis. *Surg Gynecol Obstet*. 1935;61:102-121.

46. Kumar S, Sarr MG, Kamath PS. Mesenteric venous thrombosis. *N Engl J Med*. 2001;345:1683-1688.

47. Abdu RA, Zakhour BJ, Dallis DJ. Mesenteric venous thrombosis—1911 to 1984. *Surgery*. 1987;101:383-388.

48. Amitrano L, Brancaccio V, Guardascione MA, et al. High prevalence of thrombophilic genotypes in patients with acute mesenteric vein thrombosis. *Am J Gastro*. 2001;96:146-149.

49. Rhee RY, Gloviczki P, Mendonca CT, et al. Mesenteric venous thrombosis: still a lethal disease in the 1990s. *J Vasc Surg*. 1994;20:688-697.

50. Kumar S, Kamath PS. Acute superior mesenteric venous thrombosis: one disease or two? *Am J Gastro*. 2003;98:1299-1304.

51. Rhee RY, Gloviczki P. Mesenteric venous

thrombosis. *Surg Clin North Am*. 1997;77:327-339.

52. Font VE, Hermann RE, Longworth DL. Chronic mesenteric venous thrombosis: difficult diagnosis and therapy. *Cleve Clin J Med*. 1989;56:823-828.

53. Bradbury MS, Kavanagh PV, Chen MY, Weber TM, Bechtold RE. Noninvasive assessment of portomesenteric venous thrombosis: current concepts and imaging strategies. *J Comput Assist Tomogr*. 2002;26:393-404.

54. Hagspiel KD, Leung DA, Angle JF, et al. MR angiography of the mesenteric vasculature. *Radiol Clin N Am*. 2002;40:867-886.

55. Poplausky MR, Kaufman JA, Geller SC, Waltman AC. Mesenteric venous thrombosis treated with urokinase via the superior mesenteric artery. *Gastroenterology*. 1996;110:1633-1635.

56. Wang ZG, Zhang FJ, Yi MQ, Qiang LX. Evolution of management for Budd-Chiari syndrome: a team's view from 2564 patients. *ANZ J Surg*. 2005;75:55-63.

57. Menon KVN, Shah V, Kamath PS. The Budd-Chiari syndrome. *N Engl J Med*. 2004;350:578-585.

58. Murad SD, Valla DC, De Groen PC, et al. Determinants of survival and the effect of portosystemic shunting in patients with Budd-Chiari syndrome. *Hepatology*. 2004;39:500-508.

59. Janssen HLA, Meinardi JR, Vleggaar FP, et al. Factor V Leiden mutation, prothrombin gene mutation, and deficiencies in coagulation inhibitors associated with Budd-Chiari syndrome and portal vein thrombosis: results of a case-control study. *Blood*. 2000;96:2364-2368.

60. Valla DC. The diagnosis and management of the Budd-Chiari syndrome: consensus and controversies. *Hepatology*. 2003;38:793-803.

61. Perello A, Garcia-Pagan JC, Gilaber R, et al. TIPS is a useful long-term derivative therapy for patients with Budd-Chiari syndrome uncontrolled by medical therapy. *Hepatology*. 2002;35:132-139.

62. Ryu RK, Durham JD, Krysl J, et al. Role of TIPS as a bridge to hepatic transplantation in Budd-Chiari syndrome. *J Vasc Interv Radiol*. 1999;10:799-805.

63. Lemierre A. On certain septicaemias due to anaerobic organisms. *Lancet*. 1936;40:701-703.

64. Hoehn S, Dominguez TE. Lemierre's syndrome: an unusual cause of sepsis and abdominal pain. *Crit Care Med*. 2002;30:1644-1647.

65. Kristensen LH, Prag J. Human necrobacillosis, with emphasis on Lemierre's syndrome. *Clin Infect Dis*. 2000;31:524-532.

66. Min SK, Park YH, Cho YK, et al. Lemierre's syndrome: unusual cause of internal jugular vein thrombosis. *Angiology*. 2005;56:483-487.

67. Hoehn KS. Lemierre's syndrome: the controversy of anticoagulation. *Pediatrics*. 2005;155:1415-1416.

68. Fietta P, Manganelli P. Mondor's diseases. Spectrum of the clinical and pathological features. *Minerva Med*. 2002;93:453-456.

69. Mayor M, Buron I, de Mora JC, et al. Mondor's disease. *Int J Dermatol*. 2000;39:922-925.

70. Shumaker HB, Wayson EE. Traumatic arteriovenous fistula and false aneurysms. *Am J Surg*. 1950; 79:532.

71. Lemierre A. On certain septicaemias due to anaerobic organisms. *Lancet*. 1936; 40:701-703.

72. Hoehn S, Dominguez TE. Lemierre's syndrome: an unusual cause of sepsis and abdominal pain. *Crit Care Med* 2002; 30:1644-1647.

73. Kristensen LH, Prag J. Human Necrobacillosis, with emphasis on Lemierre's syndrome. *Clin Infect Dis*. 2000; 31:524-532.

74. Min SK, Park YH, Cho YK et al. Lemierre's syndrome: unusual cause of internal jugular vein thrombosis. *Angiology*. 2005; 56:483-487.

75. Hoehn KS. Lemierre's syndrome: the controversy of anticoagulation. *Pediatrics*. 2005; 155:1415-1416.

76. Fietta P, Manganelli P. Mondor's diseases. Spectrum of the clinical and pathological features. *Minerva Med*. 2002;93:453-456.

77. Mayor M, Buron I, de Mora JC, et al. Mondor's disease. *Int J Dermatol*. 2000;39:922-925.

24

Chronic Venous Insufficiency and Varicose Veins

Steven M. Dean and Saundra S. Spruiell

An estimated 30 million to 40 million Americans have *varicose veins;* 2 million to 6 million have *chronic venous insufficiency (CVI)* with associated manifestations such as pain, swelling, and dermatitis; and approximately a half million are plagued with venous stasis ulcerations. Collectively, CVI and varicose veins constitute the most common vascular condition.

Prevalence

The prevalence and incidence of varicose veins and CVI vary by geographic location, with higher rates in Western countries and lower rates in underdeveloped societies. For example, in Mekky's[1] epidemiological study more than a 5-fold difference in prevalence existed between England and Egypt. The San Diego population study, the first investigation of venous disease within a multiethnic populace, demonstrated that varicose vein prevalence was highest in Hispanics (26%) and lowest in Asians (19%).[2] Reported prevalence and incidence variances

are probably due to variable population risk factors combined with different diagnostic criteria and assessment techniques.

The Framingham Study (n = 3822) documented a 2.6% annual incidence of varicose veins in females and 1.9% in males.[3] The prevalence of varicose veins in Western countries classically ranges between 25% and 30% in females and 10% and 20% in males[4]; yet higher rates are sometimes reported. In DaSilva's and Widmer's studies,[5,6] males and female prevalence rates were 57% and 68%, and 56% and 55%, respectively.

Smaller telangiectatic and reticular veins are more common than varicose veins. In the Duesseldorf/Essen civil servant study of 9261 employees, 27% of subjects were identified with small cutaneous and/or reticular veins, whereas only 9% had typical varicose veins.[7] In the Edinburgh Vein Study, over 80% of the studied population manifested telangiectatic and reticular veins.[8]

Clinical manifestations of CVI such as dermal hyperpigmentation, eczema, and edema vary from < 1% to 17% in males and < 1% to 20% in females.[5,8,9] The prevalence of active or

Vascular Disease: Diagnostic and Therapeutic Approaches. © 2011 Michael R. Jaff and Christopher J. White, editors. Cardiotext Publishing, ISBN: 978-1-935395-16-4.

healed venous stasis ulcerations is lower, ranging between 0.1% and 4.7% in males and between 0.2% and 4.1% in females.[9-12]

Epidemiology

Table 24.1 presents a synopsis of conventional and potential risk factors associated with varicose veins and CVI based on up-to-date evidence. Generally, both conditions have analogous risk profiles.

Age

Multiple studies have documented a nearly linear correlation between advancing age and varicose vein prevalence.[8,13-16] For instance, in the Edinburgh Vein Study, the prevalence of truncal varices increased in a linear fashion with age in both genders, ranging from 12% in 18- to 24-year-olds to 56% in 55- to 64-year-old subjects ($P < 0.001$). Similarly, the prevalence of smaller telangiectatic and reticular veins increased linearly with age in both sexes ($P < 0.001$).[8] However, in the Framingham Study age had no effect on varicosity incidence rates, which remained constant over the age of 40

years.[3] The Edinburgh Vein Study also established that the prevalence of CVI increased markedly with age ($P < 0.001$).[8]

Heredity

A family history of varicose veins increases the likelihood of varicosities within progeny.[13,17-19] In a 1990 Japanese study (n = 541), 42% of women with varicosities described a positive familial history compared with only 14% of women without varicosities.[20] A dual case-control study documented that varicose vein–affected patients were nearly 22 times more likely to convey a positive family history of varicosities as compared to controls ($P = 0.0001$).[21] Another case-control study observed that patients with CVI were significantly more likely to have a family history of the same disease (OR = 7.7).[22]

Gender

A preponderance of long-standing evidence links the female gender as a risk factor for varicose veins.[2,9,10,12,14,15,20,23,24] However, exceptions have been reported. Three contemporary investigations found a higher prevalence of

	VV	CVI
Older age	+	+
Family history	+	+
Female gender	+	–/+/0
Standing occupation	+	+
Constipation/low fiber intake	+/0	0
Obesity	+	+/0
Smoking	+/0	+/0
Oral contraceptives/HRT	-/0	-/0
Hypertension	+/0	+/0
Physical activity	-/0	-
Injury	+/0	+
History of phlebitis/clot	+	+

Table 24.1 Established and Potential Risk Factors for Varicose Veins (VV) and Chronic Venous Insufficiency (CVI) (Adapted from Beebe-Dimmer JL, Pfeifer JR, Engle JS, et al. The epidemiology of chronic venous insufficiency and varicose veins. *Ann Epidemiol.* 2005;15:175-184.) - = Negative; + = Positive; 0 = No association

truncal varicosities in males.[8,19,24] Yet in all of these studies, females were still more likely than males to be affected with telangiectatic and reticular veins.

Pregnancy, especially multiparity, is a consistent risk factor for varicose vein development.[3,6,13,18,19,25] Although Framingham data illustrated that women with 2 or more pregnancies had a higher incidence of varicose veins when compared to nulliparous women or those with 1 pregnancy, this difference did not achieve statistical significance.[3] Likewise, in the population-based study of Tecumseh, no relationship was identified between parity and varicosities.[10] Of interest, a 1960 report suggested that pregnancy was not a risk factor for varicose veins since women in underdeveloped societies have a decreased occurrence of varicosities, yet elevated parity, versus women residing in Western countries.[26]

In contrast to the predominance of varicose veins in women, this gender proclivity is less reliable in reference to CVI. In the Edinburgh Vein Study, the age-adjusted prevalence of CVI (grades 1–3) was 9% in males and 7% in females ($P < 0.05$). Nevertheless, gender variations were not statistically substantial when the grades of severity were examined independently ($P > 0.05$).[8] Scott et al[21] reported that patients with CVI were more likely to be male.[21] Still, other studies document a higher prevalence in the female population.[9,27,28]

Obesity

Obesity is one of the most consistent reasons for varicose vein development.[3,6,10,18,24,29,30] But in several of these studies, the relationship between obesity and varicosity genesis was only relevant in females.[3,6,10] Seidell et al[30] identified that women with a body mass index (BMI) > 30.0 kg/m^2 were 3 times more apt to have varicose veins when compared to women with normal weight. In a multivariate regression analysis, Kroger et al[7] showed that BMI was the most important determinant for an increase in venous cross-sectional diameter while standing, even when patients were free of visible venous

disease (CEAP class 0). Some investigations have linked obesity and CVI,[18] whereas others have not.[22,31]

Vocation

Multiple articles suggest that occupational-associated orthostatic limb stress increases the risk of varicose vein and CVI development.[3,29,32-36] For example, in the Framingham Study, men and women with varicose veins reported significantly lower levels of activity when compared to subjects without varicosities (men $P < 0.05$ and women $P < 0.001$). Women who described spending ≥ 8 hours per day in sedentary activities (sitting or standing) had a notably higher incidence of varicose veins when compared to women who spent ≤ 4 hours per day in similar activities ($P < 0.05$).[3] In a Spanish epidemiological, cross-sectional multicenter study involving 6695 patients, low physical activity was identified as a risk factor for CVI in 56% of all cases.[17] Gourgou et al[22] identified that subjects afflicted with CVI were 2.7 times more likely to stand while working for > 4 hours per day compared with a control group.

Other Possible Risk Factors

Less investigated, yet potential risk factors for venous hypertension include a low fiber, constipating diet,[18,37,38] tobacco,[3,17,22] alcohol,[17] and hypertension.[3]

Pathophysiology

Normal Venous Physiology

The calf muscles and attendant deep veins exhibit properties similar to the cardiac ventricle. Anatomically, the calf muscle "pump" is composed of the gastrocnemius and soleal muscles, whereas the "chamber" includes the deep veins and thin-walled venous sinuses. Physiologically, the calf muscle pump demonstrates both systolic and diastolic phases.

During a normal systolic phase, calf muscle contraction closes the valves of the perforating veins, which ensures that venous blood is propelled out of the deep veins and toward the heart but not into the superficial veins (Figure 24.1a). High pressures are generated within the calf muscle during systole. When the calf muscle relaxes in the diastolic phase, pressure within the deep veins and sinuses decreases; subsequently, blood flows via open perforator veins from the superficial to deep system. The calf muscle pump is "recharged" and the phases of systole and diastole can be repeated.

Macrovascular Pathophysiology

Although the diastolic phase in CVI is similar to that of a normal limb, the systolic phase is dysfunctional. When the calf muscle undergoes systolic contraction, incompetent perforating valves allow blood to flow from the deep to superficial veins. Consequently, elevated venous pressure, or *ambulatory venous hypertension,* ensues within the superficial venous system and fascial planes (Figure 24.1b). Coexisting incom-

petent superficial and/or deep veins allow additional retrograde flow, which further increases the ambulatory venous pressure. Ambulatory venous hypertension is the invariable pathophysiological feature in venous disease.

Venous valvular incompetency can be primary or secondary in etiology. Primary valvular incompetency results from either a congenital or acquired connective tissue defect with the vein wall or valve. Congenital causes of valvular incompetence include the Klippel-Trenaunay, Parkes-Weber, and Maffucci syndromes. Rarely, congenital valvular agenesis occurs, which is inherited as an autosomal dominant trait. It is unclear at present whether primary valvular incompetence or primary vein wall dilatation ultimately initiates the pathophysiological changes of venous hypertension.[39-41] A 1966 study suggested that patients with primary varicosities had veins that were more distensible than veins in normal subjects.[42] Browse et al[43] proposed that reflux is probably due to vein wall weakening and subsequent venous dilatation that eventually leads to a failure of valvular coaptation. Other studies have implicated aberrant collagen

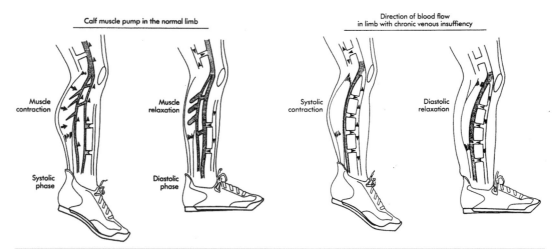

Figure 24.1 (a) Physiology of the perforating (communicating) veins in a subject with competent valves. During the systolic phase of calf muscle contraction, the one-way valves of the perforating veins are closed, thus preventing deep to superficial blood flow. In the diastolic phase, the perforating venous valves are open and allow the deep veins to fill with blood via the superficial veins. (b) Physiology of the perforating (communicating) veins in a subject with incompetent valves. During the systolic phase of the calf muscle pump, blood flows paradoxically from the deep to the superficial venous system across the incompetent valves of the perforating veins. Ambulatory venous hypertension ultimately develops. The diastolic phase is similar to that of a normal limb. (Adapted from O'Donnell TF Jr, Shepard AD. Chronic venous insufficiency. In: Jarrett F, Hirsch SA, eds. *Vascular Surgery of the Lower Extremities.* St Louis, MO: C.V. Mosby; 1985.)

configuration, smooth muscle cell proliferation, decreased elastin, and chronic inflammation with cytokine release as risk factors for primary venous valve and wall fragility. Figure 24.2 exemplifies the pathological transformation of a normal to a markedly dysfunctional valve and vein wall.

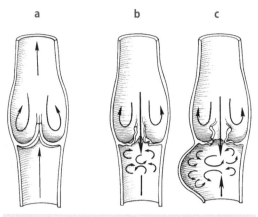

a   b   c

Figure 24.2 Antegrade flow pattern within a normal vein with competent valves that prohibit retrograde flow (a). Retrograde flow pattern within an incompetent vein due to thin, fibrotic valve cusps that fail to properly coapt. Turbulent flow occurs distal to the valve cusps (b). Protracted retrograde flow due to worsening valvular dysfunction may produce a saccular outpouching or "blowout" of the vein wall inferior to the level of the cusps (c). (Adapted and reprinted with permission from Goldman, MP. *Sclerotherapy: Treatment of Varicose and Telangiectatic Leg Veins.* 2nd ed. St. Louis: Mosby-Year Book; 1995,19.)

Secondary valvular incompetency is most often a consequence of previous venous thrombosis or trauma. Proximal outflow obstruction is another potential secondary cause of ambulatory venous hypertension. Although outflow obstruction can exist as an isolated cause of venous hypertension, it usually occurs in the setting of concurrent valvular reflux.[44] A previous deep venous thrombosis (DVT) that fails to recanalize is the most likely cause of venous outflow obstruction. Less frequently, obstruction can arise due to extramural venous compression, intrinsic vein wall abnormality, and/or intraluminal defect. Table 24.2 outlines various nonthrombotic causes of lower-extremity venous obstruction. In a significant portion

of people, the left common iliac vein is compressed between the overlying right common iliac artery and the underlying fifth lumbar vertebra. Although this configuration is usually a normal anatomic variant, in the setting of increased lumbar lordosis, trauma, or pregnancy, superimposed acute thrombosis can occur, which is referred to as the May-Thurner syndrome. Hypoplastic or aplastic anomalies of the iliocaval system should be considered as a cause

Inferior Vena Cava
Congenital hypoplasia/aplasia
Primary tumor (eg, leiomyosarcoma)
Secondary pericaval tumor
Pericaval adenopathy
Abdominal aortic aneurysm (uncomplicated *and* inflammatory)
Intraluminal membranous webs
Retroperitoneal fibrosis
Pancreatic pseudocyst
Pregnancy
Massive hydronephrosis
Iliac and Common Femoral Veins
Pelvic tumors/adenopathy
May-Thurner syndrome (LEFT-sided obstruction)
Enlarged iliopsoas bursa
Giant synovial cyst of the hip
Pregnancy
Primary venous tumor (eg, lipoma, leiomyosarcoma)
Intraluminal membranous webs
Juxtaposed arterial aneurysms (true and pseudoaneurysms)
Massive bladder enlargement
Inguinal lymphocele
Femoral and Popliteal Veins
Popliteal venous entrapment syndrome
Popliteal synovial cysts
Perivenous tumors (eg, chondrosarcoma, liposarcoma, fibrosarcoma)
Juxtaposed arterial aneurysms (true and pseudoaneurysms)

Table 24.2 Nonthrombotic Causes of Lower-Extremity Venous Obstruction

of significant venous outflow obstruction in a young patient.

Concurrent conditions that can aggravate both primary and secondary valvular incompetency include obesity, neuromuscular disease, congestive heart failure, pregnancy, and arthropathies.

Microvascular Pathophysiology

As ambulatory venous hypertension progresses, the venous blood capillary, or *microcirculation,* is ultimately impaired at a capillary, intravascular, and extravascular level.

Initially, capillaries become dilated, tortuous, and elongated. Additionally, the capillaries become more permeable. With long-standing venous hypertension, capillaries disappear and white dermal atrophy, or *atrophie blanche,* develops. Junger et al[45] observed an inverse correlation between severity of clinical symptoms and number of capillaries.

Venous hypertension also elicits a variety of microintravascular pathophysiological processes. For instance, capillary sludging eventuating in capillary thrombosis can reduce the transcutaneous PO_2 and lower the threshold for skin ulceration.[46] Capillary dilatation and associated reduction in flow velocity can reduce the shear rate.[47] This reduction in shear stress can provoke leukocyte capillary plugging and adhesion as well as leukocyte and endothelial cell activation. Subsequently, a variety of inflammatory molecules such as cytokines (eg, tumor necrosis factor, vascular endothelial growth factor), free oxygen radicals, proteolytic enzymes, and chemotactic substances are released. These leukocyte-mediated intravascular changes fulfill the *white cell trapping hypothesis* suggested by Coleridge Smith et al.[48]

Eventually, leukocyte, erythrocyte, and protein transmigration into the extravascular tissue transpires. Consequently, a pericapillary fibrin cuff is created with associated microedema, hemosiderin, and other molecules.[49] For instance, pericapillary laminin, fibronectin, and tenascin are deposited. Macrophages and T-lymphocytes invade the pericapillary space.[50]

Additionally, granulation tissue accumulates within the subepithelial layer and results in deposition of disoriented collagen fibers. Traditionally, the pericapillary fibrin cuff was thought to act as a barrier to oxygen and nutrient diffusion, which can lead to venous stasis ulceration. However, investigators using xenon-133 clearance through lipodermatosclerotic skin have failed to identify that the cuff prohibits oxygen transfer.[51]

Increased extracellular expression of matrix metalloproteinases (MMPs) 1, 2, and 9 combined with decreased activity of tissue inhibitor of metalloproteinase 2 has been identified within lipodermatosclerotic and ulcerated skin.[52,53] Over time, this multifactorial inflammatory response becomes self-perpetuating. Ultimately, the combination of decreased shear stress, intra- and extravascular inflammation, and extracellular matrix remodeling can stimulate the characteristic skin changes of CVI, including dermatitis, liposclerosis, and ulceration (Figure 24.3).

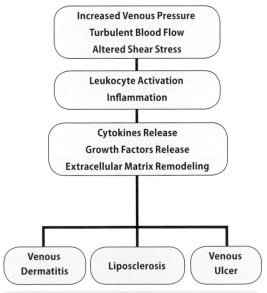

Figure 24.3 Schematic of the microvascular pathophysiology in CVI that ultimately provokes skin changes. (Adapted from Pascarella L, Schobein GW, Bergan JJ. Microcirculation and venous ulcers: a review. *Ann Vasc Surg.* 2005;19:921-927.)

Natural History

Primary Venous Insufficiency

A relative paucity of concrete data exist regarding features associated with primary disease evolution, since the ability to effectively monitor this population is problematic for a variety of reasons. To begin, the connection between varicosities, reflux, and subsequent symptoms is often uncertain. For example, the Edinburgh Vein Study (n = 1566 patients) illustrated that even in the presence of truncal varices, the majority of lower-limb symptoms were probably nonvenous in origin. Furthermore, with the exception of pruritus, there was no statistically significant relation between truncal varicosities and symptoms in men.[54] Others have suggested that a preponderance of patients with symptomatic primary disease undergo palliative treatment shortly after presentation but fail to undergo subsequent historical monitoring, thus limiting natural history data.[55]

Calculating the true prevalence of stasis ulcerations associated with *presumed* primary venous disease is potentially fraught with error since antecedent DVT is often subclinical. Moreover, the potential inconsistency between a history and actual objective documentation of DVT has been previously documented.[56]

In a longitudinal fashion, a large cohort of German children from 10 to 12 years of age were examined at baseline, 4, 8, and 19 years later via history, physical examination, and noninvasive testing. Telangiectasias and reticular veins were identified early and were independent of the existence of reflux. Larger varicosities developed in the older subjects and were frequently heralded by saphenous vein reflux.[57] In a study of 36 patients with varicosities evaluated with serial noninvasive testing over a median of 20 months (range, 15–27), 25% of initially ultrasonographically normal limbs developed new superficial venous reflux. In addition, 18% of the initially ultrasonographically abnormal limbs developed additional reflux.[58] Labropoulos et al[59] prospectively examined 116 limbs in 90 patients with varicose veins (93% primary

disease). A baseline duplex ultrasound (DU) was followed by a second study 1 to 43 months later (median, 19 months). In 85 limbs (73%), no change occurred. Thirteen limbs (11%) had progression of clinical disease. For instance, 7 limbs progressed from C2 to C3, 4 limbs from C3 to C4, and 2 limbs from C4 to C6. Thirty-one limbs (27%) had ultrasonographically documented reflux progression. Seventeen limbs (15%) had extension of preexisting reflux whereas 14 (12%) developed reflux within a new segment. The greater saphenous vein (GSV) and its tributaries were the most likely system to undergo change. Ultrasonographic or clinical progression occurred 6 months or later after the initial DU in 95% of cases. At present, there are no large, long-term studies that clearly document the rate of progression from uncomplicated varicose veins to dermatitis and ulcerations.

Secondary Venous Insufficiency

In contrast to primary venous disease, a large body of data is available to study the natural history of secondary venous reflux, or the postthrombotic syndrome. Since an acute DVT often has a symptomatic initiation point, duplex ultrasonography can be utilized to serially monitor resultant anatomic and physiologic changes. Concurrent serial clinical information can be obtained as well.

Ultrasonographic and venographic studies have revealed that the vein lumen is usually reopened after an acute DVT. Specifically, venous recanalization ultimately ensues in 50% to 80% of cases within several months to years after the index thrombotic event, with the greatest reduction in thrombotic burden occurring within the initial 3 to 6 months.[60-65] One prospective ultrasound study found that recanalization transpired in 100% of patients with postoperative DVTs, 59% of cancer-free outpatients, but in only 23% of patients with cancer ($P = 0.0001$). Statistically significant independent predictors for recanalization failure included younger age, outpatient presentation of the index DVT, thrombosis involving the entire femoropopliteal axis, and the presence of cancer.[66] Iliofemoral DVT treated with standard anticoagulant therapy is unlikely to recanalize. AbuRahma et al[67] documented a 5-year iliofemoral venous patency rate of only 18% when subjects received conventional heparin therapy.

The process of thrombosis and recanalization leads to isolated valvular damage and subsequent reflux in 33% to 59% of cases.[61] The exact determinants of postthrombotic valvular reflux are unclear but several potential factors exist, including recurrent thrombosis, slow recanalization times, and residual venous obstruction (Table 24.3).

1. Recurrent DVT
2. Slow rate of recanalization
3. Residual venous obstruction

Table 24.3 Potential Determinants of the Postthrombotic Syndrome

For instance, recurrent DVT appears to increase the probability of valvular dysfunction. In one study, the incidence of incompetence involving segments with recurrent thrombosis ranged from 36% to 73% versus 6% to 18% in segments devoid of rethrombosis.[68] Inadequate anticoagulation can increase the likelihood of recurrent thrombosis. For example, Caps et al[69] subjected 71 patients with an acute DVT to an average of 4.6 duplex scans per patient (range, 3–7) during a 3-week study period. The cumulative incidence of contiguous/noncontiguous extension of the DVT at 3 weeks was 26% (95% CI, 14%–38%). The time during which the level of anticoagulation was therapeutic (international normalized ratio [INR] $\geq$ 2.0 and/or heparin concentration $\geq$ 0.2 IU/mL) was inversely proportional to the risk of extension/new thrombi ($P = 0.01$, Cox proportional hazards analysis).

Meissner and colleagues[70] illustrated the importance of early recanalization in preserving valvular function. In their serial ultrasonographic follow-up study of 113 patients with acute DVT, the duration of recanalization was 2.3 to 7.3 times longer in segments ultimately developing reflux versus segments with preserved valvular function.

Interestingly, up to 30% of venous segments that become dysfunctional on serial exams have not been previously thrombosed.[71] Fixed, proximal venous obstruction may be involved in the pathogenesis of this latent valvular reflux in a segment without antecedent thrombosis. Inadequate anticoagulation may also play a role in residual venous obstruction. Caprini et al[72] followed 33 patients with symptomatic DVTs throughout 1 year of anticoagulation therapy with serial ultrasonography. Patients with subtherapeutic INRs were significantly more likely to manifest residual DVT at 1 year of follow-up. INR levels were significantly higher in patients with complete DVT resolution.

Finally, multiple investigations have assessed the relationship between acute DVT and the consequent clinical features of the postthrombotic syndrome. In these studies, mild to moderate manifestations developed in 29% to 79% of subjects. Severe clinical sequelae and ulceration developed in 7% to 23% and 4% to 6% of subjects, respectively.[73-76] The incidence and severity of the postthrombotic syndrome increases when the proximal (popliteal and higher) veins are initially thrombosed. Recurrent DVT is associated with a 6-fold increased risk of developing the postthrombotic syndrome.[77] Johnson et al[44] identified that patients afflicted with both fixed venous obstruction and reflux have the highest incidence of skin changes and ulceration. In their prospective follow-up study from 1 to 6 years, symptomatic postthrombotic syndrome developed in 15% of patients with isolated obstruction, in 18% with isolated reflux, but in 65% with combined obstruction and reflux. Similarly, Franzeck et al[78] prospectively followed 39 patients after a DVT for up to 12 years and ultimately demonstrated the postthrombotic syndrome in 8% of subjects with residual obstruction, in 33% with reflux, and in 50% with a combination of obstruction and reflux. In a 1-year post-DVT follow-up study, occlusive thrombi provoked the postthrombotic syndrome in 62% of patients. In contradistinction, nonocclusive thrombi were associated with the postthrombotic syndrome in only 11% of patients ($P = 0.003$).[72] Stasis ulcerations are more frequent in patients with recurrent venous thrombosis.[77]

History and Physical Examination

History

The symptoms of CVI and varicose veins are myriad and include leg pain, fatigue, aching, heaviness, and swelling (Table 24.4). Varicose veins can also cause itching, burning, stinging, and throbbing. Varicosity-associated symptoms are not always proportional to the size of the ectatic vein. For example, reticular and spider veins are sometimes more symptomatic than a large, dilated varicose vein. Symptomatology may be worse in warm and humid weather or during menstrual periods. Women are more likely than men to experience symptoms.[13,19,54] In the Edinburgh Vein Study of 1566 people (699 men and 867 women), the prevalence of symptoms tended to increase with age in both sexes. Additionally, in women, there was a significant association between truncal varices and the symptoms of heaviness ($P < 0.001$), aching ($P < 0.001$), and itching ($P < 0.005$). With the exception of itching, there was no significant association between symptoms and truncal varices in men. Last of all, the authors noted that many patients with truncal varices are asymptomatic.[54] Other patients experience a variety of venous-related symptoms with minimal or no clinical evidence of venous disease; thus suggesting either deep venous incompetence causation or a nonvenous cause for their discomfort. CVI and varicose veins are a frequently overlooked cause of restless legs syndrome and nocturnal leg cramps. Severe CVI can even lead to a peripheral neuropathy with its attendant pain and dysesthesias.

Symptoms are typically aggravated by dependency and are worse at the end of the day, especially after protracted sitting or standing. Recumbency, particularly with leg elevation, and the use of support hosiery are palliative measures.

Chronic iliac vein obstruction may cause the potentially disabling symptom of venous claudication, whereby ambulation elicits an intense cramping or bursting sensation within the calf. Relief is obtained by cessation of ambulation and elevating the affected extremity. In a recent study of 39 patients with chronic iliac vein occlusion followed for a mean of 5 years, 44% developed venous claudication with treadmill testing (initial claudication distance 130 m, range 105–268 m).[79]

Physical Examination

Dilated veins

Superficial venous hypertension can provoke telangiectatic or spider veins (0.1–1.0 mm in diameter; red or blue), venulectasias (1–2 mm diameter; blue, sometimes distended above the skin surface), reticular veins (2–8 mm in diameter; flat, blue to blue green), and varicose veins (> 8 mm in diameter; bulging, blue to blue green) in isolation or in various combinations (Figure 24.4).

Corona phlebectatica

Corona phlebectatica, or the so-called ankle flair sign, is a fan-shaped confluence of telangiectasias inferior to the medial malleolus and along the pedal instep. Corona is an early marker of superficial venous hypertension. Photo data from a recent study found that the relative risk of identifying incompetent calf perforators was 4.4 times greater in patients with corona phlebectatica.[80]

Manifestations of Chronic Venous Insufficiency	
Pain	Swelling
Stinging	Pruritus
Burning	Ulcers
Aching	Nocturnal leg cramps
Fatigue	Restless legs syndrome
Heaviness	Peripheral neuropathic symptoms
Throbbing	Venous claudication

Table 24.4 Symptoms of Chronic Venous Disease (Varicose Veins and CVI)

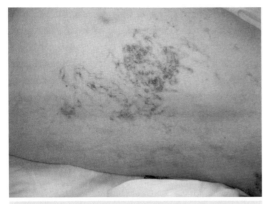

Figure 24.4 Classic lateral thigh pattern of both telangiectasias (0.1–1.0 mm in diameter; red or blue) and venulectasias (1–2 mm in diameter; blue, and sometimes bulging). Although not well visualized in this photograph, a feeding reticular vein is present. This lateral thigh distribution of ectatic superficial veins is referred to as the lateral subdermic venous system of Albanese.

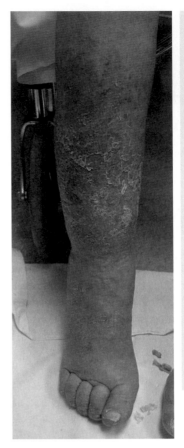

Figure 24.5 A swollen limb with a combination of CVI and secondary lymphedema. Uncomplicated CVI-associated swelling should spare the foot; however, patients with long-standing reflux complicated by dermatitis, cellulitis, panniculitis, and/or ulcerations can develop concurrent secondary lymphedema with associated foot/toe swelling.

Edema

Ankle *edema* is often the first manifestation of CVI. In the early stages of venous hypertension, edema tends to be distal and localized to the malleolar region. As CVI progresses, swelling can ascend the calf. An orthostatic provocation can occur. In contrast to lymphedema, simple CVI-associated swelling should spare the foot; however, patients with reflux complicated by skin changes and infection can develop concurrent secondary lymphedema with associated foot/toe swelling (Figure 24.5). Initially, the edema may pit with pressure but long-standing CVI with associated dermal and subcutaneous fibrosis or "woody induration" may not exhibit pitting.

Hyperpigmentation

Brownish *hyperpigmentation* within the gaiter or sock distribution (ankle to midcalf) occurs as CVI worsens. Cutaneous hyperpigmentation denotes extravasated intact or fragmented erythrocytes and hemosiderin-laden macrophages scattered between tortuous and dilated capillaries. Minor blunt trauma may provoke capillary rupture and subsequent hyperpigmentation. Early red blood cell extravasation appears stippled and red. With time, the staining fades to brown and the stippling can change to confluence. Discoloration is typically concentrated on the posteromedial gaiter region due to the presence of underlying incompetent perforator veins that communicate with a large GSV tributary (posterior arch vein). In the presence of SSV incompetence, hyperpigmentation affects the posterolateral calf and ankle.

Dermatitis

Similar to hyperpigmentation, stasis *dermatitis* usually involves the posteromedial gaiter zone. The dermatitis is typically well demarcated, erythematous, dry, and scaly. However, a weeping transudative eczematous stasis dermatitis can also occur. Chronic pruritus leading to lichenification may ensue. Rarely, stasis dermatitis can be complicated by a generalized autosensitization dermatitis or "ID" reaction.

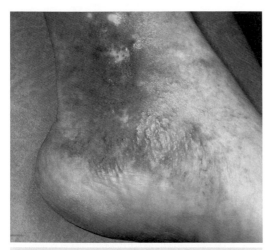

Figure 24.6 Medial malleolar photograph illustrating several classic features of advanced CVI including corona phlebectatica (ankle flair sign), hyperpigmentation, and atrophie blanche (white atrophy). Duplex ultrasonography confirmed the presence of 2 underlying incompetent perforating veins between the posterior arch vein (GSV tributary) and 1 of the posterior tibial veins.

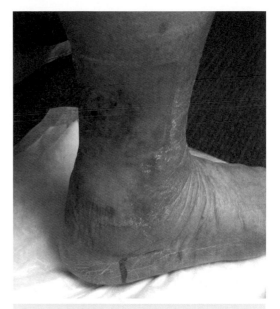

Figure 24.7 Although venous stasis ulcerations usually occur within the distal medial gaiter area, they can involve the posterolateral calf when SSV incompetency exists. In this subject, duplex ultrasonography confirmed the presence of reflux within the saphenopopliteal junction, SSV, lateral arch vein, and a lateral-based perforating vein.

Atrophie blanche

Atrophie blanche, or "white atrophy," is a morphologic term that signifies white, stellate plaques that overlie the distal lower extremity in advanced CVI. The plaque border is hyperpigmented and sometimes eczematous. Dilated, red capillaries are sometimes interspersed within the avascular, white plaques (Figure 24.6). Atrophie blanche can be either a harbinger or sequela of venous stasis ulceration.

Ulceration

The venous stasis *ulceration* is the end stage manifestation of CVI. Similar to hyperpigmentation and eczema, a venous stasis ulceration usually occurs within the distal medial calf and medial malleolar region. The base is beefy red, shallow, edematous, moist, and friable. The border is mildly irregular and well defined, with surrounding hyperpigmentation and eczematous scaling. Secondary infection may complicate the ulceration. Uncontrolled ankle edema is often present. Significant reflux within the short saphenous vein can elicit stasis ulcerations on posterolateral calf (Figure 24.7).

Lipodermatosclerosis

Lipodermatosclerosis or stasis associated sclerosing panniculitis (SASP) is an often underdiagnosed sign of advanced CVI and refers to strikingly "bound down" or sclerotic skin involving the gaiter region of the calf. Lipodermatosclerosis is more common in middle-aged, obese females.[81] Both acute and chronic forms exist. In the acute phase, a tender erythematous and edematous plaque develops within the distal anteromedial gaiter distribution. Over time, a chronic phase occurs whereby the plaque becomes increasingly well demarcated, indurated, and depressed, and erythema transforms into hyperpigmentation. Concurrent atrophie blanche and/or venous stasis ulcerations may complicate lipodermatosclerosis. Finally, progressive dermal and subcutaneous atrophy impart a concave appearance to the mid-/distal calf, which resembles an "inverted champagne bottle" or "bowling pin" (Figure 24.8).

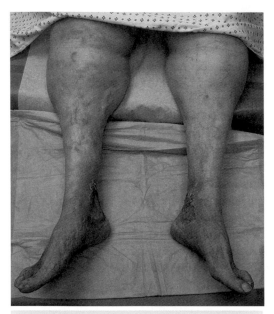

Figure 24.8 Lower extremities illustrating multiple signs of long-standing venous hypertension. Marked atrophy due to chronic stasis panniculitis is present within the gaiter distribution and an inverted "champagne bottle" or "bowling pin" appearance is evident. Bipedal venulectasias and scattered telangiectasias and reticular veins overlie the calves. Severe bilateral stasis dermatitis, ulcerations, and mild hyperpigmentation are also present.

Noninvasive Evaluation
Tourniquet testing

The classic, 2-part *Trendelenburg tourniquet test* can be utilized in the office to obtain rudimentary information on the competence of the superficial and perforating valves. To begin, the veins are emptied of blood by elevating the leg above the heart for approximately 1 minute. A tourniquet (eg, 0.5-in Penrose drain) or the hand is subsequently applied at the proximal thigh. The patient is asked to stand and the examiner observes the leg for superficial venous filling. The 4 possible test results are shown in Figure 24.9. Additional tourniquets can be applied throughout the limb in an attempt to further localize the level of disease. The tourniquet test is sometimes difficult to interpret in the absence of bulging varicosities.

Handheld continuous-wave Doppler

Large truncal veins can be interrogated for re-

flux with a simple handheld continuous-wave Doppler instrument. With the patient standing and placing the majority of the weight on the unexamined extremity, the instrument is placed directly over the vein of interest and angled at 45°. The extremity is compressed distal to the probe and a brief flow signal should be audible. When calf compression is released in the setting of a competent valve, no venous flow is heard. However, release of compression in the presence of an incompetent valve results in an audible, sustained flow signal. Reflux can be terminated by repeat calf compression but every time compression is released, a persistent signal will again be heard. The GSV-saphenofemoral junction, SSV-saphenopopliteal junction, as well as large bulging truncal varicosities can be sequentially assessed in their entirety with the aforementioned technique. Abnormal results warrant follow-up venous duplex ultrasonography.

Duplex ultrasonography

Over the last 2 decades, venous duplex ultrasonography has become the test of choice for diagnosing the majority of patients with suspected CVI. Duplex ultrasonography is generally regarded as being superior to venography for diagnosing venous incompetency. Duplex ultrasonography yields both an anatomic and physiologic venous valvular assessment. Anatomically, precise segments of valvular dysfunction can be located and system involvement (eg, superficial, deep, perforating venous systems) defined. Physiologically, duplex scanning can assess for the presence and severity of reflux.

Routine imaging is conducted with a 4- to 7-MHz multifrequency linear array transducer. However, when superficial veins are interrogated, a 10-MHz transducer can be utilized. The patient is usually examined in the recumbent position with the bed in a 15° reverse Trendelenburg position. However, if a detailed examination for superficial and/or perforating vein reflux is required, then a 45° reverse Trendelenburg position is more helpful. Alternatively, the veins can be insonated with the subject standing and holding onto a frame with the major-

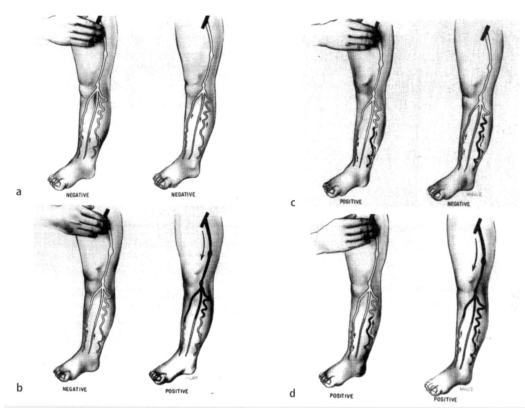

Figure 24.9 Two-part Trendelenburg (tourniquet) test. (a) Negative-negative response: Part I is negative with gradual filling of the veins at the ankle over a 30-second period indicative of competent perforating veins. Part II Is negative following release of compression (hand or tourniquet) demonstrating a competent saphenofemoral junction. (b) Negative-positive response: Part I is negative with gradual filling of the veins at the ankle over a 30-second period indicative of competent perforating veins. Part II is positive following release of compression (hand or tourniquet) with rapid retrograde filling of the GSV due to an incompetent saphenofemoral junction. (c) Positive-negative response: Part I is positive despite GSV compression with rapid filling of the superficial veins indicative of incompetent perforators. Part II is negative following release of compression (hand or tourniquet) demonstrating a competent saphenofemoral junction. (d) Positive-positive response: Part I is positive despite GSV compression with rapid filling of the superficial veins indicative of incompetent perforators. Part II is positive following release of compression (hand or tourniquet) with rapid retrograde filling of the GSV due to an incompetent saphenofemoral junction. (Adapted from DeWeese JA. Venous and Lymphatic Disease. In: Schwartz SI, ed. *Principles of Surgery*. 4th ed. New York: McGraw-Hill; 1984.)

ity of the weight on the unexamined limb. The primary veins of the deep system from the distal tibioperoneal veins to the external iliac vein and of the superficial system from the distal greater/short saphenous veins to the saphenofemoral junction are assessed. If clinically relevant, the perforating veins can also be interrogated.

The Valsalva maneuver is used to exaggerate and quantitate reflux within the proximal thigh veins. However, an effective Valsalva maneuver requires a cooperative patient. Manual compression of the thigh and calf veins with abrupt release is also used to demonstrate and

quantitate reflux. A reflux time (or valve closure time) is traditionally defined as significant when it exceeds 0.5 seconds (Figure 24.10). Other investigators have suggested that the conventional cutoff value of > 0.5 second is applicable for the superficial and deep calf veins, yet values of > 1.0 second and 0.35 second should be used for defining reflux within the femoropopliteal and perforating veins, respectively.[82] Neglen et al[83] questioned the value of reflux time and suggested that parameters such as the peak reflux velocity (m/sec) and time of average rate of reflux (mL/min) are better correlates of venous incompetency. Color-flow duplex imaging provides additional information regarding venous hemodynamics and anatomy. In color-flow imaging, venous flow is traditionally blue and arterial flow is red. When a red color is identified within the vein after release of muscle compression, reflux is present. An incompetent perforating vein within Cockett's distribution is ultrasonographically shown in Figure 24.11. Duplex ultrasonography also distinguishes between primary and secondary venous insufficiency. For instance, the presence of recanalized thrombus is consistent with secondary CVI, whereas the absence of remote thrombus suggests primary reflux disease. Duplex scanning is both operator and interpreter dependent and may yield suboptimal information when utilized on the markedly swollen limb or while attempting to assess the iliac veins.

Air plethysmography

Although less commonly utilized and available than duplex ultrasonography, *air plethysmogra-*

phy remains a viable option for noninvasively evaluating valvular reflux. In air plethysmography, an air chamber placed over the leg provides a functional assessment of the calf muscle pump, venous reflux, and venous obstruction. The plethysmographic data correlate favorably with the severity of venous disease and can also document postintervention improvement.

Other

Other less-available and uncommonly used noninvasive venous testing modalities include dynamic foot volumetry, strain gauge plethysmography, liquid crystal thermography, photoplethysmography, and light reflection rheography.

Invasive Evaluation

Venography (phlebography)

Prior to the advent of duplex ultrasonography, ascending venography was the diagnostic test

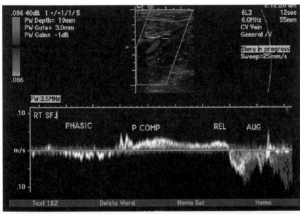

Figure 24.10 Duplex ultrasonography demonstrating nearly 4 seconds of retrograde flow, or "reflux," within an incompetent saphenofemoral junction.

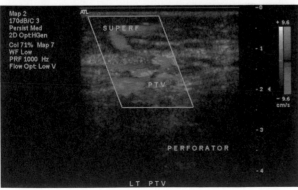

Figure 24.11 Duplex ultrasonography of an incompetent perforating vein within the Cockett's distribution traversing the fascia between the left posterior arch vein (major below-knee GSV tributary) and the posterior tibial vein.

of choice for defining anatomy, confirming venous patency, and distinguishing between primary and secondary venous pathology. Testing indications are now limited to situations where venous duplex ultrasonography is not available, generates equivocal results, or is technically inadequate. For instance, when compared to suprainguinal venous duplex ultrasonography, ascending femoral venography provides a superior assessment of the iliocaval system (Figure 24.12). Additionally, ascending venography continues to function as the gold standard in comparison studies with novel venous investigational modalities. Limitations include poor visualization of the profunda femoral and internal iliac veins. If the pedal vein is cannulated (versus the femoral vein), the iliocaval system is often suboptimally evaluated. Although ascending venography provides an anatomic venous assessment, it fails to yield functional information.

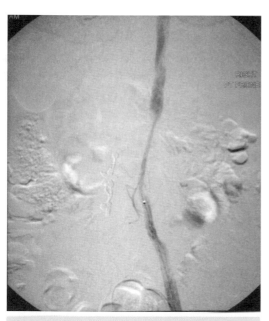

Figure 24.12 Venography (prone position) from an 18-year-old girl with right thigh swelling demonstrating a congenitally hypoplastic inferior vena cava and proximal right common iliac vein. Although duplex ultrasonography is the preferred test for the diagnosis of infrainguinal venous disease, it is less sensitive in evaluating the suprainguinal veins; consequently, venography is still a useful modality for iliocaval imaging.

In contrast to ascending venography, descending venography can give functional information by demonstrating the location and severity of reflux. Although rarely utilized, descending venography is indicated before repeat varicose vein surgery when duplex ultrasonography is inconclusive or prior to complicated deep venous reconstructions (eg, valvuloplasty, valvular transposition, or venous bypass surgery).

Potential complications of venography include patient discomfort, anaphylactoid reactions, superficial and deep venous thrombophlebitis, nephrotoxicity, and cutaneous extravasation. The procedure is costly as well.

Normal Venous Anatomy

The veins of the lower extremity comprise 3 types: superficial, deep, and perforating veins.

Superficial Veins

The *superficial venous system* lies under the skin, above the deep fascia, and consists of the great and small saphenous veins with their tributaries. The *great* (greater, long, magna) *saphenous vein (GSV)* is the longest vein in the body. It begins in the medial marginal pedal vein, ascends anterior to the medial malleolus, along the medial calf and thigh, and eventually terminates in the common femoral vein at the foramen ovale. The average diameter of a normal GSV is 3.5 to 4.5 mm (range 1–7 mm) and contains 10 to 13 valves. The GSV receives numerous tributaries along its path. The major below-knee tributary is the posterior arch vein, which connects to the GSV at the proximal calf. The largest above-knee tributaries are the anterolateral and posteromedial branches, which join the GSV in the proximal thigh. Constant inguinal GSV tributaries include the inferior superficial epigastric, superficial circumflex iliac, and external pudendal veins (Figure 24.13).

The *small* (lesser, short, parva) *saphenous vein (SSV)* begins in the lateral marginal pedal vein and ascends posterior to the lateral malleo-

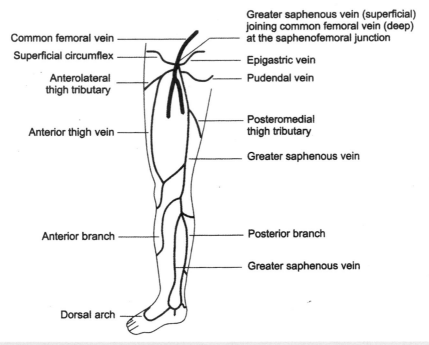

Figure 24.13 Anatomy of the GSV and its primary tributaries. (Reprinted with permission from Weiss RA, Feied CF, Weiss MA. *Vein Diagnosis and Treatment: A Comprehensive Approach.* New York: McGraw-Hill; 2001.)

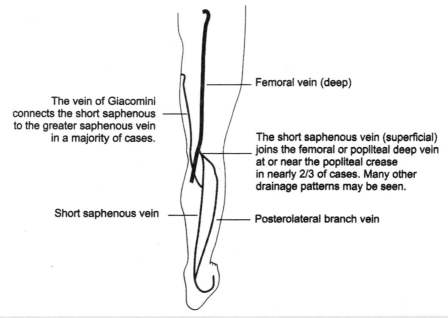

Figure 24.14 Anatomy of the SSV and its primary tributaries. (Reprinted with permission from Weiss RA, Feied CF, Weiss MA. *Vein Diagnosis and Treatment: A Comprehensive Approach.* New York: McGraw-Hill; 2001.)

lus and up the midposterior calf between the lateral and medial gastrocnemius heads. The SSV eventually penetrates the deep fascia and enters the popliteal fossa and ultimately terminates within the popliteal vein or GSV. The normal SSV diameter is 3 mm and contains anywhere from 7 to 13 closely placed valves. The major tributary is the lateral arch vein, which traverses along the lateral calf and joins the SSV distal to the popliteal fossa (Figure 24.14).

Deep Venous System

The majority of venous egress occurs through the deep veins. Within the calf, there are 3 sets of paired deep veins that parallel the course of the associated named arteries. Venous bridges join the paired veins along the length of the tibioperoneal arteries. The proximal tibioperoneal veins converge within the inferior popliteal fossa to form the popliteal vein. Important popliteal vein tributaries include the gastrocnemius and SSVs. At the level of the adductor canal, the popliteal vein becomes the femoral vein. When the proximal femoral vein receives its primary tributary, the deep (profunda) femoral vein and the common femoral vein (CFV) are formed. The GSV joins the CFV roughly 3 cm distal to the inguinal ligament. The CFV becomes the external iliac vein at the level of the inguinal ligament (Figure 24.15). Hundreds of lower-extremity deep venous valves exist, which are more concentrated within the distal portions of the extremity.

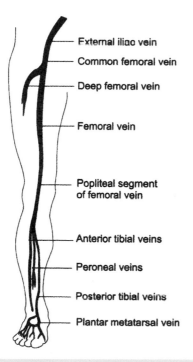

Figure 24.15 Anatomy of the deep veins of the lower extremity. (Reprinted with permission from Weiss RA, Feied CF, Weiss MA. *Vein Diagnosis and Treatment: A Comprehensive Approach.* New York: McGraw-Hill; 2001.)

Perforating Veins

Perforating (communicating) veins with one-way valves connect and transfer blood from the superficial to the deep veins and are present from the ankle to the inguinal region. Anatomically, perforating veins are classified as either direct or indirect. Direct perforating veins unite the superficial and deep veins with no interruption. Indirect perforating veins allow deep and superficial vein communication through muscular channels. Perforating veins are more numerous in the distal aspect of the lower extremity and normally range from < 1 to 2 mm in diameter. Table 24.5 lists the clinically significant perforating veins between the GSV and the deep system. When incompetent, 2 perforating vein distributions warrant additional discussion. First, refluxing perforating veins within the Cockett's distribution (communication between the posterior arch vein and posterior tibial vein) are the nidus for classic venous stasis ulcerations along the distal medial gaiter region (Figure 24.16). Second, incompetent Hunterian perforating veins (communication between the mid/distal femoral vein and GSV) are a common cause of distal medial calf varicose veins in the presence of a *competent* saphenofemoral junction.

Name	Location
Saphenofemoral junction	Proximal medial thigh
Hunterian	Mid/distal medial thigh
Dodd's	Distal medial thigh
Boyd's	Proximal medial calf
Cockett's	Mid/distal medial calf
Submalleolar	Medial inframalleolus

Table 24.5 Primary Named Perforating Veins Between the GSV and the Deep Veins

Important Collateral Circulation

Many unnamed superficial dermal and saphenous vein tributary collateral veins exist throughout the lower extremities. Table 24.6 lists several of the more recognized collateral venous systems.

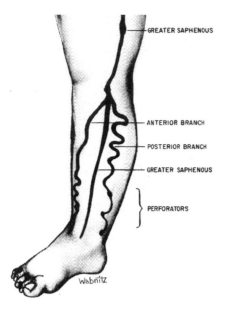

Figure 24.16 The GSV and its major below-knee branches. Three perforating veins originate from the mid/distal portion of the posterior branch or posterior arch vein (Cockett's distribution). If these communicating veins become incompetent, typical stasis dermatitis and ulcerations may occur within the medial gaiter region. (Adapted from DeWeese JA. Venous and Lymphatic Disease. In: Schwartz SI, ed. *Principles of Surgery.* 4th ed. New York: McGraw-Hill; 1984.)

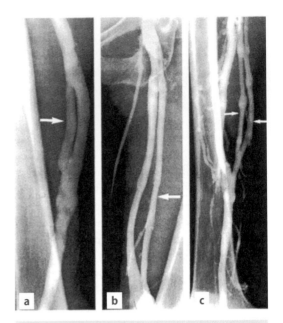

Figure 24.17 Venography of anomalous femoral veins. (a) Short segment lateral duplication (arrow) of the femoral vein. (b) Long segment lateral duplication (arrow) of the femoral vein. (c) Complex venous anatomy of the femoral vein with 3 veins (arrow) at the midthigh level. (Reprinted with permission. Quinlan DJ, Alikhan R, Gishen P, Sidhu PS. Variations in lower limb venous anatomy: implications for US diagnosis of deep venous thrombosis. *Radiology.* 2003;228:443-448.)

Vein/Pathway	Distribution
Giacomini vein	Oblique thigh vein connecting the GSV and SSV along the posteromedial thigh
Presacral venous plexus	Cross pelvic collateral veins that engorge in the setting of unilateral common/external iliac vein occlusion, including prominent internal iliac, lateral sacral, and unnamed suprapubic collateral veins
Anterior crural veins	Inferior lateral calf to medial knee
Infrageniculate veins	Drains peripatellar skin
Sciatic venous pathway	Internal iliac vein to posterior thigh
Anterolateral GSV branch	Lateral knee to saphenofemoral junction
Lateral subdermal	Lateral distal thigh and proximal calf vein plexus

Table 24.6 Important Venous Collateral Systems

Common Venous Variations

Although a preponderance of anatomy texts typically illustrate the venous system as continuous and devoid of duplication, Cockett's 1954 article showed that only 1 in 6 patients had a truly normal venous anatomy.[84] The major deep venous variation involves the femoral vein, which is duplicated or multiple in 6% to 46% of cases.[85-89] In Quinlan et al's 2003 retrospective review of 404 (808 limbs) bilateral lower-extremity venograms,[90] 31% of femoral veins were duplicated (Figure 24.17). This study also found that 5% of popliteal veins were duplicated; however, 2 veins were identified within the popliteal fossa in 42% of venograms, reflecting

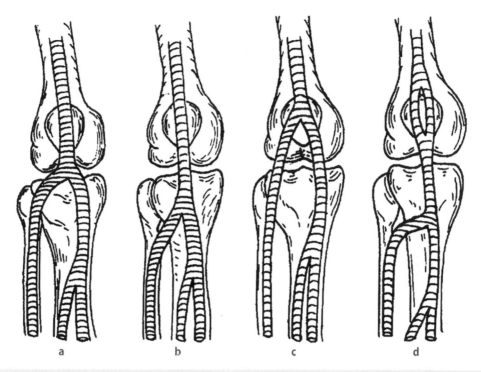

Figure 24.18 Variations in the formation of the popliteal vein at the knee joint (a), distal to knee joint (b), proximal to knee joint (c), and true duplication of the popliteal vein (d). (Reprinted with permission. Quinlan DJ, Alikhan R, Gishen P, Sidhu PS. Variations in lower limb venous anatomy: implications for US diagnosis of deep venous thrombosis. *Radiology*. 2003;228:443-448.)

variable confluence of the veins that ultimately form the popliteal vein (Figure 24.18). Lastly, only single anterior tibial, posterior tibial, and peroneal veins were seen in 33%, 17%, and 6% of the veins, respectively. Three or more peroneal veins were seen in 8% of patients.

The prevalence of GSV duplication ranges from 8% to 35%.[91-94] Although the SSV usually terminates within the popliteal vein, multiple variations exist. In a study of 528 limbs, anatomical variations in the saphenopopliteal junction and SSV occurred in 30% of cases.[95] For example, terminations within the GSV, other deep veins, both the popliteal vein and the GSV, the vein of Giacomini, and the gluteal vein are possible (Figure 24.19).

CEAP Classification

Once the diagnosis of chronic venous disease is ascertained, a patient with this disorder can be graded and categorized in accordance with the comprehensive *CEAP classification*.[96] In this scheme, a limb with CVI is assessed for clinical manifestations (C), etiological factors (E), anatomic distribution of involvement (A), and underlying pathophysiology (P) as outlined in Table 24.7. Of these 4 classes, the clinical nomenclature is the easiest to utilize in an office-based practice. The CEAP classification format facilitates interinstitutional communication and investigation of chronic venous disease in a standardized fashion.

Medical Therapy

The primary goal of medical treatment is to reduce or reverse the effects of ambulatory venous hypertension. Various complementary nonsurgical methods have been employed to achieve

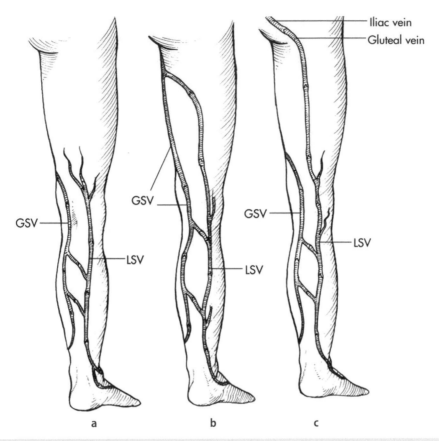

Figure 24.19 Anatomical variations in the termination of the SSV. Termination of the saphenopopliteal junction (a); termination into the GSV (b); termination into the gluteal vein (c). (Reprinted with permission from Goldman, MP. *Sclerotherapy: Treatment of Varicose and Telangiectatic Leg Veins.* 2nd ed. St. Louis; Mosby-Year Book; 1995.)

Clinical signs (grades 0–6):	Class supplemented by (A) for asymptomatic and (S) for symptomatic presentation
Etiologic classification:	Congenital, primary, or secondary
Anatomic distribution:	Superficial, deep, perforating, alone or in combination
Pathophysiological dysfunction:	Reflux or obstruction, alone or in combination
Class	**Clinical Definition**
0	No visible or palpable signs of venous disease
1	Telangiectasias or small reticular veins
2	Varicose veins
3	Edema
4	Skin changes related to hyperpigmentation, eczema, and/or lipodermatosclerosis
5	Skin changes (as above) with healed venous ulceration
6	Skin changes (as above) with active venous ulceration

Table 24.7 CEAP Classification System

this goal and include the use of supportive care, compression, and pharmacotherapy (Table 24.8).

Supportive Care

A supportive measure such as simple leg elevation is an effective tool to reduce edema. Ideally, a sitting patient should have the feet higher than the hips and a recumbent patient's feet should be above the heart. Adjunctive active calf exercises with flexion and extension movements at the level of the ankle should be encouraged. Nevertheless, strict bed rest with leg elevation is unrealistic for many patients.

Meticulous skin care is an integral component of supportive care for venous hypertension. The regular use of a nonirritating lotion or cream should be encouraged. Hyperkeratotic and ichthyotic skin may require exfoliation via a urea or α-hydroxy acid–containing lotion. A pruritic eczematous stasis dermatitis can provoke scratching. Resultant excoriations can potentially evolve into ulcerations. Consequently, the episodic use of a topical glucocorticoid may be required.

Weight loss in the obese subject is helpful. Regular exercise with a graduated compression stocking in place should be promoted. Aggressive antimicrobial therapy is warranted for soft tissue infections to prohibit secondary lymphedema and its attendant swelling burden.

Compression

Compression has long been the mainstay of therapy for the medical management of CVI

Supportive Care
Leg elevation
Meticulous skin care
Weight loss
Exercise
Compression
Elastic compression stockings
Compression bandages—elastic or inelastic, Unna's boot
Other—sequential pneumatic compression boots, CircAid wraps, manual lymphatic drainage, impulse compression of the plantar venous plexus
Systemic Pharmacotherapy
Phlebotropic agents
Horse chestnut seed extract (HCSE)
Hydroxyrutosides (Venoruton, Paroven)
Micronized purified flavonoid fraction (MPFF) or Daflon
Other—maritime pine bark extract, calcium dobesilate, centella asiatica, aminaftone, and grape seed extract
Fibrinolytic agents
Anabolic steroids—stanozolol, oxandrolone
Danazol
Defibrotide
Sulodexide
Mesoglycan
Hemorheologic agent
Pentoxifylline
Antiplatelet agent
Aspirin

Table 24.8 Medical Therapy of Chronic Venous Disease (CVI and varicose veins)

and varicose veins. Several types of external compression are available, including both elastic and inelastic wraps, elastic graduated compression stockings, and sequential pneumatic compression pumps. The physiological benefits of compression are diverse (Table 24.9). Extrinsic compression increases the subcutaneous interstitial pressure, which inhibits Starling forces, which promote transcapillary fluid leakage into the interstitium, thereby decreasing peripheral edema. Regardless of the type of compression employed, several tenets regarding their use exist. First, the applied pressure should be graduated. Specifically, maximal at the malleolar level but decreasing with ascension to the proximal limb. Second, the compression device should be correctly fitted and applied in an accurate and appropriate fashion. Third, the amount of applied compression should be commensurate to the degree of venous dysfunction and patient somatotype. Fourth, caution should be exercised when utilizing compression in the setting of severe peripheral artery disease.

Elastic compression stockings

Graduated elastic compression hosiery is the most widely used and standard therapy for venous hypertension. Elastic hose are available in a variety of compositions, lengths (below and above knee, panty hose), and compression (class 1–4, 20–60 mm Hg). A preponderance of data have established the salutary effects of elastic compression stockings in treating the complications of CVI and varicose veins. Substantial evidence exists that the regular use of a below-knee graduated stocking supplying 30 to 40 mm Hg for 2 years reduces the risk of developing postthrombotic syndrome after a DVT by ap-

proximately 50%.[97,98] One survey identified that patients who developed a DVT were amenable to the relatively costly purchase and use of compression stockings.[99] A few inquiries have questioned the benefit of compression hosiery. One crossover randomized controlled trial found no significant difference in symptoms when 30 to 40 mm Hg compression stockings and no stockings were compared during a 4-week period in patients with varicose veins.[100] In a controversial randomized study, a 30 to 40 mm Hg compression stocking was no more effective than a loosely applied placebo stocking in treating postthrombotic syndrome.[101] Finally, stockings have been criticized as being difficult to apply, hot in warmer temperatures, cosmetically disagreeable, and moderately expensive.

Compression bandages

Wrapping the limb with elastic or inelastic compression bandages is an inexpensive modality to reduce edema. However, attaining and preserving appropriate pressure gradients with compression wraps is decidedly dependent on operator proficiency. Compression bandages are advantageous in the following scenarios:

- for treating active venous stasis ulcerations, especially when they are weeping and require frequent dressing changes;
- when providing initial compressive therapy of edema prior to undergoing fitting with a graduated compression hose;
- for abnormally contoured lower extremities;
- with patients who lack the ability to self-apply and remove firm compression stockings.

Increase	Decrease
Plasminogen activator release	Edema
Interstitial pressure	Ambulatory venous pressure
Superficial vein compression	Superficial venous distension
Capillary clearance	Superficial venous pressure
Calf muscle pump volume	

Table 24.9 Physiologic Benefits of Compression

Elastic wraps employed in a figure-8 fashion yield superior and more sustained compression than conventionally applied spiral wraps. In a 2006 Cochrane database review of compression for venous leg ulcers, 22 trials reporting 24 comparisons were identified and the following conclusions were reached: compression increases ulcer healing rates compared to no compression, multilayered systems are more effective than single-layered systems, and high compression is more effective than low compression but there are no clear differences in the effectiveness of different types of high compression.[102] A parallel Cochrane review noted that compression stockings might *prevent* recurrent venous ulcers, yet the evidence is not particularly compelling.[103]

Other compression therapies

Other less frequently used compression therapies include sequential intermittent pneumatic compression of the calf and thigh, CircAid wraps (circumferential inelastic bands secured by Velcro), manual lymphatic drainage, and impulse compression of the plantar venous plexus.

Systemic Pharmacotherapy

Pharmacologic treatment of CVI and varicose veins has principally been investigated and utilized in Europe but not in the United States. The precise role of pharmacotherapy for venous reflux is not well defined, but these agents may be a useful adjunct to supportive care and compression. Alternatively, these medications could be an attractive therapeutic substitute when compression is not tolerated. Some of the more widely utilized agents are listed next.

Phlebotropic agents

Horse chestnut seed extract (HCSE), the active component of which is escin, inhibits the enzymes hyaluronidase and elastase. Both of these enzymes are involved in proteoglycan degradation. HSCE may prevent leukocyte activation as well.[104] Multiple reviews suggest that HSCE is superior to placebo in mitigating manifestations of CVI and varicose veins, such as edema, leg pain, and pruritus.[105,106] The medication is well tolerated with rare side effects such as headache, dizziness, increasing pruritus, and gastrointestinal upset occurring in ≤ 3%.

Hydroxyrutosides (Venoruton, Paroven: O-[β-hydroxyethyl]rutoside) are a class of venoactive medications that decrease capillary filtration rate and permeability. Several studies have confirmed the effectiveness of hydroxyrutosides in decreasing the clinical signs and symptoms of venous hypertension.[107-109] This agent is generally well tolerated as well.

Micronized purified flavonoid fraction (MPFF), or Daflon, is a well-investigated, phlebotrophic, micronized flavonoid of 90% diosmin and 10% hesperidin that reduces bradykinin-mediated capillary permeability and inhibits leukocyte activation and migration.[110,111] In addition to significantly improving mild to moderate reflux-associated manifestations, Daflon has also been shown to significantly expedite healing of venous stasis ulcers when compared to placebo.[112,113] Gastrointestinal side effects occur in up to 10% of patients.[112,113]

Other phlebotropic agents include maritime pine bark extract, calcium dobesilate, centella asiatica, aminaftone, and grape seed extract.

Fibrinolytic agents

Stanozolol is an anabolic steroid that decreases the level of tissue plasminogen activator inhibitor, resulting in improved fibrinolysis. Several small analyses have illustrated that stanozolol is an effective therapy for lipodermatosclerosis[114-116] Conversely, stanozolol has neither provided benefit in healing venous stasis ulcerations nor prevented them.[116,117] Oxandrolone[118] and danazol[119] are other androgenic compounds with fibrinolytic properties that have been used in the setting of lipodermatosclerosis with success.

Defibrotide is an antithrombotic medication that enhances prostacyclin production and activates fibrinolysis. In a randomized, double-blind, placebo-controlled trial of 288 patients with CVI, oral defibrotide significantly reduced the primary end point of ankle circumference.

Additionally, defibrotide significantly reduced venous thromboembolic events.[120] Another small trial (n = 32 patients) showed that defibrotide plus compression was significantly more effective than placebo plus compression in improving venous stasis ulcers.[121] Defibrotide is not commercially available in the United States.

Sulodexide, a glycosaminoglycan, is a drug with profibrinolytic and antithrombotic activity. Two relatively recent randomized controlled trials involving 330 patients have demonstrated that the addition of oral sulodexide to compression significantly reduced ulcer healing time when compared to adding placebo to compression.[122,123] Sulodexide is well tolerated but is not currently commercially available in the United States.

Mesoglycan, a polysaccharide, has both fibrinolytic and antithrombotic properties. In a randomized, placebo-controlled, double-blind study of 183 patients, sequential intramuscular (21-day therapy) and oral (21-week therapy) Mesoglycan was significantly more effective than placebo in decreasing the healing time of venous ulcerations.[124] The use of a daily intramuscular injection may be objectionable to some patients. Mesoglycan is not available in the United States.

Hemorheologic agents

Pentoxifylline is a widely studied medication with both hemorheologic and anti-inflammatory properties that appreciably expedites the healing of venous stasis ulcerations. Two randomized control trials[125,126] and one 2001 systematic review[127] found that pentoxifylline was significantly more effective than placebo in healing venous stasis ulcerations. Side effects include diarrhea and gastrointestinal upset.

Antiplatelet agents

Only one small, randomized controlled trial of 20 patients determined that aspirin (300 mg daily, enteric coated) increased ulcer healing rates compared with placebo (38% with aspirin vs. 0% with placebo).[128] In addition to small sample size, this trial had several methodological weaknesses that limit the significance of the conclusion.

Ulcer Therapy

A comprehensive discussion of venous ulcer therapy is beyond the scope of this chapter; however, multiple cardinal issues should be addressed when caring for ulcer-affected patients (Table 24.10). It is worth emphasizing that the mainstay of therapy involves the use of compression. Table 24.11 summarizes the randomized, controlled trials that have compared compression treatments for venous stasis ulcerations.[129-135] The definitive compression pres-

The mainstay of therapy is adequate compression.
The wound base should be kept moist, free of contamination, and excessive exudates should be appropriately managed—there is no definitive agent or dressing that constitutes "best topical therapy."
Local wound debridement may be needed to remove devitalized tissue, thus reducing surface bacterial burden as well as senescent cells, which are unresponsive to growth factors. Debridement can be surgical, enzymatic, autolytic (via moisture-containing dressings), or biological (maggot therapy).
Reserve topical (eg, iodine or silver impregnated dressings) and/or systemic antibiotic therapy for overt concurrent soft tissue infection or wounds that have been present for > 30 days.
Corrective superficial and/or perforating vein therapy via surgery, endovascular repair, or sclerotherapy may be warranted.
Larger ulcers (eg, > 10 cm² in diameter) may require animal or artificial skin grafts.
Consider a trial of adjunctive systemic pharmacotherapy.

Table 24.10 Cardinal Principles of Venous Stasis Ulceration Therapy

Type of Compression Study	Study	Study Number	Interventions	Outcomes/Healing Rates
Elastic compression vs. no compression	O'Brien et al[130]	n = 200		Completely healed at 3 months
			1. 4-layer (Profore) n = 100	1. 54%
			2. "Usual care" range of dressings chosen in community care n = 100	2. 34%
Unna's boot vs. no compression	Kikta et al[131]	n = 84		Completely healed at 6 months
			1. Unna's boot; n = 42	1. 70%
			2. DuoDERM hydrocolloid dressing; n = 45	2. 38%
Elastic compression vs. inelastic short stretch compression	Callam et al[132]	n = 132		Completely healed at 12 weeks
			1. Elastic compression (orthopedic wool, Tensopress + Tensoshape) n = 65	1. 54%
			2. Nonelastic compression (orthopedic wool, Elastocrepe + Tensoplus Forte) n = 67	2. 28%
Multilayer vs. single-layer elastic compression	Nelson et al[133]	n = 200		Completely healed in 6 months
			1. Single-layer compression bandage (Granuflex Adhesive) n = 100	1. 49%
			2. 4-layer: wool, crepe, Elset, Coban; n = 100	2. 69%
Multilayer high-compression vs. inelastic short-stretch compression	Nelson et al[134]	n = 387		Completely healed in 6 months
			1. 4-layer bandage (Profore or System 4)	1. 67.5%
			2. Short stretch system (Comprilan or Rosidal K)	2. 55.4%
Unna's boot vs. multilayer elastic compression vs. single-layer elastic compression	Colgan et al[135]	n=30		Completely healed in 12 weeks
			1. Modified Unna's boot (paste bandage, Elastocrepe, Elastoplast, class 2 compression sock) n = 10	1. 60%
			2. 4-layer bandage (Profore) n = 10	2. 70%
			3. Lyofoam dressing + Setopress bandage n = 10	3. 20%

Table 24.11 Summary of Randomized Controlled Trials Comparing Compression Treatments for Venous Leg Ulcers
(Adapted from Clarke-Moloney M, Lyons GM, Burke PE, et al. A review of technological approaches to venous ulceration. *Critical Reviews in Biomedical Engineering.* 2005;33[6]:511-556.)

sure for ulcer treatment is not well defined but a pressure of 35 to 40 mm Hg at the ankle appears necessary to inhibit capillary exudation in limbs with venous disease.[136,137]

Despite following the aforementioned guidelines, convalescent rates for venous ulcerations remain a discouraging 50% to 70% (depending on initial ulcer size and chronicity) after 12 weeks of therapy.[138] In the 2005 *Clinical Evidence* review of venous leg ulcer therapy, only compression bandages and oral pentoxifylline received a "beneficial" rating.[139] Cultured allogenic bilayer skin replacement, oral flavonoids, oral sulodexide, periulcer injection of granulocyte-macrophage colony stimulating factor, and systemic Mesoglycan were classified as "likely to be beneficial." Table 24.12 lists these therapies in a number needed to treat (NNT) fashion. Compression stockings were the only therapy to achieve a "beneficial" rating in preventing ulcer recurrence. Superficial vein surgery was "likely to be beneficial" in preventing relapse.[139]

Surgical Therapy

Ligation and Stripping

Combination *ligation* and *stripping* is the gold standard treatment for saphenous vein insufficiency with involvement of the saphenofemoral or saphenopopliteal junction. Decades of ex-perience and refinement have borne this out. Treatment of GSV insufficiency by stripping is superior to treatment by high ligation and sclerotherapy combined.[143] Saphenofemoral junction reflux treated by high ligation alone is associated with a high rate of persistent and recurrent disease,[144,145] whereas simultaneous stripping of the GSV has been shown to reduce the risk of recurrent disease by two-thirds.[146] There is an ongoing debate regarding the source of recurrence at the groin. Dilatation of existing collaterals has fallen into disfavor. Neovascularization is the more favored theory at this time.[147-149]

The goal of stripping is to reduce axial load and separate the GSV from its perforators. The diminution of the hydrostatic forces at play is accomplished with above-knee stripping. Indication for stripping the GSV or SSV is symptomatic axial reflux. Although considered the standard in this country, whether or not high ligation is added, remains an area of controversy. Most recent research indicates high ligation may not be necessary.[150] Traditionally, each of the 5 major branches at the saphenofemoral junction is dissected and reflected to its own first or second tributary and ligated. Short- and midterm results of multicenter and individual reports utilizing outpatient radiofrequency and laser endovenous thermal ablation techniques show promising evidence that junctional ligature is not crucial. Long-term studies are needed to adopt this change as a standard. Contraindications to saphenous stripping include arterial

Intervention	NNT (95% CI)
Multilayer elastomeric compression vs. nonelastomeric compression bandages	5 (3–12)[140]
Multilayer high-compression vs. single-layer compression bandages	6 (4–18)[140]
Pentoxifylline 400 mg 3 times daily vs. placebo (concurrent use of compression)	6 (4–14)[127]
Periulcer injection of granulocyte-macrophage colony stimulating factor (400 μg) vs. placebo	2 (1–7)[141]
Cultured allogenic bilayer skin equivalent vs. nonadherent dressing	7 (4–41)[142]
Sulodexide plus compression vs. compression alone	4 (3–9)[122,123]

Table 24.12 Number Needed to Treat (NNT) for Healing of Leg Ulcerations (Adapted from Nelson EA, Cullum N, Jones J. Venous leg ulcers. *Clin Evid.* 2005;13:2507-2526)

occlusive disease, nonambulatory status, severe postphlebitic leg, infected ulcer, morbid obesity, and pregnancy. Coexisting deep venous insufficiency is not an absolute contraindication to treatment.[148,151] Secondary deep venous insufficiency is known to improve following adequate treatment of superficial venous incompetence.

Side effects and adverse sequelae of ligation and stripping include bruising and hematoma. These usually are not seen until 3 to 5 days after surgery. Technique modifications have reduced the incidence of hematomas requiring surgical evacuation. Nerve injury caused by removal of the distal GSV, which is closely associated with its nerve below the knee, has been reduced by stripping the thigh portion only. Stripping of the SSV often proves more difficult than stripping saphena magna. Difficult and varied anatomy at the saphenopopliteal junction is culpable. The SSV is intimately associated with the sural nerve, especially in its more distal course. Proximity dictates injury is possible. If so, a localized area of hypoesthesia or dysesthesia may occur. These may be temporary or permanent in nature. Less frequently, injuries to the peroneal nerve with resultant foot drop have been reported. Wound infection is reported as < 1%. Additional reported side effects are induration along the stripper tract, damage to lymphatic channels, seroma, and phlebitis. DVT is less concerning due to simultaneous high ligation. However, both DVT and pulmonary embolism have been reported. Major side effects are considered unusual when consideration of contraindications, whether absolute or relative, occurs.

As a procedure, stripping has undergone many refinements. These changes have decreased morbidity to allow treatment in the outpatient setting. Two randomized trials compare conventional and perforate invaginate stripping (PIN). It seems intuitive that PIN stripping,[152] by allowing the vein to be pulled inside out, would minimize trauma. Interestingly, neither trial supports one method over the other as superior.[153,154]

Stripping from the groin to just below the knee has reduced the incidence of saphenous nerve injury. In many cases GSV stripping below the knee is unnecessary. Medial calf perforators associated with ulceration are more likely to be in the Cockett's distribution as opposed to paratibial in location. Cockett's perforators are associated with the posterior arch vein, whereas paratibial perforators may communicate directly or indirectly with the GSV.

The impact of venous surgery on quality of life has been assessed. Significant positive differences in the areas of physical functioning and pain 2 years postoperatively have been noted.[155] Since the chance for recurrence in genetically susceptible individuals is high, a longer look may not be truly warranted. Irrespective of genetic susceptibility, when patients with uncomplicated varicose veins are treated surgically, treatment provides symptomatic relief and significant improvements in quality of life compared to conservative treatment. The randomized controlled trial evaluating the impact of surgical intervention compared to conservative therapy was limited by evaluating only uncomplicated venous disease. Also, at midterm evaluation a significant portion (51.6%) of the conservative treatment group had elected to undergo surgery.[156]

Treatment of primary varicose veins by surgical methods that avoid stripping remains controversial.[144,157a,157b,157c] However, there are some instances when this may be appropriate. Symptomatic medial calf varicosities associated with an incompetent GSV and saphenofemoral junction may be treated by high ligation and stab avulsion of varicosities if the saphenous vein is minimally dilated on standing duplex examination. Ultrasound confirmation of competent medial thigh and knee perforators is also helpful. This allows preservation of the saphenous vein for later use in cardiac or peripheral vascular surgery.

As a treatment method, ligation and stripping remain the cornerstone of current thought regarding treatment of hydrostatic, gravitational reflux. It is the procedure with which we have the most experience and the most accumulated data. In spite of this, it has fallen by the wayside as more gentle, less invasive technologies gain popularity. Long-term observations of replacement modalities are needed. If favorable, the results may lower the final curtain on ligation and stripping as the standard of care.

Ambulatory Phlebectomy

Ambulatory phlebectomy dates back to Roman times and the Middle Ages.[158] Robert Muller, a Swiss dermatologist, is responsible for its 1940s renaissance with further refinement by AA Ramelet in the early 1950s.[159] Their technique introduces small vein hooks under the skin through tiny incisions to avulse abnormal veins. Considered a gentle and cosmetically pleasing technique, it is often used as an adjunct to the various methods employed to eradicate saphenous vein reflux. It is utilized for primary and adjunctive treatment of incompetent reticular and varicose veins > 3 mm in diameter. Also known as *microphlebectomy,* it is especially good for varicose saphenous tributaries and for refluxing reticular veins in the popliteal crease, lateral thigh, and leg. It is used on pudendal veins, in addition to the ankles and feet, with satisfactory results.[160] Ambulatory phlebectomy has been used on arms, hands, and periorbital and temporal veins with good results by skilled practitioners.[161]

Excellent results in categories of safety, cosmesis, and low complication rates are attributed to tumescent anesthesia, preoperative markings by transillumination,[159] small 1- to 3-mm incisions or 18-gauge needle punctures, gentle traction extirpation of the vein, compression, and early ambulation (Figure 24.20).

Indications for ambulatory phlebectomy are symptomatic incompetence of the GSV and SSV and symptomatic varicose veins of CEAP classification 2 to 6, varicosities in difficult locations such as foot, ankle, or popliteal fossa in the setting of failed conservative therapy. If incompetence of the GSV or SSV or their deep anastomoses is present this should be treated first. Note there are case reports of skilled physicians utilizing standard ambulatory phlebectomy or stab avulsion phlebectomy for refluxing GSVs and SSVs.[162,163] Use in this fashion is not common.

Contraindications of stab avulsion venectomy are saphenofemoral or saphenopopliteal junction reflux, cellulitis, localized infection, severe peripheral edema, uncontrolled insulin-dependent diabetes mellitus, serious chronic illness, and inability to ambulate, wear compression, or follow postoperative instructions. Deep venous insufficiency is a relative contraindication. Secondary deep venous insufficiency may improve following treatment of primary superficial disease. The decision to perform ambulatory phlebectomy in this setting should be made on a case-by-case basis only with the benefit of thorough reflux mapping by venous duplex. Additional relative contraindications include chronic dermatosis involving the treatment area or arthritide with associated skin disease such as scleroderma. The largest risk associated with ambulatory phlebectomy is patient access to poorly trained or inexperienced practitioners.[164] Aside from this instance untoward reactions are considered more bothersome than worrisome as they are usually minimal and transient in nature. Furthermore, they are avoidable as experience generates refinement of personal technique. Reported complications associated with phlebectomy are cutaneous, vascular, neurologic, and anesthetic related. Blister formation associated with compressive bandaging is the most common complication.[165] Hyperpigmentation, hematoma, telangiectatic matting, skin necrosis, seroma,[166] neuroma, dermal scar, tat-

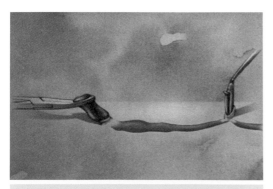

Figure 24.20 Ambulatory phlebectomy, multifocal pull-through technique. (Reprinted courtesy of Neil S. Sadick, MD.)

too, thrombophlebitis, paresthesia, dysesthesia, lymphocele—particularly near the tibia and in the foot and ankle—lymphorrhea, anesthetic overdose, anesthetic delayed reaction, and, rarely, DVT[164] are reported. Contact dermatitis to compressive wrap and topical medications has been reported, as has an unusual talc granuloma. Skin perforation and subdermal scarring have been reported specific to the resector used in transilluminated-powered phlebectomy.[167]

A small, single-blind, randomized controlled trial compared ambulatory phlebectomy and compression sclerotherapy addressing the risk for recurrence by treatment method. Statistically significant differences were noted at 1- and 2-year follow-up. The risk for recurrence was less with ambulatory phlebectomy at 2.1% at both year 1 and year 2 compared with 25.0% and 37.5%, respectively, for compression sclerotherapy. The relative risk for recurrence at year 1 was 12 and at year 2 equaled 18 (95% CI). When analyzed by logistic regression, $P < 0.001$ for both years.[168] An additional finding was the presence of a residual varicose vein 4 weeks *post procedure* as a significant indicator of future recurrence.

Current literature makes mention of alterations in ambulatory phlebectomy which have allowed practitioners to decrease the incidence of complications. One is the addition of tumescent anesthesia with versus without epinephrine. The use of tumescent is seemingly intuitive because it can decrease ecchymosis and hematoma formation. It may subsequently minimize the risk that hemosiderin deposition will cause hyperpigmentation. Another benefit, the addition of epinephrine, slows down the absorption of lidocaine thereby minimizing the chance of significant response to this cardiosensitive drug. Inadvertent intravenous injections of tumescent have been associated with systemic symptoms that are cardiac and neurologic in nature. Another alteration, a modified pull-thorough technique, has been reported to decrease operative time and improve cosmesis.[169] Soft tissue probes, for example, a circumcision probe, are useful when the vein is adhered to overlying skin.

Power-Assisted Phlebectomy

Power-assisted ambulatory phlebectomy or transilluminated powered phlebectomy (TIPP), commercially known as TRIVEX (InaVein), became available in the United States in 1999. An endoscopic technique, TRIVEX, is performed under general or spinal anesthesia as an outpatient (Figure 24.21). Direct visualization of the varicose vein is accomplished by a transilluminator placed in the subcuticular space posterior to the vein to be treated. Hydrodissection is accomplished via tumescent fluid delivered through the transilluminating handpiece. Next, a powered resector carefully follows a lighted path. Equipped with suction and an oscillating nonreusable blade, the resecting handpiece morcellates and aspirates the vein. Second-stage tumescent is applied to minimize postoperative complications.[170]

Proposed advantages of this method over conventional stab avulsion technique are the ability to efficiently remove large varicose clusters and extensive varicosities spanning the upper and lower leg, reduction in the number of surgical incisions, and subsequent reduction in postoperative pain. An additional assumed benefit, in the case of extensive disease, is reduced operative time.

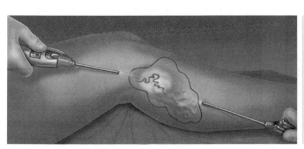

Figure 24.21 TRIVEX, or power-assisted ambulatory phlebectomy. This is an endoscopic technique that involves placement of a transilluminating handpiece and a powered resector within the subcuticular space for targeted removal of large and extensive varicosities. Tumescent fluid is delivered through the transilluminating handpiece. (Reprinted with permission from InaVein LLC, Lexington, MA.)

The disadvantages of this technique are increased expense over the traditional method and the need for a higher-skilled operative assistant compared to standard ambulatory phlebectomy. Arguably, decreased operative time may be a cost-saving measure. However, 2 randomized trials did not find statistically significant differences in operative times between the conventional and powered phlebectomy.[170,171]

The same 2 studies report conflicting information regarding the significance of postoperative pain and hematoma formation by method. However, both trials found the decreased number of incisions associated with TRIVEX to be significant ($P < 0.00001$, $P < 0.001$). Both found comparison of procedure-related paresthesia to be insignificant. Differences in cosmesis and patient satisfaction between power-assisted and conventional ambulatory phlebectomy were not significant. Most case reports indicate a significant learning curve associated with this procedure.[167,172] Overall, TIPP appears to be safe and effective without significant adverse events. It is best utilized for extensive varicosities. More randomized trials of significant participation are necessary to assess long-term impact on recurrent disease and quality of life.

Subendofascial Perforator Procedure

The surgical treatment of perforator disease was first performed by Linton[173] in 1938. An open technique, it was associated with a high rate of wound complications and has been widely abandoned. Multiple modifications have been made to the original procedure. It was not until 1985 when Hauer[174] developed an endoscopic method of perforator division that surgical treatment of incompetent perforators was revolutionized.[174] Subendofascial perforator surgery (SEPS) involves the placement of an endoscope into the subfascial space. Utilizing single-port- or multiple-port-approach videoscopic instrumentation allows perforator interruption by surgical clips, electrocautery, or harmonic scalpel.[175] All incompetent perforators influencing the medial calf cannot be visualized from this plane.[176] The posterior deep

compartment can be accessed to allow visualization of Cockett's perforators, when located in the intermuscular septum, and to allow access to proximal paratibial perforators. The limitation of this endoscopic technique when treating incompetent medial calf perforators is the frequent inability to access Cockett I due to its retromalleolar position.

SEPS is indicated for treatment of incompetent perforators of the medial calf resulting in CEAP 4 to 6 disease. Active ulceration is not a contraindication of the procedure. Active ulceration should be distinguished from an infected ulceration, which is a contraindication, just as caution should be exercised if a large circumferential ulcer is present. In this instance, careful examination of refluxing pathways by duplex ultrasonography and confirmation of diagnosis should occur. Additional contraindications are arterial occlusive disease, nonambulatory status, chronic illness, and subsequent high operative risk. Careful consideration should be given in cases involving coexisting severe rheumatologic disease, chronic dermatologic conditions such as scleroderma, severe lymphedema, extremely large and muscular legs, and recent DVT.[175] Currently, no randomized trials reporting the long-term benefit of SEPS on venous ulcer healing are available. Short-term improvement has been reported by many.[177,178] The North American SEPS (NASEPS) Registry collected data from 17 centers in the United States and Canada from 1993 to 1996.[179] The cumulative ulcer-healing rate at 1 year was 88%. The majority of healing occurred in < 8 weeks. One- and 2-year ulcer recurrence rates were 16% and 28%, respectively. Recurrence was more likely to occur by 2 years in post thrombotic limbs. It has been demonstrated that SEPS can result in rapid ulcer healing. Good results can be expected in patients suffering from *primary* valvular failure. Whether success can be attributed solely to SEPS remains unknown as the contribution of concomitant GSV ablation, when indicated, has not been assessed. Advances in ultrasound imaging have lead to ultrasound-guided open perforator ligation as an alternative to SEPS. Ultrasound guidance provides precise pre-procedure mapping resulting in smaller incisions than older open techniques. A nonsurgical alternative performed with duplex guidance, *foam sclerotherapy*, may also be used to treat incompetent perforator veins. The newest technologic development is a radiofrequency catheter specifically designed for perforators. The procedure is known as *transluminal occlusion of perforators (TRLOP)*. The use of laser as opposed to the radiofrequency probe is often referred to as *percutaneous ablation of perforators (PAPs)*.

Endovenous Therapy

Sclerotherapy

Sclerotherapy, a form of endovenous chemical ablation, is the targeted destruction of incompetent superficial veins whether they are dermal, subcuticular, extrafascial, transfascial (perforators), or epifascial, by the injection of sclerosing solution. The goal of sclerotherapy (*sclero* = hard) is to induce irreversible panluminal endofibrosis utilizing a minimal volume and minimal concentration of sclerosant without damaging interrelated normal veins or adjacent structures. Multiple agents can be injected to induce endothelial damage. The aim is to induce enough injury to result in fibrosis rather than thrombosis as the latter leads to recanalization.[180]

Sclerosants are categorized in 3 broad categories according to their mechanism of action: osmotic, detergent, or chemical irritant in nature (Table 24.13).

Properties of commonly used sclerosants

Sclerotherapy is the gold standard treatment of leg veins *less* than 3 mm in diameter, referred to as *microsclerotherapy*. Microsclerotherapy is often used as an adjunct following surgical and endovascular procedures on incompetent

Category	Osmotic	Detergent	Chemical Irritant
Agents	Hypertonic saline (HS), Sclerodex (25% dextrose + 10% hypertonic saline), polyiodinated iodine (Variglobin and Sclerodine)	Sodium morrhuate, ethanolamine oleate, sodium tetradecyl sulfate (STS), and polidocanol (POL)	Chromated glycerin (CG)
Intended Use	Vessels < 1.5–2.0 mm	Large and small vessels	Vessels < 0.5 mm
Advantage[194]	Hypertonic saline has no allergic potential	STS and POL-FDA approved for leg veins, POL unlikely necrosis with extravasation, both effective at low concentrations and minimal to no pain with injection	Hyperpigmentation and matting rare
Disadvantage[194]	Painful, significant extravasation necrosis, cramping related to salt load, hyperpigmentation	Anaphylactic reactions reported but low incidence,[195] caution asthmatics, prone to hyperpigment if [ ] too high	Viscosity causes painful injection, chromate moiety allergenic, ureteral colic and hematuria reported secondary to high dosages
Maximum Dose per Session[194,213]	HS: 8 cc at 23.4% concentration Sclerodex—10 cc Variglobin: 3 cc at 12%	Liquid STS: 10 cc of 3% solution (300 mg) Liquid POL: 4 cc at 3% solution (2 mg/kg) Microfoam: STS and POL 10 cc of 1%–3% concentration	5–10 cc

Table 24.13 Properties of Commonly Used Sclerosants

saphenous stems and truncal varicosities. Table 24.14 reviews the relative potencies of commonly used sclerosants.

Sotradecol 2%–3%	■■■■■
Polidocanol 3%–5%	■■■■■
Sotradecol 1%–2%	■■■■
Polidocanol 2%	■■■■
Sotradecol 0.5%–1%	■■■
Polidocanol 1%–2%	■■■
Hypertonic saline 23.4%	■■
Sotradecol 0.25%	■■
Polidocanol 0.75%	■■
Hypertonic Saline 11.7%	■
Sotradecol 0.1%	■
Polidocanol 0.25%–0.50%	■
Chromated Glycerin 50%–72%	■

Table 24.14 Relative Strengths of Commonly Used Liquid Sclerosants

In the era before duplex ultrasonography, sclerotherapy of vessels > 4 mm in diameter, referred to as *macrosclerotherapy*, was associated with high failure rates.[181,182] For this reason it was considered inferior to ligation and stripping or stab avulsion for large veins and was largely abandoned by US physicians. The advent of high-resolution duplex ultrasonography has improved diagnostic ability in the form of reflux mapping, and yields improved decision making.[183,184] The ability to monitor needle placement and vessel response during ultrasound-guided macrosclerotherapy heightens treatment efficacy. Ultrasound-guided sclerotherapy is considered a safe and effective procedure for ambulatory patients with 2-year outcomes comparable to that of surgery.[185]

Indications

Regardless of vessel size, treatment is indicated for symptomatic venous reflux when conservative measures fail. Sclerotherapy is performed to relieve pain or swelling and to prevent spontaneous hemorrhage, recurrent superficial thrombophlebitis, and ulceration. Treatment is also performed for cosmetic concerns.

Contraindications

Generalized severe systemic diseases such as diabetes, kidney, liver, cardiac, pulmonary, and collagen vascular disease and malignancies are contraindications to injection sclerotherapy. Advanced rheumatologic disease is a contraindication if it interferes with mobility or the ability to don compression hose. Fragile, senile skin and severe chronic dermatologic conditions that are not of venous origin are contraindications if they will interfere with the ability to comply with post treatment compression. Patients who suffer from peripheral artery disease with an ankle-brachial index below 0.7 should not be injected. Milder forms of arterial insufficiency coexisting with CVI may not preclude treatment if segmental and located in an area remote to the site of sclerotherapy. Nonambulatory status, severe obesity, thrombophilia, allergies to sclerosing agents, or intense urticaria after previous treatment are contraindications. Polidocanol induces an immediate urticaria, which should be distinguished from an abnormal or exaggerated urtication following sclerotherapy. Sclerotherapy is contraindicated during pregnancy since this is considered a hypercoagulable state and polidocanol is known to cross the placenta.[186] However, small doses of localized treatment may be cautiously considered for pregnant patients in the setting of intensely painful pudendal or vulvar varicosities, burning venulectasias, threatened spontaneous venous hemorrhage, and recurrent superficial thrombophlebitis *only* if these conditions are refractory to conservative treatment. Hypercoagulable states are considered a relative contraindication to treatment. Pretreatment identification of thrombophilia risks based on personal and family history must be evaluated and should include consideration of historical thrombotic events, age-appropriate cancer screenings, spontaneous abortions, postpartum state, and thrombophilia labs if indicated. Risk analysis comparing the need for sclerotherapy against potential anticoagulation-related dangers should be made. If sclerotherapy is warranted in the thrombophilic patient or one who is chronically anticoagulated for other reasons, anticoagulation may be bridged utilizing low-molecular-weight heparin in the standard fashion. Hormonal treatments with estrogen and progesterone are relative contraindications.[187] Patients on tamoxifen should be considered. DVT and telangiectatic matting[188] while on hormonal therapy have been incident to sclerotherapy. Severe obesity is considered a contraindication due to difficulty with post-treatment compression on massive legs. Any suspected noncompliance with support hose contraindicates treatment. Nonambulatory status and conditions predisposing to immobility contradict treatment. Acute DVT is an obvious contraindication. However, history of uncomplicated DVT is considered only a relative contraindication. Treatment of primary superficial venous insufficiency is known to improve secondary deep venous insufficiency.

Risks and complications

Risks associated with sclerotherapy are inadvertent intra-arterial injection and unexpected anaphylaxis. The most frequently noticed complication is hyperpigmentation, which has a reported incidence of 10% to 30%.[189,190] Extravasation necrosis is unlikely to occur with today's popular detergent sclerosants. Telangiectatic matting has been reported as high as 30% but is probably less than this.[188] Complications of liquid and foam sclerotherapy are listed in Table 24.15.

A resurgence of interest in macrosclerotherapy has occurred in the past decade. Instead of injecting liquid, ultrasonography is used to inject a combination of air and liquid known as sclerosant foam (sclerofoam). Trials comparing the 2 have found macrosclerotherapy with liquid inferior to foam sclerotherapy in multiple areas: successful obliteration ($P < 0.01$),[191] recurrence ($P = 0.048$),[192] and quality of life.[193]

Foam Sclerotherapy

The use of sclerotherapy to treat veins ≥ 4 mm has seen a renaissance in recent years due to the advent of *foam sclerosants*.[200] This latest era of sclerotherapy seeks to minimize dilutional fac-

tors and increase sclerosant contact time by combining gas with liquid to create sclerosant foam (Figure 24.22). The most widely utilized foams are microfoams created by the double syringe system (DSS) and the Tessari method. The Tessari method mixes gas to sclerosant in a 1:1 or 8:1 ratio[201] and is known to create microbubbles ≤ 100 μm in diameter (Figure 24.23).[202] Presently, room air containing 21% oxygen and 79% nitrogen is the most widely used gas but growing evidence supports an admixture of O_2/CO_2 may be advantageous in terms of safety and possibly efficacy.[219,220,223,225] The perfect gaseous mixture for microfoam application aims to maintain physical properties such as bubble size, density, and durability while simultaneously speeding the absorption of bubbles in blood.

Hyperpigmentation
Telangiectatic matting
Coagula formation
Superficial thrombophlebitis
Temporary swelling
Compression bandage friction blisters
Compression bandage–induced folliculitis
Cutaneous extravasation necrosis
Vasovagal reactions secondary to panic
Localized hirsutism
Urticaria
Anaphylaxis
Inadvertent arterial injections leading to muscle and skin necrosis, amputation
Deep venous thrombosis
Pulmonary embolism
Air embolism
Scintillating scotoma
Membranous fat necrosis
Myocardial infarction[233]
Cerebrovascular accident[224,198]
Transient ischemic attack[235]
Seizure[233,199]
Headache[233]
Septicemia[235]

Table 24.15 Known Adverse Sequlae and Complications Following Liquid and Foam Sclerotherapy[196,197]

More rapid absorption is theorized to decrease the potential of gas emboli.

The indications for foam sclerotherapy are the same as those for liquid sclerotherapy with a few caveats. Several randomized controlled studies support the sclerosing action of microfoam, which has increased efficacy compared to liquid sclerosant.[191,203-205] For this reason it is a superior choice when treating saphenous incompetence, large varicosities, venous ulcers, and perforator veins[206] by injection. A randomized controlled trial of 88 GSVs treated by 3% polidocanol liquid versus 3% microfoam reported absence of reflux in 40% of the liquid group compared with 84% of the foam group ($P < 0.01$).[191] The same study found equivalent volume dose of foam versus liquid occluded a longer segment of the GSV (average 28 cm for foam vs. 15 cm for liquid). When analyzed through the lens of recurrence, efficacy of duplex-guided foam over liquid was demonstrated by Yamaki et al[192] with 8.1% of the foam group and 25.0% of the liquid group showing recurrent varicose veins at 1 year ($P = 0.48$).[192] Debate exists regarding diameter limitations of foam sclerotherapy. In skilled hands diameters of ≥ 20 cm[207] have been successfully treated, deflat-

ing previously held notions[208] that larger veins should be reserved for either surgery or thermal endovenous vascular ablation.

Microfoam administered under ultrasound guidance is appropriate for GSVs, SSVs, tributaries, and recurrent varicose veins. Sclerotherapists favor the foam method for treatment of GSV aneurysms particularly when near the saphenofemoral junction. Foam sclerotherapy has been used successfully for treatment of venous malformations.[209-211] Direct injection of incompetent perforators can be performed under duplex guidance. This is rarely necessary as secondary perforator sclerosis usually occurs when the associated saphenous or varicose tributary is injected. Treatment of telangiectasias and reticular veins with foam sclerosant is considered appropriate by some and inappropriate by others.[212,213]

Contraindications of foam sclerotherapy parallel those of liquid sclerotherapy but also include considerations related to the intravenous administration of gas. A large prospective randomized trial documented no perfusion defects on lung scintigraphy after 10 mL of foam injected.[214] Another study indicated detergent sclerosant is 97% gone by the time it reaches

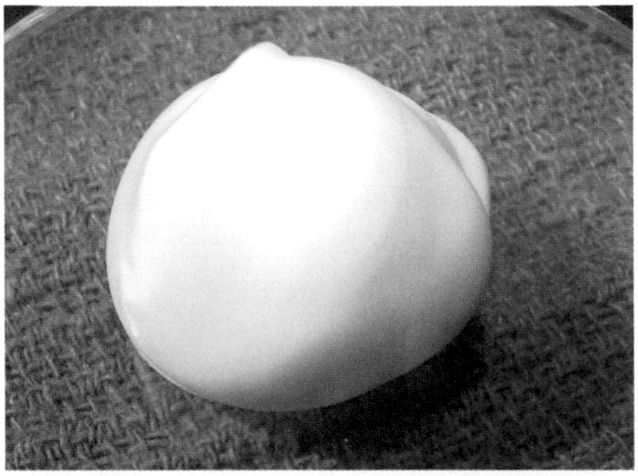

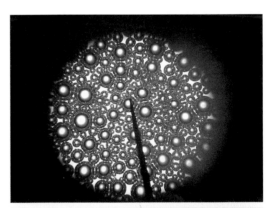

Figure 24.22 Microfoam created by the Tessari method as visualized immediately after preparation. Note its dense, homogenous nature. The properties inherent in sclerofoam impart its success. These are compactness, density, durability, and adhesiveness, which are determined by sclerosant concentration, quantity or ratio of sclerosant and gas, type of gas, temperature, pH, and method of agitation or preparation.

Figure 24.23 Microfoam bubble as viewed through a high-powered microscope. Diameter is less than 100 to 150 μm. Each small bubble carries on it the exact concentration of the sclerosant with which it is mixed. Thus, small bubbles allow more sclerosant contact than larger bubbles. Uniformly sized bubbles have greater internal surface tensions and improved durability allowing for increased sclerosant endothelial contact time.[290] (Image courtesy of Alessandro Frullini, MD, Florence, Italy.)

pulmonary circulation.[215] An analysis of patented polidocanol endovenous microfoam (PEM) confirms the agent does not result in remote sclerosis of the lung.[216] Hence, following intravenous injection of microfoam sclerosants, circulating gas bubbles reach the right heart and are filtered by the lung without consequence (Figure 24.24). If a right-to-left cardiac shunt is present, gaseous microbubbles may enter arterial circulation. Cautious application must therefore be considered in certain patient populations known to have increased risk of patent foramen ovale (PFO) compared to the general population.[217] Specifically, migraine cephalgia with or without aura is not contraindicated. Known asymptomatic PFO is only a relative contraindication, whereas known symptomatic PFO is an absolute contraindication. Prescreening for the presence of PFO is not considered necessary.[212] Table 24.16 lists some of the relative contraindications of foam sclerotherapy.

Known thrombophilia
Migraine cephalgia with and without aura
Visual, mental, or neurological symptoms after previous foam sclerotherapy session
Known asymptomatic PFO
History of thromboembolism

Table 24.16 Relative Contraindications of Ultrasound-Guided Foam Sclerotherapy According to a Consensus of Experts in the Technique (From Breu FX, Guggenbichler S, Wollmann JC. Second European consensus meeting on foam sclerotherapy, 2006. Tegernsee, Germany. Vasa. 2008;37:S71.)

The incidence of PFO in the general population is established. A pooled analysis of autopsy studies yielded an average prevalence of PFO of 26% (range 17%–35%).[218,219] Interestingly, 2 recently reported pilot studies demonstrate a higher prevalence of right-to-left shunt in CVI patients. In the first, 25 of 66 (42.7%; 95% CI, 31.5%–55.9%) had a PFO by transcardiac echo (TCE).[220] In the second, 130 of 221(58.8%; 95% CI, 52.5%–65.1%) demonstrated right-to-left shunt as evidenced by transcranial Doppler (TCD).[221] TCD cannot distinguish intracardiac from intrapulmonary shunt, which may account for the unusually high incidence noted in this study. Yet, a third pilot study[222] makes brief mention of a 29% incidence of middle cerebral artery (MCA) bubbles in shunt-negative CVI patients, raising the question of their etiology and the role of vasoactive mediators elaborated post injection. Further research is needed to identify the role of vasoactive mediators specific to this population.

Multiple studies document intracardiac emboli and middle cerebral artery (MCA) emboli following the administration of microfoam within peripheral leg veins.[220,223-226] MCA bubbles detected during treatment with proprietary low-nitrogen polidocanol microfoam were associated with no elevation of cardiac markers, no new abnormal neurological exam or visual field defects, and no new MRI lesions in a study of patients with known right-to-

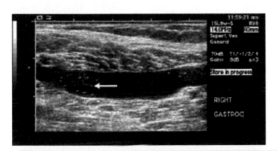
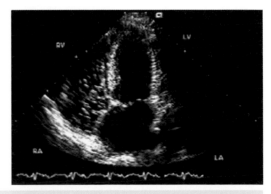

Figure 24.24 (a) Longitudinal ultrasound image of the gastrocnemius vein with brightly echogenic emboli circulating within the dilated lumen during ultrasound–guided microfoam sclerotherapy. (b) Apical four chamber view of an echocardiographic ultrasound image with brightly echogenic emboli circulating within the right ventricle. (Royal Society of Medicine Press)

left shunt and MCA bubbles detected during treatment.[227]

Emboli, which serve to deliver medication to the endothelium, endure beyond that delivery regardless of the gaseous composition utilized in foam preparation (O_2, CO_2, O_2/CO_2 combined)[228] and in spite of techniques engaged to prevent their migration.[229] The rate at which bubbles disintegrate is related to gas composition; the more soluble the gas in blood the more quickly it disintegrates,[201] theoretically decreasing the possibility of significant cerebral microemboli. A prospective cohort study reported the absence of migraine symptoms in patients with known migraine cephalgia with or without aura.[230] The sample size of this study is small and may reflect the overall low incidence of migraine cephalgia related to foam sclerotherapy. Alternatively, the low incidence may reflect the proprietary composition of the gases utilized and should not be extrapolated to other foams. The findings of this prospective cohort study lend evidence not only to the safety of foam but also give further credence to the use of physiologic gases to decrease side effects. Others have suggested an increased safety profile with the use of O_2, CO_2, and O_2/CO_2 combination.[231,232] The injection of gaseous microbubbles versus macrobubbles is believed to be safe. Characteristics bestowing safety rely on the physical properties of foam. Its hyperechoic nature enhances duplex guidance and allows visualization of medication within the target vein or veins, as well as visualization of foam as it clears the deep system (Figure 24.25). Extravasation of foam is known to be less harmful than liquid extravasation. The compactness, density, and durability allow direction of the foam to a desired segment of vein. Homogenous foam allows utilization of sclerosants at higher concentrations and lower volumes. This translates to fewer injection sites and fewer treatment sessions.

The potentially serious risks associated with foam sclerotherapy are intra-arterial injection, stroke, myocardial infarction, thromboembolism, and anaphylaxis. A meta-analysis of 69 studies including over 9000 patients treated with foam sclerotherapy found the overall inci-

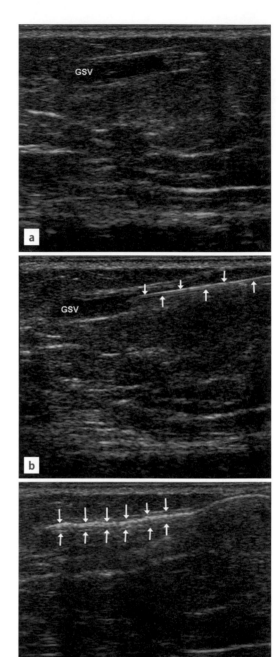

Figure 24.25 (a) Great saphenous vein (GSV) before injection of 3% sotradecyl sulfate microfoam created by Tessari method 4:1 (air to sclerosant). (b) Ultrasound-guided percutaneous access of GSV with 25-gauge, 1.5-in needle, longitudinal view. (c) GSV immediately after injection of hyperechoic microfoam. Note intense vessel spasm signifying treatment end point. (Images courtesy of Mark N. Isaacs, MD, FACPh, FAAFP)

dence of serious adverse events to be low (Table 24.17).[233] The same meta-analysis demonstrated matting/skin staining or hyperpigmentation and pain at the site of injection to be the most frequent adverse events (Table 24.18). Neurologic side effects including transient visual disturbance, acute confusional state, and stroke have been reported. Of these, transient visual disturbance is the most common with a reported incidence as high as 5.8% and predominance among migraine cephalgia sufferers.[234] Septicemia is rare but 1 case related to foam sclerotherapy is reported bringing the total to 3 cases in 30 years for liquid and foam sclerotherapy combined.[235] The most commonly reported side effects overall are pain at injection site, hyperpigmentation, headache, painful phlebitis, and scotoma. They are considered minor in nature.

The thrombogenicity of microfoamed sclerosants has not been directly investigated. The reported incidence of DVT varies (Table 24.19). In a large retrospective observational study of 500 veins with saphenofemoral and great saphenous incompetence the incidence of DVT was reported as zero.[236] Yet, other smaller studies have reported incidences ranging from 0.007% to 5.9%.[193,237,238] Pulmonary embolism has been reported but is rare.[235] The aforementioned meta-analysis further supports DVT and pulmonary embolism (PE) as rare occurrences post foam.[233]

Event	Median Rate (%)
Visual disturbance	1.4
Transient confusion	0.5
Headache	4.2
Other systemic symptoms: cough, chest tightness, panic attack, malaise, vasovagal event	0.5
Thrombophlebitis	4.7
Matting/skin pigmentation	17.8
Pain at injection site	25.6

Table 24.18 Summary of Nonserious Adverse Events Related to Foam Sclerotherapy for Varicose Veins on over 9000 Patients According to a Meta-Analysis of 69 Studies Conducted in Europe and the United States from 1999 to 2006 (From Jia X, Mowatt J, Burr M, et al. Systematic review of foam sclerotherapy for varicose veins. *Br J Surg.* 2007;94:925-936.)

Study	Incidence DVT (%)
Barrett	2.7
Frulinni and Cavezzi	0.66
Alos	0
Bountouroglou	0
Cabrera[236,239]	0
Bhowmick	5.7
McCollum	4.8
Gillet et al[235]	0.98
Hamel-Desnos et al[240]	0
Rabe et al[204]	0
Wright et al[241]	4.5

Table 24.19 Reported Incidence of DVT Associated with Foam Sclerotherapy in Randomized Controlled Trials and Observational Studies from 2000 to 2009

Foam sclerotherapy has many advantages. It requires no general or regional anesthesia, and it does not require hospitalization and no time is lost from work. Patients remain ambulatory, and fewer sessions are required. Patients report high satisfaction with this technique.[193] Ultrasound-guided compression foam sclerotherapy is reported to heal ulcers more rapidly than compression alone.[242] A 2006 randomized study[243] comparing combined surgical techniques of

Event	Median Rate (%)
Anaphylaxis	0
Arterial events	0
Pulmonary embolus	0.0–0.3
Deep venous thrombosis	0.4–0.7
Cutaneous necrosis	0.0–1.3
Cutaneous ulceration	0–4
Intra-arterial injection	0

Table 24.17 Summary of Serious Adverse Events Related to Foam Sclerotherapy Performed on over 9000 Patients According to a Meta-Analysis of 69 Studies Conducted in Europe and the United States from 1999 to 2006 (From Jia X, Mowatt J, Burr M, et al. Systematic review of foam sclerotherapy for varicose veins. *Br J Surg.* 2007;94:925-936.)

high ligation, stripping, and stab avulsion for saphenofemoral, great saphenous, and tributary incompetence with high ligation plus ultrasound-guided foam found short-term success at 3 weeks in 87% of the high ligation plus foam patients compared with 93% for the surgical-only patients. Success was defined as complete obliteration or partial obliteration without reflux on follow-up venous duplex examination. At 3 months, 86% of high ligation with foam veins and 82.6% of the surgery-only veins remained closed. Mean time to return to work or back to normal activity was 2 days for foam sclerotherapy and 8 days for surgery patients ($P < 0.001$). Patient reports of quality-of-life scores improved by 46% and 40%, respectively ($P < 0.001$). A randomized multicenter trial was conducted with 656 patients randomized to Varisolve polidocanol endovenous microfoam (Provensis/BTG plc) versus alternative therapy. Alternative therapy was defined as either sclerotherapy utilizing homemade foam or surgery. The primary end point of complete obliteration and elimination of reflux > 500 ms determined by duplex ultrasonography was evaluated at month 3 and 12. Findings were analyzed against a noninferiority hypothesis. The Varisolve/surgery cohort response rates at 3 months (Varisolve 68.2%, surgery 87.2%) and at 12 months (Varisolve 63.1%, surgery 86.2%) confirm the superiority of surgery over polidocanol microfoam at 12 months.[241] It is plausible noninferiority of polidocanol microfoam to surgery might be found if a 3- to 5-year observation had occurred.

Larger studies are needed to further validate safety, but presently it appears from a combination of consensus statements, case reports, prospective and retrospective observational studies, and randomized controlled trials that foam sclerotherapy is safe in experienced hands, efficacious, less expensive, less painful, and less time consuming than other treatments. It is known to significantly improve quality of life and enjoys high satisfaction rates among patients.

Future applications
Foam sclerotherapy is expected to play an expanded role in the treatment of venous malformations. In addition, male varicocele, pelvic congestion syndrome, and popliteal cysts are future considerations.

Endovenous Thermal Ablation
Attempts to decrease down time, cost, and morbidity associated with traditional surgical treatment of axial reflux have spawned development of minimally invasive percutaneous methods to thermally ablate the endothelium. These are catheter-based techniques that utilize the physics of radio waves and laser beams to generate and apply heat to the saphenous veins, *in situ* (Figure 24.26). Designed for the outpatient setting, they are performed under duplex guidance utilizing tumescent anesthesia.

Radiofrequency Ablation
The first method to obtain FDA approval for endovenous thermal ablation, known as *radiofrequency ablation (RFA)*, utilized a bipo-

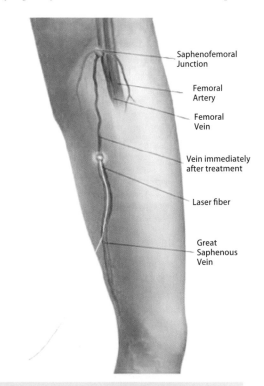

Figure 24.26 Diagram of endovenous laser ablation. Following ultrasound-guided placement of the laser fiber and administration of tumescent anesthesia, energy is delivered endovenously as the fiber is withdrawn.[272] (Courtesy of Wiley-Blackwell.)

lar radiofrequency catheter with expandable electrodes in direct contact with the vein wall (Closure, VNUS/Covidien Vascular Therapies) (Figure 24.27). A direct feedback mode or thermocouple allows operator-controlled continuous heating in the range of 85 to 120°C. This is sufficient temperature to cause collagen contraction and endothelial denudation.[244] Subsequent to this stimulus, a fibrotic cord forms causing complete sealing of the vein lumen at 6 weeks (Figure 24.28).[245]

Indications and contraindications

Indications for endovenous thermal ablation by radiofrequency technique include symptomatic GSV or SSV reflux with or without reflux at their corresponding deep system junctions; nontortuous major saphenous tributaries such as the accessory saphenous, anterior thigh circumflex branch, and vein of Giacomini may also be treated.

Contraindications include inability to ambulate, nonpalpable pedal pulses, or ABI < 0.7, pregnancy, lactation, active local or systemic infection, aneurysmal segment, or arteriovenous malformation involving the proposed treatment vein. Current guidelines for RFA no longer limit maximum vein dilatation at 12 mm.[246] The necessity of direct contact between electrodes and the vein wall limiting treatment of larger veins was specific to the first-generation Closure catheter. RFA is not contraindicated in the presence of a pacemaker. The theoretic risk of inadvertent electromagnetic interference is considered minimal.[247]

Outcomes: side effects, success

Complications of endovenous thermal ablation by radiofrequency technique include paresthesia, skin burns, phlebitis, DVT, pulmonary embolism, hematoma, ecchymosis, and hyperpigmentation. Table 24.20 outlines the reported success rates following this technique. Table 24.21 outlines reported side effects.

Of these side effects, paresthesia is the most common with a reported incidence as high as 8.5% to 21% during the first week after treatment.[248,249] Increased incidence is associated with below-knee ablation. Spontaneous

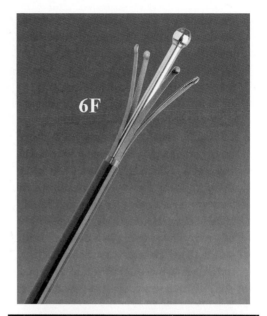

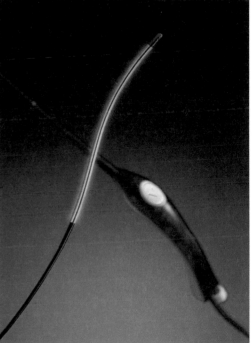

Figure 24.27 (a) Original Radiofrequency or Closure® catheter. Endovenous delivery of radiofrequency energy via expandable, insulated electrodes allows resistive heating of the vein wall. A thermocouple allows continuous monitoring of the temperature at the vessel wall. Controlled heating results in contraction of vein collagen and induces endoluminal fibrosis. (b) Radiofrequency ClosureFAST® catheter. Catheter improvements circa 2006 allow continuous and sequential heating of 7cm vein segments. Diameter limitations of 12mm are no longer contraindicated. (Product image copyright © Covidien. Used with permission.)

weeks is known to occur (Figure 24.29). Individual authors have reported a DVT incidence as high as 16%.[250] Hingorani's study[250] found no statistically significant differences in the age or gender of patients with or without post procedure DVT. There was no significant difference in pretreatment CEAP classification, addition

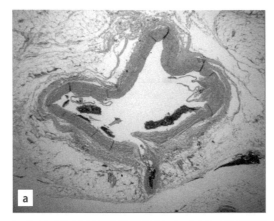

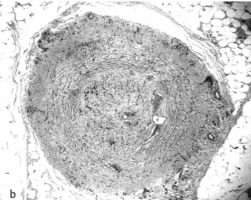

Figure 24.28 Radiofrequency-generated thermal injury to the vein wall causes immediate histologic changes, which progress to complete fibrotic sealing of the vessel at 6 weeks post ablation. (a) Vein pretreatment and (b) 6 weeks post treatment. (Product image copyright ©Covidien. Used with permission.)

resolution over 6 to 12 months is expected for the majority. Thermal injury or burn is reported with an incidence of 1.7% to 9.0% prior to the administration of tumescent anesthesia. Perivenous tumescent fluid provides a thermal heat sink around the vessel serving not only to protect nearby structures but also to compress the vein. Reports of paresthesia and thermal injury substantially decreased with its adoption. DVT is a rare occurrence. When present it is often described as a thrombus extension into the common femoral vein, which suggests procedure-related genesis. Timeline protocol variations for post procedure ultrasonography may miss DVT if not performed soon after treatment; regression within 1 to 4

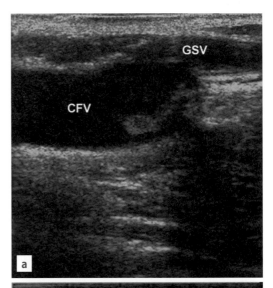

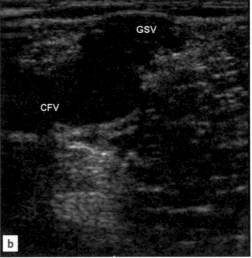

Figure 24.29 (a) Terminal valve thrombus floating in common femoral vein as seen immediately post endovenous laser ablation. Thrombus formation is attributed to guide-wire trauma near the terminal valve. A learning curve is associated with this procedure. (b) Terminal valve thrombus resolved 4 weeks post procedure. Patient was treated with anticoagulation for 4 weeks without additional sequelae.

First Author	Year	N	Method	F/U	Success	Recan	rVV
Chandler et al[254]	2000	301	RFA + HL[a] RFA + AP[b]	4.9 months	96.0%		3.4%
Goldman et al[255]	2000	12	RFA + AP	3 months 6 months	100.0%		0.0%
Hinchliffe et al[256]	2006	19	RFA + AP	6 weeks 12 months	84.0%		
Hingorani et al[250]	2004	73	RFA + Adjunct[c]	2–30 days (mean 10 days)	96.0%		
Lurie et al[257]	2003	46 40 S&L	RFA	Immediate 72 hours	95.0% 83.7%		
Lurie et al[258]	2005	46 40 S&L	RFA	2 years	95.0%		14.3%
Manfrini[249]	2000	152	RFA	1 weeks 6 months	93.0% 91.0%		
Merchant et al[259]	2002	319	RFA	1 week 1 year 2 years	93.4% 83.6% 85.2%	11.3%	
Merchant et al[248]	2005	1078	RFA + AP (5%)	4 weeks 6 months 1 year 2 years 3 years 4 years	97.4% 91.0% 88.8% 86.2% 84.2% 88.8%		
Puggioni et al[260]	2005	130 53 77	 RFA EVLT		 90.9% 94.4%		
Sybrandy et al[261]	2002	26	RFA	1 year	88.0%		
Spruiell[d]	2006	44	RFA	6 weeks 6 months 12 months	100.0% 97.7% 95.4%		2.2%
Weiss et al[262]	2002	140	RFA	1 week 6 weeks 1 year 2 years (21/140)	98.0% 96.0% 96.0% 90.0%		

Table 24.20 Endovenous RFA: Rates of Success, Recanalizataion, and Recurrence by Study

a, High ligation; b, Ambulatory phlebectomy; c, Ambulatory phlebectomy or subendofascial perforator procedure as indicated; d, Unpublished data

of adjunctive procedure, or type of anesthesia—general versus tumescent. The largest radiofrequency study to date (N = 1078) reports a DVT incidence of 0.5%.[248] The combined experience of 3 large treatment centers yields a thrombus extension rate of 0.4% (5 of 1150).[251] The latter suggests the incidence of DVT following radiofrequency is not unlike that reported following surgery, of 0.15% to 5.7%.[25]

Successful endovenous obliteration is inconsistently defined as the absence of reflux with partial or complete occlusion of the treated axial segment on post treatment duplex examination. Immediate success, 93% to 100%; early success, 91% to 100%; midterm, 84% to 90%; and near long term, 4-year reporting of 88% all implicate the viability of radiofrequency-induced thermal occlusion as an alternative to ligation and stripping for combined saphenofemoral and great saphenous insufficiency. Figure 24.30 demonstrates fibrotic occlusion of the GSV 6 weeks following RFA.

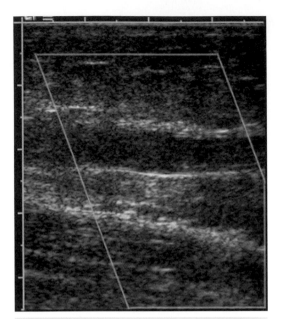

Figure 24.30 Longitudinal image of GSV with wall thickening and endoluminal fibrotic change 6 weeks post endovenous ablation by radiofrequency method.

Clinical trials: registries, case reports, randomized controlled trials

Two randomized studies compared radiofrequency obliteration with stripping and ligation (S&L).[263] The larger of the 2, the EVOLVeS Study,[257,258] randomized 44 limbs to RFA and 36 to S&L. Patients were followed over 2 years. In the RFA group, 80.5% of patients returned to routine activities of daily living within 1 day, compared with 46.9% of the S&L group ($P < 0.01$). Patients in the RFA group returned to work in 4.7 days (95% CI, 1.16–8.17), compared with 12.4 days (95% CI, 8.66–16.23) for the S&L group ($P < 0.05$). Early analysis of pre- and post treatment quality-of-life measurements significantly favored RFA ($P < 0.0001$). Ultrasonography follow-up occurred at multiple intervals over 2 years. Definition of complete occlusion was < 5 cm of proximal patent GSV and no reflux in the patent segment. Successful occlusion progressively increased over time existing in 95% of treated limbs at 2 years. In addition, 41% of the GSVs were undetectable on ultrasonography at the 2-year follow-up. Cumulative rates of recurrent varicose veins combined at 1 and 2 years were 14.3% for RFA and 20.9% for S&L ($P >$

0.05 Long Rank test). Although the recurrence rate was numerically lower it did not reach the level of statistical significance. Within the same study, neovascularization was observed at 2 years in 1 RFA patient and 4 S&L patients. The only case of neovascularization in the RFA group occurred in a patient who was an initial treatment failure. By contrast, the absence of neovascularization in the successfully obliterated RFA group is worthy of contemplation. It contradicts a long-held surgical belief that all saphenofemoral junction tributaries must be properly reflected and ligated to their own first tributaries to influence future disease state. A cohort of the EVOLVeS Study studied by Pichot et al[264] specifically looked at ultrasonography findings for 2 years after GSV radiofrequency obliteration. They found no evidence of groin neovascularity and > 90% of GSVs occluded. It may very well be that preservation of prograde flow through patent groin tributaries protects against neovascularization. An earlier study explored patients undergoing RFA with and without saphenofemoral ligation.[150] No statistically significant difference in recurrent varicose veins was noted ($P > 0.156$). However, they were only followed for 1 year. A suggestion that neovascularity at the groin following ligation as the likely culprit of recurrent disease was made. The exact mechanism of neovascularity has not been confirmed. To determine this, Labropoulos et al[265] looked at the prevalence, distribution, and flow characteristics of intraluminal neovascularization in patients undergoing GSV ablation by radiofrequency (n = 46) compared to laser obliteration with an 810-nm wavelength (n = 56). Post treatment multiple small vessels adjacent to the involved vein formed small arteriovenous fistulae (AVF) within the obliterated vein (n = 5). It is postulated that small AVF undetected by initial duplex examination may be a source of recanalization or recurrence following endovenous ablation.

Recanalization with subsequent reflux of the obliterated saphenous segment and the development of new varicose veins are seen after RFA. The pathophysiology involved is likely multifactorial. Further studies of sufficient

First Author	Year	N	Method	DVT	PE	Paresthesia	Burn	STP
Chandler et al	2000[254]	301	RFA + HL[a] RFA + AP[b]	1.4%	0.45%	19.0% overall 28.0% GSV BK[c]	2.7%	6.7%
Goldman et al	2000[255]	12	RFA + AP	0.0%	0.0%	0.0%	0.0%	
Hingorani et al	2004[250]	73	RFA + Adjunct[d]	16.0%	0.0%	NR	NR	NR
Manfrini et al	2000[249]	152	RFA	3.5%	0.6%	21.0%	9.0%	NR
Merchant et al	2002[259]	319	RFA	1.0%	0.35%	15.0% (1 week) 30.9% (1 year) 56.0% (2 years)	4.2%	2.1%
Merchant et al	2005[248]	1078	RFA + AP (5%)	0.5%	0.6%	12.1% (1 week) 7.2% (6 months) 2.0% (4 years)	1.7%[e]	3.3%
Puggioni et al	2005[260]	130 53 77	RFA EVLT	0.0% 2.3%	0.0% 0.0%	NR	NR	3.1%
Spruiell	2006[f]	44	RFA	0.0%	0.0%	2.3% (1 week) 0.0% (12 months)	0.0%	2.3%
Weiss et al	2002[262]	140	RFA	0.0%	0.0%	8.5% (1 week) 1.0% (6 months)	0.0%	0.0%

Table 24.21 Incidence of Reported Side Effects Following RFA by Study

a, High ligation; b, Ambulatory phlebectomy; c, Below the knee; d, Ambulatory phlebectomy or subendofascial perforator procedure as indicated; e, Pretumescent; f, Unpublished data; NR, not reported.

size and duration are necessary to understand the processes at play. Early and midterm findings for this method of treatment are sufficient to confirm its alternative role in the treatment of saphenous insufficiency. Long-term results may support supplantation of high ligation and stripping as the gold standard treatment for saphenous insufficiency.

Endovenous Laser Ablation (EVLA)

Laser affinity for target chromophores hemoglobin, deoxyhemoglobin, melanin, and water is not new science (Figure 24.31).[266] The application of selective photothermolysis from *within* an incompetent vein is novel. A small laser fiber, placed within incompetent axial veins, can sufficiently injure the endothelium to result in permanent fibrosis. The mechanism of destruction for hemoglobin-specific wavelengths is believed to be thrombotic occlusion mediated by steam bubbles from heated blood.[267] Disagreement exists in this area. Others believe inflammation and swelling, nonthrombotic occlusion, play a role in successful lumen fibrosis.[268] Currently, 7 wavelengths are available for endovenous laser techniques: 810 nm (VenaCure EVLT, AngioDynamics), 940 nm (ELAS, Dornier MedTech GmbH), 980 nm (VenaCure, AngioDynamics), 1064 nm (EVLP), 1319nm (Pro-V, Sciton), 1320 nm (CTEV, CoolTouch) and 1470 nm (ELVeS, biolitec). Available wavelengths have varying affinity for hemoglobin and water. The target chromophore for 810-, 940-, 980-, and 1064-nm wavelengths is red blood cell hemoglobin. The 980- and 1064 nm wavelengths also have some affinity for water. The 1320-nm and 1470-nm wavelengths are the only ones that bypass red blood cells to specifically target water in vein wall collagen. These properties of laser biophysics have been explored for each wavelength in hope of producing superior results with fewer side effects.

Indications, contraindications

After thorough mapping of reflux pathways by duplex ultrasonography, EVLA may be employed to treat superficial venous incompetence. Indications are identical to those for

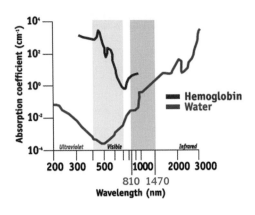

Absorption coefficients at 810nm and 1470 nm wavelengths for hemoglobin and water

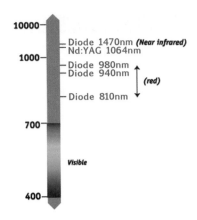

Wavelengths of lasers adapted for endovenous thermal ablation

Figure 24.31 Absorption coefficients at various wavelengths for water, oxyhemoglobin, and melanin. (Adapted from Cotton AM, A review of the principles and use of lasers in lower limb problems, *Lower Extremity Wounds*, 2004;3[3]:134.)

RFA with one exception: there is no diameter limitation for endolaser ablation. Venous diameters in excess of 30 mm have been successfully obliterated.[268] Contraindications for endolaser ablation are indistinguishable from those of RFA with one stipulation. Treatment of venous aneurysms of large diameter is not limited by catheter size as seen with radiofrequency.

Outcomes: side effects, success

Untoward effects following EVLA are similar to those encountered with RFA. Transient bruising and pain requiring medication are more frequently reported following endolaser ablation. Minor events of bruising, pain, hyperpigmentation, paresthesia, burns, phlebitis, and induration along the treated vein secondary to endovenous ablation by lasers are reported. An undesirable complication, arteriovenous fistula, may result (Table 24.22).[269] The incidence of paresthesia ranges from 1.1% to 36.5%, thermal injury from 0.9% to 4.8%, and phlebitis from 1.6% to 33%. DVT is unusual—incidence varies from 0.9% to 7.7%. No reports of pulmonary embolus have been noted. Techniques utilized to minimize complications and impart success are:

- *vein emptying:* Increased understanding of energy transfer has lead to emptying the vein to decrease thrombotic occlusion and increase nonthrombotic occlusion

- *tumescent anesthesia:* Ultrasound-guided circumferential application of 1 cm compresses the vein and provides a thermal barrier for surrounding tissue

- *optimal laser energy parameters:* Nonocclusion and early reopening are believed to be fluence dependent.[270] Multiple regression analysis indicated pretreatment vein diameter, laser energy per centimeter of vein length, and distance of the thrombus to the saphenofemoral junction at day 1 after treatment had no bearing on obliteration failures ($P = 0.004$).

- *direct wall contact:* The sterling occlusion rates reported by the originators of EVLT imply their belief that direct contact between laser fiber and vein wall may be germane to their success.[268]

Clinical data of the mid- and long-term results in the use of EVLA imply success. In the first 1000 limbs treated with an 810-nm diode laser, 99% occlusion was seen at 2 years and 98% at up to 5 years of follow-up.[268] Table 24.23 summarizes the results of several clinical studies utilizing various lasers. The data reflect successful vein occlusion by all wavelengths.

Author	Year	N	Wavelength	DVT	PE	Paresthesia	Burn	STP
Chang et al[271]	2002	252	1064 + HL	0.0%	0.0%	36.5% (3 weeks) 28.0% (6 months)	4.8%	1.6%
Goldman et al[272]	2004	24	1320	0.0%	0.0%	0.0%	0.0%	0.0%
Kabnick[273]	2006	30	810	0.0%	0.0%	0.0%	0.0%	33.0%
		30	980	0.0%	0.0%	0.0%	0.0%	10.0%
Min et al[274]	2001	90	810	0.0%	0.0%	1.1%	0.0%	0.0%
Mozes et al[275]	2005	56	810 + AP	7.7%	0.0%	NR	NR	NR
Navarro et al[276]	2001	40	810	0.0%	0.0%	0.0%	0.0%	0.0%
Oh et al[277]	2003	15	980	0.0%	0.0%	NR	0.0%	NR
Perkowski et al[278]	2004	203	940 + AP	0.0%	0.0%	0.0%	NR	NR
Proebstle et al[279]	2003	109	940[a]	0.0%	0.0%	NR	NR	10.0%
Proebstle et al[280]	2003	39	940	3.0%[b]	0.0%	11.0%	NR	8.0%
Spruiell et al[281]	2007	100	1320	0.0%	0.0%	1.0%	0.0%	1.0%
Timperman et al[282]	2004	111	810	0.9%	0.0%	0.0%	0.9%	0.0%

Table 24.22 Incidence of Reported Complications Following EVLA by Study

a, Prophylactic low-molecular-weight heparin given; b, Noted 5 weeks postablation in patient with history of multiple DVT and polycythemia vera; HL = high ligation; AP = ambulatory phlebectomy; NR = not reported.

Variance appears more technique dependent than wavelength dependent.

Clinical trials: registries, case reports, randomized controlled trials

A single-center series analyzed ablation of the saphenous system using 810-nm, 940-nm, and 1320-nm lasers. Ultrasonography follow-up over 3 years confirmed 97.7% of veins were successfully ablated. Ninety-seven percent of patients were satisfied with their procedure. No significant differences in lasers stood out.[286] Direct comparison between 810-nm and 980-nm lasers by the same author revealed less bruising ($P < 0.005$) at 1 week (980 nm) with more itching at 3 weeks (810 nm), less pain and lower varicose vein ratings (980 nm) at 4 months of follow-up ($P < 0.05$).[273] Direct comparison of 1320-nm with 940-nm lasers found significantly less pain and bruising in the CTEV patients ($P < 0.005$).[285]

Only 2 randomized trials comparing laser and surgery exist. Both are small in number and report only short-term results. In the De Medeiros study,[287] methodology for blinding and randomization is sparse. The study compares high ligation of saphenofemoral junction tributaries followed by EVLT, 810 nm (n = 20) with high ligation followed by ankle to groin surgical stripping (n = 20). There were no significant differences in procedure-related pain. Seven days post treatment significant differences were noted in the areas of swelling and bruising. Two months post treatment, blinded patients reported the laser-treated side as the limb deriving the most benefit from treatment ($P = 0.0184$). Successful obliteration between the 2 groups was comparable. Rasmussen et al[288] randomized 137 limbs representing CEAP C2 to C4 to either high ligation and stripping or EVLA of the GSV. Post procedure pain was higher in the surgical group compared to laser ablation ($P < 0.01$). However, there were no significant differences in use of analgesics or time to resume normal activity. Short-term efficacy for the 2 groups was similar. Long-term studies are needed to derive meaningful treatment decisions.

Author	Year Published	Number Treated Limbs	Wavelength	Duplex Ultrasonography Interval Follow-up	Rate Successful Obliteration
Alencar et al[283]	2006	190	810	2 weeks	92.4%
Bush[284]	2003	350	940	18 months	96.0%
Chang et al[271]	2002	252	1064 + HL	6 months (mean 19 months)	96.8%
Goldman et al[272]	2004	24	1320	6–12 months	100.0%
Kabnick[273]	2006	30 30	810 980	1 year 1 year	93.3% 93.3%
Min et al[274]	2001	90	810	1 week 1–9 months	97.0% 99.0%
Navarro et al[276]	2001	40	810	mean 4.2 months (up to 14 months)	100.0%
Oh et al[277]	2003	15	980	1 week 4 weeks 12 weeks	100.0% 100.0% 100.0%
Perkowski et al[278]	2004	203	940 + AP	2 weeks	87.0%
Proebstle et al[285]	2005	33 136	1320 940[a]	3 months 3 months	0.0% 97.0%
Proebstle et al[270]	2004	106	940	1 day 1 month 3 months	94.0% 91.0% 90.0%
Proebstle et al[267]	2002	31	940	1 day 7 day 28 day	97.0% 97.0% 97.0%
Proebstle et al[279]	2003	109	940	1 year	90.4%
Proebstle et al[280]	2003	39	940	3–12 months (median 6 months)	100.0%
Spruiell et al[281]	2007	100	1320	3 days 6 weeks 6 months 12 months	100.0% 100.0% 95.0% 95.0%
Timperman et al[282]	2004	111	810	1 week 3–78 weeks (mean 29.5 weeks)	100.0% 77.5%

Table 24.23 Endovenous Laser Ablation: Summary of Reported Clinical Success at Various Intervals in Time
a, Continuous pullback @ 30 W; HL = high ligation; AP = ambulatory phlebectomy.

A meta-analysis of 64 studies conducted between 1994 and 2007 involved a total of 12,320 treated limbs. Success rates of S&L, ultrasound-guided foam sclerotherapy, EVLA, and endovenous RFA were compared. EVLA was superior to all other treatment modalities. After adjusting for follow-up, ultrasound-guided foam sclerotherapy and RFA were as effective as surgical stripping. RFA treatments used the first-generation thermal probe, which may account for EVLA's superiority to RFA. In the absence

randomized, long-term studies on large patient populations, new treatment modalities for saphenous insufficiency appear deserving of their role in the treatment armamentarium.

The treatment of superficial venous insufficiency by minimally invasive endovenous techniques is a rapidly evolving field. As the numbers of treating physicians and well-informed patients grow, the need for larger studies and more definitive answers will abound. At this time there is a paucity of definitive information regarding long-term results. Due to favorable midterm results, either method of endovenous thermal ablation or ultrasound-guided chemical ablation is not only suitable but is possibly a superior alternative to ligation and stripping in the areas of safety, efficacy, downtime, cosmesis, and cost.

Procedure	Description	Target Veins
Stripping and Ligation	Ligation of femoral vein and proximal tributaries followed by GSV stripping from groin to knee	GSVs or SSVs
Ambulatory Phlebectomy	*Standard or conventional*—tributary varicosities extirpated through series of small incisions; under tumescent anesthesia *Power-assisted method (TRIVEX)*—endoscopic removal of extensive and large varicosities by transilluminated powered resector; performed under general anesthesia	*Standard or conventional*—localized areas varicose saphenous tributaries or varicose collaterals, minimally bulging reticular veins *TRIVEX*—extensive and large varicosities covering significant surface area of lower extremity; possibly adhesed due to inflammation
Subendofascial Perforator Procedure	Endoscopic disruption of calf perforator veins under general anesthesia	Below-knee perforator veins associated with posterior arch (Cockett's) or GSV (paratibial)
Endovenous Ablation by Radiofrequency	Endovenous ablation by radiofrequency-induced thermal fibrosis wavelengths	Enlarged nontortuous saphenous veins, accessory saphenous, vein of Giacomini, (2–12 mm)
Endovenous Ablation by Laser	Endovenous ablation by laser-generated thermal-induced fibrosis; blood absorption or near-infrared laser	Enlarged nontortuous saphenous veins, nontortuous saphenous tributaries such as accessory saphenous, anterior or posterior thigh branch, vein of Giacomini, posterior arch vein (1320-nm special fiber allows treatment moderately tortuous tributaries)
Transcutaneous Laser/Light	Laser vaporization by external application of laser beam or light source through skin to dermal and immediate subdermal vessels	> 2 mm diameter but < 3 mm—1064 Nd:YAG laser or RF +IPL, venulectasia or telangiectasia up to 2-mm diameter—1064 Nd:YAG laser, < 2 mm–532 nm KTP, 585- to 595-nm pulsed dye or 1064-nm Nd:YAG laser
Sclerotherapy	Injection of sclerosant, which injures endothelium resulting in luminal fibrosis	< 3 mm, *liquid micro*sclerotherapy > 3 mm, *liquid macro*sclerotherapy with possible duplex guidance ≥ 4 mm *foam* sclerotherapy utilizing duplex guidance for GSV, SSV, and their associated deep junctions, saphenous tributaries, and incompetent perforators
Transluminal Occlusion Perforator Veins	Radiofrequency-induced thermal fibrosis specific to refluxing perforators	Incompetent leg perforating veins above or below knee
Percutaneous Ablation of Perforators	Endovenous ablation by laser-generated thermal-induced fibrosis applied specifically to refluxing perforator veins	Incompetent leg perforating veins above or below the knee

Table 24.24 Procedures Utilized to Treat Incompetent Superficial and Perforator Veins

Summary

Chronic venous insufficiency, characterized by retrograde flow of blood within the lower extremities, remains a significant cause of vascular associated morbidity. Although peripheral arterial disease tends to receive more recognition, CVI is the more prevalent of the two disorders. Chronic venous disease is best evaluated via the CEAP classification scheme which yields a logical, structured method for decision making and communication. Recent studies have provided insight into the chronic inflammation that underlies this disease process. Although traditional therapy for disabling venous disease has been ligation and stripping, newer minimally invasive techniques utilizing laser energy or radiofrequency technology have revolutionized treatment. Table 24.24 (page 505) summarizes the treatment methodologies discussed in this chapter by vein type.

References

1. Mekky S, Schilling RSF, Walford J. Varicose veins in women cotton worker. An epidemiological study in England and Egypt. *BMJ*. 1969;2:591-595.

2. Criqui MH, Jamosmos M, Fronek A, et al. Chronic venous disease in an ethnically diverse population. *Am J Epidemiol*. 2003;158:448-456.

3. Brand FN, Dannenberg AL, Abbott RD, et al. The epidemiology of varicose veins: the Framingham Study. *Am J Prev Med*. 1988;4:96-101.

4. Kurz X, Kahn SR, Abenhaim L, et al. Chronic venous disorders of the leg: epidemiology, outcomes, diagnosis and management. Summary of an evidence-based report of the VEINES* task force. *Int Angiol*. 1999;18:83-102.

5. Da Silva A, Widmer LK, Martin H, et al. Varicose veins and chronic venous insufficiency: prevalence and risk factors in 4376 subjects in the Basle Study II. *Vasa*. 1974;3:118-125.

6. Widmer LK. *Peripheral Venous Disorders, Basel III Study*. Bern, Switzerland: Hans Huber; 1978:1-90.

7. Kroger K, Ose C, Rudofsky J, et al. Peripheral veins: influence of gender, body mass index, age and varicose veins on cross-sectional area. *Vasc Med*. 2003;8:249-255.

8. Evans CJ, Fowkes FG, Ruckley CV, Lee AJ. Prevalence of varicose veins and chronic venous insufficiency in men and women in the general population: Edinburgh Vein Study. *J Epidemiol Community Health*. 1999;53(3):149-153.

9. Maffei FHA, Magaldi C, Pinho SZ, et al. Varicose veins and chronic venous insufficiency in Brazil: prevalence among 1755 inhabitants of a country town. *Int J Epidemiol*. 1986;15:210-217.

10. Coon MM, Willis PW, Keller JB. Venous thromboembolism and other venous disease in the Tecumseh Community Health Study. *Circulation*. 1973;48:839-846.

11. Ruckley CV, Evans CJ, Allan PL, et al. Chronic venous insufficiency: clinical and duplex correlations. The Edinburgh Vein Study of venous disorders in the general population. *J Vasc Surg*. 2002;36:520-525.

12. Franks PJ, Wright D, Moffatt CJ, et al. Prevalence of venous disease: a community study in west London. *Eur J Surg*. 1992;158:143-147.

13. Carpentier PH, Maricq HR, Biro C, et al. Prevalence, risk factors, and clinical patterns of chronic venous disorders of lower limbs: a population–based study in France. *J Vasc Surg*. 2004;40:650-659.

14. Canonico S, Gallo C, Paoliss G, et al. Prevalence of varicose veins in an Italian elderly population. *Angiology*. 1998;49:129-135.

15. Abramson JH, Hopp C, Epstein LM. The epidemiology of varicose veins—a survey of Western Jerusalem. *J Epidemiol Community Health*. 1981;35:213-217.

16. Beaglehole R, Salmond CE, Prior IAM. Varicose veins in New Zealand: prevalence and severity. *N Z Med J*. 1976;84:396-399.

17. Callejas JM, Manasanch J, ETIC Group. Epidemiology of chronic venous insufficiency of the lower limbs in the primary care setting. *Int Angiol*. 2004;23(2):154-163.

18. Jawien A. The influence of environmental factors in chronic venous insufficiency. *Angiology*. 2003;54(Suppl 1):S19-S31.

19. Chiesa R, Marone EM, Limoni C, et al. Demographic factors and their relationship with the presence of CVI signs in Italy: the 24-Cities Cohort Study. *Eur J Vasc Endovasc Surg.* 2005;30:674-680.

20. Hirai M, Naiki K, Nakayama R. Prevalence and risk factors of varicose veins in Japanese women. *Angiology.* 1990;41:228-232.

21. Scott TE, LaMorte WW, Gorin DR, et al. Risk factors for chronic venous insufficiency: a dual case-control study. *J Vasc Surg.* 1995;22:622-628.

22. Gourgou S, Dedieu F, Sancho-Garnier H. Lower limb venous insufficiency and tobacco smoking: a case-control study. *Am J Epidemiol.* 2002;155:1007-1015.

23. Komsuoglu B, Goldelli O, Kulan K, et al. Prevalence and risk factors of varicose veins in an elderly population. *Gerontology.* 1994;40:25-31.

24. Beaglehole R, Prio IAM, Salmond CE, Davidson F. Varicose veins in the South Pacific. *Int J Epidemiol.* 1975;4:295-299.

25. Dindelli M, Parazzini F, Basellini A, et al. Risk factors for varicose disease before and during pregnancy. *Angiology.* 1993;44(5):361-367.

26. Cleave TL. *On the Causation of Varicose Veins and Their Prevention and Arrest by Natural Means.* Bristol, England: Wright; 1960.

27. Boccalon H, Janbon C, Saumet JL, et al. Characteristics of chronic venous insufficiency in 895 patients followed in general practice. *Int Angiol.* 1997;16:226-234.

28. Lacroix P, Abuyans V, Preux PM, et al. Epidemiology of venous insufficiency in an occupation population. *Int Angiol.* 2003;22(2):172-176.

29. Laurikka JO, Sisto T, Tarkka MR, et al. Risk indicators for varicose veins in forty- to sixty-year-olds in the Tampere varicose veins study. *World J Surg.* 2002;26:648-651.

30. Seidell JC, Bakx KC, Deurenberg P, et al. Overweight and chronic illness—a retrospective cohort study with a follow-up of 6-17 years, in men and women of initially 20-50 years of age. *J Chronic Dis.* 1986;39:585-593.

31. Berard A, Abenhaim L, Platt R, et al. Risk factors for the first time development of venous ulcers of the lower limbs: the influence of heredity and physical activity. *Angiology.* 2002;53:647-657.

32. Tuchsen F, Krause N, Hannerz H, et al. Standing at work and varicose veins. *Scan J Work Environ Health.* 2000;26:414-420.

33. Krijnen RM, de Boer EM, Ader HJ, Bruynzeel DP. Venous insufficiency in male workers with a standing profession: part 1: epidemiology. *Dermatology.* 1997;194:111-120.

34. Guberan E, Widmer LK, Martin H, et al. Causative factors of varicose veins: myths and facts. An epidemiological study of 610 women. *Vasa.* 1973;2:115-120.

35. Kontosic I, Vukelic M, Drescik I, et al. Work conditions as risk factors for varicose veins of the lower extremities in certain professions of the working population of Rijeka. *Acta Med Okayama.* 2000;54:33-38.

36. Fowkes FGR, Lee AJ, Evans CJ, et al. Lifestyle risk factors for lower limb venous reflux in the general population: Edinburgh Vein Study. *Int J Epidemiol.* 2001;30:846-852.

37. Malhotra SL. An epidemiological study of varicose vein sin Indian railroad workers from the South and North of India, with special reference to the causation and prevention of varicose veins. *Int J Epidemiol.* 1972;1:177-183.

38. Burkitt DP. A deficiency in dietary fiber may be one cause of certain colonic and venous disorders. *Am J Dig Dis.* 1976;21:104-108.

39. Clarke GH, Vasdekis SN, Hobbs JT, et al. Venous wall function in the pathogenesis of varicose veins. *Surgery.* 1992;111:402-408.

40. Cooper DB, Hillmon-Cooper CS, Barker SGE, Hollingsworth SJ. Primary varicose veins: the sapheno-femoral junction, distribution of varicosities, and patterns of incompetence. *Eur J Vasc Endovasc Surg.* 2003;25:53-59.

41. Ibrahim S, MacPherson DR, Goldhaber SZ. Chronic venous insufficiency: mechanisms and management. *Am Heart J.* 1996;132:856-860.

42. Zsoter, R, Cronin RF. Venous distensibility in patients with varicose veins. *Can Med Assoc J.* 1966;94:1293-1297.

43. Browse NL, Burnand KG, Irvine AT, Wilson NM. Varicose veins: pathology. In: *Diseases of Veins.* New York: Oxford University Press; 1999:145-162.

44. Johnson BF, Manzo RA, Bergelin RO, et al. Relationship between changes in the deep venous system and the development of the postthrombotic syndrome after an acute episode of lower limb deep vein thrombosis: a one- to six-year follow-up. *J Vasc Surg.* 1995;21:307-313.

45. Junger M, Steins A, Hahn M, Hafner HM. Microcirculatory dysfunction in chronic venous insufficiency (CVI). *Microcirculation.* 2000;7(6 Pt2):S3-S12.

46. Bollinger A, Leu AJ. Evidence for microvascular thrombosis obtained by intravital fluorescence videomicroscopy. *Vasa.* 1991;20:252-255.

47. Schmid-Schoenbein GW, Fung YC, Zweifach BW. Vascular endothelium-leukocyte interaction; sticking shear force in venules. *Cir Res.* 1975;36:173-184.

48. Coleridge Smith PD, Thomas P, Scurr JH, Dormandy JA. Causes of venous ulceration: a new hypothesis. *BMJ.* 1988;296:1726-1728.

49. Browse NL, Gray L, Jarrett PE, Morland M. Blood and vein-wall fibrinolytic activity in health and vascular disease. *BMJ.* 1977;1:478-481.

50. Wilkinson LS, Bunker C, Edwards JC, et al. Leukocytes: their role in the etiopathogenesis of skin damage in venous disease. *J Vasc Surg.* 1993;17:669-675.

51. Cheatle TR, McMullin GM, Farrah J, et al. Three tests of microcirculatory function in the evaluation of treatment for chronic venous insufficiency. *Phlebology.* 1990;5:165-172.

52. Tarlton JF, Bailey AJ, Crawford E, et al. Prognostic value of markers of collagen remodeling in venous ulcers. *Wound Repair Regen.* 1999;7:347-355.

53. Herouy Y, May AE, Pronschlegel G, et al. Lipodermatosclerosis is characterized by elevation expression and activation of matrix metalloproteinase: implications for venous ulcer formation. *J Invest Dermatol.* 1998;111:822-827.

54. Bradbury A, Evans C, Allan P, et al. What are the symptoms of varicose veins? Edinburgh Vein Study cross sectional population survey. *BMJ.* 1999;318:353-356.

55. Tran NT, Meissner MH. The epidemiology, pathophysiology, and natural history of chronic venous disease. *Semin Vasc Surg.* 2002;15(1):5-12.

56. Darke SG, Penfold C. Venous ulceration and saphenous ligation. *Eur J Vasc Surg.* 1992;6:4-9.

57. Schultz-Ehrenburg U, Reich, S, Robak-Pawelczyk B, et al. Twenty-year prospective epidemiologic study from childhood to adulthood on the development of varicose veins. Abstract presented at the 16th annual meeting of the American Venous Forum, February 26-29, 2004, Kissimmee, FL.

58. Sarin S, Shields DA, Farrah J, et al. Does venous function deteriorate in patients waiting for varicose vein surgery? *J R Soc Med.* 1993;86:21-23.

59. Labropoulos N, Leon L, Kwon S, et al. Study of the venous reflux progression. *J Vasc Surg.* 2005;41:291-295.

60. Killewich LA, Bedford GR, Beach KW, et al. Spontaneous lysis of deep venous thrombi: rate and outcome. *J Vasc Surg.* 1989;9:89-97.

61. Markel A, Manzo RA, Bergelin RO, et al. Valvular reflux after deep vein thrombosis: incidence and time of occurrence. *J Vasc Surg.* 1992;15:377-384.

62. Rosfors S, Eriksson M, Leijd B, et al. A prospective follow-up study of acute deep venous thrombosis using colour duplex ultrasound, phlebography and venous occlusion plethysmography. *Int Angio.* 1997;16:39-44.

63. Arcelus JI, Caprini JA, Hoffman KN, et al. Laboratory assays and duplex scanning outcomes after symptomatic deep vein thrombosis: preliminary results. *J Vasc Surg.* 1996;23(4):616-621.

64. O'Shaughnessy AM, FitzGerald DE. Organisation patterns of venous thrombus over time as demonstrated by duplex ultrasound. *J Vasc Invest.* 1996;2:75-81.

65. O'Shaughnessy AM, FitzGerald DE. Natural history of proximal deep vein thrombosis assessed by duplex ultrasound. *Int Angio.* 1997;16:45-49.

66. Piovella F, Crippa L, Barone M, et al. Normalization rates of compression ultrasonography in patients with a first episode of deep vein thrombosis of the lower limbs: association with recurrence and new thrombosis. *Haematologica.* 2002;87(5):515-522.

67. AbuRahma AF, Perkins SE, Wulu JT, Ng, HK.

Iliofemoral deep venous thrombosis: conventional therapy versus lysis and percutaneous transluminal angioplasty and stenting. *Ann Surg.* 2001;233(6):752-760.

68. Meissner MH, Caps MT, Bergelin RO, et al. Propagation, rethrombosis, and new thrombus formation after acute deep venous thrombosis. *J Vasc Surg.* 1995;22:558-567.

69. Caps MT, Meissner MH, Tullis MJ, et al. Venous thrombus stability during acute phase of therapy. *Vasc Med.* 1999;4(1):9-14.

70. Meissner MH, Manzo, Bergelin RO, et al. Propagation, rethrombosis, and new thrombus formation after acute deep venous thrombosis. *J Vasc Surg.* 1993;18:596-608.

71. Caps MT, Manzo RA, Bergelin RO, et al. Venous valvular reflux in veins not involved at the time of acute deep vein thrombosis. *J Vasc Surg.* 1995;22:524-531.

72. Caprini JA, Arcelus JI, Reyna JJ, et al. Deep vein thrombosis and the level of oral anticoagulation therapy. *J Vasc Surg.* 1999;30(5):805-811.

73. Prandoni P, Villalta, S, Polistena P, et al. Symptomatic deep-vein thrombosis and the post-thrombotic syndrome. *Haematologica.* 1995;80:42-48.

74. Monreal M, Martorell A, Callejas J, et al. Venographic assessment of deep vein thrombosis and risk of developing post-thrombotic syndrome: a prospective trial. *J Intern Med.* 1993;233:233-238.

75. Lindner DJ, Edwards JM, Phinney ES, et al. Long-term hemodynamic and clinical sequelae of lower extremity deep vein thrombosis. *J Vasc Surg.* 1986;4:436-442.

76. Strandness DE, Langlois Y, Cramer M, et al. Long-term sequelae of acute venous thrombosis. *JAMA.* 1983;250:1289-1292.

77. Prandoni P, Lensing AWA, Cogo A, et al. The long-term clinical course of acute deep venous thrombosis. *Ann Intern Med.* 1996;125:1-7.

78. Franzeck UK, Schalch I, Bollinger A. On the relationship between changes in the deep veins evaluated by duplex sonography and the post-thrombotic syndrome 12 years after deep vein thrombosis. *Thromb Haemost.* 1997;77:1109-1112.

79. Delis KT, Bountouroglou D, Mansfield AO. Venous claudication in iliofemoral thrombosis: long-term effects on venous hemodynamics, clinical status, and quality of life. *Ann Surg.* 2004;239(1):118-126.

80. Uhl JF, Cornu-Thenard A, Carpentier PH, et al. Clinical and hemodynamic significance of corona phlebectatica in chronic venous disorders. *J Vasc Surg.* 2005;42(6):1163-1168.

81. Bruce, AJ, Bennett DD, Lohse CM, et al. Lipodermatosclerosis: review of cases evaluated at Mayo Clinic. *J Am Acad Dermatol.* 2002;46:187-192.

82. Labropoulos N, Tiongson J, Pryor L, et al. Definition of venous reflux in lower-extremity veins. *J Vasc Surg.* 2003;38(4):793-798.

83. Neglen P, Egger JF III, Olivier J, Raju S. Hemodynamic and clinical impact of ultrasound-derived venous reflux parameters. *J Vasc Surg.* 2004;40(2):303-310.

84. Cockett FB. Abnormalities of the deep veins of the leg. *Post Med J.* 1954;30:512-522.

85. Thomas ML. *Phlebography of the Lower Limb.* New York: Churchill Livingstone; 1982:162-163.

86. Liu GC, Ferris EJ, Reifsteck JR, Baker ME. Effect of anatomic variations on deep venous thrombosis of the lower extremity. *AMJ Am J Roentgenol.* 1986;146:845-848.

87. Screaton NJ, Gillard JII, Berman LH, Kemp PM. Duplicated superficial femoral veins: a source of error in the sonographic investigation of deep vein thrombosis. *Radiology.* 1998;206:397-401.

88. Gordon AC, Wright I, Pugh ND. Duplication of the superficial femoral vein: recognition with duplex ultrasonography. *Clin Radiol.* 1996;51:622-624.

89. Kerr TM, Smith JM, McKenna P, et al. Venous and arterial anomalies of the lower extremities diagnosed by duplex scanning. *Surg Gynecol Obstet.* 1992;175:309-314.

90. Quinlan DJ, Alikhan R, Gishen P, Sidhu PS. Variations in lower limb venous anatomy: implications for US diagnosis of deep venous thrombosis. *Radiology.* 2003;228:443-448.

91. Thompson H. The surgical anatomy of the superficial and perforating veins of the lower

limbs. *Ann R Coll Surg Engl.* 1979;61:198-205.

92. Kupinski AM, Evans SM, Khan AM, et al. Ultrasonic characterization of the saphenous vein. *Cardiovasc Surg.* 1993;1(5):513-517.

93. Shah DM, Chang BB, Leopold PW, et al. The anatomy of the greater saphenous venous system. *J Vasc Surg.* 1986;3(2):273-283.

94. Van Dijk LC, Wittens CH, Pieterman H, van Urk H. The value of peri-operative ultrasound mapping of the greater saphenous vein prior to "closed" in situ bypass operations. *Eur J Radiol.* 1996;23(3):235-237.

95. Corcos L, Macchi C, de Anna D, et al. The anatomical variable of the sapheno-popliteal junction visualization by radiological and echographic examination. *Ital J Anat Embryol.* 1996;101(1):15-28.

96. Porter JM, Moneta GL, International Consensus Committee on Chronic Venous Disease. Reporting standards in venous disease: an update. *J Vasc Surg.* 1995;21:635-645.

97. Brandjes DPM, Buller HR, Heijboer H, et al. Randomised trial of effect of compression stockings in patients with symptomatic proximal-vein thrombosis. *Lancet.* 1997;349:759-762.

98. Prandoni P, Lensing AW, Prins MH, et al. Below-knee elastic compression stockings reduced development of the postthrombotic syndrome in proximal deep venous thrombosis. *Ann Int Med.* 2004;141:249-256.

99. Kahn SR, Elman E, Rodger MA, Well PS. Use of elastic compression stockings after deep venous thrombosis: a comparison of practices and perceptions of thrombosis physicians and patients. *J Thromb Haemost.* 2003;1:500-506.

100. Anderson JH, Geraghty JG, Wilson YT, et al. Paroven and graduated compression hosiery for superficial venous insufficiency. *Phlebology.* 1990;5:271-276.

101. Ginsberg JS, Hirsh J, Julian J, et al. Prevention and treatment of postphlebitic syndrome. Results of a 3-Part-Study. *Arch Intern Med.* 2001;161:2105-2109.

102. Cullum N, Nelson EA, Fletcher AW, Sheldon TA. Compression for venous leg ulcers. The Cochrane database of systematic reviews 2006; Issue 1.

103. Nelson EA, Bell-Syer SEM, Cullum NA. Compression for preventing recurrence of venous ulcers. The Cochrane database of systematic reviews 2006; Issue 1.

104. Facino RM, Carini M, Stefani R, et al. Antielastase and anti-hyaluronidase activities of saponins and sapogenins from *Hedera helix, Aesculus hippocastanum*, and *Ruscus aculeatus*: factors contributing to their efficacy in the treatment of venous insufficiency. *Arch Pharm.* (Weinheim). 1995;328:720-724.

105. Pittler MH, Ernst E. Horse chestnut seed extract for chronic venous insufficiency (Cochrane Review). In: *The Cochrane Library,* Issue 2, 2004. Chichester, UK: John Wiley & Sons, Ltd.

106. Pittler MH, Ernst E. Horse-chestnut seed extract for chronic venous insufficiency. *Arch Dermatol.* 1998;134:1356-1360.

107. Belcaro G, Cesarone MR, Bavera, et al. HR (Venoruton1000, Paroven, 0-(beta-hydroxyethyl)-rutosides) vs. Daflon 500 in chronic venous disease and microangiopathy: an independent prospective, controlled, randomized trial. *J Cardiovasc Pharmacol Ther.* 2002;7(3):139-145.

108. Cesarone MR, Incandela L, DeSanctis MT, et al. Treatment of edema and increased capillary filtration in venous hypertension with HR (Venoruton1000, Paroven, 0-(beta-hydroxyethyl)-rutosides): a clinical, prospective, placebo-controlled, randomized, dose-ranging trial. *J Cardiovasc Pharmacol Ther.* 2002;7(Suppl 1):S21-S24.

109. Cesarone MR, Belcaro G, Pellegrini L, et al. HR, 0-(beta-hydroxyethyl)-rutosides; (Venoruton): rapid relief of signs/symptoms in chronic venous insufficiency and microangiopathy: a prospective, controlled study. *Angiology.* 2005;56(2):165-172.

110. Ramelet AA. Daflon 500 mg: symptoms and edema clinical update. *Angiology.* 2005;56(Suppl 1):S25-S32.

111. Jantet G. Chronic venous insufficiency: worldwide results of the RELIEF study. Reflux assEment and quaLity of lIfe improvEment with micronized Flavonoids. *Angiology.* 2002;53(3):245-256.

112. Glinski W, Chodynicka B, Roszkiewicz J, et al. The beneficial augmentative effect of micronised purified flavonoid fraction (MPFF) on the healing of leg ulcers: an open, multicentre, controlled randomised study. *Phlebology.* 1999;14:151-157.

113. Guilhou JJ, Dereure O, Marzin L, et al. Efficacy of Daflon 500 mg in venous leg ulcer healing: a double-blind, randomized, controlled versus placebo RCT in 107 patients. *Angiology.* 1997;48:77-85.

114. Browse NL, Jarrett PE, Morland M, Burnand K. Treatment of lipodermatosclerosis of the leg by fibrinolytic enhancement: a preliminary report. *BMJ.* 1977;2:434-435.

115. Burnand K, Lemenson G, Morland M, et al. Venous lipodermatosclerosis: treatment by fibrinolytic enhancement and elastic compression. *Br Med J.* 1980;280:7-11.

116. McMullen GM, Watkin GT, Coleridge Smith PD, Scurr JH. The efficacy of fibrinolytic enhancement with stanozolol in the treatment of venous insufficiency. *Aust NZ J Surg.* 1991;61:306-309.

117. Stacey MC, Burnand KG, Layer GT, et al. Transcutaneous oxygen tensions in assessing the treatment of healed venous ulcers. *Br J Surg.* 1990;77:1050-1054.

118. Segal S, Cooper J, Bolognia J. Treatment of lipodermatosclerosis with oxandrolone in a patient with stanozolol-induced hepatotoxicity. *J Am Acad Dermatol.* 2000;43(3):558-559.

119. Hafner C, Wimmershoff M, Landthaler M, Vogt T. Lipodermatosclerosis: successful treatment with danazol. *Acta Derm Venereol.* 2005;85(4):365-366.

120. Coccheri S, Andreozzi GM, D'Addato M, et al. Effects of defibrotide in patients with chronic deep insufficiency. The PROVEDIS study. *Int Angiol.* 2004;23(2):100-107.

121. Belcaro G, Marelli C. Treatment of venous lipodermatosclerosis and ulceration in venous hypertension by elastic compression and fibrinolytic enhancement with defibrotide. *Phlebology.* 1989;4:91-106.

122. Coccheri S, Scondotto G, Agnelli G, et al. Randomised, double blind, multicentre, placebo controlled study of sulodexide in the treat-

ment of venous leg ulcers. *Thromb Haemost.* 2002;87:947-952.

123. Scondotto G, Aloisi D, Ferrari P, et al. Treatment of venous leg ulcers with sulodexide. *Angiology.* 1999;50:883-889.

124. Arosio E, Ferrari G, Santoro F, et al. A placebo-controlled, double blind study of mesoglycan in the treatment of chronic venous ulcers. *Eur J Endovasc Surg.* 2001;22:365-372.

125. De Sanctis MT, Belcaro G, Cesarone MR, et al. Treatment of venous ulcers with pentoxifylline: a 12-month double-blind placebo controlled trial. Microcirculation and healing. *Angiology.* 2002;53:S49-S51.

126. Belcaro G, Cesarone MR, Nicolaides AN, et al. Treatment of venous ulcers with pentoxifylline: a 6-month randomized double-blind placebo controlled trial. *Angiology.* 2002;53:S45-S47.

127. Jull AB, Waters J, Arroll B. Oral pentoxifylline for treatment of venous leg ulcers. In: The Cochrane Library, Issue 3, 2004. Chichester, UK.

128. Layton AM, Ibbotson, SH, Davies JA, et al. Randomised RCT of oral aspirin for chronic venous leg ulcers. *Lancet.* 1994;344:164-165.

129. Clarke-Moloney M, Lyons GM, Burke PE, et al. A review of technological approaches to venous ulceration. *Crit Rev in Biomed Eng.* 2005;33(6):511-556.

130. O'Brien JF, Burke PE, Perry I, et al. Randomized clinical trial and economic analysis of four-layer compression bandaging for venous ulcers. *Br J Surg.* 2003;90:794-798.

131. Kikta MJ, Schuler JJ, Meyer JP, et al. A prospective, randomized trial of Unna's boots versus hydroactive dressing in the treatment of venous stasis ulcers. *J Vasc Surg.* 1988;7:478-483.

132. Callam MJ, Harper DR, Dale JJ, et al. Lothian and forth valley leg ulcer healing trial; elastic versus nonelastic bandaging in the treatment of chronic leg ulceration. *Phlebology.* 1992;7:136-141.

133. Nelson EA, Harper DR, Ruckley CV, et al. A randomized trial of single layer and multilayer bandages in the treatment of chronic venous ulceration. *Phlebology.* 1995;(Suppl 1):915-916.

134. Nelson EA, Iglesias CP, Cullum N, et al. Randomized clinical trial of four-layer and short-stretch compression bandages for venous leg

ulcers (VenUS 1). *Br J Surg.* 2004;91:1292-1299.

135. Colgan MP, Teevan M, McBride C, et al. Cost comparisons in the management of venous ulceration. In: Proceedings of the 5th European Conference on Advances in Wound Management, 1996. London: Macmillan Magazines; 1996.

136. Stemmer R, Marescaux J, Furderer C. (Compression therapy of the lower extremities particularly with compression stockings). *Hautarzt.* 1980;31:355-365.

137. Fletcher A, Cullum N, Sheldon TA. A systematic review of compression treatment for venous leg ulcers. *BMJ.* 1997;315:576-580.

138. Castineira F, Fisher H, Coleman D, et al. The Limerick Leg-Ulcer Project. *Ir J Med Sci.* 1999;168:17-20.

139. Nelson EA, Cullum N, Jones J. Venous leg ulcers. *Clin Evid.* 2005;13:2507-2526.

140. Cullum N, Nelson EA, Fletcher AW, et al. Compression for venous leg ulcers. In: *The Cochrane Library,* Issue 4, 2003. Chichester, UK.

141. Da Costa RM, Ribeiro Jesus FM, Aniceto C, et al. Randomized, double-blind, placebo-controlled, dose-ranging study of granulocyte-macrophage colony stimulating factor in patients with chronic venous leg ulcers. *Wound Repair Regen. 1999;7:17-25.*

142. Falanga V, Margolis D, Alvarez O, et al. Rapid healing of venous ulcers and lack of clinical rejection with an allogenic cultured human skin equivalent. Human Skin Equivalent Investigators Group. *Arch Dermatol. 1998;134:293-300.*

143. Rutgers PH, Kitslaar PJ. Randomized trial of stripping versus high ligation combined with sclerotherapy in the treatment of the incompetent greater saphenous vein. *Am J Surg.* 1994;168:311-315.

144. McMullen GM, Smith PD, Scurr JH. Objective assessment of high ligation without stripping the long saphenous vein. *Br J Surg.* 1991;78:1139-1142.

145. Sarin S, Scurr JH, Coleridge Smith PD. Assessment of stripping the long saphenous vein in the treatment of primary varicose veins. *Br J Surg.* 1992;79:889-893.

146. Dwerryhouse S, Davies B, Harradine K, et al.

Stripping the long saphenous vein reduces the rate of reoperation for recurrent varicose veins: five-year results of a randomized trial. *J Vasc Surg.* 1999;29:589-592.

147. Winterborn RJ, Earnshaw JJ. Crossectomy and great saphenous vein stripping. *J Cardiovasc Surg.* 2006;47:19-33.

148. van Rij AM, Jiang P. Solomon C, et al. Recurrence after varicose vein surgery: a prospective long-term clinical study with duplex ultrasound scanning and air plethysmography. *J Vasc Surg.* 2003;38:935-943.

149. van Rij AM, Jones GT, Hill GB, et al. Neovascularization and recurrent varicose veins: more histologic and ultrasound evidence. *J Vasc Surg.* 2004;30:296-302.

150. Chandler JG, Pichot O, Sessa C, et al. Defining the role of extended saphenofemoral junction ligation: A prospective comparative study. *J Vasc Surg.* 2000;32:941-944.

151. Raju S, Easterwood L, Fountain T, et al. Saphenectomy in the presence of chronic venous obstruction. *Surgery.* 1998;123:637-644.

152. Oesch A. "Pin Stripping": a novel method of atraumatic stripping. *Phlebology.* 1993;8:171-173.

153. Durkin MT, Turton EPL, Scott DJA, et al. A prospective randomized trial of PIN versus conventional stripping in varicose vein surgery. *Ann R Coll Engl.* 1999;81:171-174.

154. Lacroix H, Nevelsteen A, Suy R. Invaginating versus classical stripping of the long saphenous vein. A randomized prospective study. *Acta Chir Belg.* 1999;99:22-25.

155. Sam R, MacKenzie R, Paisley A, et al. The effect of superficial venous surgery on generic health-related quality of life. *Eur J Vasc Endovasc Surg.* 2004;28:253-256.

156. Michaels JA, Brazier JE, Campbell WB, et al. Randomized controlled trial comparing surgery with conservative treatment for uncomplicated varicose veins. *Br J Surg.* 2006;93:175-181.

157a. Fligelstone L, Carolan G, Pugh N, et al. An assessment of the long saphenous vein for potential use a vascular conduit after varicose vein surgery. *J Vasc Surg.* 1993;18:836-840.

157b. Carandina S, Mari C, De Palma M, et al. (February 2008). "Varicose vein stripping vs haemo-dynamic correction (CHIVA): a long term random-ised trial". *Eur J Vasc Endovasc Surg* 35 (2): 230–7.

157c. Lurie F (February 2009). "Venous haemody-namics: what we know and don't know." *Phlebology* 24 (1): 3–7.

158. Olivencia JA. Ambulatory phlebectomy turned 2400 years old. *Dermatol Surg.* 2004;30:704-708.

159. Weiss RA, Goldman MP. Transillumination mapping prior to ambulatory phlebectomy. *Dermatol Surg.* 1998;24:447-450.

160. Ramelet AA. Phlebectomy—cosmetic indications. *J Cosmetic Dermatol.* 2002;1:13-19.

161. Weiss RA, Ramelet A. Removal of blue peri-ocular lower eyelid veins by ambulatory phlebectomy. *Dermatol Surg.* 2002;28:43-45.

162. Ricci S, Georgiev M. Office varicose surgery under local anesthesia. *J Dermatol Surg Oncol.* 1993;18:55-58.

163. Georgiev M, Ricci S, Carbone D, et al. Stab avulsion of the short saphenous vein. Technique and duplex evaluation. *J Dermatol Surg Oncol.* 1993;19:456-464.

164. Ramelet AA. Complications of ambulatory phlebectomy. *Dermatol Surg.* 1997;23:947-954.

165. Olivencia JA. Complications of ambulatory phlebectomy. Review of 1000 consecutive cases. *Dermatol Surg.* 1997;23:51-54.

166. Dortu Y, Raymond-Martimbeau P. *Ambulatory Phlebectomy.* Houston, TX: PRM Editions; 1993;12:111-112.

167. Shamiyeh A, Schrenk P, Huber E, et al. Transilluminated powered phlebectomy: advantages and disadvantages of a new technique. *Dermatol Surg.* 2003;29:616-619.

168. De Roos K, Nieman F, Neumann H. Ambulatory phlebectomy versus compression sclerotherapy: results of a randomized controlled trial. *Dermatol Surg.* 2003;29:221-226.

169. Sadick NS. Multifocal pull-through endovascular cannulation technique of ambulatory phlebectomy. *Dermatol Surg.* 2002;28:32-37.

170. Aremu MA, Mahendran B, Butcher W, et al. Prospective randomized controlled trial: conventional versus powered phlebectomy. *J Vasc Surg.* 2004;39:88-94.

171. Chetter IC, Mylankal KJ, Hughes H, et al. Randomized clinical trial comparing multiple stab incision phlebectomy and transilluminated powered phlebectomy for varicose veins. *Br J Surg.* 2006;93:169-174.

172. Scavee V, Theys S, Schoevaerdts JC. Surgery of varicose veins with transilluminated powered mini-phlebectomy: clinical experience. *Phlebology.* 2003;18:97-99.

173. Linton RR. The operative treatment of varicose veins and ulcers, based upon a classification of these lesions. *Ann Surg.* 1938;107:582-593.

174. Hauer G. Endoscopic subfascial discussion of perforating veins-preliminary report. (German) *Vasa.* 1985;14:59-56.

175. Gloviczki P. Subfascial endoscopic perforating vein surgery. In: *Handbook of Venous Disorders.* London: Arnold; 2001:391-398.

176. van Rij AM, Hill G, Christie R, et al. A prospective study of the fate of venous leg perforators after varicose vein surgery. *J Vasc Surg.* 2005;42:1156-1162.

177. Bergan JJ, Murray J, Greason K. Subfascial endoscopic perforator surgery (SEPS): a preliminary report. *Ann Vasc Surg.* 1996;10:211-219.

178. Gloviczki P, Bergan JJ, Menawat SS, et al. Safety, feasibility, and early efficacy of subfascial endoscopic perforator surgery: a preliminary report from the North American Registry. *J Vasc Surg.* 1997;25:94-105.

179. Gloviczki P, Bergan JJ, Rhodes JM, et al. Mid-term results of endoscopic perforator vein interruption for chronic venous insufficiency: lessons learned from the North American subfascial endoscopic perforator surgery registry. The North American Study Group. *J Vasc Surg.* 1999;29:489-502.

180. Kahle B, Leng K. Efficacy of sclerotherapy in varicose veins—a prospective, blinded, placebo-controlled study. *Dermatol Surg.* 2004;30:723-728.

181. Hobbs JT. Surgery and sclerotherapy in the treatment of varicose veins. *Arch Surg.* 1974;190:793-796.

182. Einarrsson E, Eklof B, Neglen P. Sclerotherapy or surgery as treatment for varicose veins: a prospective randomized study. *Phlebology.* 1993;8:22-26.

183. Kanter A, Thibault P. Saphenofemoral incompetence treated by ultrasound-guided sclerotherapy. *Dermatol Surg.* 1996;22:648-652.

184. Blomgren L, Johansson G, Bergqvist D. Randomized trial of routine preoperative duplex imaging before varicose surgery. *Br J Surg.* 2005; 92:688-692.

185. Kanter A. Clinical determinants of ultrasound-guided sclerotherapy outcome. Part I: the effects of age, gender, and vein size. *Dermatol Surg.* 1998;24:131-135.

186. Goldman MP. *Sclerotherapy: Treatment of Varicose and Telangiectatic Leg Veins.* 2nd ed. St. Louis: Mosby-Year Book; 1995:273,333.

187. Goldman MP. *Sclerotherapy: Treatment of Varicose and Telangiectatic Leg Veins.* 2nd ed. St. Louis: Mosby; 1995:336.

188. Goldman MP, Sadick NS, Weiss RA. Cutaneous necrosis, telangiectatic matting, and hyperpigmentation following sclerotherapy. *Dermatol Surg.* 1995;21:19-29.

189. Rabe E, Pannier-Fischer F, Gerlach H, et al. Guidelines for sclerotherapy of varicose veins. *Dermatol Surg.* 2004;30:687-693.

190. Duffy DM. Small vessel sclerotherapy: an overview. *Adv Dermatol.* 1998;3:221-242.

191. Hamel-Desnos C, Desnos P, Wollmann J, et al. Evaluation of the efficacy of polidocanol in the form of foam compared with liquid form in sclerotherapy of the greater saphenous vein: initial results. *Dermatol Surg.* 2003;29:1170-1175.

192. Yamaki T, Nozaki M, Owasala S. Comparative study of duplex-guided foam sclerotherapy and duplex-guided liquid sclerotherapy for the treatment of superficial venous insufficiency. *Dermatol Surg.* 2004;30:718-722.

193. Barrett JM, Allen B, Ockelford A, Goldman MP. Microfoam ultrasound-guided sclerotherapy of varicose veins in 100 legs. *Dermatol Surg.* 2004;30:6-12.

194. Weiss RA, Feied CF, Weiss MA. *Vein Diagnosis and Treatment: A Comprehensive Approach.* New York: McGraw-Hill; 2001:126-128.

195. Goldman MP. *Sclerotherapy: Treatment of Varicose and Telangiectatic Leg Veins.* 2nd ed. St. Louis: Mosby-Year Book; 1995:8:318-319.

196. Goldman MP. *Sclerotherapy: Treatment of Varicose and Telangiectatic Leg Veins.* 2nd ed. St. Louis: Mosby-Year Book; 1995;8:280-337.

197. Fronek HS. The fundamentals of phlebology: venous disease for clinicians. *Am Coll Phlebology.* 2004;10:75-85.

198. Hanisch F, Muller T, Krivokuca M, et al. Stroke following variceal sclerotherapy. *Eur J Med Res.* 2006;9(5):282-284.

199. Bush RG, Derrick M, Manjoney D. Major neurological events following foam sclerotherapy. *Phlebology.* 2008;23:189-192.

200. Cavezzi A. Sclerosant foam: renaissance of sclerotherapy of varicose veins. *Phlebologie.* 2003;32(4):A34-A35.

201. Eckman D. Polidocanol for endovenous microfoam sclerosant therapy. *Expert Opin Investig Drugs.* 2009;18:1919-1927.

202 Tessari L. Presented at the 18thAnnual Congress of the American College of Phlebology, Marco Island, 2004.

203. Alos J, Carreno JA, Lopez M, et al. Efficacy and safety of sclerotherapy using polidocanol foam: a controlled clinical trial. *Eur J Vasc Endovasc Surg.* 2006;31:1010-1107.

204. Rabe E, Otto J, Schliephake D. Efficacy and safety of great saphenous vein sclerotherapy using standardised polidocanol foam (ESAF): a randomized controlled multicentre clinical trial. *Eur J Vasc Endovasc Surg.* 2008;35:238-245.

205. Ouvry F, Allaert A, Hamel-Desnos C. Efficacy of plidocanol foam versus liquid in sclerotherapy of the great saphenous vein: a multicentre randomised controlled trial with a 2-year follow-up. *Eur J Vasc Endovasc Surg.* 2008;36:366-370.

206. Van Neer PA. Perforans varicosis: treatment of the incompetent perforating vein is important. *Dermatol Surg.* 2004;30:754-755.

207. Cabrera-Garrido JR, Cabrera-Garcia-Olmedo JR, Garcia-Olmedo Dominguez MA. Elargissement des limites de la schlerotherapie: noveaux produits scelrosants. *Phlebologie.* 1997;50:181-188.

208. Guex J. Foam sclerotherapy: an overview of use for primary venous insufficiency. *Semin Vasc Surg.* 2005;18:25-29.

209. Yamaki T, Nozaki M, Sasaki K. Color duplex-

guided sclerotherapy for the treatment of venous malformations. *Dermatol Surg.* 2000;26:323-328.

210. Bergan JJ, Parcarella L, Mekenas L. Venous disorders: treatment with sclerosant foam. *J Cardiovasc Surg.* 2006;47:9-18.

211. Cabrera J, Cabrera JR, Garcia-Olmedo MA, Redondo P. Treatment of venous malformations with sclerosant in microfoam form. *Arch Dermatol.* 2003;139:1409-1416.

212. Breu FX, Guggenbichler S, Wollmann JC. Second European consensus meeting on foam sclerotherapy, 2006. Tegernsee, Germany. *Vasa.* 2008;37:S71.

213. Breu FX, Guggenbichler S. European consensus meeting on foam sclerotherapy, 2003. Tegernsee, Germany. *Dermatol Surg.* 2004;30:709-717.

214. Belcaro G, Cesarone MR, Di Renzo A, et al.M. Foam-sclerotherapy, surgery, sclerotherapy, and combined treatment for varicose veins: a 10-year, prospective, randomized, controlled, trial (VEDICO* trial). *Angiology.* 2003;54:307-315.

215. Morrison N. Foam. Presented at the19th Congress of the American College of Phlebology. San Francisco, 2005.

216. Wright D. Polidocanol microfoam does not cause remote sclerosis in the lung. Presented at the 23rd Congress of the American College of Phlebology. Palm Desert, 2009.

217. Raymond-Martimbeau R. Transient adverse events positively associated with patent foramen ovale after ultrasound-guided foam sclerotherapy. *Phlebology.* 2009; 24:114-119.

218. Meier B, Lock JE. Contemporary management of patent foramen ovale. *Circulation.* 2003;107:5-9.

219. Windecker S, Meier B. Patent foramen ovale and atrial septal aneurysm: when and how should they be treated. *ACC Curr J Rev.* 2002;11:97-101.

220. Wright D, McCollum C, Rush JE. A single-centre pilot study of polidocanol endovenous microfoam (PEM) treatment to evaluate presence and durability of gas emboli using echocardiography. Presented at the 22nd Congress of the American College of Phlebology. Marco Island, November 2008.

221. Wright DD, Gibson KD, Barclay J, et al. High prevalence of right-to-left shunts in patient with symptomatic great saphenous incompetence and varicose veins. *J Vasc Surg.* 2010;51(1):104-107.

222. Gibson KD, Regan JD, Shortell CK, et al. Proprietary polidocanol endovenous microfoam bubble embolization does not cause cerebral injury. Presented at the 22nd Congress of the American College of Phlebology. Marco Island, 2008.

223. Neuhardt D, Morrison N, Rogers C, et al. Emboli detection in the middle cerebral artery concurrent with treatment of lower extremity superficial venous insufficiency with foam sclerotherapy. *Phlebology.* 2009; 24:85-95.

224. Forlee M, Grouden M, Moore D, et al. Stroke after varicose vein foam injection sclerotherapy. *J Vasc Surg.* 2006; 43:162-163.

225. Ceulen RP, Sommer A, Vernooy KJ. Microembolism during foam sclerotherapy of varicose veins. *N Engl J Med.* 2009;358:1525-1526.

226. Rush JE, Wright DD. More on microembolism and foam sclerotherapy. *N Engl J Med.* 2008;359:656-657.

227. Regan JD, Gibson KD, Ferris JE, et al. Safety of proprietary sclerosant microfoam for saphenous incompetence in patients with R to L shunt: interim report. *J Vasc Interv Radiol.* 2008:19:S35.

228. Wright DD, McCollum CN, Tristram S, et al. A single-centre pilot study of polidocanol endovenous microfoam treatment to evaluate the presence and durability of gas emboli using echocardiography. *Phlebology.* 2009;24:87-88.

229. Morrison N, Neuhardt D, Rogers C, et al. Studies on foam migration. *Phlebology.* 2009;24:88.

230. Shortell CK, Regan JD, Gibson KD, et al. Endovenous microfoam ablation in patients with migraine headache with and without right-to-left cardiac shunt. Presented at the 23rd Congress of the American College of Phlebology. Palm Desert, 2009.

231. Morrison N, Neuhardt DL, Rogers CR. Comparisons of side effects using air and carbon dioxide foam for endovenous chemical ablation. *J Vasc Surg.* 2008;48:830-836.

232. http://clinicaltrials.gov/ct2/results?term=vanish. Efficacy and safety of Varisolve polidocanol endovenous microfoam (PEM) for the treatment of saphenofemoral junction (SFJ) incompetence. Accessed May 4, 2010.

233. Jia X, Mowatt J, Burr M, et al. Systematic review of foam sclerotherapy for varicose veins. *Br J Surg.* 2007;94:925-936.

234. Kern O, Ramlett AA, Wutschart R, et al. Single-blind, randomized study comparing chromated glycerin, polidocanol solution, and polidocanol foam for treatment of telangiectatic leg veins. *Dermatol Surg.* 2004;30:367-372.

235. Gillet J-L, Guedes JM, Guex JJ, et al. Side-effect and complications of foam sclerotherapy of the great and small saphenous veins: a controlled multicentre prospective study including 1025 patients. *Phlebology.* 2009;24:131-138.

236. Cabrera J. Treatment of varicose long saphenous veins with sclerosant microfoam form: Long-term outcomes. *Phlebology.* 2000;15:19-23.

237. Frullini A, Cavezzi A. Sclerosing foam in the treatment of varicose veins and telangiectases: History and analysis of safety and complications. *Dermatol Surg.* 2002;28:11-15.

238. Bhowmick A, Harper D, Wright D, McCollum CN. Polidocanol microfoam sclerotherapy for long saphenous varicose veins. *Phlebology.* 2001;16:41-50.

239. Cabrera J. Dr J. Cabrera is the creator of the patented polidocanol microfoam. *Dermatol Surg.* 2004;30:1605-1606.

240. Hamel-Desnos C, Ouvry P, Bengini JP, et al. Comparison of 1% and 3% polidocanol foam in ultrasound guided sclerotherapy of the great saphenous vein: a randomized, double-blind trial with 2 year-follow-up. "The 3/1 Study." *Eur J Endovasc Surg.* 2007;34:723-729.

241. Wright D, Gobin JP, Bradbury AW, et al. Varisolve polidocanol microfoam compared with surgery or sclerotherapy in the management of varicose veins in the presence of trunk vein incompetence: European randomized controlled trial. *Phlebology.* 2006;21:180-190.

242. Bergan JJ, Pascarella L. severe chronic venous insufficiency: primary treatment with sclerofoam. *Semin Vasc Surg.* 2005;18:49-56.

243. Bountouroglou D, Azzam M, Kakkos S, et al. Ultrasound-guided foam sclerotherapy combined with sapheno-femoral ligation compared to surgical treatment of varicose veins: Early results of a randomized controlled trial. *Eur J Vasc Endovasc Surg.* 2006;31:93-100.

244. Weiss RA. Comparison of endovenous radiofrequency versus 810 nm diode laser occlusion of large veins in an animal model. *Dermatol Surg.* 2002;28:56-61.

245. Weiss RA, Feied CF, Weiss MA. *Vein Diagnosis and Treatment: A Comprehensive Approach.* New York: McGraw-Hill; 2001:214.

246. Proebstle TM, Vago B, Alm J, et al. Treatment of the incompetent saphenous vein by endovenous radiofrequency powered segmental thermal ablation: first clinical experience. *J Vasc Surg.* 2008;47:151-156.

247. Yu SS, Tope WD, Grekin RC. Cardiac devices and electromagnetic interference revisited: new radiofrequency technologies and implications for dermatologic surgery. *Dermatol Surg.* 2005;31:932-940.

248. Merchant RE, Pichot O, Myers KA. Four-year follow-up on endovascular radiofrequency obliteration of great saphenous reflux. *Dermatol Surg.* 2005;31:129-134.

249. Manfrini S, Gasbarro V, Danielson M, et al. Endovenous management of saphenous vein reflux. *J Vasc Surg.* 2000;32:330-342.

250. Hingorani A, Enrico A, Markevich N, et al. Deep venous thrombosis after radiofrequency ablation of greater saphenous vein: a word of caution. *J Vasc Surg.* 2004;40:500-504.

251. Merchant R, Kistner R, Kabnick L. Regarding "Is there an increased risk for DVT with the VNUS closure procedure?" *J Vasc Surg.* 2003;38:628-629.

252. Hagmuller GW. Complications in surgery of varicose veins. *Lagenbecks Arch Chir Suppl Kongressbd.* 1992;377:470-474.

253. van Rij AM, Chai J, Hill GB, et al. Incidence of deep vein thrombosis after varicose vein surgery. *Br J Surg.* 2004;91;1582-1585.

254. Chandler JG, Pichot O, Sessa C, et al. Treatment of primary venous insufficiency by endovenous saphenous vein obliteration. *Vasc Surg.* 2000;34:201-214.

255. Goldman MP, Amiry S. Closure of the greater saphenous vein with endoluminal radiofrequency thermal heating of the vein wall in combination with ambulatory phlebectomy: 50 patients with more than 6-month follow-up. *Dermatol Surg.* *2002;28:29-31.*

256. Hinchliffe RJ, Ubhi J, Beech A, et al. A prospective randomized controlled trial of VNUS closure versus surgery for the treatment of recurrent long saphenous varicose veins. *Eur J Vasc Endovasc Surg.* 2006;31:212-218.

257. Lurie F, Creton D, Eklof B, et al. Prospective randomised study of endovenous radiofrequency obliteration (closure procedure) versus ligation and stripping in a selected patient population (EVOLVeS Study): two-year follow-up. *J Vasc Surg.* 2003;38:207-214.

258. Lurie F, Creton D, Eklof B, et al. Prospective randomised study of endovenous radiofrequency obliteration (closure) versus ligation and vein stripping (EVOLVeS): two year follow-up. *Eur J Vasc Endovasc Surg.* 2005;29:67-73.

259. Merchant RF, DePalma RG, Kabnick LS. Endovascular obliteration of saphenous reflux: a multicenter study. *J Vasc Surg.* 2002;35:1190-1196.

260. Puggioni A, Kalra M, Carmo M, et al. Endovenous laser therapy and radiofrequency ablation of the great saphenous vein: analysis of early efficacy and complications. *J Vasc Surg.* 2005;42:488-493.

261. Sybrandy J, Wittens CH. Initial experiences in endovenous treatment of saphenous vein reflux. *J Vasc Surg.* 2002;36:1207-1212.

262. Weiss RA, Weiss MA. Controlled radiofrequency endovenous occlusion using a unique radiofrequency catheter under duplex guidance to eliminate saphenous varicose vein reflux: a 2-year follow-up. *Dermatol Surg.* 2002;28:38-42.

263. Perala J, Rautio T, Biancari F, et al. Radiofrequency endovenous obliteration versus stripping of the long saphenous vein in the management of primary varicose veins: 3-year outcome of a randomized study. *Ann Vasc Surg.* 2005;19:669-672.

264. Pichot O, Kabnick LS, Creton D, et al. Duplex ultrasound scan findings two years after great

saphenous vein radiofrequency endovenous obliteration. *J Vasc Surg.* 2004;39:189-195.

265. Labropoulos N, Bhatti A, Leon L, et al. Neovascularization after great saphenous vein ablation. *Eur J Vasc Endovas Surg.* 2006;31:219-222.

266. Roggan A, Friebel M, Dorschel K, et al. Optical properties of circulating human blood in the wavelength range 400-2500 nm. *J Biomed Opt.* 1999;4:36-46.

267. Proebstle TM, Lehr HA, Kargl A, et al. Endovenous treatment of the greater saphenous vein with a 940-nm diode laser: thrombotic occlusion after endoluminal thermal damage by laser-generated steam bubbles. *J Vasc Surg.* 2002;35:729-736.

268. Min J, Khilnani M. Endovenous laser ablation of varicose veins. *J Cardiovasc Surg.* 2005;46:395-405.

269. Timperman PE. Arteriovenous fistula after endovenous laser treatment of the short saphenous vein. *J Vasc Interv Radiol.* 2004;15:625-627.

270. Proebstle T, Krummenauer F, Gui D, et al. Nonocclusion and early reopening of the great saphenous vein after endovenous laser treatments fluency dependent. *Dermatol Surg.* 2004;30:174-178.

271. Chang C, Chua J. Endovenous laser photocoagulation (EVLP) for varicose veins. *Lasers Surg Med.* 2002;31:257-262.

272. Goldman MP, Mauricio M, Rao J. Intravascular 1320-nm laser closure of the great saphenous vein: a 6- to 12-month follow-up study. *Dermatol Surg.* 2004;30:1380-1385.

273. Kabnick LS. Outcome of different endovenous laser wavelengths for great saphenous vein ablation. *J Vasc Surg.* 2006;43:88.c.1-88.c.7.

274. Min RJ, Zimmet SE, Isaacs MN, et al. Endovenous laser treatment of the incompetent greater saphenous vein. *J Vasc Interv Radiol.* 2001;12:1167-1171.

275. Mozes G, Kalra M, Carmo M, et al. Extension of saphenous thrombus into the femoral vein: a potential complication of new endovenous ablation techniques. *J Vasc Surg.* 2005;41:130-135.

276. Navarro L, Min R, Bone C. Endovenous laser: a new minimally invasive method of treatment for varicose veins—preliminary observations

using an 810 nm diode laser. *Dermatol Surg.* *2001;27:117-122.*

277. Oh CK, Jung DO, Jang HS, et al. Endovenous laser surgery of the incompetent greater saphenous vein with a 980-nm diode laser. *Dermatol Surg.* 2003;29:1135-1140.

278. Perkowski P, Ravi R, Gowda R, et al. Endovenous laser ablation of the saphenous vein for treatment of venous insufficiency and varicose veins:early results from a large single center experience. J Endovasc Ther. 2004;11:132-138.

279. Proebstle TM, Gul D, Lehr HA, et al. Infrequent early recanalization of greater saphenous vein after endovenous laser treatment. *J Vasc Surg.* 2003;38:511-516.

280. Proebstle TM, Gsul D, Kargl A, et al. Endovenous laser treatment of the lesser saphenous vein with a 940-nm diode laser: early results. *Dermatol Surg.* 2003;29:357-361.

281. Spruiell S, Stanbro M. Blood versus water. Does laser wavelength influence success of endovenous thermal ablation? Presented at the 21st Congress of the American College of Phlebology. Tuscon 2007.

282. Timperman PE, Sichlau M, Ryu RK. Greater energy delivery improves treatment success of endovenous laser treatment of incompetent saphenous veins. *J Vasc Interv Radiol.* 2004;15:1061-1063.

283. Alencar H, Baum R, Binkert C, et al. Endovenous laser treatment (EVLT) for varicose veins: experience in a large academic institution. Presented at the 31st Society of Interventional

Radiology Annual Scientific Meeting. Toronto, 2006.

284. Bush RG. Regarding endovenous treatment of the greater saphenous vein with a 940-nm diode laser: thrombolytic occlusion after endoluminal thermal damage by laser generated steam bubbles. *J Vasc Surg.* 2003;37:242.

285. Proebstle TM, Moehler T, Gul D, et al. Endovenous treatment of the great saphenous vein using a 1320 nm Nd:YAG laser causes fewer side effects than using a 940 nm diode laser. *Dermatol Surg.* 2005;31:1678-1684.

286. Kabnick LS, Moritz MW, Agis H, et al. Endolaser venous system treatment for the ablation of the saphenous system using 810 nm, 980 nm, or 1320 nm. 31st Society of Interventional Radiology Annual Scientific Meeting. Toronto, Canada, March 2006.

287. De Medeiros CA, Luccas GC. Comparison of endovenous treatment with an 810 nm laser versus conventional stripping of the great saphenous vein in patients with primary varicose veins. *Dermatol Surg.* 2005;31:1685-1694.

288. Rasmussen LH, Bjoern L, Lawaetz M, et al. Randomized trial comparing endovenous laser ablation of the great saphenous vein with high ligation and stripping in patients with varicose veins: short-term results. *J Vasc Surg.* 2007;46:308-315.

289. Eckmann DM. Intravascular foams and bubbles: surface interactions with endothelium and provocation of cellular responses. Presented at the 19th Annual Congress of the American College of Phlebology. San Francisco, 2005.

Part 8

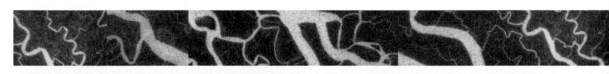

Hypercoagulability and Uncommon Vascular Diseases

25

Hypercoagulable States

Julia A. M. Anderson and Jeffrey I. Weitz

Arterial and venous thromboses are common problems facing vascular medicine specialists. Some patients with thrombosis have an underlying *hypercoagulable state.* These states can be divided into 3 categories; inherited disorders, acquired disorders, and those that are mixed in origin.[1,2]

Inherited hypercoagulable states, which are also known as *thrombophilic disorders,* can be due to loss of function of natural anticoagulant pathways or gain of function in procoagulant pathways (Table 25.1). *Acquired hypercoagulable states* represent a heterogeneous group of disorders in which the risk of thrombosis appears to be higher than that in the general population. These include such diverse risk factors as a prior history of thrombosis, obesity, pregnancy, cancer and its treatment, antiphospholipid syndrome, heparin-induced thrombocytopenia, and myeloproliferative disorders, among others. The pathogenesis of thrombosis in these situations is largely unknown and, in many cases, is likely multifactorial in origin. Finally, *mixed disorders* are those with both an inherited and an acquired component. One such example is hyperhomocysteinemia. Although severe hyperhomocysteinemia and associated homocysteinuria are rare genetic disorders, most cases of mild to moderate hyperhomocysteinemia result from acquired folate and/or vitamin B_{12} deficiency superimposed on common genetic mutations in biochemical pathways involved in methionine metabolism.[2]

Genetic hypercoagulable states and acquired risk factors combine to establish an intrinsic risk of thrombosis for each individual.[3,4] This risk can be modified by extrinsic or environmental factors, such as surgery, immobilization, or hormonal therapy, which also increase the risk of thrombosis. When the intrinsic and extrinsic forces exceed a critical threshold, thrombosis occurs (Figure 25.1). Appropriate thromboprophylaxis can prevent the thrombotic risk from exceeding this critical threshold, but breakthrough thrombosis can occur if procoagulant stimuli overwhelm protective mechanisms.

Focusing on hypercoagulable states, this chapter (1) details the inherited, acquired, and mixed hypercoagulable states; (2) explains how these disorders trigger thrombosis; (3) discusses the laboratory evaluation of hypercoagulable

Vascular Disease: Diagnostic and Therapeutic Approaches. © 2011 Michael R. Jaff and Christopher J. White, editors. Cardiotext Publishing, ISBN: 978-1-935395-16-4.

Hereditary	Mixed	Acquired
Loss of Function	Hyperhomocysteinemia	Previous VTE
Antithrombin deficiency		Obesity
Protein C deficiency		Cancer
Protein S deficiency		Pregnancy, puerperium
		Drug-induced:
		Heparin-induced thrombocytopenia
Gain of Function		Prothrombin complex concentrates
Factor V Leiden		L-asparaginase
Prothrombin FII20210A		Hormonal therapy
Elevated factor VIII, IX, or XI		Postoperative
		Myeloproliferative disorders

Table 25.1 Classification of Hypercoagulable States

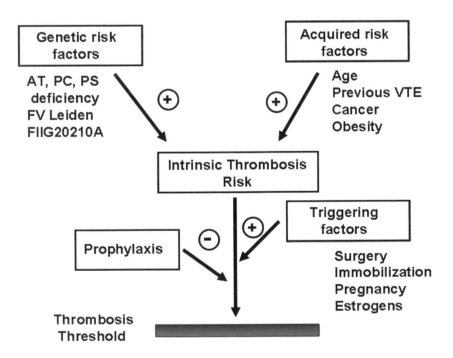

Figure 25.1 Thrombosis threshold. Genetic and acquired risk factors combine to determine an intrinsic risk of thrombosis for each individual. This risk is increased by extrinsic or environmental factors and decreased by thromboprophylaxis. If the intrinsic and extrinsic forces exceed a critical threshold where thrombin generation overwhelms the protective mechanisms, thrombosis will result. (AT, antithrombin; PC, protein C; PS, protein S)

states; (4) identifies those patients who deserve laboratory evaluation for an underlying hypercoagulable state; and (5) outlines the treatment of patients with hypercoagulable states.

Inherited Hypercoagulable States

Inherited disorders are found in up to half of patients who present with *venous thromboembolism (VTE)* before the age of 45, particularly those whose event occurred either in the absence of well-recognized risk factors, such as surgery or immobilization, or with minimal provocation, such as after minor trauma, after a long-haul airplane flight, or after taking estrogens.[5] Patients with inherited thrombophilic disorders often have a family history of thrombosis. Of greatest significance is a family history of sudden death due to pulmonary embolism or a history of multiple family members requiring long-term anticoagulation therapy because of recurrent thrombosis. Patients who present with venous thrombosis in unusual sites, such as the cerebral venous sinuses or mesenteric veins, those with recurrent thrombosis, and patients who develop skin necrosis upon initiation of warfarin therapy also should be suspected of having an inherited hypercoagulable state.[6,7]

From a pathophysiological perspective, inherited hypercoagulable states fall into 2 categories. First are those associated with loss of function of endogenous anticoagulant proteins. These include deficiencies of antithrombin, protein C, and protein S. The second category involves gain of function in procoagulant pathways. These disorders include Factor V Leiden and the prothrombin gene mutation, as well as increased levels of procoagulant proteins, such as factors VIII, IX, and XI. Each of these conditions will be briefly described.

Loss of Function of Endogenous Anticoagulants

Antithrombin deficiency

Antithrombin, a member of the serine protease inhibitor (serpin) superfamily, is synthesized in the liver.[8] Antithrombin plays a critical role in regulating coagulation by forming a 1:1 covalent complex with thrombin, factor Xa, and other activated clotting factors. Once covalent complexes are generated, they are cleared from the circulation via the liver. The rate of antithrombin interaction with its target proteases is accelerated by heparin.[9] Heparan sulfate, which coats the vasculature, is the physiological counterpart of medicinal heparin.[10]

Antithrombin deficiency can be inherited or acquired.[11] Inherited antithrombin deficiency is relatively rare, occurring in about 1 in 2000.[12,13] Inherited antithrombin deficiency can be 1 of 2 types (Table 25.2), both of which are inherited in an autosomal dominant fashion[11] and affect both sexes equally.[14,15] Type I deficiency, which represents the classic deficiency state, is the result of reduced synthesis of biologically normal antithrombin.[16] Heterozygotes with this condition have parallel reductions in antithrombin antigen and activity with levels reduced to about 50% those of normal. Nonsense mutations, small deletions, insertions, or single base substitutions are the molecular cause of most cases, although gene deletions also can be responsible. In total, more than 250 mutations

Type	Antigen	Activity (no heparin)	Activity (with heparin)
I	Reduced	Reduced	Reduced
II (reactive center loop mutation)	Normal	Reduced	Reduced
II (heparin-binding domain mutation)	Normal	Normal	Reduced

Table 25.2 Types of Inherited Antithrombin Deficiency

have been identified as causes of type I antithrombin deficiency.[17]

Type II antithrombin deficiencies are characterized by normal levels of antithrombin with reduced functional activity. This condition is caused by missense mutations that result in single amino acid substitutions.[11] The clinical consequences of type II antithrombin deficiency depend on the location of the mutation.[18,19] For example, some mutations in the reactive center loop of antithrombin slow its interaction with target proteases and are characterized by reduced antithrombin activity in the absence or presence of heparin. In contrast, mutations in the heparin-binding domain are associated with reduced antithrombin activity in the presence of heparin but normal activity in its absence.[20] Unlike other inherited forms of antithrombin deficiency, which are embryonic lethal in the homozygous state, mutations in the heparin-binding domain only have clinical consequences in individuals homozygous for these mutations.[21]

Acquired antithrombin deficiency can reflect decreased antithrombin synthesis, increased consumption, or enhanced clearance (Table 25.3). Decreased synthesis can occur in patients with severe hepatic disease, particularly cirrhosis, or in those given L-asparaginase.[22] Increased activation of coagulation can result in antithrombin consumption. Disorders associated with excessive clotting include acute thrombosis, disseminated intravascular coagulation, severe sepsis, multiple trauma, disseminated malignancy, extensive burns, or prolonged extracorporeal circulation.[23,24] Finally, heparin treatment can reduce antithrombin levels up to 20% by enhancing its clearance.[25] Severe antithrombin deficiency can occur in some patients with nephrotic syndrome due to loss of protein in the urine.[26]

Protein C deficiency

The protein C pathway is an important natural anticoagulant pathway.[27] This on-demand pathway is activated when thrombin is generated (Figure 25.2). Thrombin binds to thrombomodulin, a transmembrane thrombin receptor found on the surface of endothelial cells. Once bound to thrombomodulin, the substrate specificity of thrombin is altered such that it no longer serves as a procoagulant enzyme but becomes a potent activator of protein C. Thus, thrombin bound to thrombomodulin activates protein C 1000-fold more efficiently than free thrombin.[28] The endothelial cell protein C receptor (EPCR), another transmembrane receptor on the endothelial cell surface, binds protein C and presents it to the thrombin-thrombomodulin complex for activation.[29,30]

Activated protein C (APC) dissociates from this activation complex and then acts as an anticoagulant by proteolytically degrading and inactivating factor Va, thereby attenuating thrombin generation. For efficient inactivation of factor Va, APC must bind to protein S, its cofactor. This interaction facilitates APC binding to activated cell surfaces, particularly the

Decreased Synthesis	Increased Consumption	Enhanced Clearance
Hepatic cirrhosis	Major surgery	Heparin
Severe liver disease	Acute thrombosis	Nephrotic syndrome
L-asparaginase	Disseminated intravascular coagulation	
	Severe sepsis	
	Multiple trauma	
	Malignancy	
	Prolonged extracorporeal circulation	

Table 25.3 Causes of Acquired Antithrombin Deficiency

Protein C Pathway

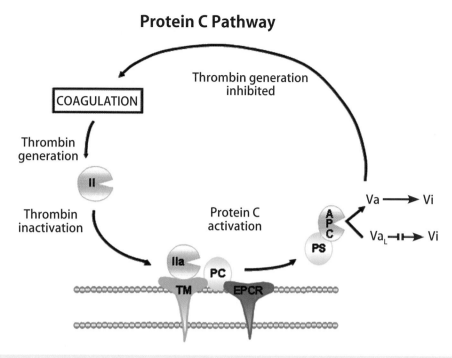

Figure 25.2 Protein C pathway. Activation of coagulation triggers thrombin (IIa) generation. Excess thrombin binds to thrombomodulin (TM) on the endothelial cell surface. Once bound, the substrate specificity of thrombin is altered so that it no longer acts as a procoagulant but becomes a potent activator of protein C (PC). Endothelial protein C receptor (EPCR) binds protein C and presents it to thrombomodulin-bound thrombin where it is activated. Activated protein C (APC), together with its cofactor, protein S (PS), binds to the activated platelet surface and proteolytically degrades factor Va into inactive fragments (Vi). Because factor Va is a critical component of the prothrombinase complex, factor Va inactivation by APC attenuates thrombin generation. Because factor Va Leiden (VaL) is resistant to inactivation by APC, patients with the factor V Leiden mutation have reduced capacity to regulate thrombin generation.

platelet surface, where factor Va is localized.[27,28]

APC has a half-life in the circulation of about 15 minutes, whereas thrombin has a half-life of about 10 seconds. APC is inhibited by protein C inhibitor and α1-antitrypsin, both of which are relatively slow inhibitors. Only the activity of protein C inhibitor is enhanced by heparin, but both inhibitors appear to contribute to APC inhibition *in vivo*.

Protein C deficiency can be inherited or acquired. Like antithrombin deficiency, protein C deficiency is inherited in an autosomal dominant fashion.[31] Heterozygous protein C deficiency can be found in up to 1 in 200 of the adult population,[32] but many of these individuals do not have a history of thrombosis. Thus, the phenotypic expression of hereditary protein C deficiency is highly variable and may depend on

other, as yet unrecognized, modifying factors.[5] In contrast to antithrombin deficiency, where the homozygous state is embryonic lethal, homozygous, or doubly heterozygous, protein C deficiency can occur. Newborns with these disorders often present with purpura fulminans characterized by widespread thrombosis.

Individuals with heterozygous protein C deficiency can develop skin necrosis upon initiation of warfarin therapy.[33-35] Typically, skin lesions are found on the extremities, breasts, or trunk. Starting as erythematous macules, the central regions of the cutaneous lesions become purpuric and then necrotic. Biopsies reveal fibrin thrombi within the vessels of the skin associated with interstitial hemorrhage. The skin lesions, which are clinically and histologically similar to those seen in infants with purpura fulminans, are attributable to a transient hy-percoagulable state induced by warfarin. The half-life of protein C is short, and similar to that of factor VII. Starting warfarin in patients with protein C deficiency causes a further reduction in protein C levels, particularly if loading doses of warfarin are given. Thus, the activity of the natural anticoagulant protein C pathway is compromised before warfarin lowers the levels of the vitamin K procoagulant proteins into the range required for its antithrombotic effects.

Hereditary protein C deficiency can be further delineated into 2 subtypes using immuno-logical and functional assays (Table 25.4). Most functional assays use Protac, a snake venom protease, to activate protein C in plasma.[36] The enzymatic activity of APC can then be assayed directly using an APC-directed synthetic substrate, or it can be indirectly quantified by measuring the extent of prolongation of the activated partial thromboplastin time (aPTT).[37] The most common form of hereditary protein C deficiency is the classic, or type I, deficiency state. This disorder reflects reduced synthesis of a normal protein and is characterized by a parallel reduction in protein C antigen and activity. A variety of genetic defects can produce type I protein C deficiency, but missense or nonsense mutations are the most common.

Type	Antigen	Activity
I	Reduced	Reduced
II	Normal	Reduced

Table 25.4 Types of Inherited Protein C Deficiency

Type II protein C deficiency reflects synthesis of a dysfunctional protein and is characterized by normal protein C antigen with reduced functional activity. Most type II protein C deficiency states are caused by point mutations. Mutations in the active site of APC reduce its activity against synthetic substrates and decrease its capacity to prolong the aPTT. In contrast, mutations that affect other protein C domains essential for its activity may reduce its anticoagulant activity but may not affect its am-

idolytic activity. Therefore, coagulation-based functional assays are preferred when screening patients for protein C deficiency.

Diagnosis of protein C deficiency is complicated. Protein C antigen levels are log normally distributed in healthy adults such that 95% of the values range from 70% to 140%. Furthermore, protein C levels increase with age by about 4% per decade. The wide range of values makes it difficult to establish a normal range. Levels less than 55%, however, are likely to reflect deficiency, while those between 55% and 70% are considered borderline.[7,36,38]

Acquired protein C deficiency can be due to decreased synthesis or increased consumption. Decreased synthesis can occur in patients with liver disease or in those given warfarin.[39] Warfarin decreases functional activity more than immunological activity. Newborns have protein C levels 20% to 40% lower than those of adults, and premature infants have even lower levels.[40] Protein C consumption can occur with severe sepsis, with disseminated intravascular coagulation, and after surgery. In contrast to antithrombin, which is lost in the urine of patients with nephrotic syndrome, the levels of protein C are normal or elevated in patients with nephrotic syndrome.[41]

Protein S deficiency

Protein S serves as a cofactor for APC and enhances its capacity to inactivate factors Va and VIIIa.[29,42] In addition, protein S may have direct anticoagulant activity by inhibiting prothrombin activation through its capacity to bind factor Va or factor Xa, components of the prothrombinase complex.[28,43] The importance of the direct anticoagulant activity of protein S is uncertain.

In the circulation, about 60% of total protein S is bound to C4b-binding protein, a complement component. Only the 40% of the protein S that is free is functionally active. The diagnosis of *protein S deficiency,* therefore, requires measurement of both free and bound forms of protein S.[7] Total protein S levels can be measured immunologically under conditions that dissociate protein S from C4b-binding protein.[44] A monoclonal antibody that only recognizes uncomplexed protein S can then be used to measure free protein S.[45] The functional activity of protein S can be measured using an APC cofactor assay. This assay depends on prolongation of the aPTT when diluted patient plasma is added to protein S–depleted plasma containing APC and factor Va.[37,46]

Protein S deficiency can be inherited or acquired. Based on measurements of total and free protein S antigen and protein S activity, 3 types of inherited protein S deficiency have been identified (Table 25.5). Type I, or classical, deficiency results from decreased synthesis of a normal protein and is characterized by reduced levels of total and free protein S antigen together with reduced protein S functional activity. Molecular analysis of protein S deficiency is complicated because there are 2 homologous protein S genes, one of which is likely a pseudogene. Nonetheless, most cases of type I protein S deficiency are caused by partial gene deletions.[47]

Type	Total Protein S	Free Protein S	Protein S Activity
I	Reduced	Reduced	Reduced
II	Normal	Normal	Reduced
III	Normal	Reduced	Reduced

Table 25.5 Types of Inherited Protein S Deficiency

Type II protein S deficiency is characterized by normal levels of total and free protein S, associated with reduced protein S activity. This type of deficiency is uncommon and most of the causative mutations encode protein S domains involved in its interaction with APC.[48]

Type III protein S deficiency is characterized by normal levels of total protein S, but low levels of free protein S associated with reduced protein S activity. The molecular basis of this type of deficiency appears to be similar to that of the type I deficiency states.[49,50] In fact, type I and type III protein S deficiency may be manifestations of the same disease because they often coexist in families. Thus, younger family members present with type I deficiency, whereas older family members have type III deficiency because protein S levels increase with age.

Acquired protein S deficiency can be due to decreased synthesis, increased consumption, loss, or shift of free protein S to the bound form. Decreased synthesis can occur in patients with severe liver disease,[51] in those given L-asparaginase,[52] and in patients given vitamin K antagonists.[51] Increased consumption of protein S occurs in patients with acute thrombosis or in those with disseminated intravascular coagulation. Patients with nephrotic syndrome can lose free protein S in their urine, causing decreased protein S activity.[53] Total protein S levels in these patients are often normal because the levels of C4b-binding protein increase, shifting more protein S to the bound form. C4b-binding protein levels also increase in pregnancy and with the use of estrogen-containing oral contraceptives. This shifts more protein S to the bound form and lowers the levels of free protein S and protein S activity.[54] The pathophysiological consequences of this phenomenon are uncertain.

Gain-of-Function Mutations

Gain-of-function mutations include Factor V Leiden, FIIG20210A, elevated levels of procoagulant proteins, and other less-well-characterized genetic disorders.

Factor V Leiden

In 1993, Dahlback and colleagues[55,56] described 3 families with a history of VTE. Affected family members exhibited limited prolongation of the aPTT when APC was added to their plasma. Accordingly, this phenotype was designated APC resistance (APCR). Bertina et al[57] demonstrated that APCR cosegregated with the *FV* gene and was due to a single base substitution, guanine to adenine at position 1691, that produced an Arg 506 Gln mutation at one of the APC cleavage sites on factor Va.[58,59] This mutation, which is designated Factor V Leiden, endows activated Factor V Leiden with a 10-fold longer half-life in the presence of APC than its wild-type counterpart.

The Factor V Leiden mutation is responsible for most cases of APCR.[60] Other causes are mutations at Arg 306, another APC cleavage site. Arg 306 is replaced by a Gly residue in Factor V Hong Kong[61] and by a Thr residue in Factor V Cambridge.[62] Neither of these mutations is associated with thrombosis.

The Factor V Leiden mutation is inherited in an autosomal dominant fashion. The prevalence of the mutation ranges from 2% to 5% in Caucasians,[63] but it is rare in Asians and Africans.[64,65] This racial difference likely reflects a founder effect with the mutation arising 20,000 to 30,000 years ago, after the divergence of non-Africans from Africans and Caucasoids from Mongoloid subpopulations.[66] The prevalence of Factor V Leiden homozygosity is about 1 in 2500.[7] The risk of thrombotic complications is lower with Factor V Leiden than it is with deficiencies of antithrombin, protein C, or protein S.[67-69] Heterozygotes with the Factor V Leiden mutation have a yearly risk of 0.1% to 0.3%, whereas the risk with deficiencies of antithrombin, protein C, or protein S ranges from 0.5% to 1.5% per year.

A diagnosis of APCR is established using a functional assay based on the ratio of the aPTT after APC addition divided by that determined before APC addition.[70] Second-generation tests, which add dilute patient plasma to factor V–deficient plasma, are more specific for Factor V Leiden.[71] An equivocal functional test for APCR should be confirmed with a genetic test for the Factor V Leiden mutation.[72]

Prothrombin gene mutation

After extensive screening of 28 families with unexplained VTE, Poort and colleagues[73] identified a heterozygous G to A nucleotide transition at position 20210 in the 3'-untranslated region of the prothrombin gene in 5 of the probands. This mutation, *FIIG20210A*, results in elevated levels of prothrombin. Elevated levels of prothrombin, in turn, may increase the risk of thrombosis by enhancing thrombin generation[74,75] or by inhibiting factor Va inactivation by APC.[76]

The mechanism by which the *FIIG20210A* mutation causes increased prothrombin levels appears to vary. Enhanced protein synthesis may result from more efficient 3'-end

formation, increased messenger RNA stability, increased translation efficiency, or some combination of these mechanisms.[77] An intronic *FII* gene polymorphism, A19911G, which influences splicing efficiency, may modulate the effect of the *FIIG20210A* mutation such that heterozygous carriers of both mutations have a greater risk of thrombosis than those with only the *FIIG20210A* mutation.[78]

Like the Factor V Leiden mutation, the prevalence of the *FIIG20210A* mutation is high in Caucasians but low in Asians, American Indians, and African Americans.[79] A founder effect likely explains the higher prevalence in Caucasians. The mutation may have provided a survival advantage based on a protective prenatal effect.[80,81]

FIIG20210A is found in 1% to 6% of Caucasians.[73,82] The mutation is more common in southern than in northern Europe, a gradient opposite to that of Factor V Leiden.[83] Rare individuals homozygous for the *FIIG20210A* mutation have been identified.[84,85]

Laboratory diagnosis of *FIIG20210A* depends on genetic screening after PCR amplification of the 3'-untranslated region of the *FII* gene.[37] Although *FIIG20210A* heterozygotes have 30% higher levels of prothrombin than noncarriers, the wide range of prothrombin levels in healthy individuals precludes the use of this phenotype to identify carriers.[86]

Elevated levels of procoagulant proteins

Elevated levels of factor VIII and other coagulation factors, including factors X and XI, have been implicated as independent risk factors for thrombosis.[87-90] Although the molecular bases for the high levels of these coagulation factors have yet to be identified, genetic mechanisms are likely responsible because the hereditability of these quantitative abnormalities is high.

Other hereditary disorders

Polymorphisms in the gene for EPCR, an endothelial cell surface receptor that binds protein C and presents it to the thrombin-thrombomodulin complex for activation, have been associated with thrombosis. An EPCR polymorphism associated with high levels of soluble EPCR has been identified. By binding circulating APC, soluble EPCR prevents it from functioning as an anticoagulant.[91,92]

Polymorphisms in factor XIII are associated with a reduced risk of thrombosis. Replacement of Val134 by Leu in the α-chain of factor XIII results in more rapid factor XIII activation by thrombin.[93] In case-control studies, this polymorphism had a paradoxical protective effect on the risk of myocardial infarction in some studies and possibly also on the risk of VTE.[94] The mechanism responsible for this protection is unclear.[95]

Acquired Hypercoagulable States

Acquired hypercoagulable states include antiphospholipid syndrome and cancer, as well as pregnancy and estrogen therapy (oral contraception or hormone replacement therapy). These disorders can occur in isolation or can be superimposed on hereditary hypercoagulable states. Heparin-induced thrombocytopenia is an immune-mediated adverse drug reaction and is a strong, independent risk factor for arterial and venous thrombosis.

Antiphospholipid Syndrome

First described in a study by Wassermann and colleagues[96] in 1906 among patients with positive serologic tests for syphilis, antiphospholipid antibodies are a heterogeneous group of autoantibodies directed against proteins that bind phospholipid.[97] Antibodies can be categorized into those that prolong phospholipid-dependent coagulation assays, known as a lupus anticoagulant (LA), or an anticardiolipin antibody (ACA), which targets cardiolipin. A subset of ACAs recognize other phospholipid-bound proteins, particularly β_2-glycoprotein I.

Patients who have thrombosis in association with an LA and/or ACA are diagnosed with *antiphospholipid syndrome (APS)*. APS is considered primary when it occurs in isolation and secondary when it is associated with autoimmune disorders, such as systemic lupus erythematosis or other connective tissue diseases. Thrombosis in APS patients can be arterial, venous, or placental.[98] Placental thrombosis is hypothesized to be the root cause of the pregnancy-related complications that characterize APS. These include fetal loss before 10 weeks gestation and unexplained fetal death after 10 weeks gestation.[99] Intrauterine growth retardation, pre-eclampsia, and eclampsia also have been associated with APS.

Laboratory diagnosis of APS requires the presence of a LA or an ACA on tests taken at least 6 weeks apart.[100] LA is detected using phospholipid-dependent clotting tests. Most screening assays are based on the aPTT. aPTT reagents differ in their sensitivity for detection of LA and many laboratories have adopted less-sensitive aPTT reagents for routine aPTT testing. LA is suspected when the aPTT is prolonged. To explore the cause of the prolonged aPTT, patient plasma is then mixed with normal plasma and the aPTT is again determined. If the aPTT remains prolonged, LA is suspected. The diagnosis is confirmed by demonstrating that addition of excess hexagonal phase phospholipid normalizes the aPTT, thereby documenting the phospholipid-dependence of the abnormal test result. In addition to the aPTT, a battery of phospholipid-dependent clotting tests are often used for diagnosis of LA. These include the dilute Russell viper venom time and kaolin clotting time.[101]

ACAs are detected using immunoassays.[102] Only ACAs of medium to high titer and of the IgG or IgM subclass are associated with thrombosis. The amount of IgG or IgM antibody binding to cardiolipin-coated plates is expressed in standardized GPL or MPL units, with 1 unit representing the cardiolipin-binding capacity of 1 µg/mL affinity-purified antiphospholipid antibody from reference sera. The extent of antibody binding is influenced by both the titer of the antibody and its affinity for cardiolipin. Lack of standardization of ACA assays makes it difficult to compare results between laboratories.[103,104]

ACAs are found in 3% to 10% of healthy individuals. They also are common with certain infections, such as mycobacterial pneumonia, malaria, or parasitic disorders, and after exposure to some medications. Often, these antibodies are of low titer and are transient. ACAs are detected in about 30% to 50% of patients with systemic lupus erythematosis.[105] Of these, 10% to 20% also have a LA.[106]

The mechanism by which antiphospholipid antibodies trigger thrombosis is unclear. In cell culture systems, these antibodies can directly activate endothelial cells and induce the expression of adhesion molecules that can tether tissue factor–bearing leukocytes or microparticles onto their surface. Tissue factor can then trigger clotting *in vitro*. Antiphospholipid antibodies also have been shown to (1) interfere with the protein C pathway, (2) inhibit antithrombin catalysis by vessel wall heparan sulfate, and (3) impair fibrinolysis.[104,107-109] Whether these mechanisms are operative *in vivo* has yet to be established.

In contrast to most hypercoagulable states, APS can be associated with spontaneous arterial thrombosis as well as with VTE.[6] Arterial thrombosis can manifest as a stroke or transient ischemic attack.[110,111] Thrombosis of the sagittal sinus, a form of venous thrombosis, also can cause stroke in these patients.[112]

Heparin-induced Thrombocytopenia

A clinicopathologic syndrome, *heparin-induced thrombocytopenia (HIT)* is diagnosed on the basis of clinical features (Table 25.6) and laboratory detection of HIT antibodies. The risk of HIT is higher with unfractionated heparin than with low-molecular-weight heparin. HIT is more common in surgical patients than in medical patients and occurs more frequently in women.

Typical clinical features of HIT include thrombocytopenia and thrombosis (arterial or venous). Less-common features include necrotic skin lesions at the site of subcutaneous heparin injection, acute systemic reactions to heparin, and, rarely, disseminated intravascular coagulation.[113,114] Thrombocytopenia is the most common finding, occurring in 90% of patients. Typically, the platelet count falls 5 to 10 days after heparin is started. However, thrombocytopenia can occur earlier if the patient has been exposed to heparin in the past 3 months.[115] Rarely, the onset of HIT can be delayed and occurs several days after stopping heparin.[116]

HIT is an autoimmune-like disorder and is caused by heparin-dependent, platelet-activating antibodies of the IgG subclass. These antibodies are directed against neoantigens that are exposed on platelet factor 4 (PF4) when it is complexed by heparin.[114] By binding to FcγII receptors on platelets, these antibodies trigger platelet activation. Activated platelets and platelet-derived microparticles provide an anionic phospholipid surface on which coagulation factors assemble and promote thrombin generation. This produces a hypercoagulable state and explains why 30% to 70% of HIT patients develop thrombosis.[117,118]

The diagnosis of HIT is supported by assays that capitalize on the platelet-activating properties of HIT antibodies. The platelet serotonin release assay is the gold standard for the diagnosis of HIT.[119] Enzyme immunoassays for detection

Feature	Details
Thrombocytopenia	Platelet count of ≤ 100,000/μL or a decrease in platelet count of ≥ 50%
Timing	Platelet count falls 5–10 days after starting heparin
Type of heparin	More common with unfractionated heparin than low-molecular-weight heparin
Type of patient	More common in surgical patients than medical patients; more common in women than in men
Thrombosis	Venous thrombosis more common than arterial thrombosis

Table 25.6 Features of Heparin-induced Thrombocytopenia

of antibodies against PF4 are more sensitive but less specific than the serotonin release assay.[120]

When the diagnosis of HIT is established, heparin must be stopped and an alternative anticoagulant should be given (Table 25.7). Options include direct thrombin inhibitors, such as lepirudin, argatroban, or bivalirudin, or factor Xa inhibitors, such as fondaparinux. Treatment with these agents should be continued until the platelet count returns to baseline levels, at which point low-dose warfarin can be initiated.

Stop all heparin
Give an alternative anticoagulant, such as lepirudin, argatroban, bivalirudin, or fondaparinux
Do not give platelet transfusions
Do not give warfarin until the platelet count returns to its baseline level; if warfarin is administered, give vitamin K to restore the INR to normal
Evaluate for thrombosis, particularly deep vein thrombosis

Table 25.7. Management of Heparin-induced Thrombocytopenia

Cancer

About 25% of patients who present with VTE have cancer.[121] Cancer patients who develop this condition have reduced survival compared with those who do not develop it.[122] Patients with brain tumors and advanced ovarian or prostate cancer have particularly high rates of VTE.[123] Treatment with chemotherapy, hormonal therapy, and biological agents, such as erythropoietin and antiangiogenic drugs, further increases the risk of VTE.

The pathogenesis of thrombosis in cancer patients is multifactorial in origin and represents a complex interplay among the tumor, the patient characteristics, and the hemostatic system. Tumor cells often express tissue factor or other procoagulants that can initiate coagulation.[124,125] In addition to its role in coagulation, tissue factor also acts as a cell signaling molecule that promotes tumor proliferation and spread.

Patient factors that contribute to VTE include immobility and venous stasis secondary to extrinsic compression of major veins by tumor. Surgical procedures, indwelling central venous catheters, and chemotherapy can produce vessel wall injury.[126] In addition, tamoxifen and selective estrogen receptor modulators (SERMs) induce an acquired hypercoagulable state by reducing the levels of natural anticoagulant proteins.[127]

A proportion of patients who present with unprovoked VTE have occult cancer. This observation has prompted some experts to recommend extensive screening for cancer in such patients. Any benefits of this approach, however, are offset by potential harms. These include procedure-related morbidity, the psychological impact of false-positive tests, and the cost of screening. Furthermore, early detection of cancer is only of benefit if there is potentially curative therapy. To date, only screening for breast, cervical, colon, and possibly prostate cancer has been shown to reduce mortality.[128]

Small studies comparing extensive cancer screening with no screening in patients with unprovoked VTE have yet to demonstrate that extensive screening reduces cancer-related mortality. Therefore, it is difficult to recommend extensive screening at this time.[5] Instead, a careful history should be taken to identify any symptoms suggestive of underlying cancer. If such symptoms are present, further investigation is warranted. If there are no symptoms suggestive of underlying cancer, patients should be encouraged to undergo age-appropriate screening tests for breast, cervical, colon, or prostate cancer.

Pregnancy

Pregnancy is an independent risk factor for VTE. The risk of VTE in pregnant women is 5- to 6-fold higher than that in age-matched nonpregnant women.[7] About 1 in 1000 pregnancies are complicated by VTE, and about 1 in 1000 women develop VTE in the postpartum period.[129] Thus, venous thromboembolic disease is the leading cause of maternal morbidity and mortality.[130,131]

The individual risk of VTE in pregnancy and the puerperium is influenced by patient-related factors. These include age > 35 years, body mass index > 29, Cesarean delivery, and thrombophilia or family history of VTE.[129,132] A past history of VTE,[133] ovarian hyperstimulation, and multiparity are other risk factors.

Over 90% of deep vein thrombosis in pregnancy occurs in the left leg because the enlarged uterus further compresses the left iliac vein by placing pressure on the overlying right iliac and ovarian arteries.[134,135] A similar mechanism likely explains the isolated left iliofemoral thrombosis that can occur in pregnancy.

Hypercoagulability of the blood occurs in pregnancy and reflects a combination of venous stasis and changes in the hemostatic system. The enlarging uterus reduces venous blood flow from the lower extremities. This is not the only mechanism responsible for venous stasis because blood flow from the lower extremities begins to decrease by the end of the first trimester, likely reflecting hormonally induced venous dilatation. Systemic factors also contribute to hypercoagulability. Thus, the levels of circulating procoagulant proteins increase in the third trimester of pregnancy. These include factor VIII, fibrinogen, and von Willebrand protein, among others.[136,137] Coincidentally, there is suppression of natural anticoagulant pathways. Thus, there is an acquired resistance to activated protein C related, at least in part, to reduced levels of free protein S.[138,139] The net effect of these changes is enhanced thrombin generation as evidenced by elevated levels of prothrombin fragments and thrombin-antithrombin complexes.[140,141]

About half of the episodes of VTE in pregnancy occur in women with thrombophilia.[142,143] The risk of VTE in women with thrombophilic defects depends on the type of abnormality and the presence of other risk factors.[144] The risk appears to be highest in women with antithrombin, protein C, or protein S deficiency and lower in those with Factor V Leiden or the prothrombin gene mutation.[145,146] In general, the daily risk

of VTE in these women is higher in the postpartum period than it is during pregnancy.[147,148] The risk during pregnancy is similar in all 3 trimesters.[144] Therefore, if thromboprophylaxis is given during pregnancy, it must be administered throughout the pregnancy and continued for at least 6 weeks postpartum.[149]

Hormonal Therapy

Oral contraceptives, estrogen replacement therapy, and SERMs are all associated with an increased risk of thrombosis.[150,151] The relatively high risk of VTE associated with early oral contraceptives prompted development of low-dose formulations containing reduced doses of estrogen and progestin. Currently available low-estrogen combination oral contraceptives contain 20 to 50 μg of ethinylestradiol and one of several different progestins. Even these low-dose combination contraceptives are associated with a 3- to 4-fold increased risk of VTE compared with the risk in nonusers. In absolute terms, this translates to an incidence of 3 to 4 per 10,000 compared with 5 to 10 per 100,000 in nonusers of reproductive age.[152]

Whereas smoking increases the risk of myocardial infarction and stroke in women taking oral contraceptives, it is unclear whether smoking affects the risk of VTE.[153] In contrast, obesity impacts on the risk of both arterial and venous thrombosis.[154] The risk of VTE is highest during the first year of oral contraceptive use and persists only for the duration of use.[155,156]

Case-control studies suggest that the risk of VTE is 20- to 30-fold higher in women with inherited thrombophilia who use oral contraceptives than it is in nonusers with thrombophilia or users without these defects.[152,157-159] Despite the increased risk, however, routine screening for thrombophilia is not indicated in women considering the use of oral contraceptives. Based on the estimated incidence and case fatality rate of thrombotic events, it is estimated that 400,000 women would need to be screened to detect 20,000 carriers of Factor V Leiden. Oral contraceptives would need to be withheld in all of these women to prevent a single death.[160]

For less-prevalent thrombophilic defects, even larger numbers of women would need to be screened. Based on these considerations, routine screening cannot be recommended.

There has been mounting evidence that hormonal replacement therapy with conjugated equine estrogen with or without a progestin increases the risk of myocardial infarction, ischemic stroke, and VTE.[161,162] Consequently, the use of hormone replacement therapy has markedly decreased.

SERMs are estrogen-like compounds. The prototypical SERM is tamoxifen, which serves as an estrogen antagonist in the breast but as an estrogen agonist in other tissues, such as bone and uterus.[163] Like estrogens, tamoxifen increases the risk of VTE 3- to 4-fold.[164] The risk is higher in postmenopausal women, particularly those also receiving systemic combination chemotherapy.[127] Aromatase inhibitors are replacing tamoxifen for treatment of estrogen-receptor-positive breast cancer. These newer agents are associated with a lower risk of VTE than tamoxifen.[165] Raloxifene, a SERM used to prevent osteoporosis, increases the risk of VTE 3-fold compared with placebo.[166] Therefore, this agent is contraindicated for prevention of osteoporosis in women with a prior history of VTE.[148]

Prior History of VTE

A history of previous VTE places patients at risk for recurrence.[167,168] Those with unprovoked VTE have a particularly high risk of recurrence when anticoagulant treatment is stopped.[169] Their risk of recurrence is about 10% at 1 year and 30% at 5 years. This risk appears to be independent of whether or not there is an underlying thrombophilic defect, such as Factor V Leiden or the prothrombin gene mutation.

The risk of recurrent VTE is lower in patients whose incident event occurred in association with well-recognized transient risk factors, such as major surgery or prolonged immobilization. These patients have a risk of recurrence of about 4% at 1 year and 10% at 5 years. Patients whose venous thromboembolic event oc-

curred on the background of minor risk factors, such as oral contraceptive use or a long-haul airplane flight, likely have an intermediate risk of recurrence.[170,171] Patients at highest risk for recurrence are those with inherited deficiencies of antithrombin, protein C, or protein S; APS; advanced malignancy; or those homozygous for Factor V Leiden or the prothrombin gene mutation. Their risk of recurrence is likely to be at least 15% at 1 year and up to 50% at 5 years.[67-69]

Combined Inherited and Acquired Hypercoagulable States

Hyperhomocysteinemia is the prototypical hypercoagulable state that occurs due to a combination of inherited and acquired factors.[172,173] Homocysteine is an intermediate sulfur-containing amino acid that acts as a methyl group donor during the metabolism of methionine, an essential amino acid derived from the diet. The interconversion of methionine and homocysteine depends on the availability of 5-methyltetrahydrofolate, a methyl group donor; vitamin B_{12} and folate, cofactors in the interconversion; and the enzyme methionine synthase.[174] Increased levels of homocysteine can be the result of increased production or reduced metabolism. Severe hyperhomocysteinemia and cysteinuria are rare and are usually caused by deficiency in the enzyme cystathione β-synthetase.[175] More common is mild to moderate hyperhomocysteinemia. This can be caused by genetic mutations in methyl-tetrahydrofolate reductase (MTHFR) when they are accompanied by nutritional deficiency of folate, vitamin B_{12}, or vitamin B_6.[176] Common polymorphisms in MTHFR, C677T and A1298C, are associated with reduced enzymatic activity and increased thermolability. The cofactor requirements are therefore increased with these mutations.[2] Hyperhomocysteinemia also can be associated with certain drugs, such as methotrexate, theophylline, cyclosporine, and most anticonvulsants, as well as some chronic diseases, such as end stage renal disease, severe hepatic dysfunction, and hypothyroidism.[177]

A fasting serum homocysteine level over 15 mmol/L is considered elevated. Although elevated levels were a common finding, routine fortification of flour with folic acid has resulted in lower homocysteine levels in the general population.[178,179] Elevated serum levels of homocysteine have been associated with an increased risk of arterial thrombosis (myocardial infarction, stroke, and peripheral artery disease) and VTE.[177,180]

Elevated levels of homocysteine can be reduced by administration of folate along with vitamin B_{12} and vitamin B_6.[181] Recent randomized trials, however, have shown that reduction of homocysteine levels with vitamin therapy does not reduce the risk of recurrent cardiovascular events in patients with coronary artery disease or stroke,[182] nor does it lower the risk of recurrent VTE. Based on these negative trials and the declining incidence of hyperhomocysteinemia, the enthusiasm for screening for this condition has rapidly declined.

Treatment of Thrombosis in Patients with Hypercoagulable States

Thrombosis treatment is usually divided into 2 overlapping stages: *initial treatment* and *extended therapy*. The impact of hypercoagulable states on these 2 stages is discussed separately, as is their impact on duration of anticoagulant therapy and recommendations for prevention of recurrence.

Initial Treatment

With few exceptions, management of initial thrombotic events in patients with hypercoagulable states is no different from the management of these events in patients without underlying hypercoagulable disorders.[71] The exceptions are purpura fulminans in newborns with homozygous protein C or protein S deficiency and thrombosis in patients with severe antithrombin deficiency. Newborns with purpura fulminans require protein C or protein S concentrates or sufficient amounts of plasma to increase the levels of protein C or protein S.[183,184] Patients with severe antithrombin deficiency require antithrombin concentrates to increase plasma levels of antithrombin to a point where heparin or low-molecular-weight heparin can be used for treatment.[83,185]

Extended Therapy

Extended treatment of thrombosis also is similar in patients with hypercoagulable states as it is in those without these underlying disorders. Caution is needed when starting patients with protein C or protein S deficiency on warfarin or other vitamin K antagonists to prevent skin necrosis.[186] Warfarin should not be started in these patients until therapeutic anticoagulation has been achieved with heparin or low-molecular-weight heparin. Once started, low doses of warfarin should be given to prevent precipitous decreases in the levels of protein C or protein S.

Randomized trials have shown that usual-intensity warfarin (target INR of 2–3) is as effective as higher-intensity warfarin in patients with antiphospholipid syndrome. The risk of major bleeding is lower with usual-intensity warfarin than it is with higher-intensity regimens.[187,188] A target INR of 2 to 3 is appropriate for patients with other hypercoagulable states as well.[189]

Patients with thrombosis on the background of metastatic cancer may do better with extended treatment with low-molecular-weight heparin than with warfarin. Randomized clinical trials have shown that, compared with warfarin, low-molecular-weight heparin reduces the risk of recurrent VTE without increasing bleeding.[190] Furthermore, low-molecular-weight heparin simplifies treatment because it can be given subcutaneously once daily without coagulation monitoring. The drug can be held before invasive procedures and the dose reduced if there is thrombocytopenia. The major drawback of low-molecular-weight heparin is cost, although the drug has been shown to be cost-effective in patients at high risk of recurrent VTE.[191]

Duration of Treatment

The presence of a hypercoagulable state has no influence on the duration of anticoagulant treatment in patients whose venous thromboembolic event occurred in the setting of a well-recognized and transient risk factor, such as major surgery or prolonged immobilization due to medical illness. These patients are treated with anticoagulants for at least 3 months.[192] For those with unprovoked VTE, long-term anticoagulation treatment is often recommended.[169,193] Heterozygosity for Factor V Leiden or the prothrombin gene mutation does not influence the risk of recurrence. In contrast, patients with deficiency of antithrombin, protein C, or protein S or those homozygous for Factor V Leiden or the prothrombin gene mutation appear to be at higher risk for recurrence and likely should receive longer-term anticoagulation treatment.[194-196] Likewise, patients with APS with a persistent ACA or LA also are at high risk for recurrence and require long-term treatment.[97]

Treatment and Prevention of Thrombosis During Pregnancy

Thrombophilic disorders have no influence on the treatment of venous thrombosis during pregnancy. Pregnant women require therapeutic doses of subcutaneous heparin or low-molecular-weight heparin throughout pregnancy.[149,197] Heparin is given twice daily with the dose titrated to achieve a therapeutic mid-interval aPTT. Low-molecular-weight heparin can be given once or twice daily in a weight-adjusted fashion.[144] Monitoring with anti–factor Xa levels is recommended, particularly in the third trimester. Fondaparinux can also be used in pregnancy, but data are limited. The drug is given once daily. It is uncertain whether monitoring is required. After delivery, low-molecular-weight heparin or warfarin should be given for at least 4 to 6 weeks. In total, treatment should be given for 6 months from the time of diagnosis. Warfarin can be safely administered in nursing mothers, with no detectable anticoagulant effect in breast milk.[198]

Women with a past history of unprovoked or recurrent VTE; those with deficiencies of antithrombin, protein C, or protein S; and those homozygous for Factor V Leiden or the prothrombin gene mutation should receive antepartum prophylaxis with heparin or low-molecular-weight heparin.[149] Postpartum, low-molecular-weight heparin or warfarin should be given for 4 to 6 weeks.[199] Postpartum treatment with low-molecular-weight heparin or warfarin for 4 to 6 weeks is likely adequate for women with a history of VTE secondary to a well-defined risk factor.[200] Prophylaxis during pregnancy, as well as postpartum, should be considered for women who developed VTE after taking oral contraceptives, particularly if they have underlying thrombophilia. Women with thrombophilic defects and no prior history of VTE likely do not require antepartum prophylaxis or postpartum treatment, but definitive data are lacking.[149] A summary of these recommendations is provided in Table 25.8.

Thrombophilia and Fetal Loss

About 30% of women have at least one fetal loss, and approximately 5% of women of reproductive age experience recurrent fetal loss.[201] Women with hereditary thrombophilia have a 2- to 5-fold increased risk of fetal loss.[202] Acquired hypercoagulable states, particularly APS, also increase the risk of fetal loss.[203-205] The use of once-daily heparin or low-molecular-weight heparin in prophylactic doses, with or without aspirin, is often prescribed for women with recurrent fetal loss on the background of an underlying thrombophilic defect, although clinical trials assessing the efficacy of such an approach are lacking.[199]

Clinical History	Thrombophilia	Antepartum	Postpartum*
Prior venous thrombosis secondary to a transient risk factor	No	Surveillance	Yes
Prior venous thrombosis secondary to pregnancy or estrogens	Yes or no	Prophylactic heparin or LMWH	Yes
Prior idiopathic venous thrombosis	Yes or no	Prophylactic heparin or LMWH	Yes
Recurrent venous thrombosis	Yes or no	Treatment-dose heparin or LMWH	Resume long-term anticoagulation
No prior venous thrombosis	antithrombin deficiency; FIIG20210A or Factor V Leiden; double heterozygosity for both mutations	Prophylactic or full dose heparin or LMWH; antithrombin concentrates for severe antithrombin deficiency	Yes

Table 25.8 Management of Women with a History of Venous Thrombosis During Pregnancy and the Puerperium

*Postpartum prophylaxis involves a 4- to 6-week course of warfarin with the dose adjusted to achieve an INR of 2 to 3. Prophylactic doses of low-molecular-weight heparin can be used as an alternative. LMWH = low-molecular-weight heparin.

Thrombophilia Screening

The indications for *thrombophilia screening* remain controversial.[206,207] For patients with a first episode of VTE, screening is indicated if the results influence the duration of treatment or impact on family counseling regarding use of estrogen-containing compounds.[37] It is reasonable to screen patients whose first episode of thrombosis occurred before the age of 45; those with recurrent thrombosis, particularly if unprovoked; patients with thrombosis in an unusual site,[208] such as cerebral or mesenteric veins; those with 2 or more first-degree relatives with thrombosis; and women who develop thrombosis during pregnancy or in association with estrogen treatment. It also is reasonable to screen women with a history of second-trimester pregnancy loss or intrauterine death.[7]

Screening should include functional assays for antithrombin and protein C, a free protein S level, testing for activated protein C resistance using the modified APC sensitivity ratio with DNA testing for the Factor V Leiden mutation if the screening test is equivocal, DNA testing for the prothrombin gene mutation, phospholipid-based clotting tests to detect a LA, and an enzyme immunoassay for ACA.[5]

Summary

With increased understanding of the regulation of coagulation, inherited or acquired hypercoagulable states can now be identified in up to 50% of patients with VTE. The role of these disorders in the pathogenesis of arterial thrombosis is less clear. Therefore, more work is needed to identify patients who are vulnerable to arterial thrombosis after plaque rupture.

Although our ability to diagnose hypercoagulable states has improved, the impact of this information on clinical decisions remains limited. Common congenital hypercoagulable states increase the risk of a first episode of VTE but have little impact on the risk of recurrence. Identification of patients at risk for recurrent VTE and elucidating new hypercoagulable states are goals for the future.

References

1. Crowther MA, Kelton JG. Congenital thrombophilic states associated with venous thrombosis: a qualitative overview and proposed classification system. *Ann Intern Med*. 2003;138(2):128-134.

2. Jacques PF, Bostom AG, Williams RR, Ellison RC, Eckfeldt JH, Rosenberg IH. Relation between folate status, a common mutation in methylenetetrahydrofolate reductase, and plasma homocysteine concentrations. *Circulation*. 1996;93(1):7-9.

3. Salomon O, Steinberg DM, Zivelin A, et al. Single and combined prothrombotic factors in patients with idiopathic venous thromboembolism: prevalence and risk assessment. *Arterioscler Thromb Vasc Biol*. 1999;19(3):511-518.

4. Vandenbroucke JP, Koster T, Briet E, Reitsma PH, Bertina RM, Rosdendaal FR. Increased risk of venous thrombosis in oral-contraceptive users who are carriers of factor V Leiden mutation. *Lancet*. 1994;344(8935):1453-1457.

5. Walker ID, Greaves M, Preston FE, on behalf of the Haemostasis and Thrombosis Task Force, British Committee for Standards in Haematology. Investigation and management of heritable thrombophilia. *Br J Haematol*. 2003;114:512-528.

6. Kitchens CS. Thrombophilia and thrombosis in unusual sites. In: Colman RW, Hirsh J, Marder VJ, Salzman EW, eds. *Hemostasis and Thrombosis: Basic Principles and Practice*. 3rd ed. Philadelphia: J.B. Lippincott Company; 1994:1255-1273.

7. Aiach M, Emmerich J. Thrombophilia genetics. In: Colman RW, Marder VJ, Clowes AW, George JN, Goldhaber SZ, eds. *Hemostasis and Thrombosis. Basic Principles and Clinical Practice*. 5th ed. Philadelphia: Lippincott Williams and Wilkins; 2006:779-793.

8. Petersen TE, Dudek-Wojciechowska G, Sottrup-Jensen L, Magnusson S. Primary structure of antithrombin III (heparin cofactor). In: Collen D, Wiman B, Verstrate M, eds. *The Physiological Inhibitors of Coagulation and Fibrinolysis*. Amsterdam: Elsevier,1979:43-54.

9. Olson ST, Bjork I. Regulation of thrombin activity by antithrombin and heparin. *Semin Thromb Hemost*. 1994;20(4):373-409.

10. Marcum JA, Atha DH, Fritze LM, Nawroth P, Stern D, Rosenberg RD. Cloned bovine aortic endothelial cells synthesize anticoagulantly active heparan sulfate proteolglycan. *J Biol Chem*. 1986;261(16):7507-7517.

11. Bock SC. Antithrombin III and heparin cofactor II. In: Colman RW, Marder VJ, Clowes AW, George JN, Goldhaber SZ, eds. *Hemostasis and Thrombosis. Basic Principles and Clinical Practice*. 5th ed. Philadelphia: Lippincott Williams and Wilkins; 2006:235-248.

12. Tait RC, Walker ID, Perry DJ, et al. Prevalence of antithrombin deficiency in the healthy population. *Br J Haematol*. 1994;87(1):106-112.

13. Wells PS, Blajchman MA, Henderson P, Wells MJ, Demers C, Bourque R. Prevalence of antithrombin deficiency in healthy blood donors: a cross-sectional study. *Am J Hematol*. 1994;45:321-324.

14. Perry D, Carrell R. Molecular genetics of human antithrombin III deficiency. *Hum Mutat*. 1996;7(1):7-22.

15. Perry DJ. Antithrombin and its inherited deficiencies. *Blood Reviews*. 1994;8(1):37-55.

16. Ambruso DR, Leonard BD, Bies RD, Jacobson L, Hathaway WE, Reeve EB. Antithrombin III deficiency: decreased synthesis of a biochemically normal molecule. *Blood*. 1982;60:78-83.

17. Lane DA, Bayston T, Olds RJ, et al. Antithrombin mutation database: 2nd (1997) update. For the Plasma Coagulation Inhibitors Subcommittee of the Scientific and Standardization Committee of the International Society on Thrombosis and Haemostasis. *Thromb Haemost*. 1997;77(1):197-211.

18. Finazzi G, Caccia R, Barbui T. Different prevalence of thromboembolism in the subtypes of congenital antithrombin III deficiency: review of 404 cases. *Thromb Haemost*. 1987;58(4):1094.

19. Girolami A. The incidence of thrombotic manifestations in AT III abnormalities. *Thromb Haemost*. 1987;57(1):123-124.

20. van Boven HH, Lane DA. Antithrombin III and its inherited deficiency states. *Semin Hematol*. 1997;34(3):188-204.

21. Bauters A, Zawadzki C, Bura A, Thery C, Watel A, Subtil D. Homozygous variant of antithrombin with lack of affinity for heparin: management of severe thrombotic complications associated with intrauterine fetal demise. *Blood Coag Fibrinolysis*. 1996;7(7):705-710.

22. Buchanan GR, Holtkamp CA. Reduced anti-

thrombin III levels during L-asparaginase therapy. *Med Pediatr Oncol.* 1980;8(1):7-14.

23. de Boer AC, van Riel LAM, den Ottolander GJH. Measurement of antithrombin III, alpha-macroglobulin and alpha-antitrypsin in patients with deep venous thrombosis and pulmonary embolism. *Thromb Res.* 1979;15(1-2):17-25.

24. Damus PS, Wallace GA. Immunologic measurement of antithrombin III-heparin cofactor and alpha2-macroglobulin in disseminated intravascular coagulation and hepatic failure coagulopathy. *Thromb Res.* 1975;6(1):27-38.

25. Marciniak E, Gockerman JP. Heparin induced decrease in circulating antithrombin III. *Lancet 2.* 1977;8038:581-584.

26. Kauffman RH, Veltkamp JJ, van Tilburg NH, Van Es LA. Acquired antithrombin III deficiency and thrombosis in the nephrotic syndrome. *Am J Med.* 1978;65(4):607-613.

27. Esmon CT. The protein C pathway. *Chest.* 2003;124(3 Suppl):26S-32S.

28. Dahlback B, Villoutreix BO. The anticoagulant protein C pathway. *FEBS Lett.* 2005;579(15):3310-3316.

29. Esmon CT. The endothelial cell protein C receptor. *Thromb Haemost.* 2000;83(5):639-643.

30. Taylor F Jr, Peer GT, Lockhart MS, Ferrell G, Esmon CT. Endothelial cell protein C receptor plays an important role in protein C activation in vivo. *Blood.* 2001;97(6):1685-1688.

31. Griffin JJ, Evatt B, Zimmerman TS, Kleiss AJ, Wideman C. Deficiency of protein C in congenital thrombotic disease. *J Clin Invest.* 1981;68(5):1370-1373.

32. Tait RC, Walker ID, Reitsma PH, et al. Prevalence of protein C deficiency in the healthy population. *Thromb Haemost.* 1995;73(1):87-93.

33. Monagle P, Andrew M, Halton J, et al. Homozygous protein C deficiency: description of a new mutation and successful treatment with low molecular weight heparin. *Thromb Haemost.* 1998;79(4):756-761.

34. Alhenc-Gelas M, Emmerich J, Gandrille S, et al. Protein C infusion in a patient with inherited protein C deficiency caused by two missense mutations: Arg 178 to Gln and Arg-1 to His. *Blood Coag Fibrinolysis.* 1995;6(1):35-41.

35. Pescatore P, Horellou HM, Conard J, Piffoux M, Van Dreden P, Ruskone-Fourmestraux A. Problems of oral anticoagulation in an adult with homozygous protein C deficiency and late onset of thrombosis. *Thromb Haemost.* 1993;69(4):311-315.

36. Miletich JP. Laboratory diagnosis of protein C deficiency. *Semin Thromb Haemost.* 1990;16(2):169-176.

37. Tripodi A. A review of the clinical and diagnostic utility of laboratory tests for the detection of congenital thrombophilia. *Semin Thromb Hemost.* 2005;31(1):25-32.

38. Broze GJ Jr, Warren LA, Novotny WF, Higuchi DA, Girard JJ, Miletich JP. The lipoprotein-associated coagulation inhibitor that inhibits the factor VII-tissue factor complex also inhibits factor Xa: insight into its possible mechanism of action. *Blood.* 1988;71(2):335-343.

39. Weiss P, Soff GA, Halkin H, Seligsohn U. Decline of protein C and S and factors II, VII, IX and X during the initiation of warfarin therapy. *Thromb Res.* 1987;45(6):783-790.

40. Manco-Johnson MJ, Marlar RA, Jacobson LY, Hays T, Warady BA. Severe protein C deficiency in newborn infants. *J Pediatr.* 1988;113(2):359-363.

41. Citak A, Emre S, Sairin A, Bilge I, Navir A. Hemostatic problems and thromboembolic complications in nephrotic children. *Pediatr Nephrol.* 2000;14(2):138-142.

42. Walker FJ. Regulation of activated protein C by a new protein: a role for bovine protein S. *J Biol Chem.* 1980;255(12):5521-5524.

43. Heeb MJ, Mesters RM, Tans G, et al. Binding of protein S to factor Va associated with inhibition of prothrombinase that is independent of activated protein C. *J Biol Chem.* 1993;268(4):2872-2877.

44. Comp P. Laboratory evaluation of protein S status. *Thromb Haemost.* 1990;16(2):177-181.

45. Amiral J, Grosley B, Boyer-Neumann C, et al. New direct assay of free protein S antigen using two distinct monoclonal antibodies specific for the free form. *Blood Coagul Fibrinolysis.* 1994;5(2):179-186.

46. Wolf M, Boyer-Neumann C, Martinoli JL,

et al. A new functional assay for human protein S activity using activated factor V as substrate. *Thromb Haemost.* 1989;62:1144-1145.

47. Borgel D, Gandrille S, Aiach M. Protein S deficiency. *Thromb Haemost.* 1997;78:351-356.

48. Gandrille S, Borgel D, Sala N, et al. Protein S deficiency: a database of mutations—summary of the first update. Plasma coagulation inhibitors Subcommittee of the Scientific and Standardization Committee of the International Society on Thrombosis and Haemostasis. *Thromb Haemost.* 2000;84(5):918.

49. Zoller B, Garcia de Frutos P, Dahlback B. Evaluation of the relationship between protein S and C4-binding protein isoforms in hereditary protein S deficiency demonstrating type I and type III deficiencies to be phenotypic variants of the same genetic disease. *Blood.* 1995;85(12):3524-3531.

50. Castoldi E, Maurissen LF, Tormene D, Spiezia L, Gavasso S, Radu C, Hackeng TM, Rosing J, Simioni P. Similar hypercoagulable state and thrombosis risk in type I and type III protein S-deficient individuals from families with mixed typeI/III protein S deficiency. *Haematologica.* 2010;95(9):1563-1571.

51. d'Angelo A, Vigano-D'Angelo S, Esmon CT, Comp PC. Acquired deficiencies of protein S. Protein S activity during oral anticoagulation, in liver disease, and in disseminated intravascular coagulation. *J Clin Invest.* 1988;81(5):1445-1454.

52. Pui CH, Chesney CM, Bergum PQ, Jackson CW, Rapaport SI. Lack of pathogenic role of protein C and S in thrombosis associated with asparaginase prednisone-vincristine therapy for leukemia. *Br J Haematol.* 1986;64(2):283-290.

53. Vigano-D'Angelo S, d'Angelo A, Kaufman CE Jr, Sholer C, Esmon CT, Comp PC. Protein S deficiency occurs in the nephrotic syndrome. *Ann Intern Med.* 1987;107(1):42-47.

54. Malm J, Laurell M, Dahlback B. Changes in the plasma levels of vitamin K-dependent proteins C and S and of C4b-binding protein during pregnancy and oral contraception. *Br J Haematol.* 1988;68(4):437-443.

55. Dahlback B, Carlsson M, Svensson PJ. Familial thrombophilia due to a previously unrecognized mechanism characterized by poor anticoagulant response to activated protein C: prediction of a cofactor to activated protein C. *Proc Natl Acad Sci. USA.* 1993;90(3):1004-1008.

56. Dahlback B. The discovery of activated protein C resistance. *J Thromb Haemost.* 2003;1(1):3-9.

57. Bertina RM, Koeleman BP, Koster T, et al. Mutation in blood coagulation factor V association with resistance to activated protein C. *Nature.* 1994;369(6475):64-67.

58. Kalafatis M, Bertina RM, Rand MD, Mann KG. Characterisation of the molecular defect in factor VR506Q. *J Biol Chem.* 1995;270(8):4053-4057.

59. Camire RM, Kalafatis M, Cushman M, Tracy RP, Mann KG, Tracy PB. The mechanism of inactivation of human platelet factor Va from normal and activated protein C-resistant individuals. *J Biol Chem.*1995; 270(35):20794-20800.

60. Nicolaes G, Dahlback B. Activated protein C resistance (FV (Leiden)) and thrombosis: factor V mutations causing hypercoagulable states. *Hematol Oncol Clin N Am.* 2003;17(1):37-61.

61. Chan WP, Lee CK, Kwong YL, Lam CKLR. A novel mutation of Arg 306 of factor V gene in Hong Kong Chinese. *Blood.* 1998;91(4):1135-1139.

62. Williamson D, Brown K, Luddington R, Baglin C, Baglin T. FV: Cambridge: a new mutation (Arg306 → Thr) associated with resistance to activated protein C. *Blood.* 1998;91(4):1140-1144.

63. Lee DH, Henderson PA, Blajchman MA. Prevalence of Factor V Leiden in a Canadian blood donor population. *CMAJ.* 1996;155(3):285-289.

64. Ridker PM, Hennekens CH, Lindpaintner K, Stampfer MJ, Eisenberg PR, Miletich JP. Mutation in the gene coding for coagulation Factor V and the risk of myocardial infarction, stroke, and venous thrombosis in apparently healthy men. *N Engl J Med.* 1995;332(14):912-917.

65. Rees DC, Cox M, Clegg JB. World distribution of Factor V Leiden. *Lancet.* 1995;346(8983):1133-1134.

66. Zivelin A, Griffin JH, Xu X. A single genetic origin for a common Caucasian risk factor for

venous thrombosis. *Blood.* 1997;89(2):397-402.

67. Rodegheiro F, Tosetto A. Activated protein C resistance and Factor V Leiden mutation are independent risk factors for venous thromboembolism. *Ann Intern Med.* 1999;130(8):643-650.

68. Martinelli I, Mannucci PM, De Stefano V, Taioli E, Rossi V, Crosti F. Different risks of thrombosis in four coagulation defects associated with inherited thrombophilia: a study of 150 families. *Blood.* 1998;92(7):2353-2358.

69. Bucciarelli P, Rosendaal FR, Tripodi A, et al. Risks of venous thromboembolism and clinical manifestations in carriers of antithrombin, protein C, protein S deficiency, or activated protein C resistance: a multicenter collaborative family study. *Arterioscler Thromb Vasc Biol.* 1999;19(4):1026-1033.

70. Dahlback B, Hildebrand B. Inherited resistance to activated protein C is corrected by anticoagulant cofactor activity found to be a property of factor V. *Proc Natl Acad Sci. USA* 1994;91(4):1396-1400.

71. Spencer F, Becker RC. Diagnosis and management of inherited and acquired thrombophilias. *J Thromb Thrombolysis.* 1999;7(2):91-104.

72. Hertzberg MS. Genetic testing for thrombophilia mutations. *Semin Thromb Hemost.* 2005;31(1):33-38.

73. Poort SR, Rosendaal FR, Reitsma PH, Bertina RM. A common genetic variation in the 3'-untranslated region of the prothrombin gene is associated with elevated plasma prothrombin levels and an increase in venous thrombosis. *Blood.* 1996;88(10):3698-3703.

74. Wolberg AS, Monroe DM, Roberts HR, Hoffman M. Elevated prothrombin results in clots with an altered fiber structure: a possible mechanism of the increased thrombotic risk. *Blood.* 2003;101(8):3008-3013.

75. Kyrle PA, Mannhalter C, Beguin S, et al. Clinical studies and thrombin generation in patients homozygous or heterozygous for the G20210A mutation in the prothrombin gene. *Arterioscler Thromb Vasc Biol.* 1998;18(8):1287-1291.

76. Smirnov MD, Safa O, Esmon NL, Esmon CT. Inhibition of activated protein C anti-coagulant activity by prothrombin. *Blood.* 1999;94(11):3839-3846.

77. Ceelie H, Spaargaren-van Riel CC, Bertina RM, Vos HL. G20210A is a functional mutation in the prothrombin gene; effect on protein levels and 3'-end formation. *J Thromb Haemost.* 2004;2(1):119-127.

78. von Ahsen N, Oellerich M. The intronic prothrombin 19911A>G polymorphism influences splicing efficiency and modulates effects of the 20210G>A polymorphism on mRNA amount and expression in a stable reported gene assay system. *Blood.* 2004;103(2):586-593.

79. Rosendaal FR, Doggen CJ, Zivelin A, Arruda VR, Aiach M, Siscovick DS. Geographic distribution of the 20210G to A prothrombin variant. *Thromb Haemost.* 1998;79:706-708.

80. Zivelin A, Mor-Cohen R, Kovalsky V, et al. Prothrombin 20210G>A is an ancestral prothrombotic mutation that occurred in whites approximately 24,000 years ago. *Blood.* 2006;107(12):4666-4668.

81. Hundsdoerfer P, Vetter B, Stover B, et al. Homozygous and double heterozygous Factor V Leiden and Factor II G20210A genotypes predispose infants to thromboembolism but are not associated with an increase of foetal loss. *Thromb Haemost.* 2003;90(4):628-635.

82. Tosetto A, Missiaglia E, Frezzato M, Rodeghiero F. The VITA project: prothrombin G20210A mutation and venous thromboembolism in the general population. *Thromb Haemost.* 1999;82(5):1395-1398.

83. Bauer K. Hypercoagulable states. In: Hoffman R, Benz EJ Jr, Shattil SS, et al, eds. *Hematology: Basic Principles and Practice.* 4th ed. Orlando, FL: Elsevier Churchill Livingstone; 2005:2197-2224.

84. Zawadzki C, Gaveriaux V, Trillot N, et al. Homozygous G20210A transition in the prothrombin gene associated with severe venous thrombotic disease: two cases in a French family. *Thromb Haemost.* 1998;80(6):1027-1028.

85. Kosch A, Junker R, Wermes C, et al. Recurrent pulmonary embolism in a 13-year-old homozygous for the prothrombin G20210A mutation combined with protein S deficiency

and increased lipoprotein (a). *Thromb Res.* 2002;105(1):49-53.

86. Soria J, Almasy L, Souto JC, et al. Linkage analysis demonstrates that the prothrombin G20210A mutation jointly influences plasma prothrombin levels and risk of thrombosis. *Blood.* 2000;95(9):2780-2785.

87. Kraaijenhagen RA, in't Anker PS, Koopman MM, et al. High plasma concentration of factor VIIIc is a major risk factor for venous thromboembolism. *Thromb Haemost.* 2000;83(1):5-9.

88. Schambeck CM, Hinney K, Mansouri Taleghani B, Wahler D, Keller F. Familial clustering of high factor VIII levels in patients with venous thromboembolism. *Arterioscler Thromb Vasc Biol.* 2001;21(2):289-292.

89. Meijers JC, Tekelenburg WL, Bouma BN, Bertina RM, Rosendaal FR. High levels of coagulation factor XI as a risk factor for venous thrombosis. *N Engl J Med.* 2000;342(10):696-701.

90. van Hylckama Vlieg A, van der Linden IK, Bertina RM, Rosendaal FR. High levels of factor IX increase the risk of venous thrombosis. *Blood.* 2000;95(12):3678-3682.

91. Saposnik B, Reny JL, Gaussan P, Emmerich J, Aiach M, Gandrille S. A haplotype of the EPCR gene is associated with increased plasma levels of sEPCR and is a candidate risk factor for thrombosis. *Blood.* 2004;103(4):1311-1318.

92. Ou D, Wang Y, Song Y, Esmon NL, Esmon CT. The Ser219 - Gly dimorphism of the endothelial protein C receptor contributes to the higher soluble protein levels observed in individuals with the A3 haplotype. *J Thromb Haemost.* 2006;4(1):229-235.

93. Ariens RA, Philippou H, Nagaswami C, Weisel JW, Lane DA, Grant PJ. The factor XIII V34L polymorphism accelerates thrombin activation of factor XIII and affects cross-linked fibrin structure. *Blood.* 2000;96(3):988-995.

94. Van Hylckama Vlieg A, Komanasin N, Ariens RA, et al. Factor XIII Val34Leu polymorphism factor XIII Antigen levels and activity and the risk of deep venous thrombosis. *Br J Haematol.* 2002;119(1):169-175.

95. Kobbervig C, Williams E. FXIII polymorphisms, fibrin clot structure and thrombotic risk. *Biophys Chem.* 2004;112(2-3):223-228.

96. Wassermann A, Neisser A, Bruck C. Eine seri-diagnistiche Reaction bei syphilis (German). *Dtsch MedWochenschr.* 1906;32:745-746.

97. Lim W, Crowther MA, Eikelboom JW. Management of antiphospholipid antibody syndrome. *JAMA.* 2006;295(9):1050-1057.

98. Derksen RH, de Groot PG, Kater L, Nieuwenhuis HK. Patients with antiphospholipid antibodies and venous thrombosis should receive long term anticoagulant treatment. *Ann Rheum Dis.* 1993;52(9):689-692.

99. Rai RS, Clifford K, Cohen H, Regan L. High prospective fetal loss rate in untreated pregnancies of women with recurrent miscarriage and antiphospholipid antibodies. *Hum Reprod.* 1995;10(12):3301-3304.

100. Levine JS, Branch DW. The antiphospholipid antibody syndrome. *N Engl J Med.* 2002;346(10):752-763.

101. Brandt JT, Barna LK, Triplett DA. Laboratory identification of lupus anticoagulants: results of the Second International Workshop for Identification of Lupus Anticoagulants. *Thromb Haemost.* 1995;77(4):1597-1603.

102. Harris EN, Gharavi AE, Boey ML, et al. Anti-cardiolipin antibodies: detection by radioimmunoassay and association with thrombosis in systemic lupus erythematosus. *Lancet.* 1983;2(8361):1211-1214.

103. Reber G, Arvieux J, Comby E, et al. Multicenter evaluation of nine commercial kits for the quantitation of anticardiolipin antibodies. The Working Group on Methodologies in Haemostasis from the GEHT (Groupe Etudes sur l'Hemostase et la Thrombose). *Thromb Haemost.* 1995;73(3):444-452.

104. Rand JH, Senzel L. Antiphospholipid antibodies and the antiphospholipid antibody syndrome. In: Colman RW, Marder VJ, Clowes AW, George JN, Goldhaber SZ, eds. *Hemostasis and Thrombosis. Basic Principles and Clinical Practice.* 5th ed. Philadelphia: Lippincott Williams and Wilkins; 2006:1621-1636.

105. Long A, Ginsberg JS, Brill-Edwards P. The relationship of antiphospholipid antibodies to thromboembolic disease in systemic lupus

erythematosus: a cross-sectional study. *Thromb Haemost.* 1991;66(5):520-524.

106. Sammaritano LR, Gharavi AE, Lockshin MD. Antiphospholipid antibody syndrome: immunologic and clinical aspects. *Semin Arthritis Rheum.* 1990;20(2):81-96.

107. de Groot PG, Horbach DA, Derksen RH. Protein C and other cofactors involved in the binding of antiphospholipid antibodies: relation to the pathogenesis of thrombosis. *Lupus.* 1996;5(5):488-493.

108. Shibata S, Harpel PC, Gharavi A, Rand J, Fillit H. Autoantibodies to heparin from patients with antiphospholipid antibody syndrome inhibit formation of antithrombin III-thrombin complexes. *Blood.* 1994;83(9):2532-2540.

109. Ames PR, Tommasino C, Iannaccone L Brillante M, Cimino R, Brancaccio V. Coagulation activation and fibrinolytic imbalance in subjects with idiopathic antiphospholipid antibodies—a crucial role for acquired free protein S deficiency. *Thromb Haemost.* 1996;76(2):190-194.

110. Brey RL, Chapman J, Levine SR. Stroke and the antiphospholipid syndrome: consensus meeting Taormina 2002. *Lupus.* 2003;12(7):508-513.

111. Brey RL, Escalante A. Neurological manifestations of antiphospholipid antibody syndrome. *Lupus.* 1998;7(Suppl 2):S67-S74.

112. Carhuapoma JR, Mitsias P, Levine SR. Cerebral venous thrombosis and anticardiolipin antibodies. *Stroke.* 1997;28(12):2363-2369.

113. Warkentin TE. Heparin-induced thrombocytopenia. In: Colman RW, Marder VJ, Clowes AW, George JN, Goldhaber SZ, eds. *Hemostasis and Thrombosis. Basic Principles and Clinical Practice.* 5th ed. Philadelphia: Lippincott Williams and Wilkins; 2006:1649-1661.

114. Warkentin TE. Heparin-induced thrombocytopenia: pathogenesis and management. *Br J Haematol.* 2003;121(4):535-555.

115. Warkentin TE, Kelton JG. Temporal aspects of heparin-induced thrombocytopenia. *N Engl J Med.* 2001;344(17):1286-1292.

116. Warkentin TE, Kelton JG. Delayed-onset heparin-induced thrombocytopenia and thrombosis. *Ann Intern Med.* 2001;135(7):502-506.

117. Lee DH, Warkentin TE. Frequency of heparin-induced thrombocytopenia. In: Warkentin TE, Greinacher A, eds. *Heparin-Induced Thrombocytopenia.* 3rd ed. New York: Marcel Dekker; 2004;107-148.

118. Warkentin TE, Roberts RS, Hirsh J, Kelton JG. An improved definition of immune heparin-induced thrombocytopenia in postoperative orthopedic patients. *Arch Intern Med.* 2003;163(20):2518-2524.

119. Sheridan D, Carter C, Kelton JG. A diagnostic test for heparin-induced thrombocytopenia. *Blood.* 1986;67(1):27-30.

120 Greinacher A, Amiral J, Dummel V, Vissac A, Kiefel V, Mueller-Eckhardt C. Laboratory diagnosis of heparin-associated thrombocytopenia and comparison of platelet aggregation test, heparin-induced platelet activation test, and platelet factor 4/heparin enzyme-linked immunosorbent assay. *Transfusion.* 1994;34(5):381-385.

121. Lee AY, Levine MN. Venous thromboembolism and cancer: risks and outcomes. *Circulation.* 2003;107(23 Suppl 1):I17-121.

122. Sorensen HT, Mellemkjaer L, Steffensen FH, Olsen JH, Nielsen GL. The risk of a diagnosis of cancer after primary deep venous thrombosis or pulmonary embolism. *N Engl J Med.* 1998;338(17):1169-1173.

123. Lee AYY. Management of thrombosis in cancer: primary prevention and secondary prophylaxis. *Br J Haematol.* 2006;128:291-302.

124. Ruf W. Molecular regulation of blood clotting in tumor biology. *Haemostasis.* 2001;31(Suppl 1):5-7.

125. Gale AJ, Gordon SG. Update on tumor cell procoagulant factors. *Acta Haematol.* 2001;106(1-2):25-32.

126. Bertomeu MC, Gallo S, Lauri D, et al. Chemotherapy enhances endothelial cell reactivity to platelets. *Clin Exp Metastasis.* 1990;8(6):511-518.

127. Pritchard KI, Paterson AH, Paul NA, et al. Increased thromboembolic complications with concurrent tamoxifen and chemotherapy in a randomized trial of adjuvant therapy for women with breast cancer. *J Clin Oncol.* 1996;14(10):2731-2737.

128. Levine MN, Lee AY, Kakkar AK. Cancer and

thrombosis. In: Colman RW, Marder VJ, Clowes AW, George JN, Goldhaber SZ, eds. *Hemostasis and Thrombosis. Basic Principles and Clinical Practice.* 5th ed. Philadelphia: Lippincott, Williams and Wilkins; 2006:1251-1262.

129. Greer IA. Thrombosis in pregnancy: maternal and fetal issues. *Lancet.* 1999;353(9160):1258-1265.

130. The National Institute for Clinical Excellence, Scottish Executive Health Department and Department of Health, Social Services and Public Safety: Northern Ireland. Confidential Enquiries into Maternal Deaths in the United Kingdom 1997–1999. London: TSO; 2001.

131. Sachs B, Brown DAJ, Driscoll SG, et al. Maternal mortality in Massachusetts. Trends and prevention. *N Engl J Med.* 1987;316(11):667-672.

132. McColl MD, Ramsay JE, Tait RC, et al. Risk factors for pregnancy associated venous thromboembolism. *Thromb Haemost.* 1997;78(4):1183-1188.

133. Anderson FA Jr, Wheeler HB, Goldberg RJ, et al. A population-based perspective of the hospital incidence and case-fatality rates of deep vein thrombosis and pulmonary embolism: the Worcester DVT study. *Arch Intern Med.* 1991;151(5):933-938.

134. Cockett FB, Thomas ML. The iliac compression syndrome. *Br J Surg.* 1965;52(10):816-821.

135. Ginsberg JS, Brill-Edwards P, Burrows RF, et al. Venous thrombosis during pregnancy: leg and trimester of presentation. *Thromb Haemost.* 1992;67(5):519-520.

136. Clark P. Changes of hemostasis variables during pregnancy. *Semin Vasc Med.* 2003;3(1):13-24.

137. Bremme K. Haemostatic changes in pregnancy. *Best Pract Res Clin Haematol.* 2003;16(2):153-168.

138. Comp P, Thurnau GR, Welsh J, Esmon CT. Functional and immunologic protein S levels are decreased during pregnancy. *Blood.* 1986;68(4):881-885.

139. Clark P, Brennand J, Conkie JA, McCall F, Greer IA, Walker ID. Activated protein C sensitivity, protein C, protein S and coagulation in normal pregnancy. *Thromb Haemost.* 1998;79(6):1166-1170.

140. Stirling Y, Woolf L, North WR, Seghatchian MJ, Meade TW. Haemostasis in normal pregnancy. *Thromb Haemost.* 1984;52(2):176-182.

141. Eichinger S, Weltermann A, Philipp K, et al. Prospective evaluation of hemostatic system activation and thrombin potential in healthy pregnant women with and without factor V Leiden. *Thromb Haemost.* 1999;82(4):1232-1236.

142. Martinelli I, Legnani C, Bucciarelli P. Risk of pregnancy-related venous thrombosis in carriers of severe inherited thrombophilia. *Thromb Haemost.* 2001;86(3):800-803.

143. Greer IA. Inherited thrombophilia and venous thromboembolism. *Best Pract Res Clin Obstet Gynaecol.* 2003;17(3):413-425.

144. Ginsberg JS, Bates SM. Management of venous thromboembolism during pregnancy. *J Thromb Haemost.* 2003;1(7):1435-1442.

145. Gerhardt A, Scharf R, Beckmann MW, et al. Prothrombin and factor V mutations in women with a history of thrombosis during pregnancy and the puerperium. *N Engl J Med.* 2000;342(6):374-380.

146. Friederich PW, Sanson BJ, Simioni P, et al. Frequency of pregnancy and related venous thromboembolism in anticoagulant deficient women: implications for prophylaxis. *Ann Intern Med.* 1996;125(12):955-960.

147. DeStefano V, Mastrangelo S, Paciaroni K, et al. Thrombotic risk during pregnancy and puerperium in women with APC resistance—effective subcutaneous heparin prophylaxis in a pregnant patient. *Thromb Haemost.* 1995;74(2):793-794.

148. Simpson EL, Lawrenson RA, Nightingale AL, Farmer RD. Venous thromboembolism in pregnancy and the puerperium: incidence and additional risk factors from a London perinatal database. *BJOG.* 2001;108(1):56-60.

149. Bates SM, Greer IA, Hirsh J, Ginsberg JS. Use of antithrombotic agents during pregnancy: the Seventh ACCP Conference on Antithrombotic and Thrombolytic Therapy. *Chest.* 2006;126(3):Suppl:627S-644S.

150. Daly E, Vessey M, Hawkins M, Carson JL, Gough P, Marsh S. Risk of venous thromboembolism in users of hormone replacement therapy. *Lancet.* 1996;348(9033):977-980.

151. Vandenbroucke JP, Rosing J, Bloemen-kamp KW, et al. Oral contraceptives and the risk of venous thrombosis. *N Engl J Med*. 2001;344(20):1527-1535.

152. Martinelli I. Risk factors in venous thromboembolism. *Thromb Haemost*. 2001;86(1):395-403.

153. Castelli WP. Cardiovascular disease: pathogenesis, epidemiology and risk among users of oral contraceptives who smoke. *Am J Obstet Gynecol*. 1999;180(6 pt 2):S349-S356.

154. Tanis BC, Rosendaal FR. Venous and arterial thrombosis during oral contraceptive use: risks and risk factors. *Semin Vasc Med*. 2003;3(1):69-84.

155. Lidegaard O, Edstrom B, Kreiner S. Oral contraceptives and venous thromboembolism: a five-year national case-control study. *Contraception*. 2002;65(3):187-196.

156. WHO Scientific Group on Cardiovascular Disease and Steroid Hormone Contraception. Cardiovascular disease and steroid hormone contraception: Report of a WHO Scientific Group. *WHO Technical Report Series*. 1998;877:1-89.

157. Bloemenkamp KW, Rosendaal FR, Helmerhorst FM, Vandenbroucke JP. Higher risk of venous thrombosis during early use of oral contraceptives in women with inherited clotting defects. *Arch Intern Med*. 2000;160(1):49-52.

158. Pabinger I, Schneider B. Thrombotic risk of women with hereditary antithrombin III, protein C- and protein S-deficiency taking oral contraceptive medication. The GTH Study Group on natural Inhibitors. *Thromb Haemost*. 1994;71(5):548-552.

159. Martinelli I, Taioli E, Bucciarelli P, Akhavan S, Mannucci PM. Interaction between the G20210A mutation of the prothrombin gene and oral contraceptive use in deep vein thrombosis. *Arterioscler Thromb Vasc Biol*. 1999;19(3):700-703.

160. Rosendaal FR. Oral contraceptives and screening for factor V Leiden. *Thromb Haemost*. 1996;75(3):524-525.

161. Perez Gutthann S, Garcia Rodriguez LA, Castellsague J, Duque Oliart A. Hormone replacement therapy and risk of venous thromboembolism: population based case control study. *BMJ*. 1997;314(7083):796-800.

162. Jick H, Derby LE, Meyers MW, Vasilakis C, Newton KM. Risk of hospital admission for idiopathic venous thromboembolism amongst users of postmenopausal oestrogens. *Lancet*. 1996;348(9033):981-983.

163. Love RR. Tamoxifen therapy in primary breast cancer: biology, efficacy, and side effects. *J Clin Oncol*. 1989;7(6):803-815.

164. Decensi A, Maisonneuve P, Rotmensz N, et al: the Italian Tamoxifen Study Group. Effect of tamoxifen on venous thromboembolic events in a breast cancer prevention trial. *Circulation*. 2005;111(5):539-541.

165. Goss PE, Ingle JN, Martino S, et al. A randomized trial of letrozole in postmenopausal women after five years of tamoxifen therapy for early-stage breast cancer. *N Engl J Med*. 2003;349(19):1793-1802.

166. Martino S, Disch D, Dowsett SA, Keech CA, Mershon JL. Safety assessment of raloxifene over eight years in a clinical trial setting. *Curr Med Res Opin*. 2005;21(9):1441-1452.

167. Prandoni P, Lensing AW, Cogo A, et al. The long-term clinical course of acute deep venous thrombosis. *Ann Intern Med*. 1996;125(1):1-7.

168. Heit JA, Silverstein MD, Mohr DN, Petterson TM, O'Fallon WM, Melton LJ III. Risk factors for deep vein thrombosis and pulmonary embolism: a population-based case-control study. *Arch Int Med*. 2000;160(6):809-815.

167. Kearon C, Gent M, Hirsh J, et al. A comparison of three months of anticoagulation with extended anticoagulation for a first episode of idiopathic venous thromboembolism. *N Engl J Med*. 1999;340(12):901-907.

170. Farmer RD, Lawrenson RA, Thompson CR, Kennedy JG, Hambleton IR. Population-based study of risk of venous thromboembolism associated with various oral contraceptives. *Lancet*. 1997;349 (9045):83-88.

171. Prandoni P. Acquired risk factors for venous thromboembolism in medical patients. *Hematology Am Soc Hematol Educ Program*. 2005:458-461.

172. Cattaneo M. Hyperhomocysteinemia, athero-

sclerosis and thrombosis. *Thromb Haemost.* 1999;81(2):165-176.

173. Ray JG. Meta-analysis of hyperhomocysteinemia as a risk factor for venous thromboembolic disease. *Arch Intern Med.* 1998;158(19):2101-2106.

174. Finkelstein JD. Methionine metabolism in mammals. *J Nutr Biochem.* 1990;1(5):228-237.

175. Mudd SH, Skovby F, Levy HL, et al. The natural history of homocysteinuria due to cystathionine beta-synthase deficiency. *Am J Hum Genet.* 1985;37(1):1-31.

176. Kluijtmans LA, van den Huevel LP, Boers GH, et al. Molecular genetic analysis in mild hyperhomocysteinemia: a common mutation in the methylenetetrshydrofolate reductase gene is a genetic risk factor for cardiovascular disease. *Am J Hum Genet.* 1996;58(1):35-41.

177. Cattaneo M. Hyperhomocysteinemia and Venous Thromboembolism. *Sem Thromb Hemost.* 2006;32(7):716-723.

178. Jacques PF, Selhub J, Bostom AG, Wilson PW, Rosenberg IH. The effect of folic acid fortification on plasma folate and total homocysteine concentrations. *N Engl J Med.* 1999;340(19):1449-1454.

179. Molloy AM, Scott JM. Folates and prevention of disease. *Public Health Nutr.* 2001;4(2B):601-609.

180. Fermo I, Vigano-D'Angelo S, Paroni R, Mazzola G, Calori G, D'Angelo A. Prevalence of moderate hyperhomocysteinemia in patients with early-onset venous and arterial occlusive disease. *Ann Intern Med.* 1995;123(10):747-753.

181. Homocysteine Lowering Trialists' Collaboration. Lowering blood homocysteine with folic acid based supplements: meta-analysis of randomised trials. *BMJ.* 1998;316:894-898.

182. Lonn E, Yusuf S, Arnold MJ, et al. Heart Outcomes Prevention Evaluation (HOPE) 2 Investigators. Homocysteine lowering with folic acid and B vitamins in vascular disease. *N Engl J Med.* 2006;354(15):1567-1577.

183. Dreyfus M, Magny JF, Bridey F, et al. Treatment of homozygous protein C deficiency and neonatal purpura fulminans with a purified protein C concentrate. *N Engl J Med.* 1991;325(22):1565-1568.

184. Monagle P, Chan A, Massicotte P, Chalmers E, Michelson AD. Antithrombotic therapy in children: the Seventh ACCP Conference on Antithrombotic and Thrombolytic Therapy. *Chest.* 2004;126(3):645S-687S.

185. Lechner K, Kyrle PA. Antithrombin III concentrates—are they clinically useful? *Thromb Haemost.* 1995;73(3):340-348.

186. McGehee WG, Klotz TA, Epstein DJ, Rapaport SI. Coumarin necrosis associated with hereditary protein C deficiency. *Ann Intern Med.* 1984;101(1):59-60.

187. Crowther MA, Ginsberg JS, Julian J, et al. A comparison of two intensities of warfarin for the prevention of recurrent thrombosis in patients with the antiphospholipid antibody syndrome. *N Engl J Med.* 2003;349(12):1133-1138.

188. Finazzi G, Marchioli R, Brancaccio V, et al. A randomised clinical trial of high-intensity warfarin vs conventional antithrombotic therapy for the prevention of recurrent thrombosis in patients with the antiphospholipid antibody syndrome (WAPS). *J Thromb Haemost.* 2005;3(5):848-853.

189. Buller HR, Prins MH. Secondary prophylaxis with warfarin for venous thromboembolism. *N Engl J Med.* 2003;349(7):702-704.

190. Lee AY, Levine MN, Baker RI, et al. Randomized comparison of low-molecular-weight heparin versus oral anticoagulant therapy for the prevention of recurrent venous thromboembolism in patients with cancer (CLOT) Investigators. Low-molecular-weight-heparin versus a coumarin for the prevention of recurrent venous thromboembolism in patients with cancer. *N Engl J Med.* 2003;349(2):146-153.

191. Marchetti M, Pistorio A, Barone M, Serafini S, Barosi G. Low-molecular-weight heparin versus warfarin for secondary prophylaxis of venous thromboembolism: a cost-effectiveness analysis. *Am J Med.* 2001;111(2):130-139.

192. Levine MN, Hirsh J, Gent M, et al. Optimal duration of oral anticoagulant therapy: a randomized trial comparing four weeks with three months of warfarin in patients with proximal deep vein thrombosis. *Thromb Haemost.* 1995;74(2):606-611.

193. Agnelli G, Prandoni P, Santamaria MG, et al. Three months versus one year of oral anticoagulant therapy for idiopathic deep vein thrombosis. Warfarin Optimal Duration Italian Trial Investigators. *N Engl J Med.* 2001;345(3):165-169.

194. Buller HR, Agnelli G, Hull RD, Hyers RD, Prins MH, Raskob GE. Antithrombotic therapy for venous thromboembolic disease: the Seventh ACCP Conference on Antithrombotic and Thrombolytic Therapy. *Chest.* 2004;126(3):401S-428S.

195. Ridker PM, Goldhaber SZ, Danielson E, et al. Long-term, low-intensity warfarin therapy for the prevention of recurrent venous thromboembolism. *N Engl J Med.* 2003;348(15):1425-1434.

196. Gallus AS. Management options for thrombophilias. *Semin Thromb Hemost.* 2005;31(1):118-126.

197. Mazzolai L, Hohlfeld P, Spertini F, Hayoz D, Schapira M, Duchosal MA. Fondaparinux is a safe alternative in case of heparin intolerance during pregnancy. *Blood.* 2006;108(5):1569-1570.

198. McKenna R, Cole ER, Vasan U. Is warfarin sodium contraindicated in the lactating mothers? *J Pediatr.* 1983;103(2):325-327.

199. Martinelli I. Thromboembolism in women. *Semin Thromb Hemost.* 2006;32(7):709-715.

200. Brill-Edwards P, Ginsberg JA, Gent M, et al. Recurrence of clot in this pregnancy group. Safety of withholding heparin in pregnant women with a history of venous thromboembolism. *N Engl J Med.* 2000;343(20):1439-1444.

201. Brenner B, Sarig G, Weiner Z, Younis J, Blumenfield Z, Lanir N. Thrombophilic polymorphisms are common in women with fetal loss without apparent cause. *Thromb Haemost.* 1999;82(1):6-9.

202. Rey E, Kahn SR, David M, et al. Thrombophilic disorders and fetal loss: a meta-analysis. *Lancet.* 2003;361(9361):901-908.

203. Nelen WL, Blom HJ, Steegers EA, den Heijer M, Eskes TK. Hyperhomocysteinemia and recurrent early pregnancy loss: a meta-analysis. *Fertil Steril.* 2000;74(6):1196-1199.

204. Ginsberg JS, Brill-Edwards P, Johnston M, et al. Relationship of antiphospholipid antibodies to pregnancy loss in patients with systemic lupus erythematosus: a cross-sectional study. *Blood.* 1992;80(4):975-980.

205. Laskin CA, Bombardier C, Hannah ME, et al. Prednisone and aspirin in women with autoantibodies and unexplained recurrent fetal loss. *N Engl J Med.* 1997;337(3):148-153.

206. Greaves M, Baglin T. Laboratory testing for heritable thrombophilia; impact on clinical management of thrombotic disease. *Br J Haematol.* 2000;109(4):699-703.

207. Mannucci PM. Genetic hypercoagulability: prevention suggests testing family members. *Blood.* 2001;98(1):21-22.

208. Heron E, Lozinguez O, Alhenc-Gelas M. Emmerich J, Fiessinger JN. Hypercoagulable states in primary upper-extremity deep vein thrombosis. *Arch Intern Med.* 2000;160(3):382-386.

26

Environmental and Hereditary Vascular Disorders

Juzar Lokhandwala and John R. Bartholomew

Environmental (Figure 26.1) and hereditary vascular disorders (Table 26.1) are clinical conditions that cardiovascular physicians may be unfamiliar with, however these are important to their practice. Many of these disorders mimic other more commonly seen diseases and therefore awareness of these disorders is essential when formulating a differential diagnosis and managing patients.

Environmental Disorders

Erythromelalgia

Erythromelalgia is an uncommon disorder that generally affects middle-aged women but may also be seen during early childhood or adolescence. Several different terms have been used to describe this syndrome, including erythermalgia or erythralgia. Most physicians prefer the term erythromelalgia, now classified as primary or secondary. The primary form is idiopathic, although a familial form (autosomal dominant) has recently been described, known as Weir Mitchell's disease.[1] A number of the different

disorders and/or medications associated with secondary erythromelalgia are listed in Table 26.2.

Pathophysiology

Most patients are believed to have a neuropathy and a vasculopathy contributing to their symptoms, although the exact cause remains unknown. A predominately small-fiber (occasionally large-fiber) neuropathy has been reported, and decreased oxygenation of the affected area (due to shunting) despite increased blood flow during attacks has been described as contributing to the vasculopathy.[2,3]

Studies also show that the familial form of erythromelalgia is a neuropathic disorder of sodium channel dysfunction.[4] In these patients, a mutation involving the gene encoding the $Na_v1.7$ sodium channel (located on chromosome 2q) has been identified.[5] Disorders of these channels, known as *hereditary channelopathies,* are also known to cause epilepsy, periodic paralysis, and certain arrhythmias.

Natural history

Erythromelalgia is a debilitating illness. In a review of 98 of 168 patients with erythromelalgia

Vascular Disease: Diagnostic and Therapeutic Approaches. © 2011 Michael R. Jaff and Christopher J. White, editors. Cardiotext Publishing, ISBN: 978-1-935395-16-4.

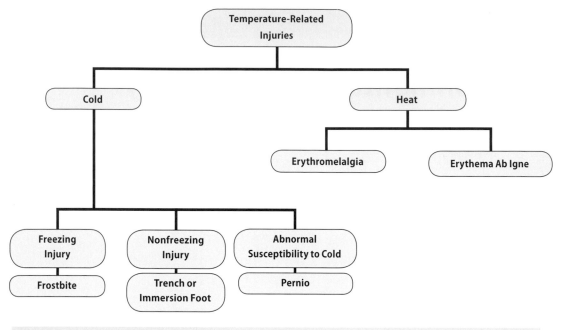

Figure 26.1 Environmental vascular disorders

Type	Cardiovascular Features
Marfan's syndrome	Aortic root dilatation, aneurysmal formation, aortic regurgitation, and aortic dissection
MASS (mitral, aortic, skin, and skeletal manifestations)	Mitral valve prolapse, borderline/nonprogressive aortic root enlargement
Ehlers-Danlos syndrome type IV	Mitral valve prolapse, thoracic aortic aneurysms and dissections; potential rupture of any medium- or large-sized arteries
Pseudoxanthoma elasticum	Coronary artery disease and peripheral artery disease
Turner's syndrome	Bicuspid aortic valve, aortic stenosis and aortic coarctation, aortic root dilatation and dissection
Bicuspid aortic valve	Aortic dilatation, ascending thoracic aortic aneurysm
Familial thoracic aortic aneurysm syndrome	Ascending thoracic aortic aneurysm or dissection

Table 26.1 Hereditary Vascular Disorders

who responded to a health status questionnaire, Davis et al[3] reported a significantly reduced quality of life and a decrease in survival compared to that for age- and sex-matched controls.

Diagnostic evaluation

The diagnosis of erythromelalgia is based on the history and a normal physical examination unless the patient is examined during an attack or has the secondary form. A triad of clinical findings including erythema, increased warmth, and burning pain of the extremities (usually symmetrical) is characteristically seen (Figure 26.2). The soles of the feet and hands are most commonly involved although the knees, elbows, ears, and face may be affected. Attacks are intermittent, may last hours to days, and are aggravated by alcohol, warm temperatures (sum-

Primary Erythromelalgia
Idiopathic
Hereditary (Weir Mitchell's disease)

Secondary Erythromelalgia
Myeloproliferative disorders:
Polycythemia rubra vera
Essential thrombocythemia
Chronic myelogenous leukemia
Hypertension
Diabetes mellitus
Multiple sclerosis
Spinal cord disease
Connective tissue disorders:
Systemic lupus erythematosus
Rheumatoid arthritis
Viral infections:
HIV
Hepatitis B
Drugs:
Calcium channel blockers
Bromocriptine, pergolide
Cyclosporine

Table 26.2 Disorders Associated with Erythromelalgia

Clinical Evaluation
History and physical examination

Vascular Evaluation
Color change
Skin temperature
Blood flow (laser Doppler flowmetry)
Oxygen saturation (transcutaneous oximetry)
Ankle-brachial index (ABI)

Neurologic Evaluation
Electromyography
Autonomic reflex screen
Quantitative sudomotor axon reflex test (QSART)
Heart rate response to deep breathing and
Valsalva ratio (cardiovagal functioning)
Adrenergic function testing
Consultation with a neurologist

Table 26.3 Tests Recommended to Aid in the Diagnosis of Erythromelalgia (Adapted from Davis MP, Sandroni P, Rooke TW, Low PA. Erythromelalgia: Vasculopathy, Neuropathy, or Both? Prospective Study of Vascular and Neurophysiologic Studies in Erythromelalgia. *Arch Dermatol.* 2003;139:1337-1343)

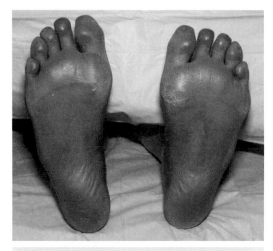

Figure 26.2 Painful erythematous and hot feet classically seen in an individual with erythromelalgia.

mer heat or warm rooms), exercise, or wearing shoes and socks. Ulceration, gangrene, and abnormal peripheral pulses may be found in some secondary forms.

No objective laboratory tests exist to help confirm the diagnosis, although the studies listed in Table 26.3 may prove beneficial to confirm or exclude the diagnosis.[2]

The differential diagnosis includes a peripheral neuropathy, complex regional pain syndrome, cellulitis, dermatitis, Raynaud's phenomenon, chronic venous insufficiency, lipodermatosclerosis, and arterial insufficiency.

Therapeutic options

Patients obtain relief cooling the affected area by immersing it in ice water or sitting in front of a fan. A number of different medications aimed at both the neuropathy and vasculopathy have been tried with varying degrees of success. Vasodilators (sodium nitroprusside and nitroglycerin), beta-blockers, tricyclic antidepressants, anticonvulsants, intravenous prostaglandins, and an antiarrhythmic agent (mexiletine), as well as capsaicin, biofeedback, sympathetic nerve block, clonidine, and narcotics have all been shown to be helpful in some patients. Aspirin or NSAIDs may help individuals with an underlying myeloproliferative disorder. The use of a lidocaine patch (a sodium channel blocker) has been found effective in relieving the pain in some patients.[6]

Education is important. The individual must understand that the illness is chronic and very difficult to treat. Patients should avoid aggravating conditions and learn to cool their extremities without causing tissue damage. They often need counseling and psychiatric help.

Pernio or Chilblains

Pernio, or *chilblains,* is a localized vascular disorder commonly seen in young females, however, it may also be found in other age groups including children and older adults.[7] Historically, pernio was quite common during wartime conditions in northern Europe. It is now less common but still occurs in the temperate and humid climates of northwestern Europe and the northern United States.

Pathophysiology

Pernio is believed to be due to vasospasm induced by cold exposure or cold-induced trauma. It generally develops in susceptible individuals who are exposed to nonfreezing cold.[7] Excessive cold exposure and parenteral neglect has led to cases of pernio in children, while among adolescents it has also been reported more frequently in association with thin body habitus.[8]

Cold exposure may eventually lead to structural changes in the skin due to vascular damage from tissue anoxemia and secondary inflammatory reactions. Histologically, a perivascular lymphocytic infiltration of the arterioles and venules of the dermis, thickening and edema of the blood vessel walls, fat necrosis, and chronic inflammatory reactions with giant cell formation are described.[7]

Natural history

Two types of pernio are described (acute and chronic), and their characteristics are outlined in Table 26.4.[7] The acute form develops shortly after exposure to cold and disappears within a few weeks once the precipitating cause is removed. Chronic pernio develops after repeated episodes of cold exposure, generally beginning in the late fall or early winter and lasts until spring or warmer weather returns. Patients with chronic pernio have a history of repeated episodes in previous years and are susceptible to occlusive vascular disease.

A form of chronic pernio has also been described in patients with anorexia nervosa, dysproteinemia, cold agglutinin or cryoglobulin disorders, chronic myelomonocytic leukemia, systemic lupus erythematosus (SLE), and other connective tissue disorders. This latter entity is often referred to as *chilblain lupus,* or *chilblain LE.*[9]

Diagnostic evaluation

The diagnosis of pernio is a made by a thorough history and physical examination. Patients generally present with purple, erythematous, or cyanotic skin lesions that affect their toes or fingers. Pernio usually begins in late fall or early winter (in cold or damp climates) and disappears in the spring or early summer (Figure 26.3). At times, the skin may develop a yellowish or brownish discoloration that can peel or

Characteristics	Acute	Chronic
Time of development	Develops within hours (12–24) following cold exposure	Develops after repeated exposures to cold or damp climates
Type of lesions	Erythematous—purplish edematous lesions, normal arterial examination	Brown plaques, or violet/yellow blisters
Previous history	No	Yes
Development of chronic occlusive disease	No (self-limited condition)	Yes

Table 26.4 Classification of Pernio

ulcerate. Involvement of the nose, cheeks, ears, and thighs may occur but is uncommon. Pernio lesions are generally bilateral, and females are more likely to be affected than males. Patients often complain of intense itching or a burning sensation.

A number of conditions have been described that may predispose a patient to pernio, including SLE and anorexia nervosa as well as the presence of antiphospholipid antibodies or cryoproteins, and in select individuals laboratory testing to confirm these disorders may be appropriate.

Patients may demonstrate a vasospastic response to cold-water immersion while pulse volume recordings (PVRs) generally reveal small-vessel disease unless measures are taken to warm the affected limb during the procedure.[10] There is generally no need to perform more invasive studies unless the diagnosis is in doubt.

Physicians often lack familiarity with pernio, therefore, recognition is important. Pernio should be differentiated from Raynaud's phenomenon, frostbite, leukocytoclastic vasculitis, erythema nodosum, atheroembolism, thromboembolism, or atherosclerosis due to trauma.

Therapeutic options

Prevention is the best treatment. Patients should avoid damp or cold exposure and take appropriate precautions (dress warmly) before going outside. A number of medications have been tried, but it appears that the calcium channel blocker (nifedipine or its equivalent) or the α-2 agonist and vasodilator (prazosin hydrochloride) are most helpful in alleviating symptoms and preventing new attacks.[7,10] Fluocinolone acetonide cream and topical steroids have been tried in an attempt to alleviate pain and itching. Lesions generally resolve over several weeks if these measures are taken. In cases of chronic pernio, chemical sympathectomy has been tried.[7]

Frostbite

Frostbite was once almost exclusively a military problem. It is now seen in persons engaged in winter outdoor sports (skiing, snowmobiling, ice-fishing, etc), homeless people, patients with psychiatric illness, people who consume drugs or alcohol excessively, and following vehicular trauma. Patients with peripheral artery disease (PAD) are also at increased risk. Factors that increase the risk for frostbite are listed in Table 26.5.[11]

General	advanced age, infancy, exhaustion
Drug use	alcohol, sedatives, clonidine, neuroleptics
Endocrine system	hypoglycemia, hypothyroidism, adrenal insufficiency, diabetes mellitus
Cardiovascular system	PAD, nicotine use
Neurologic system	peripheral neuropathy, spinal cord damage
Trauma	falls with head or spinal injury, fractures causing immobility
Infection	sepsis

Table 26.5 Factors Increasing the Likelihood of Developing Frostbite (Adapted from Biem J, Koehncke N, Classen D, Dosman J. Out of the cold; management of hypothermia and frostbite. *Can Med Assoc J.* 2003;168:305-311.)

Pathophysiology

Frostbite is a local cold-induced injury that can potentially result in death of an individual. It occurs when patients are exposed to temperatures below the freezing point of intact skin, and its

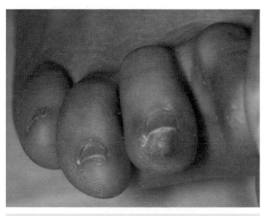

Figure 26.3 Typical bluish discoloration and a small blister seen in a patient with Pernio.

severity appears related to the duration of exposure. Injury ranges from reversible to irreversible cellular destruction.[11] Two mechanisms are responsible for the tissue injury: cellular death resulting from cold exposure, and necrosis due to progressive dermal ischemia.[12]

Natural history

Frostbite is classified as superficial or deep (Table 26.6). Patients with superficial frostbite who have retained sensation, normal skin color, and clear blisters usually have a favorable prognosis, while individuals with deep frostbite and cyanosis, firm skin, and dark, fluid-filled blisters generally have a poor prognosis.[11]

Some victims develop chronic sequelae following an episode of frostbite. These symptoms may persist for years and include cold insensitivity, sensory disturbances, hyperhidrosis, swelling, and chronic pain.[12]

Mortality generally depends on underlying risk factors.[7,12] For example, the mortality rate was 17% in a multicenter study involving 428 patients. The majority of deaths were due to an underlying cause (alcohol, psychiatric medications, inappropriate clothing for the conditions, physical exhaustion, and trauma) rather than frostbite.[13]

Diagnostic evaluation

The diagnosis of frostbite is made by a history of cold exposure and characteristic clinical findings. The extremities (hands and feet) account for approximately 90% of injuries, although the ears, nose, and cheeks may be involved (Figure 26.4).[11] Men outnumber women approximately 10:1.

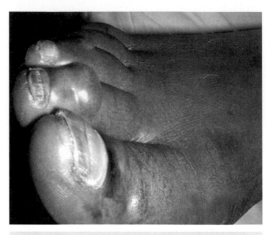

Figure 26.4 Blisters are seen in this patient with frostbite.

Patients generally complain of numbness in the affected area and may report a clumsiness or lack of fine coordination if the hands are involved. The frozen area initially appears white due to vasospasm, but as the patient is warmed, thawing leaves the area hyperemic. Edema and blisters follow. They are eventually replaced by a black eschar that ultimately heals, unless the frostbite is deep.

The diagnosis is made by the history and physical examination. In attempts to provide assessment of tissue viability, several radiographic procedures have been utilized. These include plain radiographs, radioisotope scanning, and digital plethysmography to assess perfusion. Magnetic resonance imaging (MRI) and magnetic resonance angiography (MRA) have also been used to visualize blood vessels directly in an attempt to provide better delineation of ischemic soft tissue and provide

Superficial	Deep
Affects skin and subcutaneous tissue	Affects bone, joints, and tendons
Pallor, edema, and blisters seen Transient stinging, burning, throbbing, and aching	Anesthesia followed by hyperesthesia with burning, throbbing, aching "Block of wood sensation"
Blisters are clear	Skin necrosis, blisters are hemorrhagic (violaceous), little edema

Table 26.6 Classification of Frostbite

assistance for future surgical procedures if necessary.[13]

Therapeutic options

Proper recognition and uninterrupted re-warming is essential to treatment of frostbite. Immediate care revolves around protecting the injured area from trauma. Rewarming should begin only if refreezing will not occur while the patient is being transferred to the hospital.

Rapid rewarming in a water bath between 40°C and 42°C for 15 to 30 minutes may help minimize tissue loss. Splinting and elevation of the affected limb may also be helpful to reduce edema and promote tissue perfusion. Wet clothing must be removed if nonadherent. Rubbing the affected areas is not advised. Patients should receive tetanus toxoid and analgesics, and antibiotics may be needed. Additional options include hydrotherapy, which allows for wound debridement and encourages active and passive range of motion.

Surgical therapy

Surgical care should be limited to debridement of necrotic tissue. It is generally advised not to remove blisters; however, if they rupture the area should be cleansed and covered with a topical antibiotic. Amputation and aggressive debridement is delayed until demarcation of tissue is complete, a process that can take many weeks to months.

Trench Foot and Immersion Foot

Trench foot and *immersion foot* are usually associated with damp and cold surroundings. These conditions are also known as *sea-boat foot* or *foxhole foot*.[14] Trench foot got its name from the soldiers of World War I, who stood for days in their boots in wet or damp trenches. Immersion foot was first described because of conditions that occurred during World War II, when individuals were forced to spend time in wet or damp lifeboats. These 2 conditions are generally considered to be the same disease, although they are found under different conditions.[7] A warm-water variety of trench foot

was described during the Vietnam War and the Falkland conflict, while more recently trench foot has been recognized in the elderly and in alcoholic or homeless patients.[14-16]

Pathophysiology

Trench foot and immersion foot are caused by prolonged exposure of the foot to a nonfreezing, moist environment. The conditions are made worse by higher altitudes, prolonged immobility, and dependency of the limbs. Smoking and underlying vascular problems aggravate it. Injury is believed due to cold-induced vasospasm and repeated cooling and rewarming leading to a cycle of ischemia and reperfusion. Experimental work also indicates that large, myelinated nerve fibers are damaged in this condition.[16]

Four stages of trench foot have been described: (1) exposure to cold, (2) a prehyperemic phase, (3) a hyperemic phase, and (4) a posthyperemic phase.[14]

Natural history

Although complications include gangrene, as well as nerve and muscle injury, recovery is generally complete if properly recognized and treated appropriately.[15] However, long-term sequelae related to vasospasm can develop.

Diagnostic evaluation

Trench foot and immersion foot have generally been considered uncommon outside of war time, therefore, awareness is the most important step in the diagnosis. It is now appreciated that either of these disorders should be considered in the elderly, alcoholic, or homeless person who has been immobile in cool or wet surroundings and presents with cold, patchy blue, numb, or painful feet and diminished or absent pulses. In patients who present in later stages, blistering, ulceration, increased warmth, swelling, hyperemia, or gangrene may be found. Cold sensitivity, numbness, and persistent pain that may last for years are part of the chronic sequelae.[7]

No specific tests can confirm the diagnosis, other than a thorough history and physical examination. Trench foot and immersion foot must be differentiated from other cold- or heat-induced injuries, including frostbite, pernio, erythromelalgia, and other conditions including atheroemboli, thromboembolism, peripheral neuropathy, and atherosclerosis with trauma.

Therapeutic options

Prevention is the most important aspect in the management of these conditions. Treatment revolves around recognition, removal of wet and cold footwear, and providing the patient with a warm environment, although rapid rewarming is not advisable. Elevation of the affected extremities to reduce edema and the use of analgesics for pain control are also important.[7] Pentoxifylline has been found helpful in some cases, and there are reports of benefit using vasodilators, including oral prostaglandin E1.[14] Surgery should be delayed if gangrene is present until complete demarcation of tissue occurs.[7]

Erythema Ab Igne

Erythema ab igne (EAI) is a hyperpigmented condition that results from repeated exposure to hot water bottles, space heaters, or electric heating pads not warm enough to produce a burn. It was once a common condition seen in individuals who sat too close to a fireplace, but in present time the condition may be found in persons who sit too near to space heaters, wood burning stoves, or car heaters.[17] EAI is also an occupational hazard for persons who work as bakers, or foundry or kitchen workers whose arms are repeatedly exposed to fire.

Pathophysiology

The skin discoloration appears as a reticular, telangiectatic, erythematous, hyperpigmented (brownish) pattern. It is due to chronic exposure to moderate levels of infrared radiation insufficient to produce a burn. Dysplastic changes can develop predisposing the patient to actinic keratoses and squamous cell and neuroendocrine carcinomas. Biopsy is recommended if there is suspicion for cutaneous malignancy.[17]

Natural history

The prognosis for EAI is excellent if the offending agent is removed. If not, cutaneous atrophy and a potential for the development of a cutaneous malignancy exist.[17]

Diagnostic evaluation

A careful history (questioning the use of heat applied to the area of concern) and physical examination should alert the clinician to this condition. Patients generally have no symptoms (other than skin discoloration, as shown in Figure 26.5), although they may complain of a slight burning sensation. Tan and Bertucci[17] reported that EAI affects the legs and upper parts of the feet more often in women. Some patients report using their hot water bottle or heating pad for chronic pain relief. Under these circumstances, the etiology of their pain should be further evaluated as reports of an underlying malignancy in patients with EAI have been reported.

No specific tests are needed to confirm the diagnosis, other than recognition. A biopsy

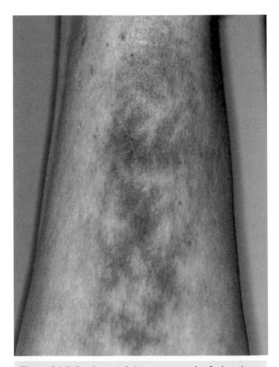

Figure 26.5 Erythema ab igne as a result of a heating pad burn.

should be performed, however, if there is a suspicion of malignancy.

Therapeutic options

Prevention is the best form of treatment. Removing the offending source is generally all that is required, although some investigators have tried 5-fluorouracil cream, which is reported to clear epithelial atypia.[17]

Hereditary Disorders

Cardiovascular physicians should be acquainted with number of hereditary disorders that can result in dilation, aneurysmal disease, or dissection of the arteries, as well as valvular disorders and peripheral and coronary artery disease. These disorders have the potential for devastating complications if not properly recognized and/or treated.

Marfan's Syndrome

Marfan's syndrome is among the most common inherited connective tissue disorders, with an estimated incidence of around 1 to 3 per 10,000 individuals.[18] It is inherited in an autosomal dominant manner, although about 25% of the cases are due to *de novo* mutations. Marfan's syndrome typically involves the cardiovascular, musculoskeletal, and ocular systems but may also affect the lungs, skin, and central nervous system.[18]

Pathophysiology

Most cases of Marfan's syndrome are caused by mutations in one of the genes for fibrillin 1. Fibrillin 1 is a major component of microfibrils which are the structural elements of the lens, cornea, skin, lung, and media of the aorta. The gene for fibrillin 1 is located on chromosome 15q21.1.[18,19] Fibrillin1 gene mutations result in a decrease in elastin in the aortic wall, leading to increased stiffness and dilatation.[20]

Murine models have indicated that fibrillin 1 also plays a key role in the regulation of transforming growth factor-beta (TGFB).[18,21] This leads to an overabundance of activated TGFB and subsequent matrix destruction, resulting in cystic medial necrosis of the aortic wall.[18,21]

Natural history

Cardiovascular complications are the leading cause of death in Marfan's syndrome. Approximately 90% of patients develop changes in their aorta and heart valves, leading to significant morbidity and mortality. Early implementation of medical and surgical measures in the current era, however, has given patients a nearly normal life expectancy.[18,19,22]

Diagnostic evaluation

Marfan's syndrome is a multisystem disorder characterized by proximal aortic aneurysm, dislocation of the ocular lens, and long-bone overgrowth. Strict criteria proposed in 1996[23] for the diagnosis rely on recognition of both major and minor clinical manifestations involving the skeletal, cardiovascular, or ocular systems and the dura.

The echocardiogram and eye examination are important for the diagnosis, while the role of genetic testing remains limited.[18] Enlargement of the aorta, aneurysms, and dissections as well as lumbosacral dural ectasia can be identified by MRI or CTA.

Many patients do not meet the full diagnostic criteria for Marfan's syndrome. The MASS phenotype, which stands for a combination of mitral valve, aortic, skin, and skeletal manifestations, is used for this group. It may be difficult to differentiate MASS from Marfan's syndrome; therefore, careful follow-up is needed in these individuals.[18]

Patients with homocystinuria often have tall stature, long-bone overgrowth, and ectopia lentis, but they do not typically have aortic enlargement or dissection. These individuals can be distinguished by an elevated plasma homocysteine level. Other disorders that must be considered in the differential diagnosis include familial thoracic aortic aneurysm syndrome and a bicuspid aortic valve.[18]

Therapeutic options

Due to the risk of aortic dissection, patients with Marfan's syndrome should be counseled not to engage in contact sports or isometric exercise (body building or weightlifting). Activities involving low to moderate intensity such as bowling, golf, snorkeling, and hiking should be encouraged.

Early detection and treatment of aortic dilatation is important in preventing dissection or rupture. Yearly assessment of the proximal aorta with a transthoracic echocardiogram is recommended. Both the absolute size of the greatest diameter and the rate of growth of the aorta are used to decide the appropriate time of surgery.

Beta-blockers are the standard of care for patients with Marfan's syndrome.[18] They are beneficial as a result of negative inotropic and chronotropic affects that decrease aortic shear stress. Beta-blockers should be titrated to maintain the heart rate at 110 beats per minute after submaximal exercise. None of the current medical treatments halt or reverse aortic dilatation; however, they may slow aortic growth.[18]

Elective surgery is recommended when the maximum aortic diameter is ≥ 5 cm. Earlier intervention may be considered if there is an increase in the aortic diameter by more than 1 cm/year, or if there is a family history of aortic dissection at a size < 5 cm.

Ehlers-Danlos Syndrome Type IV

Ehlers-Danlos syndrome (EDS) represents a group of connective tissue disorders recognized by their easy bruising, skin hyperextensibility, joint hypermobility, and tissue fragility.[24-26] There are a number of types of EDS, however, the risk of premature death occurs only in type IV (known as the vascular type). Ehlers-Danlos syndrome should be considered in any young person who suffers uterine rupture during pregnancy or in cases where there is arterial or visceral rupture.[19]

Epidemiology/prevalence

EDS has an estimated prevalence of 1 in every 25,000 births. Type IV EDS is autosomal dominant and accounts for less than 4% of all EDS patients.[27]

Pathophysiology

The mutation in EDS involves the gene for type III collagen, which is found in abundance in the arterial wall and visceral organs, especially the intestine and uterus.[28] *De novo* mutations account for half of all the reported cases.

Natural history

In a study of 419 EDS patients, arterial rupture and intestinal perforation were found in about 25% of individuals before age 20 and in 80% of patients before they reached 40 years of age. The median survival in this group was 48 years.[19] Approximately one-half of the arterial complications occurred in the thoracic or abdominal arteries, with a predilection for middle-sized arteries.[19] In pregnant women with EDS type IV, uterine rupture is an important cause of mortality.

Diagnostic evaluation

The clinical diagnosis of EDS is made from 4 criteria: (1) easy bruising, (2) thin skin with visible veins, (3) characteristic facial features, and (4) rupture of arteries, uterus, or intestines.[26] Patients may also have characteristic features seen in other EDS types, including skin hyperextensibility and fragility.

The best diagnostic test is biochemical analysis of type III collagen from a skin fibroblast culture.[26]

Therapeutic options

Patients should be advised to avoid contact sports, isometric exercises, and anti-inflammatory medications. Treatment of vascular complications is often limited as surgery or endovascular procedures are complicated by tissue friability and poor wound healing. Early recognition of this disorder in young patients (especially those presenting with arterial rupture or visceral perforation) is important in anticipating and preventing further complications of invasive diagnostic tests or subsequent surgical repair.

Pseudoxanthoma Elasticum

Pseudoxanthoma elasticum (PXE) is a rare inherited disorder of connective tissue that primarily affects the skin, retina, and occasionally the cardiovascular system. There is a female to male ratio of around 2:1.

Pathophysiology

PXE is characterized pathologically by elastic fiber mineralization and fragmentation. It is associated with mutations in the gene that encodes for ABCC6 (on chromosome 16), a member of the large ATP-dependent transmembrane transporter family.[27]

Natural history

PXE is characterized by marked clinical heterogeneity, even between siblings, in relation to age of onset and the extent and severity of organ system involvement. Most patients have a normal life span.

Diagnostic evaluation

The primary skin lesions of PXE are yellowish papules of 2 to 5 mm in diameter located on the neck and axillary folds as well as the inner lower lip. There is also generalized laxity. Angioid streaks are seen in the eye, which are grayish, irregular lines radiating outward from the optic papilla. Visual loss occurs in up to 8% of patients.

PXE can involve elastic fibers in small- and medium-sized arteries. The gradual time course of arterial narrowing is associated with collateral formation, and consequently, severe vascular symptoms are infrequent. The diagnosis of PXE should be suspected in young individuals who present with intermittent claudication of the lower limbs or tiredness of the upper limbs, and absence or decreased peripheral pulses. In a young person who presents with cardiac involvement (angina pectoris or acute myocardial infarction) without other cardiovascular risk factors, PXE should also be considered.[28]

Angioid streaks are not specific for PXE and have also been encountered in the inherited hemoglobinopathies, Marfan's syndrome, EDS, or Paget's disease of the bone. Cutaneous and articular hyperlaxity may occur in PXE but is less severe than in EDS.

The clinical findings and histologic examination of the involved skin should confirm the diagnosis. ABCC6 genotyping is only available in specialized centers, and its value for diagnosis remains to be determined.

Therapeutic options

Combat sports are contraindicated to reduce the occurrence of facial trauma and risk of retinal hemorrhages. Reduction of cardiovascular risk factors has been recommended if there is cardiac involvement.

Surgical reduction of excessive and redundant skin may be needed for cosmetic improvement. Laser has been used to treat neovascularization in the retina. Surgical revascularization may be beneficial in patients with coronary artery involvement.

Additional Hereditary Disorders

Turner's Syndrome

Turner's syndrome is a disorder of females characterized by the absence of all or part of a normal second sex chromosome. It occurs in approximately 1 in 2500 to 3000 live-born girls and is associated with an increased risk for cardiovascular malformations.[29,30] Bicuspid aortic valve and coarctation of the aorta are the most common findings, while thoracic aortic dilatation and ascending aortic aneurysmal formation as well as dissection and rupture have also been described. Hypertension, mitral valve prolapse, and conduction defects are other cardiac defects that can occur. Congenital lymphedema, short stature, and gonadal dysgenesis are part of this syndrome and often present.

Bicuspid Aortic Valve

Bicuspid aortic valve (BAV) may be the most common congenital anomaly resulting in aortic dilatation. It occurs in approximately 0.5%

to 2.0% of the general population, making it the most common cardiovascular malformation.[19,31] BAV is recognized in association with coarctation of the aorta, ascending aortic root dilatation, thoracic aortic aneurysms, and aortic dissection. Cystic medial degeneration appears to be responsible for the aortic dilatation.[20]

Familial Thoracic Aortic Dissection and Aneurysms

As many as 19% of patients referred for repair of thoracic aneurysm or dissection will have another affected family member.[32] These patients do not meet the clinical criteria for Marfan's syndrome or EDS, however, they are often familial and are now referred to as the *familial thoracic aortic aneurysm syndrome*.[20] Mutations to several genes have been identified, including 3p24.2-25, 5q13-14, and 11q23.2-q24, although routine genetic screening is not yet possible.[20]

Summary

Hereditary and environmental vascular disorders, while not as common as other vascular disorders, represent a group of conditions that should always be kept in the differential diagnosis when evaluating patients with vascular disease, due to the markedly different prognostic and therapeutic implications associated with these disorders. Prompt recognition and treatment of environmental vascular disorders associated with extremes of temperature, such as frostbite, is important, as are measures to prevent them. Continued progress in the understanding of the genetic and molecular alterations in hereditary vascular disorders holds promise for the future development of targeted therapies for these multi-system disorders.

References

1. Waxman SG, Dib-Hajj SD. Erythromelalgia: a hereditary pain syndrome enters the molecular era. *Ann Neurol*. 2005;57:785-788.

2. Davis MP, Sandroni P, Rooke TW, Low PA. Erythromelalgia: Vasculopathy, Neuropathy, or Both? Prospective Study of Vascular and Neurophysiologic Studies in Erythromelalgia. *Arch Dermatol*. 2003;139:1337-1343.

3. Davis MD, O'Fallon WM, Rogers R, Rooke TW. Natural history of erythromelalgia. *Arch Dermatol*. 2000;136:330-336.

4. Michiels JJ, te Morsche RHM, Jansen JBMJ, Drenth JPH. Autosomal dominant erythermalgia associated with a novel mutation in the voltage-gated sodium channel α subunit Nav1.7. *Arch Neurol*. 2005;62:1587-1590.

5. Burns TM, te Morsche RHM, Jansen JBMJ, Drenth JPH. Genetic heterogeneity and exclusion of a modifying locus at 2q in a family with autosomal dominant primary erythermalgia. *Br J Dermatology*. 2005;153:174-177.

6. Davis MP, Sandroni P. Lidocaine patch for pain of erythromelalgia: follow up of 34 patients. *Arch Dermatol*. 2005;141:1320-1321.

7. Olin JW, Arrabi W. Vascular diseases related to extremes in environmental temperature. In: Young JR, Olin JW, Bartholomew JR, eds. *Peripheral Vascular Diseases*, St. Louis: CV Mosby; 1996:607-620.

8. Simon TD, Soep JB, Hollister R. Pernio in pediatrics. *Pediatrics*. 2005;116:472-475.

9. Viguier M, Pinquier L, Cavelier-Balloy B, et al. Clinical and histopathologic features and immunologic variables in patients with severe chilblains. *Medicine*. 2001;80:180-188.

10. Spittel JA Jr, Spittell PC. Chronic pernio: another cause of blue toes. *Int Angiol*. 1992;11:46-50.

11. Biem J, Koehncke N, Classen D, Dosman J. Out of the cold; management of hypothermia and frostbite. *Can Med Assoc J*. 2003;168:305-311.

12. Petrone P, Kuncir EJ, Asensio JA. Surgical management and strategies in the treatment of hypothermia and cold injury. *Emerg Med Clin N Amer*. 2003;21:1165-1178.

13. Danzi DF, Pozos RS, Auerbach PS, Glazer S, et al. Multicenter hypothermia survey. *Ann Emerg Med.* 1987;16:1042-1055.

14. Oumeish OY, Parish LC. Marching in the army: common cutaneous disorders of the feet. *Clin Dermatol.* 2002;20:445-451.

15. Williams GL, Morgan AE, Harvey JS. Trench foot following a collapse: assessment of the feet is essential in the elderly. *Age and Ageing.* 2005;34:651-652.

16. Irwin Ms, Sanders R, Green CJ, Terenghi G. Neuropathy in non-freezing cold injury (trench foot). *J Royal Soc Med.* 1997;90;433-438.

17. Tan S, Bertucci V. Erythema ab igne: an old condition new again. *Can Med Assoc J.* 2000;162:77-78.

18. Judge DP, Dietz HC. Marfan's syndrome. *Lancet.* 2005;366:1965-1976.

19. Baxter BT. Heritable diseases of the blood vessels. *Cardiovasc Pathol.* 2005; 14:185-188.

20. Ng CM, Cheng A, Myers LA, et al. TGF-beta-dependent pathogenesis of mitral valve prolapse in a mouse model of Marfan syndrome. *J Clin Invest.* 2004;114:1586-1592.

21. Silverman DI, Burton KJ, Gray J, et al. Life expectancy in the Marfan syndrome. *Am J Cardiol.* 1995;75:157-160.

22. Yeowell HN, Pinnell SR. The Ehlers-Danlos syndromes. *Semin Dermatol.* 1993:12:229-240.

23. De Paepe A, Devereux RB, Dietz HC, Hennekam RC, Pyeritz RE. Revised diagnostic criteria for the Marfan syndrome. *Am J Med Genet.* 1996;62:417–426.

24. Pepin M, Schwarze U, Superti-Furga A, Byers PH. Clinical and genetic features of Ehlers-Danlos syndrome type IV, the vascular type. *N Engl J Med.* 2000;342:673-680.

25. Pyeritz RE. Ehlers-Danlos syndrome. *N Engl J Med.* 2000;342:730-732.

26. Oderich GS, Panneton JM, Bower TC, et al. The spectrum, management and clinical outcome of Ehlers-Danlos syndrome type IV: A 30 year experience. *J Vasc Surg.* 2005;42:98-106.

27. Bergen AA, Plomp AS, Schuurman EJ, et al. Mutations in ABCC6 cause pseudoxanthoma elasticum. *Nat Genet.* 2000;25:228-231.

28. Kevorkian JP, Masquet C, Kural-Menasche S, Le Dref O, Beaufils P. New report of severe coronary artery disease in an eighteen-year-old girl with pseudoxanthoma elasticum. Case report and review of the literature. *Angiology.* 1997;48:735-741.

29. Ostberg JE, Brookes JA, McCarthy C, Halcox J, Conway GS. A comparison of echocardiography and magnetic resonance imaging in cardiovascular screening of adults with Turner syndrome. *J Clin Endocrinol Metab.* 2004;89:5966-5971.

30. Lin AE, Lippe B, Rosenfeld RG. Further delineation of aortic dilation, dissection, and rupture in patients with Turner syndrome. *Pediatrics.* 1998;102:e12.

31. Cripe L, Andelfinger G, Martin LJ, Shooner K, Woodrow Benson D. Bicuspid aortic valve is heritable. *JACC.* 2004;44:138-143.

32. Coady MA, Davies RR, Roberts M, et al. Familial patterns of thoracic aortic aneurysms. *Arch Surg.* 1999;134:361-367.

Index

Figures are indicated by f
and tables by t following the page number.